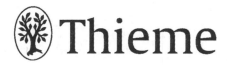

Textbook of Ophthalmology

Sanjeev Kumar Mittal, MS, FICO (Japan)
Professor and Head
Department of Ophthalmology
All India Institute of Medical Sciences
Rishikesh, Uttarakhand, India

Raj Kumar Agarwal, MS
Consultant Ophthalmologist
Saharanpur, Uttar Pradesh, India

Thieme
Delhi • Stuttgart • New York • Rio de Janeiro

Publishing Director: Ritu Sharma
Development Editor: Dr Gurvinder Kaur
Director-Editorial Services: Rachna Sinha
Project Managers: Prakash Naorem, Jyothi Sriram
Vice President, Sales and Marketing: Arun Kumar Majji
Managing Director & CEO: Ajit Kohli

Thieme Medical and Scientific Publishers Private Limited.
A - 12, Second Floor, Sector - 2, Noida - 201 301, Uttar Pradesh, India, +911204556600
Email: customerservice@thieme.in
www.thieme.in

Cover design: Thieme Publishing Group
Typesetting by RECTO Graphics, India

Printed in India by Nutech Print Services - India

5 4 3 2 1

ISBN: 978-93-88257-78-7

Dedicated to
The Almighty

Contents

Preface   ix

Acknowledgments   xi

Note from the Authors   xiii

Competency Mapping Chart   xv

1. Anatomy and Embryology of the Eye   1

2. Vision– Its Physiology, Neurology, and Assessment   14

3. Optics and Refraction   35

4. Ocular Therapeutics   60

5. The Conjunctiva   83

6. The Cornea   117

7. The Sclera   164

8. The Uveal Tract   173

9. The Pupil   213

10. The Lens   219

11. The Glaucoma   257

12. Vitreous Humor   316

13. The Retina   323

14. The Optic Nerve   393

15. The Afferent (Sensory) System   421

16. The Efferent (Motor) System   434

17. Strabismus (Squint)   449

18. Ocular Tumors   481

19. Ocular Injuries 495

20. The Lids 513

21. The Lacrimal Apparatus 545

22. The Orbit 565

23. Ocular Manifestations in Neurological Disorders 591

24. Ocular Manifestations of Systemic Diseases 636

25. Cryotherapy and Lasers in Ophthalmology 654

26. Eye Surgery 660

27. Ocular Symptoms and Examination 708

28. Community Ophthalmology 728

Index 739

Preface

The goal of this book is to provide a clinical overview of the major areas of ophthalmology in a simplified way. Although this book is essentially meant for undergraduate students, it will not only be of great use for Postgraduation aspirants but also serve as a foundation book for residents in ophthalmology.

To make it more student friendly, illustrations, tables and flow charts have been generously used to give it the form of a conceptual book.

We had started working on this book about 8 years ago. Now, we are happy to complete this and bring it to our readers. In fact, some part of the text is in more detail than required, but this feature of the book makes the text more attractive and explanatory in nature. The undergraduate course is not as extensive as the one earmarked for postgraduate entrance examinations. The contents of this book, however, cover the latter requirement. MBBS students should keep this fact in mind. Nevertheless, in spite of our efforts, the book is not likely to be free from human errors and mistakes. Therefore, any feedback and suggestions from the readers will be appreciated.

Sanjeev Kumar Mittal, MS, FICO (Japan)   **Raj Kumar Agarwal, MS**

Acknowledgments

With blessings of my parents, I, Dr. Sanjeev Kumar Mittal, acknowledge the motivation provided by my spouse Dr. Sunita Mittal and daughters Dr. Gauri Mittal and Pooja Mittal in writing this textbook of ophthalmology.

This book owes its existence to the help, support, and inspiration of several people as well as the blessings of my parents. I, Dr. Raj Kumar Agarwal, would like to express my sincere gratitude toward my spouse Dr. Renu Agarwal and daughters Dr. Akshi Raj and Dr. Archi Raj in writing the book of ophthalmology.

We extend our heartiest appreciation to our alma mater where we built a passion for teaching and writing. The students, too, have proved to be a perennial source of inspiration.

The contributions of the entire publication team at Thieme and Ms. Yukti Tyagi toward compiling the manuscript are peerless.

Sanjeev Kumar Mittal, MS, FICO (Japan)   **Raj Kumar Agarwal, MS**

Note from the Authors

We thank our contributors, listed below, for offering valuable content contribution to the following book chapters:

Chapter 2: Vision- Its Physiology, Neurology, and Assessment
Sunita Mittal, MBBS, MD
Additional Professor
Department of Physiology
All India Institute of Medical Sciences
Rishikesh, Uttarakhand, India

Gauri Mittal, MBBS
MD Resident
Department of Pharmacology
All India Institute of Medical Sciences
Rishikesh, Uttarakhand, India

Chapter 4: Ocular Therapeutics
S. S. Handu, MBBS, MD, DM
Professor and Head
Department of Pharmacology
All India Institute of Medical Sciences
Rishikesh, Uttarakhand, India

Chapter 11: The Glaucoma
Ajai Agarwal, MBBS, MS, MAMS, FICS
Additional Professor
Department of Ophthalmology
All India Institute of Medical Sciences
Rishikesh, Uttarakhand, India

Chapter 13: The Retina
Ramanuj Samantha, MBBS, MS, FICO
Assistant Professor
Department of Ophthalmology
All India Institute of Medical Sciences
Rishikesh, Uttarakhand, India

Chapter 17: Strabismus (Squint)
Anupam, MBBS, MS
Additional Professor
Department of Ophthalmology
All India Institute of Medical Sciences
Rishikesh, Uttarakhand, India

We thank the following fellow doctors for helping with providing clinical photographs:

Chapters 5 and 6: The Conjunctiva and the Cornea
Neeti Gupta, MBBS, MS, Fellow-Cornea LVPEI
Associate Professor
Department of Ophthalmology
All India Institute of Medical Sciences
Rishikesh, Uttarakhand, India

Chapters 20 and 22: The Lids and the Orbit
Rimpi Rana, MBBS, MS
Senior Resident
Department of Ophthalmology
All India Institute of Medical Sciences
Rishikesh, Uttarakhand, India

Competency Mapping Chart

Competency Code	COMPETENCY The student should be able to	Page No.
Visual Acuity Assessment		
OP1.1	Describe the physiology of vision	15
OP1.2	Define, classify, and describe the types and methods of correcting refractive errors	45, 718
OP1.3	Demonstrate the steps in performing the visual acuity assessment for distance vision, near vision, color vision, the pin hole test, and the menace and blink reflexes	22
OP1.4	Enumerate the indications and describe the principles of refractive surgery	59, 659, 680
OP1.5	Define and enumerate the types and the mechanism by which strabismus leads to amblyopia	467
Lids and Adnexa, Orbit		
OP2.1	Enumerate the causes; describe and discuss the etiology, clinical presentations, and diagnostic features of common conditions of the lid and adnexa including Hordeolum externum/internum, blepharitis, preseptal cellulitis, dacryocystitis, hemangioma, dermoid, ptosis, entropion, lid lag, and lagophthalmos	481, 519, 522, 524, 526, 532, 535, 539, 558, 574
OP2.2	Demonstrate the symptoms and clinical signs of conditions enumerated in OP2.1	481, 519, 522, 524, 526, 532, 535, 539
OP2.3	Demonstrate under supervision clinical procedures performed in the lid including: Bell's phenomenon, assessment of entropion/ectropion, regurgitation test of lacrimal sac, massage technique in congenital dacryocystitis, and trichiatic cilia removal by epilation	553
OP2.4	Describe the etiology and clinical presentation; discuss the complications and management of orbital cellulitis	574
OP2.5	Describe the clinical features on ocular examination and management of a patient with cavernous sinus thrombosis	578
OP2.6	Enumerate the causes and describe the differentiating features, clinical features, and management of proptosis	570, 578
OP2.7	Classify the various types of orbital tumors; differentiate the symptoms and signs of the presentation of various types of ocular tumors	564, 569, 582
OP2.8	List the investigations helpful in diagnosis of orbital tumors; enumerate the indications for appropriate referral	569, 582
Conjunctiva		
OP3.1	Elicit document and present an appropriate history in a patient presenting with a "red eye" including congestion, discharge, and pain	85, 187
OP3.2	Demonstrate document and present the correct method of examination of a "red eye" including vision assessment, corneal luster, pupil abnormality, and ciliary tenderness	85
OP3.3	Describe the etiology, pathophysiology, ocular features, differential diagnosis, complications, and management of various causes of conjunctivitis	89

Competency Code	COMPETENCY The student should be able to	Page No.
OP3.4	Describe the etiology, pathophysiology, ocular features, differential diagnosis, complications, and management of trachoma	98
OP3.5	Describe the etiology, pathophysiology, ocular features, differential diagnosis, complications, and management of vernal catarrh	108
OP3.6	Describe the etiology, pathophysiology, ocular features, differential diagnosis, complications, and management of pterygium	115
OP3.7	Describe the etiology, pathophysiology, ocular features, differential diagnosis, complications, and management of symblepharon	536
OP3.8	Demonstrate correct technique of removal of foreign body from the eye in a simulated environment	499
OP3.9	Demonstrate the correct technique of instillation of eye drops in a simulated environment	Practical
Corneas		
OP4.1	Enumerate, describe, and discuss the types and causes of corneal ulceration	127
OP4.2	Enumerate and discuss the differential diagnosis of infective keratitis	127
OP4.3	Enumerate the causes of corneal edema	121
OP4.4	Enumerate the causes and discuss the management of dry eye	559
OP4.5	Enumerate the causes of corneal blindness	115, 121, 122, 123, 156, 161
OP4.6	Enumerate the indications and the types of keratoplasty	676
OP4.7	Enumerate the indications and describe the methods of tarsorrhaphy	140, 143, 151, 153, 536, 539, 563, 607
OP4.8	Demonstrate technique of removal of foreign body in the cornea in a simulated environment	499
OP4.9	Describe and discuss the importance and protocols of eye donation and eye banking	676, 706
OP4.10	Counsel patients and family about eye donation in a simulated environment	Practical
Sclera		
OP5.1	Define, enumerate, and describe the etiology, associated systemic conditions, clinical features, complications, indications for referral, and management of episcleritis	165
OP5.2	Define, enumerate, and describe the etiology, associated systemic conditions, clinical features, complications, indications for referral, and management of scleritis	167
Iris and Anterior Chamber		
OP6.1	Describe clinical signs of intraocular inflammation and enumerate the features that distinguish granulomatous from nongranulomatous inflammation; identify acute iridocyclitis from chronic condition	177, 180
OP6.2	Identify and distinguish acute iridocyclitis from chronic iridocyclitis	177, 180
OP6.3	Enumerate systemic conditions that can present as iridocyclitis and describe their ocular manifestations	177, 180
OP6.4	Describe and distinguish hyphema and hypopyon	183, 505

Competency Code	COMPETENCY The student should be able to	Page No.
OP6.5	Describe and discuss the angle of the anterior chamber and its clinical correlates	2
OP6.6	Identify and demonstrate the clinical features, and distinguish and diagnose common clinical conditions affecting the anterior chamber	180, 265, 288, 292, 293, 298, 311, 716
OP6.7	Enumerate and discuss the etiology and the clinical distinguishing features of various glaucomas associated with shallow and deep anterior chamber; choose appropriate investigations and treatment for patients with above conditions	265, 288, 292, 293, 298, 311
OP6.8	Enumerate and choose the appropriate investigation for patients with conditions affecting the uvea	177, 180
OP6.9	Choose the correct local and systemic therapy for conditions of the anterior chamber and enumerate their indications, adverse events, and interactions	187
OP6.10	Counsel patients with conditions of the iris and anterior chamber about their diagnosis, therapy, and prognosis in an empathetic manner in a simulated environment	Practical
Lens		
OP7.1	Describe the surgical anatomy and the metabolism of the lens	218, 223
OP7.2	Describe and discuss the etiopathogenesis, stages of maturation, and complications of cataract	229, 230, 231, 235, 241
OP7.3	Demonstrate the correct technique of ocular examination in a patient with a cataract	233, 244
OP7.4	Enumerate the types of cataract surgery and describe the steps, and intraoperative and postoperative complications of extracapsular cataract extraction surgery	244, 686, 694
OP7.5	To participate in the team for cataract surgery	Practical
OP7.6	Administer informed consent and counsel patients for cataract surgery in a simulated environment	Practical
Retina and Optic Nerve		
OP8.1	Discuss the etiology, pathology, clinical features, and management of vascular occlusions of the retina	339, 341, 346, 351, 372, 375, 377, 378, 386
OP8.2	Enumerate the indications for laser therapy in the treatment of retinal diseases (including retinal detachment, retinal degenerations, diabetic retinopathy, and hypertensive retinopathy)	337, 339, 341, 346, 351, 372, 375, 377, 378, 386
OP8.3	Demonstrate the correct technique of fundus examination, and describe and distinguish the funduscopic features in a normal condition and in conditions causing an abnormal retinal examination	725
OP8.4	Enumerate and discuss treatment modalities in management of diseases of the retina	339, 341, 346, 351, 372, 375, 377, 378, 386, 701
OP8.5	Describe and discuss the correlative anatomy, etiology, clinical manifestations, diagnostic tests, imaging, and management of diseases of the optic nerve and visual pathway	392, 394, 395, 403, 411, 415

Competency Code	COMPETENCY The student should be able to	Page No.
Miscellaneous		
OP9.1	Demonstrate the correct technique to examine extraocular movements (uniocular and binocular)	439
OP9.2	Classify, enumerate the types, methods of diagnosis, and indications for referral in a patient with heterotropia/strabismus	450, 452, 459
OP9.3	Describe the role of refractive error correction in a patient with headache and enumerate the indications for referral	45, 59, 450, 451, 453, 631
OP9.4	Enumerate, describe, and discuss the causes of avoidable blindness and the National Programmefor Control of Blindness (including Vision 2020)	728, 729, 730, 731, 734
OP9.5	Describe the evaluation and enumerate the steps involved in the stabilization, initial management, and indication for referral in a patient with ocular injury	495
Integration		
Human Anatomy		
AN30.5	Explain effect of pituitary tumors on visual pathway	421
AN31.3	Describe anatomical basis of Horner's syndrome	593
AN31.5	Explain the anatomical basis of oculomotor, trochlear, and abducent nerve palsies along with strabismus	596, 597, 598
AN41.1	Describe and demonstrate parts and layers of eyeball	1
AN41.2	Describe the anatomical aspects of cataract, glaucoma, and central retinal artery occlusion	257
Physiology		
PY10.17	Describe and discuss functional anatomy of eye, physiology of image formation, physiology of vision including color vision, refractive errors, color blindness, physiology of pupil, and light reflex	15, 213, 257, 259
PY10.18	Describe and discuss the physiological basis of lesion in visual pathway	424
PY10.19	Describe and discuss auditory and visual evoked potentials	15
PY10.20	Demonstrate testing of visual acuity, color, and field of vision in volunteer/simulated environment	15
Pathology		
PA36.1	Describe the etiology, genetics, pathogenesis, pathology, presentation, sequelae, and complications of retinoblastoma	491
Pharmacology		
PH1.58	Describe drugs used in ocular disorders	60, 280
General Medicine		
IM24.15	Describe and discuss the etiopathogenesis, clinical presentation, identification, functional changes, acute care, stabilization, management and rehabilitation of vision, and visual loss in the elderly	57, 154, 235, 372, 733

Anatomy and Embryology of the Eye

Anatomy of Eyeball 1
Blood Supply of Eyeball 3
Innervation of Eyeball 5
Embryology of Eyeball 6

■ Anatomy of Eyeball (AN41.1)

Each eyeball is situated in a bony cavity known as the orbit. It is protected by eyelids and soft tissues. In the orbit, it is suspended by extraocular muscles and their facial sheaths.

■ Dimensions

- Anteroposterior diameter: at birth— 17.5 mm; in adults—24 mm.
- Horizontal diameter: 23.5 mm.
- Vertical diameter: 23 mm.

■ Shape

Being flattened in vertical diameter, its shape resembles an oblate spheroid.

■ Structure

Eyeball consists of three coats (tunics, **Fig. 1.1**):
1. Outer fibrous coat.
2. Intermediate vascular coat (uveal tissue).
3. Innermost nervous layer (retina).

Outer Fibrous Coat

It consists of cornea and sclera. Cornea is the anterior 1/6th, *transparent and avascular* part of the fibrous coat. Sclera is the posterior 5/6th opaque part of the fibrous coat. The anterior part of the sclera is covered by a mucous membrane, the conjunctiva, which is reflected over the inner surface of the eyelids. The junction of sclera and cornea is called the *sclerocorneal junction* or limbus. Conjunctiva is firmly adherent at the limbus.

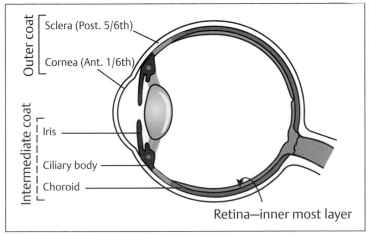

Fig. 1.1 Tunics (coats) of eyeball. Abbreviations: Ant., anterior; Post., posterior.

Outer coat
- Sclera (Post. 5/6th)
- Cornea (Ant. 1/6th)

Intermediate coat
- Iris
- Ciliary body
- Choroid

Retina—inner most layer

Intermediate Vascular Coat (Uveal Tissue)

It consists of three parts:

1. Iris: It is the anterior most part of the uveal tissue.
2. Ciliary body: It extends from iris to ora serrata and is subdivided into two parts: anterior (pars plicata, 2 mm) and posterior (pars plana, 4 mm).
3. Choroid: It is the posterior most part of the uveal tissue. It lies in contact with sclera on its outer surface and with retina on its inner surface.

Innermost Nervous Layer (Retina)

It extends from optic disc to ora serrata. It ends abruptly just behind the ciliary body as a dentate border called ora serrata. It is concerned with visual functions.

■ Segments

The eyeball is divided into anterior and posterior segments (**Fig. 1.2**) by the lens, which is suspended from the ciliary body by fine delicate fibrils called zonules (suspensory ligaments of lens). Both anterior and posterior chambers communicate with each other through the pupil.

Anterior Segment

This includes structures anterior to the lens, that is, cornea, iris, lens, and part of ciliary body. The anterior segment is divided by the iris into an *anterior chamber* and *a posterior chamber.*

Anterior Chamber (OP6.5)

- *Boundaries*: The posterior surface of cornea *forms the* anterior boundary, while the iris, part of ciliary body, and surface of lens in the pupillary *area forms the* posterior boundary of the anterior chamber.
- *Depth*: It is 2.5 mm in center. It is shallower in hypermetropes and deeper in myopes.
- It *contains* a clear watery fluid called **aqueous humor** (0.25 mL).
- *Angle*: *Angle of anterior chamber* is a peripheral recess of the anterior chamber through which drainage of aqueous humor takes place.

Posterior Chamber

- It is a triangular space and *contains* aqueous humor.
- *Boundaries*: The posterior surface of iris and part of ciliary body forms the anterior boundary, while the lens, zonules, and ciliary body forms the posterior boundary.

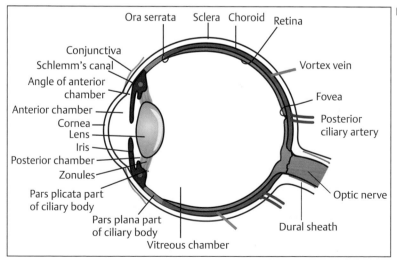

Fig. 1.2 Structure of eyeball.

Ora serrata Sclera Choroid Retina
Conjunctiva
Schlemm's canal
Angle of anterior chamber
Anterior chamber
Cornea
Lens
Iris
Posterior chamber
Zonules
Pars plicata part of ciliary body
Pars plana part of ciliary body
Vitreous chamber
Vortex vein
Fovea
Posterior ciliary artery
Optic nerve
Dural sheath

Both anterior and posterior chambers communicate with each other through the **pupil.**

Posterior Segment

This includes structures posterior to the lens, that is, vitreous humor, retina, choroid, and optic nerve.

Vitreous humor is a gel-like material which fills the cavity behind the lens. The detailed anatomy of various parts of the eyeball and ocular adnexa (eyelids, lacrimal apparatus, and orbit) is described in respective chapters.

■ Blood Supply of Eyeball

The eye has two separate systems of blood vessels (**Table 1.1**):

1. Retinal vessels: These supply part of the retina.
2. Ciliary blood vessel: These supply rest of the eye.

■ Arterial Supply

Both retinal and ciliary arteries branch from the ophthalmic artery, which is a branch of the internal carotid artery (ICA), and gives rise to the following branches (**Fig. 1.3** and **Fig. 1.4**):

- *Lacrimal artery*: It supplies the lacrimal gland.
- *Central retinal artery*: Supplies the retina.
- *Short posterior ciliary arteries* (10–20 in number): Supply the uveal tract.
- *Long posterior ciliary arteries* (two in number).
- *Muscular arteries:* Supply four recti muscles which give rise to anterior ciliary arteries.

Short posterior ciliary arteries pierce the sclera in a ring around the optic nerve and give rise to the intrascleral circle of Zinn. These end as choriocapillaris and supply the entire choroid.

Long posterior ciliary arteries pierce sclera in horizontal meridian and pass forward in suprachoroidal space (between sclera and choroid), without giving any branch, reach ciliary muscle and form circulus arteriosus iridis major (major arterial circle of iris) with anterior ciliary arteries. It supplies ciliary processes and iris. The recurrent branches from the circle supply the anterior part of choriocapillaris. Branches from this major arterial circle run radially through the iris, which form a circular anastomosis near the pupillary margin called the circulus arteriosus iridis minor (minor arterial circle of iris). Anterior ciliary arteries give branches to the conjunctiva, sclera, and limbus.

Central retinal artery supplies the inner layers of retina. Outer layers of retina are nourished by diffusion from choriocapillaris.

Small anastomoses between vessels of uveal origin and central retinal artery connect the uveal and retinal circulations.

Occlusion of one of the ciliary arteries usually does not produce dramatic effects because of arterial ring and manifold arterial supply to choriocapillaris.

■ Venous Drainage

Venous drainage of inner retina occurs via central retinal vein to superior ophthalmic vein after which the blood passes into cavernous sinus and out of the skull through internal jugular vein.

Table 1.1 Blood supply of the eyeball		
Part of the eye	**Arterial supply**	**Venous drainage**
• Iris and ciliary body • Choroid	• **Long posterior** ciliary arteries and **anterior** ciliary arteries. • **Short posterior** ciliary arteries.	**Vortex veins** drain blood from whole of uveal tract except outer part of ciliary muscle which is drained by **anterior ciliary veins**.

• Retina:
  ◊ outer layers of retina
  ◊ inner layers of retina
	By diffusion from **choriocapillaris**
	central retinal artery.
		Vortex veins
		via **central retinal vein** into cavernous sinus.

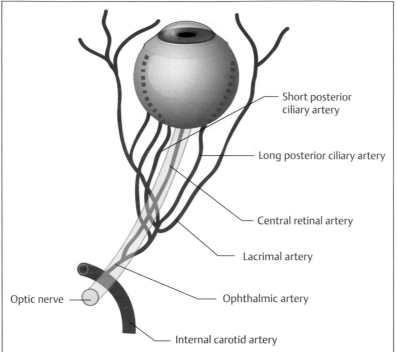

Fig. 1.3 Arterial supply of eyeball.

Short posterior ciliary artery

Long posterior ciliary artery

Central retinal artery

Lacrimal artery

Optic nerve

Ophthalmic artery

Internal carotid artery

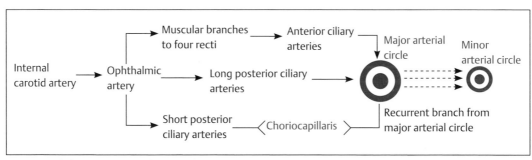

Fig. 1.4 Ophthalmic artery and its branches.

Outer retinal layers are drained by vortex veins which drain into the superior ophthalmic vein.

Uveal tract drains through three groups of ciliary veins, namely, short posterior ciliary veins, vortex veins, and anterior ciliary veins.

Short posterior ciliary veins receive blood only from sclera. They do not receive any blood from the choroid.

Vortex veins (venae vorticosae): Small veins from uveal tract join to form four vortex veins,

namely, superior temporal, inferior temporal, superior nasal, and inferior nasal veins.

These pierce sclera behind the equator and drain into superior and inferior ophthalmic veins which, in turn, drain into cavernous sinus. As ophthalmic veins communicate with cavernous sinus, they act as a route by which infections can spread from outside to inside the cranial cavity. Vortex veins drain blood from whole of the uveal tract except outer part of ciliary muscle, which is drained by anterior ciliary veins. Veins from the outer part of ciliary body form a plexus, ciliary venous plexus, which drain into anterior ciliary veins. These receive blood from only outer part of ciliary muscle.

▬ Innervation of Eyeball

Eyeball is innervated by both sensory and motor nerves.

■ Sensory Nerve Supply

It is derived from ophthalmic division of the trigeminal nerve (V1). It is *purely a sensory nerve*. It divides into three branches (**Fig. 1.5**):

- Nasociliary nerve.
- Lacrimal nerve.
- Frontal nerve.

Long ciliary nerve (a branch of nasociliary nerve) is sensory to eyeball but may also contain sympathetic fibers for pupillary dilatation. Nasociliary nerve also gives off sensory root to ciliary ganglion.

■ Motor Nerve Supply

These nerves supply extrinsic (extra ocular muscles) and intrinsic muscles.

Nerve Supply of Extrinsic Muscles (Extra Ocular Muscles)

Mnemonic—**LR$_6$ (SO$_4$)$_3$**, that is, lateral rectus is supplied by 6th nerve (Abducens nerve). Superior oblique is supplied by 4th nerve (Trochlear nerve), and rest of the muscles (i.e., superior rectus [SR], inferior rectus [IR], medial rectus [MR], and inferior oblique) are supplied by 3rd nerve (oculomotor nerve).

Oculomotor nerve (III) divides into (**Fig. 1.6**):

- *Superior branch*: It innervates SR and levator palpebrae superioris (LPS).
- *Inferior branch*: It innervates MR, IR, inferior oblique (IO), and a branch to ciliary ganglion.

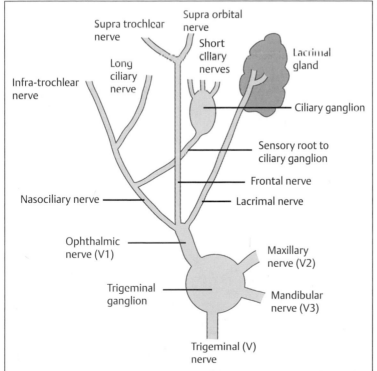

Fig. 1.5 Ophthalmic nerve and its branches.

Supra trochlear nerve

Supra orbital nerve

Short ciliary nerves

Lacrimal gland

Long ciliary nerve

Infra-trochlear nerve

Ciliary ganglion

Sensory root to ciliary ganglion

Frontal nerve

Nasociliary nerve

Lacrimal nerve

Ophthalmic nerve (V1)

Maxillary nerve (V2)

Trigeminal ganglion

Mandibular nerve (V3)

Trigeminal (V) nerve

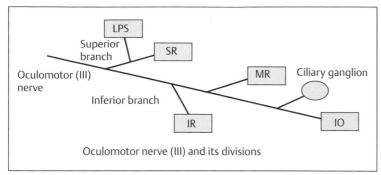

Fig. 1.6 Oculomotor nerve and its branches. Abbreviations: LPS, levator palpabrae superioris; SR, superior rectus; IR, inferior rectus; MR, medial rectus; IO, inferior oblique muscle.

Oculomotor nerve (III) and its divisions

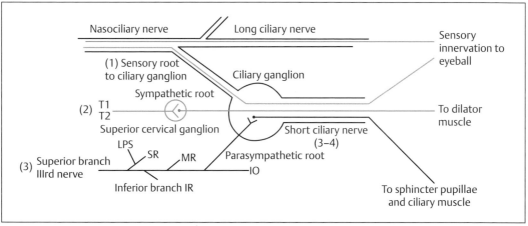

Fig. 1.7 Course of nerve supply through ciliary ganglion. Abbreviations: LPS, levator palpabrae superioris; SR, superior rectus; IR, inferior rectus; MR, medial rectus; IO, inferior oblique muscle.

Nerve Supply to Intrinsic Muscles (AN41.3)

- *Ciliary muscle* and *sphincter pupillae* are supplied by the 3rd nerve (Oculomotor nerve).
- *Dilator pupillae* is supplied by sympathetic fibers.

■ Ciliary Ganglion

It is a parasympathetic ganglion of oculomotor nerve (III), as preganglionic parasympathetic fibers from branch of oculomotor nerve (III) synapse with postganglionic parasympathetic fibers within the ganglion. Postganglionic parasympathetic fibers leave the ganglion through short ciliary nerves which enter the eyeball around optic nerve. These innervate sphincter pupillae and ciliary muscle.

A sensory root passes from the nasociliary nerve to eyeball through ganglion. These fibers are responsible for sensory innervations to all parts of the eyeball (**Fig. 1.7**).

Third branch to ganglion is the sympathetic root and contains postganglionic sympathetic fiber from the superior cervical ganglion. These fibers reach the eyeball and innervate dilator pupillae muscle. These fibers also continue along short ciliary nerves.

■ Embryology of Eyeball

In general, there are three main stages in prenatal development of the eye:
- Period of embryogenesis.
- Period of organogenesis.
- Period of differentiation.

■ Embryogenesis

Three germ layers (ectoderm, mesoderm, and endoderm) are formed after a series of divisions and proliferations in fertilized ovum.

- Ectoderm overlying notochord becomes thickened to form neural plate *(neuroectoderm)*. A ridge of cells (neural crest) develops along the edges of the neural plate. Neural crest cells subsequently migrate and give rise to various structures within the eye and orbit (**Fig. 1.8a**).
- Neural plate is converted to neural groove, which becomes deeper, and neural groove is converted into **neural tube** (**Fig. 1.8b**).
- By the end of embryogenesis, the neural tube is divided into an enlarged cranial part which develops into three primary brain vesicles: prosencephalon (forebrain), mesencephalon (midbrain), and rhombencephalon (hind brain). The narrow caudal part becomes the spinal cord (**Fig. 1.8c**).

■ Organogenesis

The period of organogenesis begins after the 3rd gestational week. On the 22nd *day of gestation*, optic pits form as lateral outpouchings of prosencephalon (**Fig. 1.8d**). *Failure of optic pit to develop into optic vesicle results in complete absence of an eye* (true anophthalmia).

- On the 25th day of gestation, optic pits enlarge and form **optic vesicles.** Proximal part of optic vesicle becomes constricted and elongated to form optic stalk. Optic vesicles grow laterally and come in contact with overlying surface ectoderm (**Fig. 1.1.8e**). *If insult to embryo occurs after outgrowth of optic vesicle, developmental arrest of ocular growth results in* microphthalmos (small eye).
- Surface ectoderm overlying the optic vesicles become thickened to form **lens placode** on the 27th day. Lens placode undergoes invagination and is converted into *lens vesicle*. Simultaneously, wall of

optic vesicle begins to invaginate and form a *double-layered optic cup* as a result of differential growth of the wall of vesicle (**Fig. 1.8f** and **Fig. 1.8g**).

- Lens vesicle becomes completely separated from the surface ectoderm on day 33 of gestation. Margins of the optic cup grow over upper and lateral sides of the lens to enclose it, but not on the inferior aspect of lens, resulting in a *choroidal or fetal fissure* under the surface of each cup and extend to the most proximal portion of the optic stalk.
- As developing neural tube is surrounded by mesoderm, this fetal fissure is the portal through which mesoderm enters the developing eye.
- Between the 5th and 7th weeks of gestation, fetal fissure closes and the globe is formed (**Fig. 1.8h**).

Embryonic fissure runs from optic nerve to margin of pupil (anterior part of optic cup). Incomplete closure of embryonic (choroidal) fissure around 5 to 8 weeks of gestation results in absence of the part of an ocular structure called **coloboma**.

As embryonic fissure is inferior and slightly nasal, typical coloboma is inferonasal in location.

If entire length of fissure is involved, coloboma is complete. If only part of fissure is involved, it may involve iris (iris coloboma), choroid (choroid coloboma), retina (retinal coloboma), and optic disc (disc coloboma).

During development of optic cup and lens vesicle, the mesoderm surrounding optic vesicle gives rise to various vascular and orbital tissues.

■ Differentiation

Differentiation begins around 8th gestational week and occurs before the eye is fully functional. For **macula,** differentiation is completed after the birth.

Various components of eyeball are derived from:

- *Optic cup* which develops from *neuroectoderm* (neural plate).
- *Mesoderm* surrounding optic vesicle.
- *Lens placode* (a specialized area of surface ectoderm).

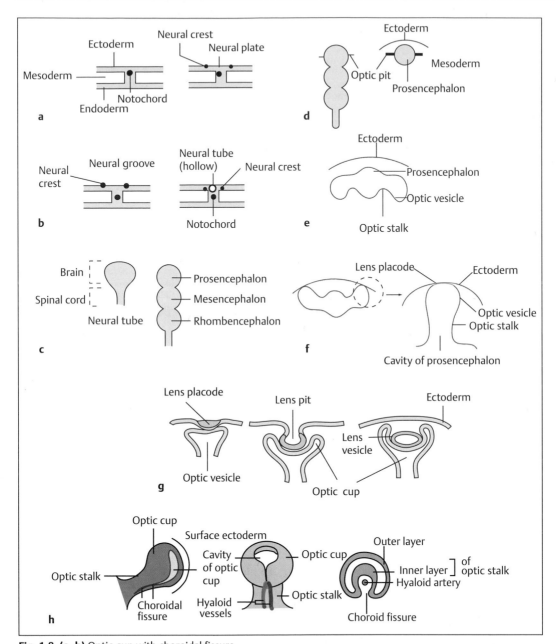

Fig. 1.8 (a–h) Optic cup with choroidal fissure.

Optic Cup

It is a double-layered embryonic tissue (**Fig. 1.9** and **Table 1.2**).

Myelination of nerve fibers begins in the 8th month. It starts at chiasm and proceeds toward optic nerve to reach lamina cribrosa just before birth and stops there. Thus, *in normal eyes, myelination stops at lamina cribrosa.*

> If myelination extends beyond lamina cribrosa, nerve fibers of retina (axons of ganglion cells) also get myelinated. The opaque nerve fibers are called myelinated (medullated) nerve fibers.

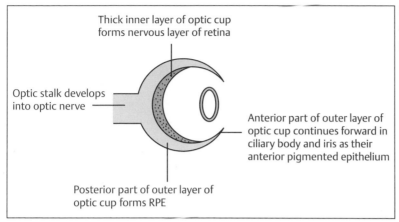

Thick inner layer of optic cup forms nervous layer of retina

Optic stalk develops into optic nerve

Anterior part of outer layer of optic cup continues forward in ciliary body and iris as their anterior pigmented epithelium

Posterior part of outer layer of optic cup forms RPE

Fig. 1.9 Layers of optic cup. Abbreviation: RPE, retinal pigment epithelium.

Table 1.2 Derivatives of optic cup

Part of optic cup	Derivative
Outer layer of optic cup The cells of outer layer contain pigment granules	• *Anterior part* of it continues forward in *ciliary body* and *iris* as their *anterior-pigmented epithelium*. • *Posterior part* of outer layer of optic cup forms RPE.
Inner layer of optic cup	• Forms *nervous layer of retina*.
Optic stalk	• It develops into *optic nerve*.
Mouth of optic cup	• It becomes a round opening, the future **pupil**.

Abbreviations: RPE, retinal pigment epithelium.

Other coats of eyeball are derived from mesoderm surrounding the optic cup. Layers of mesoderm surrounding the optic stalk form the sheaths of optic nerve.

Mesoderm

Optic cup is completely surrounded by the mesoderm. This tissue soon differentiates into outer and inner layers (**Fig. 1.10a**).

Outer layer (fibrous layer) is comparable with duramater and develops into sclera.

Inner layer (vascular layer) of mesoderm is carried into the cup through the choroidal fissure and forms **choroid, ciliary body, and iris**. Part of this mesoderm which gets invaginated into optic cup forms the **retinal vessels**.

Differentiation of mesoderm overlying the anterior aspect of eye is different. Vacuolization in mesoderm splits it into outer layer, which forms stroma and inner epithelium of cornea, and the inner layer, which forms stroma and blood vessels of iris and ciliary body. The anterior chamber forms between the two layers and correspond to the subarachnoid space of the brain (**Fig. 1.10b**).

Lens Placode

• Lens placode is converted into lens vesicle which is lined by a single layer of cubical cells surrounded by the basal lamina.
• Cells in the anterior wall of vesicle remain cubical, while cells in the posterior wall of vesicle become elongated.
• The cavity of vesicle is eventually obliterated (**Fig. 1.11**).

■ Development of Various Ocular Structures

Development of Retina

Retina is developed from two walls of optic cup (**Table 1.3**).

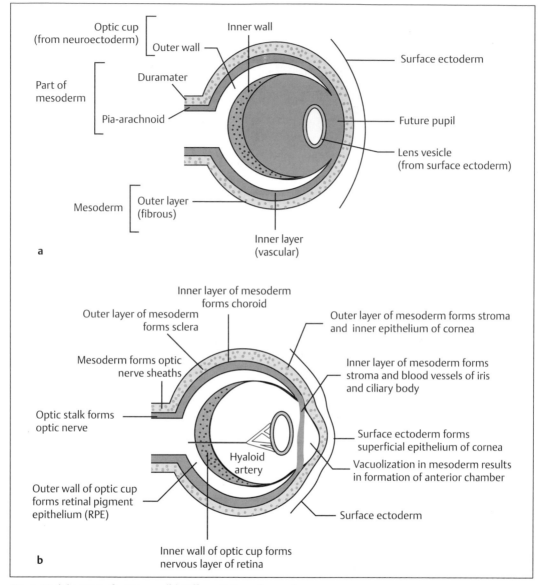

Fig. 1.10 (a) Layers of optic cup. **(b)** Differentiation of mesoderm.

Table 1.3 Development of retina

Part of optic cup	Derivative
Outer layer of optic cup The cells of outer layer contain pigment granules.	• *Anterior part* of it continues forward in *ciliary body* and *iris* as their **RPE**. • *Posterior part* of outer layer of optic cup forms RPE.
Inner layer of optic cup	• Forms *nervous layer of retina*.
Mouth of optic cup	• It becomes a round opening, the future **pupil**.
Abbreviation: RPE, retinal pigment epithelium.	

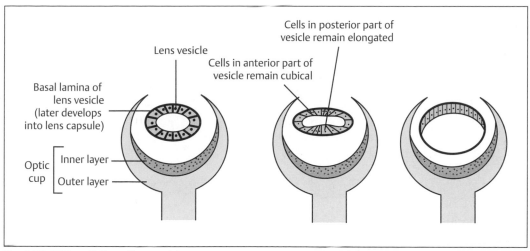

Fig. 1.11 Differentiation of lens vesicle.

Table 1.4 Development of optic nerve

Part of optic stalk	Derivative
Outer layer of optic stalk	• It gives rise to lamina cribrosa which becomes permeated by collagen fibers from sclera and choroid by 8th month.
Inner layer of optic stalk	• It develops into glial cells which separate the axons into bundles.

Table 1.5 Development of cornea and sclera

Part	Derivative
Outer layer (fibrous layer) of mesoderm *surrounding the optic cup*	• It develops into **sclera.**
Outer layer (fibrous layer) of mesoderm *anterior to optic cup*	• It forms stroma and inner epithelium of cornea.
Surface ectoderm	• It forms superficial epithelium of cornea.

Development of Optic Nerve

The optic stalk develops into the optic nerve. The nerve fiber layer (Ganglion cell axons) migrate through the vacuolization of cells in the optic stalk (**Table 1.4**).

- The hyaloid artery in the central axis of optic nerve develops into *central retinal artery.*
- *Optic nerve sheaths* are formed from the layers of mesoderm surrounding the optic stalk.
- *Myelination* of nerve fibers begins in the 8th month. It starts at chiasm and proceeds toward optic nerve to reach lamina cribrosa just before birth and stops there. Thus, *in normal eyes, myelination stops at lamina cribrosa.*

> If myelination extends beyond lamina cribrosa, myelination of nerve fibers of retina (axons of ganglion cells) results. The opaque nerve fibers are called myelinated (medullated) nerve fibers.

Development of Cornea and Sclera

Development of cornea and sclera is briefly explained in **Table 1.5**.

Development of Uveal Tissue

Development of uveal tissue is briefly explained in **Table 1.6**.

Table 1.6 Development of uveal tissue

Part	Derivative
Inner layer (vascular layer) of mesoderm	• It is carried into the cup through the choroidal fissure and forms **choroid, stroma, and blood vessels of iris and ciliary body.**
Neuroectodermally derived optic cup rim	• As the rim of optic cup grows anteriorly, it develops into **two epithelial layers.** The anterior epithelial layer becomes pigmented and is continuous with RPE posteriorly. The posterior epithelium remains nonpigmented and is continuous with the inner retinal layer of optic cup (i.e., nervous layer of retina). • **Sphincter and dilator pupillae muscles.**
Abbreviations: RPE, retinal pigment epithelium.	

Table 1.7 Derivatives of lens placode (Lens vesicle)

Parts of lens placode	Derivative
Cells in anterior wall of lens vesicles remain cubical	• Form lens **epithelium.**
Equatorial cells of anterior epithelium	• Form **secondary lens fibers.**
Cells of posterior wall become elongated and lose their nuclei	• Form **primary lens fibers.**
The basal lamina of lens vesicle	• Develops into **lens capsule.**

Development of Lens

Lens is developed from lens placode which is converted into lens vesicle (**Table 1.7**).

Development of Vitreous

Vitreous is derived from:
- *Ectoderm*—Ectodermal component is derived from optic cup (**secondary vitreous**). It is an avascular structure and surrounds the primary vitreous.
- *Mesoderm*—Mesoderm invades inside of optic cup through choroidal fissure. Here it forms hyaloid vessels (**primary vitreous**). Hyaloid artery extends toward and around lens vesicle and anastomoses with vessels in the vascular mesoderm. The Canal of Cloquet containing hyaloid artery is formed due to condensation between primary and secondary vitreous.

Fate of hyaloid artery: In the 3rd trimester, hyaloid system begins to regress, except for the portion that supplies the retina as central retinal artery. Hyaloid artery in vitreous disappears but hyaloid canal in vitreous (through which the artery passes) persists.

When secondary vitreous fills the cavity, primary vitreous with hyaloid vessels is pushed anteriorly and ultimately disappears. If primary vitreous fails to regress **persistent hyperplastic primary vitreous** (PHPV) results.

Development of Accessory Structures of Eyeball

- **Eyelids develop from both surface ectoderm and mesoderm.** Mesoderm gives rise to muscle and tarsal plates. Ingrowth of surface ectodermal cells from lids margins form tarsal glands and epithelial buds from lid margins form cilia.
- **Conjunctiva and conjunctival glands** develop from **ectoderm** lining the lids and globe.
- **Lacrimal glands** develop from a number of buds arising from the superolateral angle of the conjunctival sac.
- **Nasolacrimal system** (canaliculi, lacrimal sac, and nasolacrimal duct): Lacrimal

Table 1.8 Important events in ocular embryogenesis

Period after conception	Event
22nd day	• Appearance of optic pits.
25th day	• Formation of optic vesicles from optic pit.
27th day	• Formation of lens placoid from surface ectoderm.
28th day	• Formation of embryonic (fetal) fissure.
5th week	• Lens pit forms and deepens into lens vesicle. • Development of hyaloid vessels and primary vitreous.
6th week	• Closure of embryonic fissure. • Differentiation of retinal pigment epithelium. • Formation of secondary vitreous. • Appearance of eyelid folds and nasolacrimal duct. • Formation of primary lens fibers.
7th week	• Formation of embryonic lens nucleus. • Formation of sclera begins.
3rd month	• Differentiation of precursors of rods and cones. • Development of ciliary body and anterior chamber. • Eyelid folds lengthen and fuse.
4th month	• Regression of hyaloid vessels. • Formation of major arterial circle of iris and iris sphincter muscle. • Formation of eyelid glands and cilia.
5th month	• Eyelid separation begins. • Differentiation of photoreceptors.
6th month	• Differentiation of dilator pupillae muscle. • Nasolacrimal system becomes patent. • Differentiation of cones.
7th month	• Differentiation of rods. • Myelination of optic nerve.
8th month	• Completion of anterior chamber angle formation. • Hyaloid vessels disappear.
9th month	• Retinal vessels reach temporal periphery. • Pupillary membrane disappears.
After birth	• Development of macula.

drainage system develops from **surface ectoderm.** Nasolacrimal system becomes patent by the 6th month of gestation.

- **Extraocular muscles** develop from **mesoderm.**

In summary, the eye is formed from both ectoderm (neural and surface ectoderms) and mesoderm. Important events of development are listed in **Table 1.8**.

Vision–Its Physiology, Neurology, and Assessment

Introduction..14

Visual Process...15

Assessment of Visual Function 21

Binocular Vision..32

■ Introduction

The light falling upon the retina stimulates the sensory nerve endings, rods and cones. Histologically, retina consists of 10 distinct layers including three layers of cell (**Fig. 2.1**).

These are as follows:

- Layer of rods and cones– These are the receptors sensitive to light and serve as sensory nerve endings for visual sensations. The cell bodies of rods and cones form the outer nuclear layer (**ONL**).

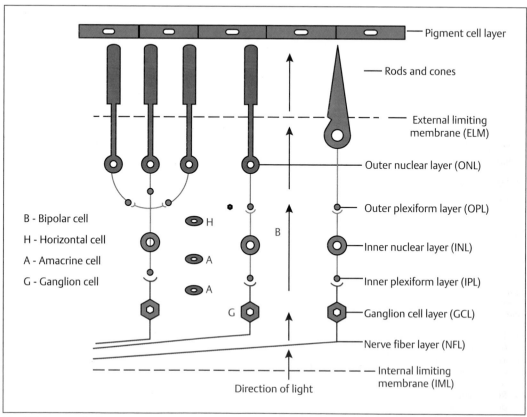

B - Bipolar cell
H - Horizontal cell
A - Amacrine cell
G - Ganglion cell

Fig. 2.1 Layers of retina.

- Layer of bipolar cells– This layer also includes horizontal cells, amacrine cells, and Muller's cells. The cell bodies of these cells form the inner nuclear layer (**INL**).
- Layer of ganglion cells– They give rise to optic nerve fibers. The cell bodies of ganglion cells form the ganglion cell layer (**GCL**).

Functionally, the retina can be subdivided into four regions, namely, optic nerve head (ONH), fovea, retina peripheral to fovea, and peripheral retina (**Table 2.1**).

■ Photoreceptors

The rods are mainly located in the periphery, whereas the cones occupy the central region (**Table 2.2**).

■ Visual Process (OP1.1, PY10.17, PY10.19, PY10.20)

It is the process by which our brain forms an image from light energy. Visual process can be divided into the following stages (**Flowchart 2.1**):

- Initiation of visual sensation.
- Transmission of visual impulse.
- Visual perception.

■ Initiation of Visual Sensation

The light falling upon retina causes two essential reactions: photochemical changes and electrical changes.

The **photochemical changes** concern visual pigments, that is, pigments in rods and cones. The photochemical changes in rods and cones

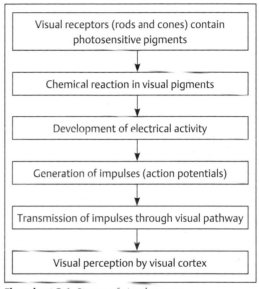

Flowchart 2.1 Stages of visual process.

Table 2.1 The regional variations of sensory nerve endings

Retinal region	Features
1 Optic nerve head (Blind spot)	Receptors are absent, i.e., *no rods and cones*. So, insensitive to light.
2 Fovea	*Only cones* are present and hence it is responsible for visual acuity. At fovea, there is one-to-one correspondence between photoreceptors and ganglion cells.
3 Retina peripheral to fovea	Here *both cones* and *rods* are present.
4 Peripheral retina	*Mainly rods* are present. This region is responsible for perception of dim light.

Table 2.2 Difference between rods and cones

Rods	Cones
• These are responsible for dim light vision (**scotopic vision**). These cannot detect color. • These predominate in extra foveal region where many rods synapse with a bipolar cell. Hence, receptive field is more with less resolution. • **Rhodopsin** (visual purple) is the visual pigment present in the rods.	• These are responsible for vision in bright light (**photopic vision**) and color vision. • These predominate at fovea and there is one-to-one correspondence between cones and bipolar cells. Hence, resolution is more and visual acuity is better. • There are three types of cones, each containing a specific pigment responsible for color discrimination and normal daylight vision.

are similar but the changes in rhodopsin have been studied in detail. **Rhodopsin** absorbs light with a peak sensitivity of **505 nm** (green light) (**Flowchart 2.2**). Rods are low-resolution detectors and consist of the following:

- An apoprotein, opsin (called scotopsin), to which the chromophore molecule (11-Cis-retinal) is attached.
- 11-Cis-retinal belongs to the carotenoid family. In the dark, it is in 11-cis form and gets converted to all-trans form in the presence of light. Retinal is derived from food sources. It is not synthesized in the body.

On exposure to light, 11-Cis-retinal is converted into all-trans-retinal isomer through short-lived intermediate products. With this change, rhodopsin loses its color (**bleaching of rhodopsin**). The all-trans-retinal is converted to all-trans-retinol and reaches the liver via blood. In liver, it is converted to 11-Cis- retinol. This is transformed to 11-Cis-retinal and combines with opsin to form rhodopsin (regeneration of rhodopsin). If subject immediately goes into dark after a brief exposure to light, all-trans-retinal is directly converted to 11-Cis-retinal by isomerase in the retina.

Only the first step in the bleaching sequence requires input of light. All subsequent reactions can proceed in the dark as well as in light.

When the intensity of background illumination remains relatively constant, rates of visual pigment bleaching and regeneration are in balance. This equilibrium between bleaching and regeneration of visual pigment is called **visual cycle**.

Electrical changes: The biochemical reactions result in generation of receptor potential. The process by which light energy is converted into receptor potential is known as **phototransduction**.

■ Transmission of Visual Impulse

The processing of visual information takes place at the following three levels:

1. At retina.
2. At LGB (lateral geniculate body).
3. At visual cortex.

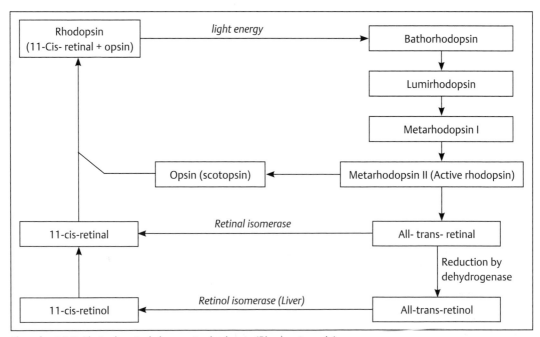

Flowchart 2.2 Photochemical changes in rhodopsin (Rhodopsin cycle).

The changes in electrical potential are transmitted through bipolar cells, ganglion cells, and optic nerve fibers to brain via visual pathway (visual pathway comprises optic nerves, optic chiasma, optic tracts, lateral geniculate bodies, optic radiations, and visual cortex in brain **Flowchart 2.3**).

Processing at Retina

Bipolar cells, horizontal cells, and amacrine cells participate in lateral inhibition (a form of inhibition in which activation of a particular neural unit is associated with inhibition of the activity of nearby units). **Lateral inhibition** prevents spreading of excitatory signal widely in the retina and improves the contrast of borders and edges of an object.

Retinal ganglion cells are of two types:
- Magno cells (M cells).
- Parvo cells (P cells).

Magno cells are larger cells and concerned with black and white response, perception of movement, and rough sketch of the object.

Parvo cells are smaller cells and predominate in the macular region. These cells are color sensitive and concerned with color vision and finer details of the object.

Two separate pathways start from ganglion cells, one from parvo cells (**parvocellular pathway**) and another from magno cells (**magnocellular pathway**). Both pathways are involved in the parallel processing of the image.

The action potentials (impulse) developed from these cells are conducted to lateral geniculate bodies (LGBs).

Processing at Lateral Geniculate Body (LGB)

The retina has point-to-point representation in a **LGB**. A LGB consists of six layers. *Magnocellular*

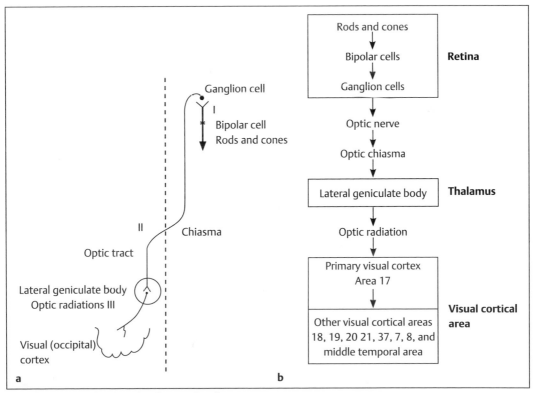

Flowchart 2.3 (a, b) Algorithm for visual pathway.

pathway from magno cells terminate *in layers 1 and 2* of LGB. *Parvocellular pathway* from parvo cells terminate *in layers 3, 4, 5 and 6* of LGB. On each side, layers 1, 4 and 6 receive input from contralateral eye, while layers 2, 3 and 5 receive input from the ipsilateral eye.

From LGB, two separate pathways project to the visual cortex. Magnocellular pathway from layers 1 and 2 carries signals for detection of movement, depth, and rough sketch of the object. Parvocellular pathway from layers 3, 4, 5, and 6 carry signals for color vision and finer details of the object (**Fig. 2.2**).

■ Visual Perception (Processing at visual cortex)

Visual cortex consists of two areas:
- Primary visual cortex or striate cortex which transforms information received from LGB and transmits it to the secondary visual cortex.
- Secondary visual cortex or extra striate cortex which transmits information received from primary visual cortex to the higher visual areas.

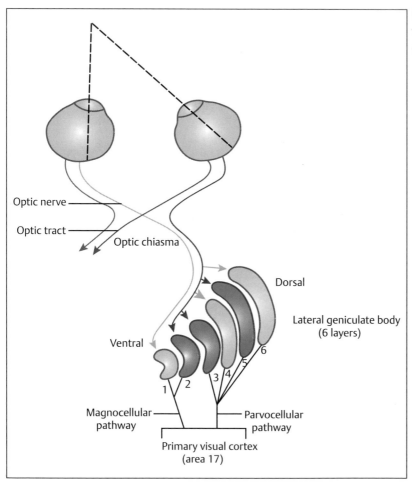

Fig. 2.2 Processing of visual impulse at lateral geniculate body.

■ Visual Sensations

Visual sensations resulting from the stimulation of retina by light are of four types:
- Light sense.
- Form sense.
- Sense of contrast.
- Color sense.

Light Sense

It is the perception of light in all its gradations of intensity. The intensity of light required to perceive it is called the *light minimum*. The light is no longer perceived if the intensity of light is reduced below the point of light minimum. The eye functions normally in a wide range of illumination by adjustment to such changes (called visual adaptation). Visual adaptation involves **dark adaptation** (adaptation to dim illumination) and **light adaptation** (adaptation to bright illumination). If we move from bright sun light into a dim light in the room, we cannot perceive the objects in the room until sometime has elapsed to adapt the amount of illumination by the eyes. The time taken to see in dim light is called *dark adaptation time*. The rods are much more sensitive to low illumination, so that rods are used in dim light at dusk (scotopic vision). The cones come into play in bright illumination (photopic vision). Bats have few or no cones; hence, it is a nocturnal animal. Squirrels have no rods and is therefore a diurnal animal. Human beings have rods and cones both.

During dark adaptation, the following changes take place in the eye:
- Pupils dilate.
- Vision changes from cones to rods (photopic vision to scotopic vision). This is called **Purkinje shift**.
- Sensitivity of receptors to light increases.
- Photopigments are resynthesized and so their concentration increases. Since vitamin A is required for the synthesis of both rod and cone pigments, deficiency of this vitamin produces visual abnormalities.
- Visual acuity decreases.

During light adaptation, the following changes take place in the eye:
- Pupils constrict.
- Vision changes from rods to cones (scotopic to photopic vision).
- Photopigments are bleached and so their concentration decreases.
- Sensitivity of receptors to light decreases. This happens due to decreased concentration of photopigments.
- Visual acuity increases. Both the photoreceptors work together at the midrange of illumination, which is the mesopic range.

Form Sense

It is the ability which enables us to perceive the shape of objects. Cones play the major role in form sense, so it is most acute at the fovea having cones. It decreases very rapidly toward the periphery due to a decrease in the number of cones. Visual acuity is the ability to see fine details of objects in the visual field. Assessment of visual acuity is discussed in the latter part of this chapter.

Sense of Contrast (Contrast Sensitivity)

It is the ability to perceive slight changes in the luminance between the regions which are not separated by definite borders. It indirectly assesses the quality of vision as loss of contrast sensitivity may disturb the patient more than the loss of visual acuity.

Color Sense

It is the ability to distinguish between different colors excited by the light of different wavelengths. The appreciation of colors (color vision) is a *function of cones*. Therefore, it occurs only in photopic vision. In dark adapted eyes, where the rod function dominates, colored objects appear as gray differing in brightness. There are three types of cones with three different pigments which absorb wavelengths of light in the spectrum corresponding to red, green, and blue colors. The three pigments are:

Pigment sensitive to red light (long wave pigment): It absorbs maximally in the yellow portion with a peak of 570 nm. The cone that contains this pigment is called "L" cone.

Pigment sensitive to green light (middle wave pigment): It absorbs maximally the green portion of spectrum with a peak of 535 nm. The cone that contains this pigment is called "M" cone.

Pigment sensitive to blue light (short wave pigment): It absorbs maximally blue violet portion of spectrum with a peak of 445 nm. The cone that contains this pigment is referred to as "S" cone (**Fig. 2.3**).

Any given cone pigment may be deficient or entirely absent.

Deficiency of red pigment is called **protanomaly** (red weakness) and its entire absence is called **protanopia** (red blindness).

Deficiency of green pigment is called **deuteranomaly** (green weakness) and its entire absence is called **deutranopia** (green blindness).

Deficiency of blue pigment is called **tritanomaly** (blue weakness) and its entire absence is called **tritanopia** (blue blindness).

Trichromats possess all three types of cones. Absence of one type of cone renders the individual dichromat, while absence of two types of cone renders the individual monochromat.

The red, green, and blue colors are called **primary colors**. These in different proportions will give a sensation of white or any other color shades. Hence, normal color vision is called trichromatic. For any given color, there is a complimentary color which when mixed will produce white. If a person stops looking at a color, he or she may continue to see it for a short time (positive after image), or he or she may see its complimentary color (negative after image). When a colored light strikes the retina, the response of the cones depends on the color mixture. The response in the form of local potentials gets transmitted into the bipolar

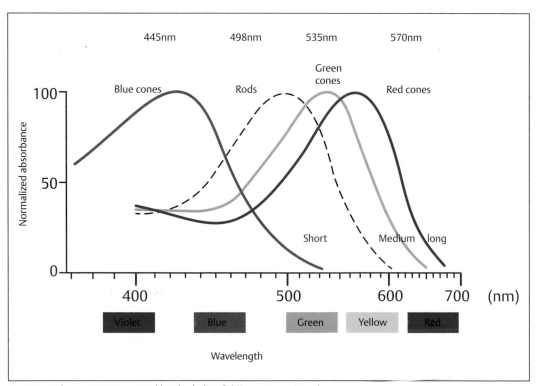

Fig. 2.3 Color sensitivity excited by the light of different wavelengths.

cells which, in turn, activates ganglion cells. The signals from the three cones after processing by the ganglion cells are conducted to LGB in three different ways:

- *Red green* pathway via parvo cells.
- *Blue yellow* pathway via parvo cells.
- Luminance (*white black*) pathway via magno cells.

The cells of LGB process the color sensation in a similar fashion as that of ganglion cells and conduct the impulses to primary visual cortex. Red–green and blue–yellow pathways take relay in the layers 3 to 6 (Parvo cells) and white–black take relay in layers 1 and 2 (Magno cells). The primary visual cortex contains clusters of color-sensitive neurons. The color information from these neurons is projected to area 37 (secondary visual cortex) which converts color input into the sensation of color.

■ Theories of Color Vision

The following theories have been proposed to explain the mechanism of color vision:

- Young-Helmholtz theory (trichromatic theory).
- Hering theory (Opponent process theory).

Young-Helmholtz Theory

- Postulates: There are three primary colors– red, green, and blue.
- There are three types of cones with different pigments, each maximally sensitive to one of the primary colors, although each color receptor also responds to the other two primary colors.
- All other colors are assumed to be perceived by combinations of these, that is, sensation of any given color is determined by the relative frequency of impulse reaching the brain from each of the three cone systems.

This theory fails to explain the sensation of black color. It also has difficulty in explaining color confusion and complimentary color after images.

Hering Theory

The Hering theory assumes three sets of receptor systems: red–green, blue–yellow, and black–white. Each system is assumed to function as an antagonistic pair. The stimulation of one results in inhibition of the opposite receptor in the pair, for example, red light stimulates the red receptors and simultaneously inhibits the green. This concept can explain color contrast (if a piece of blue paper is laid up on a yellow paper, the color of each of them is heightened due to color contrast) and color blindness.

The most widely accepted theory (stage theory) incorporates both theories which help in explaining how our color vision system works.

1. The first stage is the receptor stage. The trichromatic theory operates at the receptor level which consists of three photopigments.
2. The second stage is the neural processing stage for color vision in which signals are recorded into the opponent process form by the higher level neural system.

■ Assessment of Visual Function

Each eye must be tested separately throughout for all forms of visual perceptions (form sense, field of vision, light sense, and color sense). Visual perceptions can be assessed by:

Subjective tests– These tests require the patient's subjective expression of visual function which include:

- Assessment of visual acuity.
- Assessment of field of vision.
- Assessment of dark adaptation.
- Assessment of contrast sensitivity.
- Assessment of color vision.

Objective tests– These tests are independent of patient's expression and achieved by electro-physiological tests which include:

- Electroretinography (ERG).
- Electrooculography (EOG).
- Visual evoked potential (VEP).

■ Subjective Tests

Assessment of Visual Acuity (OP1.3)

Visual acuity of the eye is an estimation of its ability to discriminate between two points. It must be tested both for distance and near. **Distant visual acuity** is tested by:

Snellen's Test Types

The basic principle of Snellen's test types is the fact that two objects can be perceived separately only when they subtend a minimum angle of 1 minute at the nodal point of the eye. The Snellen's test type consists of a series of letters arranged in lines, each diminishing in size from above downward. Each letter is so designed that it can be placed in a square, the sides of which are 5 times the breadth of the constituent lines. Hence, at a given distance, whole letter subtends an angle of 5 minute at the nodal point of the eye. The letter of the top line subtends an angle of 5 minutes at the nodal point of eye if it is 60 m from the eye. The letters in subsequent lines subtend an angle of 5 minutes if they are 36, 24, 18, 12, 9, and 6 m away from the eye, but at 6 m, a 6/6 letters subtend an angle of 5 minutes, a 6/12 letter subtends 10 minutes, and a 6/60 letter subtends an angle of 50 minutes (**Fig. 2.4**). The illumination of chart should not fall below 20 foot candles.

Recording of Visual Acuity

The patient should be seated at a distant of 6 m from the chart. At this distance, the rays of light are practically parallel and accommodation is thus negligible. The patient is asked to read test types with each eye separately and the visual acuity is expressed as a fraction, in which the numerator is the distance of the chart from the patient (6 m) and denominator is the distance at which a person with normal vision ought to be able to read, for example, if a patient reads only the top line, his visual acuity will by 6/60 as a normal person ought to have read this line from a distance of 60 m, and when a patient reads the 7th (last) line of the chart, his visual acuity is recorded as 6/6 which is a normal person's vision.

When the top letter cannot be read, the patient is asked to move toward the chart till he reads the top line, for example, if he reads the top line from a 3 m distance, his visual acuity will be 3/60.

If the patient cannot read the top letter even from a distance of less than 1 m, he is asked to count the fingers of the examiner and visual acuity is recorded as FC- 3′, FC- 1′.

When the patient fails to count fingers, the examiner moves his or her hand and observes whether the patient appreciates hand movements (HMs) or not. If he or she appreciates HMs, his or her visual acuity is recorded as HM +ve.

In absence of the recognition of HMs, see whether the patient can perceive the light, and the visual acuity is recorded as PL +ve or PL –ve.

In illiterate individuals, "E" test types or Landolt broken ring (C) should be used.

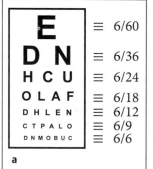
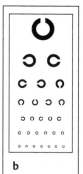
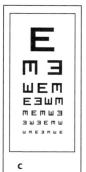
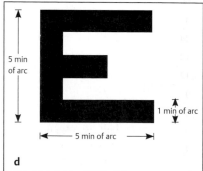

Fig. 2.4 (a) Snellen's test types; **(b)** Landolt broken ring test; **(c)** The illiterate E test; **(d)** 20/20 Snellen's letter.

In U.S.A, metric system is not usually followed and values are converted to feet (6 m = 20 ft). Therefore, 6/6 becomes 20/20 and 6/60 becomes 20/200, etc. The Snellen's fraction can also be expressed as a decimal (i.e., 6/6 = 1 and 6/12 = 0.5).

Log MAR acuity

The **Bailey-Lovie chart** is more accurate than Snellen's test type and is the standard mean of visual acuity measurement. This records the *minimum angle of resolution* (**MAR**) which relates to the resolution required to resolve the elements of a letter. At 6 m, a 6/6 letters subtend an angle of 5 minutes and each limb of the letter has an angular width of 1 minute, and then an MAR of 1 minute is needed for resolution. A 6/12 (20/40) letter subtends 10 minutes of arc and each limb of the letter has an angular width of 2 minute, so an MAR of 2 minutes is needed for resolution.

So, *Snellen's acuity is inverted and reduced to express MAR.*

Log MAR is simply the log of the MAR. Each line of the chart comprises five letters and the letter size changes by 0.1 Log MAR units per row. Thus, each letter can be assigned a score of 0.02. The final score takes account of every letter that has been read correctly. The Bailey-Lovie chart is used at 6 m testing distance.

For example, in Snellen's visual acuity of 6/6, MAR of 1 minute is needed for resolution. Therefore, Log MAR score is 0.00 as the Log of MAR value of 1 minute is 0. For Snellen's visual acuity of 6/60, MAR of 10 minute is needed for resolution. Therefore, Log MAR score is 1.00 as Log of MAR of 10 minute is 1. For Snellen's visual acuity of 6/12, MAR of 2 minute is needed for resolution. Therefore, Log MAR score is 0.30 as Log of MAR of 2 minute is 0.301 (**Fig. 2.5** and **Table 2.3**).

Pinhole Test

If the vision is subnormal, visual acuity is measured by asking the patient to read the letters through a pinhole. A pinhole is placed in front of the eye to be tested and the other eye is covered. The pinhole allows only central rays of light which are not refracted by the media.

If the vision improves by two or more lines in the chart, it indicates an underlying refractive error. The visual acuity is assessed again with the correcting glasses.

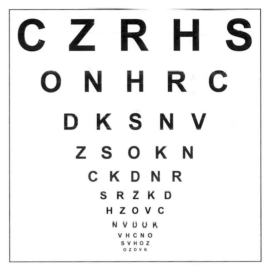

Fig. 2.5 LogMAR visual acuity chart.

Table 2.3 Notations for recording visual acuity

Visual acuity (meter)	Visual acuity (feet, 6 m = 20 ft)	Decimal equivalent	Log MAR equivalent
6/60	20/200	0.10	+1.0
6/36	20/120	0.17	+0.8
6/24	20/80	0.25	+0.6
6/18	20/60	0.33	+0.5
6/12	20/40	0.5	+0.3
6/9	20/30	0.6	+0.2
6/6	20/20	1.00	0.00
6/5	20/16	1.20	−0.1
6/4	20/12.5	1.50	−0.2

The pinhole does not improve visual acuity in the presence of macular or optic nerve diseases.

Visual Acuity in Hard/Dense Cataract

In a totally opaque cataract, testing of visual acuity is not possible by Snellen's chart/Bailey–Lovie chart. Visual acuity (likely to be regained after surgery) in the presence of dense cataract can be tested by:

- Laser interferometer.
- Potential acuity meter (PAM).

Laser interferometer is based on the phenomenon of interference. Two pin-points of a laser light are focused which interferes with each other and form a diffraction pattern of parallel lines (light and dark fringes) on the retina. The change in the distance between these two pin-points result in the alteration of fringe pattern, and the visual acuity can be estimated by asking the patient to identify the orientation of progressively finer lines.

Potential acuity meter projects a tiny Snellen's chart on to the retina. The small image of the chart passes through the defects in the media and the patient is required to read the alphabets.

Testing of Visual Acuity in Infants and Young Children

The preverbal children are tested by means of Optokinetic Nystagmus (OKN) drum and preferential looking behavior.

Optokinetic Nystagmus (OKN)

A white drum with vertical black stripes is rotated before the eyes. If vision is normal, the infant follows stripe with a slow motion. As this stripe disappears, the eyes switch suddenly back to pick up a new stripe, indicating that the infant can discriminate the stripe. By varying the distance between infant and drum or the breadth of stripes, the assessment of visual acuity can be made in children.

Preferential Looking Behavior

It is based on the fact that infants prefer to look at a pattern rather than a homogenous stimulus. The infants' preference is quantified by incorporating the patterns which vary in stripe width. The test in common use include the Teller acuity cards, which consist of 17 of them with black stripes (gratings) of varying width, and Cardiff acuity cards, which consist of familiar pictures with variable outline width. Coarse greetings or pictures with wider outline are seen more easily than fine greetings or thin outline pictures. The grating size of the card can then be converted to the equivalent of Snellen's visual acuity.

Near visual acuity is tested by:
- Jaeger test types.
- Roman test types.

In Jaeger test types, a series with print types of different sizes in increasing order is arranged and marked from 1 to 7. The patient acuity is recorded as J-1 to J-7 depending upon the print type he reads.

In Roman test types, the near vision is recorded as N6, N8, N10, N12, N18, and N36. The near vision is tested in good illumination keeping the chart at a reading distance of 14 to 16 inches (35–40 cm).

Assessment of Field of Vision

Visual fields is the space that one eye can see while remaining fixed. It is a three-dimensional area (not a flat plane) and may be described as *"island of vision surrounded by a sea of darkness."* Binocular visual field is the visual field seen simultaneously with both eyes.

Extent (of Monocular visual field)

Superiorly	60°
Nasally	60°
Inferiorly	70–75°
Temporally	> 90° (100–110°)

The extent is limited by brow superiorly, nose nasally, and the cheek inferiorly. The typical configuration of normal visual field, therefore, is horizontally oval with a shallow depression (**Fig. 2.6**).

Divisions of Visual Field

Visual field is divided into temporal and nasal halves by an imaginary vertical meridian drawn

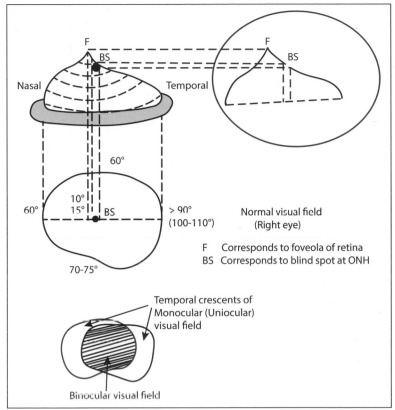

Fig. 2.6 Uniocular and binocular visual fields. Abbreviations: BS, blind spot; F, foveola of retina; ONH, Optic nerve head.

Normal visual field
(Right eye)

F   Corresponds to foveola of retina
BS   Corresponds to blind spot at ONH

Temporal crescents of Monocular (Uniocular) visual field

Binocular visual field

through fovea. It is also divided into superior and inferior halves by a horizontal meridian that passes from fovea to temporal periphery (**Fig. 2.7**).

Visual acuity is sharpest at foveola and decreases progressively toward periphery (nasal slope is steeper than temporal slope). This is described as *hill of vision*. At optic disc, there are no photo receptors. So, it is a nonvisual area and corresponds to normal blind spot. Blind spot is located 10 to 20 temporal to fixation and 1.5 degree below the horizontal meridian. Normally, a person is not aware of his blind spot because the corresponding area of other eye sees normally.

Absolute scotoma is an area of total visual loss. Even brightest and largest stimuli cannot be perceived in absolute scotoma. **Relative scotoma** is an area of partial visual loss, in which brighter or larger stimuli can be seen but smaller or dimmer targets cannot be seen. Blind spot has absolute scotoma corresponding to actual optic nerve head (Papilla) and relative scotoma surrounding the absolute scotoma which corresponds to the peripapillary retina.

Measurement of Visual Fields

1. **Confrontation test:**

   It is a rough method of assessment. In this method, patient's visual field is compared with that of the examiner; therefore, the examiner should have a normal visual field. The patient sits facing the examiner at a distance of approximately 2 feet and is asked to cover his left eye and told to look straight into the examiner's left eye with his right eye. The examiner closes his right eye and moves his finger from the periphery in the plane half way between him and the patient. The patient is asked to tell as soon as he sees the finger; the finger is moved in various parts of the field. The test is repeated for the other eye in the same way. Thus, a rough assessment is made about the visual field of the patient. If any defect is indicated by confrontation test, it must be accurately recorded by perimeter.

2. Measurement of visual field **on a flat surface:**

   Measurement of visual field on a flat surface is called **Campimetry**. Black tangent screen remains the standard tool for campimetry which was introduced by

Bjerrum (**Bjerrum's screen**). It detects localized defects or scotomas in central and paracentral visual fields. The typical arcuate scotomas seen in glaucoma still bear Bjerrum's name.

3. Measurement of visual field **on a curved surface:**

   Measurement of visual field on a curved surface is called **Perimetry**. Perimetry has largely replaced campimetry nowadays. The instrument used for perimetry is called perimeter (**Flowchart 2.4**). Both central and peripheral fields of vision can be recorded with perimeters. The perimeter is commonly a half sphere situated at the patient's near point.

The first perimeters were arc perimeters. Lister perimeter uses small round objects as test targets, while Aimark perimeter is a light projection arc perimeter. Goldmann hemispheric projection perimeter has a bowl-shaped screen. The target is projected onto the bowl and the stimulus value of test object can be varied by changing the size or intensity. Computer technology was combined with visual field testing in the mid-1970s, resulting in introduction of automated perimeters. Several automated perimeters were introduced but the two most widely used systems are octopus perimeter and Humphrey visual field analyzer.

Automated perimetry is more accurate than manual and has largely replaced manual perimetry.

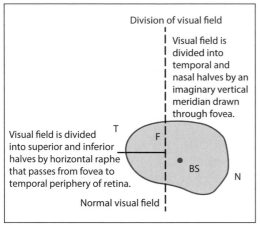

Fig. 2.7 Division of visual field. Abbreviations: BS, blind spot; F, foveola of retina.

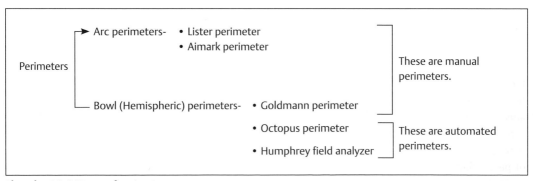

Flowchart 2.4 Types of perimeter.

Advantages of Automated Perimetry Over Manual Perimetry

- Automated perimetry is quantifiable and repeatable.
- There is constant monitoring of fixation in automated perimetry.
- Reliability of test can be verified by false +ve and false –ve results immediately.
- Abnormal points are retested automatically.

Typical stimuli used in perimetry are spots of light of various diameter (*size*) and intensity. The *factors affecting* the *perception of stimulus* include the following:

- Size of stimulus.
- Luminance of stimulus.
- Color of stimulus.
- Length of time the stimulus is presented.
- Contrast brightness of background and stimulus.

Luminance is the intensity or brightness of a light stimulus. The luminance of a given stimulus at which it is perceived 50% of the time when presented statically is known as **threshold sensitivity**. The human eye needs about a 10% change in brightness to make out a difference between light stimuli. It is highest at fovea and decreases progressively from macula to periphery. The stimulus brighter than threshold intensity is called **suprathreshold** and the dimmer one is called **subthreshold**. Differential light sensitivity measures the degree by which the luminance of the target requires to exceed the background luminance in order to be perceived by the eye.

Types of Perimetry—Perimetry Is of Two Types

- Kinetic perimetry.
- Static perimetry.

Kinetic Perimetry

In kinetic perimetry, a stimulus of a given size and intensity is moved from a nonseeing area to a seeing area until it is perceived. The stimulus is moved along various meridians and the point of perception is recorded on a chart. The points along different meridians (clock hours) are joined

and an isopter is obtained for that stimulus size and intensity. **Isopter**, therefore, *encloses an area within which a target of a given size and intensity is visible.* As the size and luminance (intensity of a light stimulus) of a target is decreased, the area within which it can be perceived becomes smaller, so that a series of ever diminishing circles (called isopters) is formed.

Using stimuli of different intensities, several different isopters can be plotted. The *brightest target will have the largest isopter* and *the dimmest target will have the smallest isopter.* Kinetic perimeter is a two-dimensional assessment of the boundaries of hills of vision. It can be performed by:

- Bjerrum's tangent screen (campimetry).
- Lister perimeter.
- Goldmann perimeter.

Static Perimetry

In static perimeter, a *nonmoving stimuli of varying luminance* is presented in the same position. It is a three-dimensional assessment of the visual field, providing the assessment of the boundary of hill of vision (area) and of differential threshold sensitivity (height). Static perimeter can be performed by using suprathreshold or threshold stimuli.

In **suprathreshold static perimetry,** visual stimuli of intensity above expected normal threshold value (suprathreshold) is presented in various locations in the visual field. Detected targets (stimuli) indicate grossly normal visual function, whereas failure to recognize the suprathreshold stimulus reflects the areas of decreased visual sensitivity. If suprathreshold intensity is too high, milder defects may be missed. Therefore, selection of appropriate suprathreshold intensity is important. This type of perimetry is used mainly for screening. If stimuli are not visible in any area, further evaluation with threshold stimuli should be conducted. **Threshold static perimetry** measures the value of threshold intensity at different locations in the visual field. The technique involves increase in the intensity of target light by large steps (4 dB) until threshold is crossed and then decreased in smaller steps (2 dB) to the point where it cannot be identified (staircase threshold determination strategy). It determines the patient's threshold for that particular point. As threshold static perimetry represents quantitative assessment, it is the most accurate method of monitoring glaucomatous visual field defects.

Static perimeter is usually carried out with computerized, automated perimeters: octopus perimeter and Humphrey visual field analyzer, as automated perimeters, use threshold static perimetry.

Physiologic Influences on Visual Fields

- Pupil size: Miosis decreases threshold sensitivities in central and peripheral visual fields and exaggerate field defects, so pupil <3 mm in diameter should be dilated prior to perimetry.
- Clarity of ocular media: In cataract change, glare is produced which can exaggerate field defects and be mistaken for glaucomatous field changes.
- Refractive errors: Refractive errors primarily influence the central field. Hypermetropia has a greater influence on perimetric results. A contact lens provides the best correction for aphakic and highly myopic eyes. Spectacles can cause ring scotomas if small aperture lenses are used, although spectacle correction can be used for central 24 degree to 30 degree of the visual field.
- Age: Increasing age is also associated with reduced retinal threshold sensitivity.

Besides standard achromatic perimetry (**SAP**), short wavelength automated perimetry (**SWAP**) and frequency-doubling technology (**FDT**) have been introduced to detect visual field defects earlier than SAP. FDT is a fast screen test to detect glaucomatous field defects. *SWAP uses a blue test object on a yellow background.* Blue–yellow ganglion cells, a sub group of retinal ganglion

cells, are sensitive to blue stimuli and lost early in glaucoma. Testing of these cells allows detection of loss of visual function at a much earlier stage of glaucoma. Therefore, SWAP is much more sensitive than white light perimetry, primarily due to neural loss.

Goals of Perimetry

- Detection of early visual field defects.
- Determination of specific patterns of visual field loss for differential diagnosis.
- Monitoring of progression of field loss.

Other Types of Perimetry

Automated perimetry is the standard way of measuring the visual field. Static targets are used in most automated perimeters. The standard stimulus in most automated perimeters is a white light on a white background (white-on-white automated perimetry). The standard white-on-white automated perimetry is commonly known as SAP. Conventionally, SAP has been used to achieve these purposes but up to 40% of retinal nerve fiber layer (RNFL) may be lost before a defect is apparent on standard white-on-white automated perimetry. Achromatic stimuli used in SAP, nonselectively stimulate ganglion cells and therefore are not always adequately sensitive to detect early glaucomatous damage.

Technique of Perimetry

Humphrey field analyzer is currently the most commonly used automated perimeter which uses a bowl-type screen. The patient is seated with the corrective lens placed in front of the eye. The other eye is occluded and the patient is instructed to fixate at a fixation target. The light stimulus can be projected onto the bowl into any location of visual field. The stimulus value of a target can be adjusted by varying target size or luminance (*brightness*) relative to that of the background. The stimulus size is set prior to the test; only luminance of stimulus is altered, and the patient is asked to respond when the target is seen. It determines the threshold level for each point tested in the visual field.

Assessment of Dark Adaptation

Dark adaptation is the ability of the eyes to adapt to decreased illumination. Dark adaptation is plotted by an adaptometer. It is plotted as the light sensitivity response against the function of time. It is particularly useful in cases of night blindness.

Technique of Adaptometry

- Retina is exposed to intense light for a sufficient time, so that more than 25% of rhodopsin in the retina is bleached and the patient is placed in the dark.
- The flashes of varying intensity are periodically presented.
- The threshold at which the patient just perceives the light is plotted versus time.

Adaptation Curve

The dark adaptation curve (**Fig. 2.8**) normally shows two successive phases:

- The first phase is rapid and is due to dark adaptation of cones. This takes place within 5 to 10 minutes and then stabilizes.
- The second phase is slow due to adaptation of rods and takes approximately 20 to 30 minutes. This phase is dependent on resynthesis of rhodopsin and, hence, takes more time. So, *both cones and rods participate in dark adaptation*. Dark adaptation is utilized evaluating retinal disorders for metabolic diseases and assessing the scotopic performance in pilots and drivers.

> Radiologists, aircraft pilots, and others who need maximal visual sensitivity in dim light can avoid waiting for 20 minutes in dark by wearing red goggles. Light wavelengths in the red end of spectrum stimulate the rods to only a slight degree while permitting the cones to function reasonably well.

Assessment of Contrast Sensitivity

Contrast sensitivity is a measure of the ability of the visual system to distinguish an object against its background. It indirectly assesses the quality of vision and must be assessed in the patient having visual problems despite a normal visual acuity. Contrast sensitivity is *reduced in* early cataract, optic nerve disease, and glaucoma. It can be assessed by letter contrast sensitivity using the visual acuity chart (Pelli–Robson chart, **Fig. 2.9**).

The **Pelli–Robson** chart is viewed at 1 m and consists of rows of letters of equal size. The letters in a group of three shows a gradual decrease in contrast down the chart. The patient is asked to the read the letters until the lowest resolvable group of three is reached.

Assessment of Color Vision

The color vision is tested by the following methods:

Ishihara's charts: These consist of colored plates with numerals in dots of primary colors printed on a background of similar dots of confusing color.

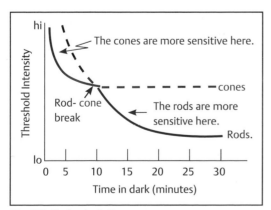

Fig. 2.8 Dark adaptation curve.

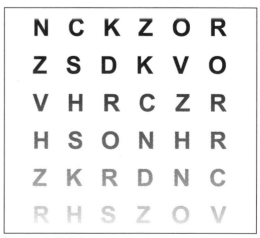

Fig. 2.9 Pelli–Robson chart.

The charts are kept at a distance of 30 cm and the patient is asked to read the numbers. Normal trichromats can easily read the numbers but a person having defective color vision is unable to read. This test is used mainly to screen for congenital protan and deutran defects (**Fig. 2.10**).

Lantern test (Edridge-green lantern): In this test, the subject is asked to name various colors shown by a lantern and the color vision defect is detected with the help of just the mistakes he or she commits.

Holmgren wool's test: In this test, the subject is asked to match the color from the heap of colored wools. A person with gross defects of color vision will make wrong matches.

Farnsworth- Munsell 100-Hue test: This test is very sensitive but time consuming. It consists of 85 hue caps in four separate racks. The subject is asked to rearrange the caps in their natural order. A normal individual will arrange them with minimum errors. A color deficient person makes the mistakes in the parts of the spectrum complimentary to his or her color defect. The score is plotted on a circular chart; greater the score the poorer is the color vision.

Nagel's anomaloscope test: In anomaloscope, a bright disc is seen divided into two halves by a horizontal line. One half is illuminated by yellow light and other half by a mixture of red and green. By turning knobs, the relative amounts of red and green in the mixture and the brightness can be varied. In this test, the subject is asked to mix red and green color in such a proportion that the mixture should match the yellow-colored disc. The color vision defect is judged by the relative amount of red and green colors and the brightness setting by the person.

City university test: It consists of 10 plates, each containing a central color and four peripheral colors. The subject is asked to select one of the peripheral colors which matches the central color most closely.

■ Objective Tests

Electroretinography tests are totally independent of patient's psyche, that is, it provides the objective recording of visual functions. These tests pick up electrical potential from retinal structures or visual cortex in response to visual stimulation. These include three basic tests:
- Electroretinography (ERG).
- Electrooculography (EOG).
- Visual evoked potential (VEP).

Electroretinography (ERG)

ERG measures changes in the resting potential of the eye produced by retina in response to stimulation by the light of adequate intensity, that is,

Light stimulus → stimulation of retina → changes in resting potential of retina → recorded as ERG.

Recording

The pupils are fully dilated and the response is recorded between two electrodes: An *active electrode* in a contact lens placed on the cornea and a *reference electrode* placed on the forehead.

ERG is recorded both in light-adapted state (photopic ERG) and in dark-adapted state (scotopic ERG). Normal ERG consists of (**Fig. 2.11**):
- **a-Wave**: It is a −ve wave generated by photoreceptors.

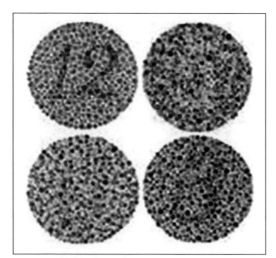

Fig. 2.10 Ishihara's charts.

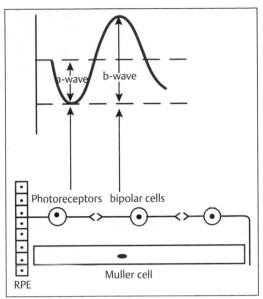

Fig. 2.11 Electroretinogram. Abbreviation: RPE, retinal pigment epithelium.

- **b-Wave:** It is a +ve deflection generated by Muller cells due to an increase in extracellular potassium from bipolar cells depolarizing the Muller cells. So, it represents electrical activity in bipolar cells (though generated by Muller cells). Amplitude of b-wave is measured from a trough of a-wave to the peak of b-wave.
- **c-wave:** It is a +ve wave related to retinal metabolism in pigment epithelium but it is not related to visual processes.

Significance

ERG gives the indication of activity of rods and cone. So, a subnormal ERG indicates that a large area of retina is not functioning and an extinguished response indicates the complete failure of rods and cones functions.

Electrooculography (EOG)

EOG measures the resting potential between electrically +ve cornea and electrically –ve back of eye (retina) with horizontal eye movements.

It reflects activity of retinal pigment epithelium (RPE) and photoreceptors, so lesions proximal to photoreceptors will have a normal EOG.

Table 2.4 Interpretation of Arden ratio

Arden ratio (%)	Interpretation
185%	Normal value
150–185%	Borderline
< 150%	Subnormal
< 125%	Flat

Recording

- Electrodes are placed over the skin near medial and lateral canthi.
- The patient is asked to move eyes from side to side and recordings are made every minute for 12 minutes. The procedure is performed in both light- and dark-adapted states. Each time the eye moves, the electrode near the cornea becomes +ve with regard to other (because of electrically +ve cornea), for example, electrode near lateral canthi becomes +ve when eye is moved laterally.
- Potential differences between two electrodes is amplified and recorded. Changes in potential thus obtained with changes of illumination are indicative of the activity of RPE and outer segments of photoreceptors.

Interpretation

The results are expressed as **Arden ratio (Table 2.4).**

$$\text{Arden ratio} = \frac{\text{maximum height of potential in light}}{\text{minimum height of potential in dark}} \times 100$$

$$\text{i.e.,} \quad \frac{\text{Light peak}}{\text{dark trough}} \times 100$$

Significance

As it is based on the activity of RPE and photoreceptors, EOG is subnormal or flat in:

- Retinitis pigmentosa.
- Degenerative myopia.
- Macular dystrophies.
- Vitamin A deficiency.

Visual Evoked Potential (VEP)

It is also called VER (visually evoked response). VEP is the recording of electrical activity of visual cortex generated by stimulation of retina (**Fig. 2.12**).

Indications

- For monitoring of visual function in babies.
- In investigation of optic neuropathy.
- To monitor macular pathway function.

VEP is the only objective test to assess functional status of visual system beyond retinal ganglion cells. So, abnormal VEP with normal ERG and EOG suggests an organic lesion in the pathway between and including ganglion cell layer (**GCL**) and visual cortex.

Technique

Visual stimulus may be:
- Flashing light (**Flash VEP**).
  or
- Patterned as in a checkerboard (Black and white) which periodically reverses polarity on a screen (**pattern reversal VEP**).

It is recorded by applying surface electrodes on the scalp over the occipital cortex.

Flash VEP: It merely indicates that light has been perceived by visual cortex. It is not affected by opacities in cornea and lens, so it is used to detect visual potential in eyes with opaque media. It can distinguish between organic and functional (Malingering) blindness and can be used in infants to assess the integrity of macula and visual pathway.

Pattern reversal VEP: In it, the pattern of stimulus is changed (i.e., black squares go white and white becomes black alternately) but overall illumination remains the same.

Interpretation

Both latency (timing of onset of response) and amplitude of VEP are assessed but latency is a more reliable and useful parameter than amplitude.
- Prolonged latency indicates conduction defects of visual pathway.
- Decreased amplitude indicates poor visual function.
- *Optic nerve lesions* cause delayed conduction (prolongation of latency) and reduced amplitude of VEP.
- *Retrochiasmal lesions* produce abnormal hemispheric responses.

> Delay in transmission time (prolonged delay) in retinobulbar neuritis (RBN) persists even when vision returns to normal. Delay (latency), therefore, suggests past attack of RBN.

■ Binocular Vision

Binocular vision is characterized by the ability to fuse the images from the two eyes and perceive a single image. It is acquired gradually in the first few years of life.

Visual input from two eyes is conveyed to the visual cortex and visual association areas. From here, impulses go to the centers controlling eye movements in the brainstem. Accordingly, eye adjust their position and a single image is seen.

Therefore, binocular vision involves the coordinated use of both eyes. The points on retina which are visually coordinated are called **corresponding retinal points**, for example, when X has stimulated the points A and B on each retina, and they have projected to the same position in space,

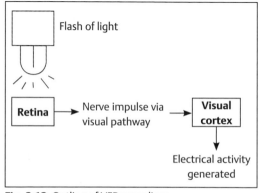

Fig. 2.12 Outline of VEP recordings.
Abbreviation: VEP, visual evoked potential.

they are said to be corresponding points. Similarly, foveae of both eyes (F1 and F2) are corresponding retinal points stimulated by Y. Points on nasal retina of one eye have corresponding points on the temporal retina of other eye and vice versa. Thus, for binocular vision, there must be a physiological relationship between two retinae; this is known as **normal retinal correspondence**. The imaginary plane in space, all points on which stimulate the corresponding retinal elements and are therefore seen singly, is known as **horopter** (**Fig. 2.13**). This plane passes through the point of intersection of two visual axes. An object which does not lie on horopter forms images on noncorresponding points and the object appears double. This diplopia of all objects which do not lie on the horopter is a normal accompaniment of vision and is seldom appreciated consciously. It may be, therefore, termed as "**physiological diplopia.**"

■ Development of Binocular Vision

At birth—no central fixation eyes move randomly.

Fixation reflexes—develop by 4th weeks after birth.

Binocular fusional reflexes—develops by age of 6 months

Well-developed binocular vision—attained by the age of 5 to 6 years.

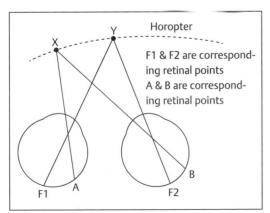

Fig. 2.13 Binocular vision and corresponding retinal points.

■ Conditions Necessary for Normal Binocular Vision

The factors which favor the development of binocular vision are concerned with the act of fusion (a sensory phenomenon) and the cortical control of ocular movements (a motor phenomenon). Thus, the conditions for normal binocular vision are:

Sensory mechanisms:
- An adequate degree of central and peripheral visions in both eyes.
- Approximately equal image size for both eyes.
- Normal retinal correspondence (NRC).

Motor mechanism: There must be precise coordination of two eyes for all directions of gaze.

Binocular visual acuity is usually better than the visual acuity obtained by each eye separately. This is due to the cortical summation of the visual input from the two eyes. Binocular vision is best measured on a Synoptophore.

■ Grades of Binocular Vision

Binocular vision is categorized into three grades, which are precisely tested on a synoptophore (**Fig. 2.14**). Grades of binocular vision are as follows:

Grade 1 Simultaneous macular perception—It is the ability of eyes to perceive two dissimilar objects simultaneously such as a lion and a cage.

Grade 2 Fusion—It is the ability of two eyes to superimpose two incomplete but similar pictures to produce a complete picture, for example, two rabbits—one lacking a tail and the other lacking a bunch of flowers. Fusion is the cortical integration and unification of two images, one from each eye. It is only possible by simultaneous stimulation of corresponding points.

Grade 3 Stereopsis—It is the perception of depth or the third dimension (the first two being height and width). It is the ability to obtain an impression of depth by superimposition of two

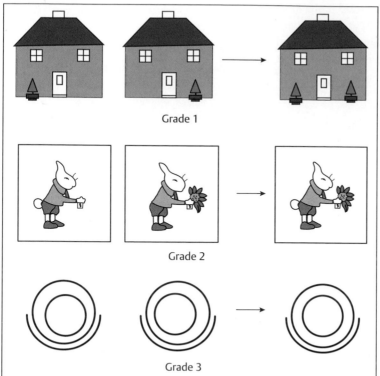

Fig. 2.14 Grades of binocular vision.

Grade 1

Grade 2

Grade 3

pictures of same object from slightly different angles.

■ Advantages of Binocular Vision

The greatest advantage of having binocular vision is stereopsis (depth perception). The binocular vision provides better exteroception of form and color. Also, if the function of one eye becomes impaired by a disease process, the advantage of visual field overlap during binocular vision becomes obvious.

■ Disorders of Binocular Vision

A lack of full binocular function is normal in infants, but it is not normal in children and adults. The binocular vision impairment results in a condition where the two eyes have difficulty working together. Reduced vision in one eye and loss of coordination of movement between the two eyes are the main reasons of loss of binocular vision. It causes vertical or horizontal (or both) misalignment of visual axes between the two eyes and includes amblyopia (lazy eye) or strabismus.

CHAPTER 3

Optics and Refraction

Elementary Optics 35
Optics of Normal Eye...39
Accommodation...41
Anomalies of Accommodation 43
Refractive Errors 45
Correction of Refractive Errors 57

Elementary Optics

Electromagnetic Spectrum

It ranges from short ionizing radiations (1×10^{-16} meter) to longest radio waves (1×10^6 m). Visible light represents a small portion of electromagnetic spectrum with wavelengths ranging between 400 and 700 nm [1 nanometer (nm) = 10^{-9} meter].

Visible light appears white but is actually composed of:

V   I   B   G   Y   O   R
Violet indigo blue green yellow orange red
(**400 nm**)   (**700 nm**)

The red end has the longest and the violet end the shortest wavelength in visible spectrum. Light with shorter wavelengths has more energy and vice versa.

- Waves of smaller wavelength <400 nm are ultraviolet (UV) rays.
- Waves of longer wavelength >700 nm are infrared (IR) rays.
- *Cornea* absorbs rays of wavelength <320 nm. *Lens* absorbs rays of wavelength <350 nm.
- *Vitreous* absorbs rays of wavelength with maximum of 270 nm (**Fig. 3.1**).

So, in normal eye, rays between 400 and 350 nm can reach the retina and also stimulate photoreceptors. But in aphakic (eyes without crystalline lens) or pseudophakic eyes (eyes with an intraocular lens) without a UV-absorbing filter, rays between 400 and 320 nm reach the retina.

Intraocular lenses (IOLs) made up of PMMA (polymethyl methacrylate) absorb only UV rays ≤320 nm, so all modern IOLs (PMMA, silicone, and foldable acrylic) are impregnated with UV-absorbing substances called chromophores which absorb wavelengths of <400 nm. Knowledge of basic optics is necessary for an understanding of the functioning of the eye.

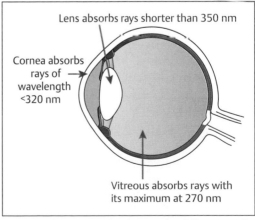

Fig. 3.1 Absorption of radiations by different ocular media.

■ Properties of Light

Speed of Light

- The speed of light in vacuum (c) = 3 × 10^8 m/s and is constant.
- The light travels slower in any medium compared with its speed in air or vacuum. The speed of light in a given medium (v) depends on the density of medium (**Table 3.1**).

Speed of light in air/vacuum, c = n × v; n = refractive index (RI)

When traveling through a substance, frequency of light remains unchanged but wavelength (and speed) becomes shorter. A medium is said to be optically denser if the speed of light becomes less in that medium.

Reflection

When light wave encounters an optical interface (boundary between two medium of different refractive index), it is partly reflected and partly refracted. The reflected ray bounces off the interface in the same medium. Greater the difference in RI between two media, the greater is the reflection and the angle of incidence is equal to the angle of reflection.

Laws of Reflection

- For all surfaces, the angle of incidence is equal to the angle of reflection.
- The rays (incident and reflected) and the normal at the point of incidence lie in the same plane.

The cornea acts as a convex mirror.

Refraction

It is the change in the direction of light traveling across an optical interface. A media with high refractive index is said to be optically denser than the media with low refractive index which is said to be optically rarer.

When a ray passes from optically rarer to a denser medium, the ray bends toward the normal. When a ray passes from optically denser to a rarer

Table 3.1 Refractive index of various media

Media	Refractive index
Air	1.0
Crown glass	1.52
Flint glass	1.65
Water	1.33

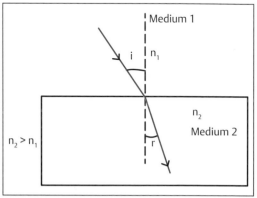

Fig. 3.2 Laws of refraction.

medium, bending of ray is away from the normal (**Fig. 3.2**). Greater the difference in optical density between the two media, greater is the deviation.

RI of crown glass which is used for optical purposes = 1.52.

For a ray traveling from optically denser to a rarer medium, if the angle of incidence is gradually increased, the angle of refraction also increases. The angle of incidence at which the incident light is bent exactly 90° away from normal (i.e., angle of refraction = 90°) is called the **critical angle** (**Fig. 3.3**).

When angle of incidence exceeds the critical angle, all light is reflected back into the same (denser) medium. This phenomenon is called **total internal reflection (TIR).** *This happens at cornea–air interface, preventing direct visualization of angle structure without a special gonioscopy lens.*

■ Prisms

In prisms, light rays are diverted toward the base, and the image is displaced toward the apex.

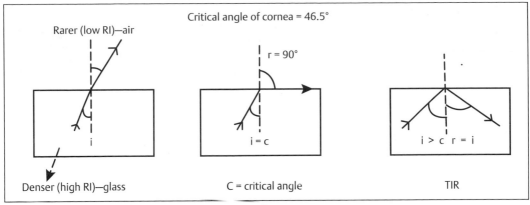

Fig. 3.3 Refraction at critical angle and total internal reflection.

The angle of deviation (D) of an ophthalmic prism is made of crown glass = (refracting angle (A) of the prism/2).

The angle of deviation is least when angles of incidence and emergence are equal (*angle of minimum deviation*).

The power of prism is measured in **prism dioptres** (Δ) (**Fig. 3.4**).

One Δ is the strength of prism which produces a linear displacement of an object by 1 cm when the object is kept at a distance of 1 m.

Two Δ **displacement** $\approx 1°$ **of arc**

If prism angle (A) = 10°, then deviation $\left(\frac{10}{2}\right)$ = 5° or 10 Δ, that is, prism has a power of 10 Δ.

Thus, *greater the angle at apex of prism (refracting angle of prism), the stronger is the prismatic effect.*

Prismatic effect also varies with wavelength. **Light of shorter wavelength is deviated more than the light of longer wavelength**. Chromatic aberration results with blue light closer to the base (short wavelength bent most) and red light closer to the apex.

Uses of Prisms in Ophthalmology

- Diagnostic uses in the following:
  - ◇ Many ophthalmic equipment such as gonioscope, keratometer, and applanation tonometer.

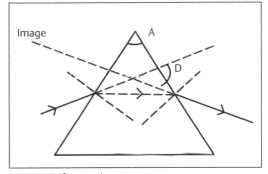

Fig. 3.4 Refraction by prism.

- ◇ Objective measurement of the angle of deviation (prism bar cover test and Krimsky test).
- ◇ Measurement of fusional reserve.
- Therapeutic use in patients afflicted with phorias and diplopia.

■ Lenses

Lenses may be spherical or cylindrical.

Spherical Lenses

A simple lens is a piece of glass with spherical surfaces. These may be:

- **Convex lens** (converging lens/plus lens): It acts like two prisms placed base to base. It may be biconvex or plano.
- Convex and concavo–convex (**Fig. 3.5**).
- **Concave lens** (diverging lens/minus lens): It acts like two prisms aligned apex to apex.

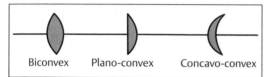

Fig. 3.5 Types of convex lenses.

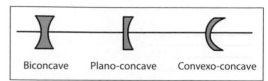

Fig. 3.6 Types of concave lenses.

It may be biconcave, plano–concave, and convexo–concave (meniscus) (**Fig. 3.6**).

On moving a lens away from the eye,
- The effective power of convex lens increases, so a *plus lens becomes stronger.*
- The effective power of concave lens decreases, so a *minus lens becomes weaker.*

To find out whether the lens is convex or concave, hold the lens near the eye and move it from side to side.
- If distant *object seems to move in the opposite direction* to that of lens, then the lens is *convex.*
- If distant *object seems to move in the same direction* as the lens, then the lens is *concave.*

To determine the refractive power (strength) of lens after determining the nature of lens by the above method, neutralize the movement of image with a lens of opposite sign. For example, if there is no movement at all with –4.0 D lens (concave lens), it means that the original lens was +4.0 D lens (convex lens).

Ophthalmic Uses of Spherical Lenses
- Convex lens is used:
  ◇ In correction of hypermetropia, aphakia, and presbyopia.
  ◇ In indirect ophthalmoscopy.
  ◇ In magnifying lens.
- Concave lens is used:
  ◇ In correction of myopia.
  ◇ As Hruby lens (with slit-lamp) for fundus examination.

Cylindrical Lenses

Cylindrical lenses are the lenses taken out from the surface of a cylinder like a tumbler. These lenses have an axis associated with them which is parallel to that of the cylinder, of which these lenses are a segment. A cylindrical lens focuses light into a line instead of a point as a spherical lens would. These may also be convex or concave.

In cylindrical lenses, one axis has zero power, while the power is incorporated in the direction at right angle to the axis. So, the object will move with/opposite to the lens only in one direction.

Ophthalmic Uses of Cylindrical Lenses

Cylindrical lenses are used:
- To correct astigmatism.
- As a cross cylinder (to check refraction).

If the object is at infinity, the image will be formed at principal focus which is very small, real, and inverted. As the object is gradually brought nearer to the lens, the image recedes further from it. The size of the image increases likewise.

■ Optical Aberrations

The lenses behave ideally near their optical axis (the line passing through the centers of curvature of the surfaces). Aberrations occur peripheral to the optical axis. Aberrations may be:
- **Spherical aberration:** It is caused by increasing the prismatic effect of the lens periphery. Peripheral rays are refracted more than paraxial ones (**Fig. 3.7a**).
- **Chromatic aberration:** It occurs between light of different wavelengths which are refracted by different amounts. Shorter wavelengths are bent more. This effect in eye, however, is small (**Fig. 3.7b**).

The eye has the following compensatory mechanisms to reduce the spherical aberrations of crystalline lens:
- *Size of pupil*: Pupillary constriction elimi-nates the peripheral rays.

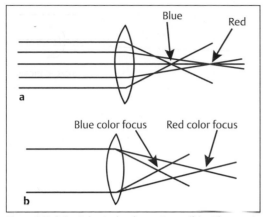

Fig. 3.7 (a) Spherical aberration. **(b)** Chromatic aberration.

Table 3.2 Refracting structures of the eye with their refractive indices	
Refracting structure	**Refractive index**
Cornea	1.376
Aqueous humor	1.336
Lens	
Anterior and posterior cortex	1.386
Nucleus (core)	1.406
Vitreous humor	1.336

- *Shape of cornea*: Cornea is progressively flatter in periphery. So, peripheral rays are refracted equal to the paraxial ones.
- *RI of lens*: RI is higher centrally in nucleus. So, paraxial rays bend more and all rays are brought to a focus at a single point.

Optics of Normal Eye

The optical system of the eye comprises several **refracting structures (Table 3.2)**:
- Cornea.
- Aqueous humor.
- Crystalline lens.
- Vitreous humor.

RI of aqueous is equal to that of vitreous and RI of air = 1.000.

Refracting interfaces in the eye are:
- Air–cornea.
- Aqueous–lens.
- Lens–vitreous.

Total dioptric power of the eye = **+ 60 D**

Out of +60 D, refractive power of the cornea = +43 D

and refractive power of the lens = +17 D.

Cornea is a major refractive component because the difference in refractive indices is maximum at anterior corneal surface interface. The centers of the corneal curvature and the two surfaces of the lens are all in the same straight line, which is called optic axis. Instead, of a simple convex lens with the same medium (air) on either side, the optical system of eye is quite complicated to understand the optics of human eye. The medium in front is air, while behind the lens, it is the vitreous having a higher RI than air.

Schematic Eye (Gullstrand)

Schematic eye is a mathematical model used to provide a basis for theoretical studies of the eye as an optical instrument. From the optical point of view, the entire system can be defined by its "cardinal points." Every optical system has six cardinal points (**Fig. 3.8** and **Table 3.3**):

1. Focal points (F_1 and F_2)–primary and secondary.
2. Principal points (P_1 and P_2)–primary and secondary.
3. Nodal points (N_1 and N_2)–primary and secondary.

When an optical system is bounded on both sides by air (same refractive index both side), the nodal points coincide with the principal points.

Listing simplified it theoretically and introduced the concept of **reduced eye**.

Reduced Eye (Listing and Donder)

In the reduced eye, the eye is regarded as one convex lens having characteristics as mentioned in **Fig. 3.9** and **Table 3.4**.

Table 3.3 Cardinal points

Cardinal points	Location
F_1 (primary focus point)	15.7 mm in front of cornea.
F_2 (secondary focus point)	24.13 mm behind the cornea.
P_1 (primary principal point)	Located in anterior chamber 1.35 mm behind the anterior surface of cornea.
P_2 (secondary principal point)	Located in anterior chamber 1.60 mm behind the anterior surface of cornea.
N_1 (primary nodal point)	Located in posterior part of lens 7.08 mm behind the anterior surface of cornea.
N_2 (secondary nodal point)	Located in posterior part of lens 7.33 mm behind the anterior surface of cornea.

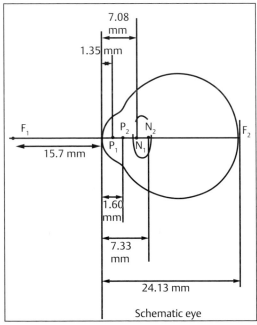

Fig. 3.8 Schematic eye.

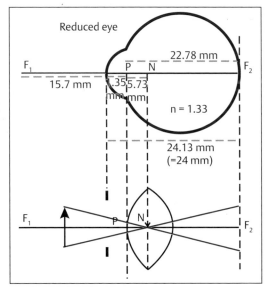

Fig. 3.9 Reduced eye.

Measured from the principal point:

- The anterior focal length (F_1) is equal to 17.05 mm (15.7 + 1.35).
- The posterior focal length (F_2) is equal to 22.78 mm (24.13–1.35).

So, the refracting system of the eye separates the two media of refractive indices 1 (air) and 1.33 (eye).

Since the rays enter and leave the refracting system through media of different refractive indices, the anterior and posterior focal distances are different. The parallel rays falling upon cornea will be brought to a focus 24 mm behind it, coinciding with position of retina/posterior focal

Table 3.4 Characteristics of reduced eye

Total power	+ 58.6 D
Radius of curvature	5.73 mm
Single principal point (P)	1.35 mm from anterior surface of cornea
Single nodal point (N)	7.08 mm from anterior surface of cornea (1.35 + 5.73 mm)
Two focal points	
• Anterior focal point (F_1) (anterior focal distance)	–15.7 mm in front of anterior surface of cornea (minus sign by sign convention)
• Posterior focal point (F_2) (posterior focal distance)	+24.13 mm behind the anterior surface of cornea
Refractive index	1.333

point in the normal eye. The optic axis passing through center of both lenticular curvatures, when produced backward, cuts the retina exactly at fovea centralis.

The reduced eye is clinically useful in:
- Calculation of IOL power.
- Localization of intra ocular foreign body.
- Designing the instruments.
- Determining the size of retinal image since nodal point (N) corresponds to the optical center of convex lens.

■ Accommodation

The parallel rays coming from infinity come to a focus on retina in the emmetropic eyes, but divergent rays falling upon cornea will not come to a focus on retina and are focused behind it. Light rays from an object within 6 m are divergent. If an object is brought nearer to the eye at reading distance (≈ 30 cm), divergent rays from object at reading distance focus behind the retina and blurred image is formed.

There are only two ways by which this image can be seen properly:
- By an increase in axial length of eye ball, which is not possible.
- Eye should increase its dioptric power to cause greater convergence of rays to focus the image of near object on retina. This is what actually happens.

This ability of eyes to change their refractive power to ensure a clear retinal image is known as accommodation.

Snellen's acuity test is traditionally performed at a distance of 20 ft (6 m). At this distance, very little accommodation is required by the patient.

■ Physiology of Accommodation

Accommodation is accomplished by increase in convexity of lens. Radius of curvature of the *anterior surface* of lens **R_1 = 10 mm** and that of *posterior surface* of lens **R_2 = 6 mm**.

At rest, the curvature of surfaces of the lens is approximately spherical.

In accommodation, the *central part of anterior lens surface becomes more convex* in relation to the peripheral part of lens because the capsule is thinner at the center and thicker at the periphery. In strong accommodation, the radius of curvature of anterior surface becomes 6 mm. The curvature of *posterior lens surface remains almost the same*. Posterior surface of lens undergoes little change in curvature as it is well-supported by the anterior face of the vitreous (**Fig. 3.10**).

■ Mechanism of Accommodation

When the eye is at rest for distant vision, the ciliary muscle is relaxed and zonules are kept tense. It keeps the lens in a flattened shape and the rays are focused on retina.

When the eye is at rest for near vision, a blurred image is formed on the retina. The blurred retinal image is the stimulus to accommodation, which is a reflex action regulated by an **accommodation reflex**.

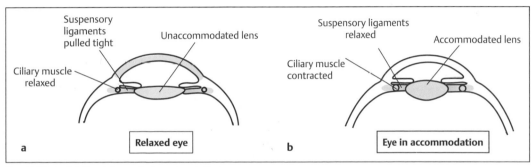

Fig. 3.10 (a, b) Physiology of accommodation.

Contraction of ciliary muscle

↓

Suspensory ligament relaxes

↓

Lens assumes conoidal shape due to *increase in anterior curvature of lens*

If a person looking at a distant object, focuses on to a near object, **three responses are associated with this accommodation reflex:**

- *Increase in anterior curvature of lens* (due to contraction of ciliary muscle).
- *Constriction of pupil* (due to contraction of sphincter pupillae).
- *Convergence of eyeballs* (due to contraction of medial recti).

The association of accommodation, convergence, and pupillary constriction in fixation at near is termed as **near response** or **near vision complex (Fig. 3.11)**.

Pathway for Near Response (Near Reflex)

Thus, a person with normal vision can see not only distant objects but also near ones. Accommodation reflex involves both skeletal muscle (medial recti) and smooth muscles (ciliary muscle and sphincter pupillae; **Flowchart 3.1** and **Fig. 3.12**).

The nearest point at which an object can be seen clearly by accommodation is called the **near point** or **punctum proximum.** *At this point, accommodation is exerted to its maximum.*

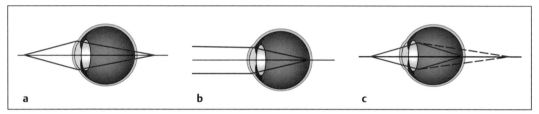

Fig. 3.11 Near vision complex. **(a)** Eye at rest with object at reading distance. **(b)** For distant objects. **(c)** Eye in accommodation for object at reading distance.

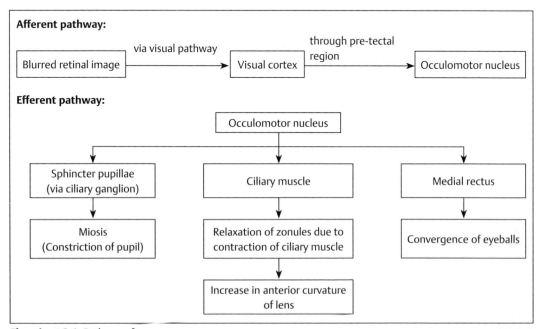

Flowchart 3.1 Pathway of near response.

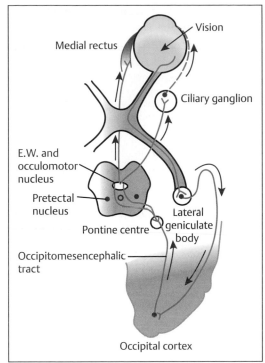

Vision

Medial rectus

Ciliary ganglion

E.W. and
occulomotor
nucleus

Pretectal
nucleus

Lateral
geniculate
body

Pontine centre

Occipitomesencephalic
tract

Occipital cortex

Fig. 3.12 Pathway of near response. Source: Clinical Features. In. Scott I, Regillo C, Flynn H et al., ed. Vitreoretinal Disease: Diagnosis, Management, and Clinical Pearls. 2nd Edition. Thieme; 2017.

The farthest point which can be brought to focus on to the retina is called the **far point** or **punctum remotum**. The distance between the near point and far point is called **range of accommodation**.

■ Amplitude of Accommodation (A)

It is the difference between refractive power of the eye at near point (**P**) and far point (**R**).

$$A = P - R$$

i.e., Amplitude of accommodation (A) = Refractive power of eye with maximum accommodation (P) − Refractive power of eye at rest (R)

$$\Rightarrow A = \frac{100}{\text{distance of near point}} - \frac{100}{\text{distance of far point (cm)}}$$

Far point and near point of eye **vary with the age** and state of **refraction.**

Variation of Accommodation with Age

With advancing age, the lens molds less to changes in the capsule due to increased nuclear sclerosis. The accommodation effort declines. Thus, near point recedes with advancing age and *amplitude of accommodation decreases as age advances. In emmetropes*, far point is at infinity and near point varies with age.

Thus, amplitude of accommodation at the age of 10 years (near point at 7 cm from the eye) is

$$A = \frac{100}{7} - \frac{100}{\infty} = 14 - 0 \rightarrow A = 14D$$

and at the age of 40 years (near point at 20 cm from the eye), accommodation will be

$$A = \frac{100}{20} - \frac{1}{\infty} = 5D$$

Variation of Accommodation with State of Refraction

Accommodation also varies with the state of refraction of eye. The amplitude of accommodation of a hypermetrope is greater than an emmetrope. A myope cannot see distant objects clearly by any effort of accommodation, but can see near object with less effort than an emmetrope or hypermetrope.

> In accommodation, the ciliary muscle contracts equally all around the circumference and simultaneously in two eyes. So, accommodation cannot correct astigmatism and anisometropia.

■ Anomalies of Accommodation

These may be due to:
- Insufficiency of accommodation:
  ◊ Physiological insufficiency—presbyopia.
  ◊ Pathological insufficiency.
- Paralysis of accommodation.
- Spasm of accommodation.

■ Insufficiency of Accommodation

Presbyopia or Physiological Insufficiency of Accommodation

It is not a refractive error but an age-related physiological insufficiency of accommodation, leading to decrease in near vision.

Causes

- Decrease in elasticity of lens capsule with age.
- Hardening (sclerosis) of lens substance with age, resulting in loss of elasticity of lens substance.
- Weakness of ciliary muscle with age.

Onset

It usually begins near the age of 40 years. Onset is early in hypermetropes and late in myopes.

Clinical Features

- Difficulty in near vision: Near point recedes and the patient prefers to keep the near objects at a greater distance than usual.
- Asthenopic symptoms (eyestrain) after reading or doing near work.

In myopes of 3 to 4D, this stage never reaches as the far point of these persons (= 33 cm or 25 cm) corresponds with comfortable working distance.

When presbyopic symptoms are seen in an individual younger than 40 years, the patient is most likely a latent hypermetrope. A cycloplegic refraction confirms the diagnosis.

Treatment

Initially, refractive error for distance is determined and corrected, if present. Then patient is asked to read the near test types at working distance and the *weakest convex lenses* are added. As the age increases, amplitude of accommodation decreases. So, power of convex lens should be increased.

No attempts should be made to overcorrect presbyopia as overcorrection reduces working distance and patient has to work at a close distance which results in discomfort.

Options for presbyopic correction include:
- *Spectacles*:
  - ◇ If distant vision is normal only, reading glasses are prescribed.
  - ◇ If distant vision needs glasses, bifocals are advised.
- *Contact lenses* (bifocal).

- *Surgery includes*:
  - ◇ Conductive keratoplasty (CK).
  - ◇ Multifocal IOLs.
  - ◇ Presbyopic LASIK.
  - ◇ Accommodative IOLs.

Pathological Insufficiency of Accommodation

Physiological insufficiency of accommodation with patient's age is called presbyopia and is normal. But when accommodation power is significantly less than normal physiological limits for patient's age, it is called **insufficiency of accommodation** which is pathological.

Causes

- Early onset of lenticular sclerosis.
- Weakness of ciliary muscle due to systemic cause, for example, anemia, toxemia, and diabetes mellitus.
- Cyclitis (inflammation of ciliary body).
- Primary open angle glaucoma, resulting in impaired function of ciliary muscle due to raised IOP.

Paralysis of Accommodation

Paralysis of accommodation is also known as *cycloplegia* (cyclo = ciliary body, plegia = paralysis).

Causes

Cycloplegic drugs: Ciliary muscle is supplied by the parasympathetic nerve (III CN). Therefore, parasympatholytic drugs cause paralysis of ciliary muscle and accommodation. *As nerve supply of sphincter pupillae is same as that of ciliary muscle, so cycloplegia is always associated with mydriasis (pupil dilatation), that is,* **cycloplegic drugs are also mydriatics**.

Clinically used cycloplegic drugs are:
- Cyclopentolate.
- Homatropine.
- Atropine.

Sympathomimetic drugs are only mydriatics and not cycloplegics, for example, phenylephrine, adrenaline.

Bilateral paresis, although less common, occurs as a complication of:

- Diphtheria.
- Syphilis.
- Diabetes.
- Alcoholism.
- Meningo encephalitis.
- Trauma involving III CN nuclei in midbrain.

Clinical Features

- *Blurring of near vision:* Symptom depends upon condition of refraction. It may not be marked in myopic patients.
- *Photophobia* due to accompanying mydriasis.

Treatment

- Recovery occurs in drug-induced cycloplegia and in cases of diphtheria.
- Dark glasses to reduce photophobia.
- Convex lenses for near work.

Prognosis

It is good in cases due to drugs or diphtheria but the condition may be permanent in traumatic cases.

> Most disorders of accommodation are bilateral in nature. The disorders that present as unilateral loss of accommodation localize to:
> - Infranuclear III CN.
> - Ciliary ganglion (Adie's syndrome).
> - Ciliary body itself.

■ Spasm of Accommodation

It is also called cyclotonia and is marked by excessive accommodation.

Ciliary muscle has a physiological tone of approximately 1 D. In spasm of ciliary muscle, this tone of ciliary muscle is increased and results in greater accommodative response than normal. Thus, emmetrope becomes myopic and the condition is called **pseudomyopia.** Apart from this, myope becomes more myopic while hypermetrope may become less hypermetropic, emmetropic, or even myopic. The condition is found only in young patients, particularly in myopes, and revealed by refraction under atropine.

Causes

- Spontaneous spasm of accommodation usually occurs when eyes are subject to excessive near work in unfavorable circumstances such as bad reading posture, bad illumination, mental stress, and anxiety.
- Spasm can be produced artificially by instillation of strong miotics.

Treatment

- Use of cycloplegic drops for several weeks to relax the spasm.
- Refraction under atropine and correction of actual refractive error are conducted.

Purkinje sanson images: There are four images:

- First image is derived formed by anterior corneal surface.
- Second image is derived formed by posterior corneal surface.
- Third image is derived formed by anterior corneal surface.
- All these three images are erect images.
- Fourth image is derived from the concave posterior lens surface, so the image is inverted and moves in opposite direction.

■ Refractive Errors (OP1.2, OP9.3)

When parallel rays of light are focused upon retina with accommodation being at rest, the condition is called **emmetropia.**

In some eyes, retina is not situated at its usual position. Parallel rays of light from a distant object may be focused either in front of or behind the retina and the condition is called **ametropia** or **errors of refraction.**

- If *eye is relatively too short,* object is focused behind retina and the condition is called **hypermetropia.**
- If *eye is relatively too long,* object is focused in front of retina and the condition is called **myopia.**

In each case, a blurred image will be formed upon retina, and vision remains subnormal.

- When refraction of two eyes is equal, the condition is called **isometropia**.
- When refraction of two eyes is different, the condition is called **anisometropia.**

■ Emmetropia (Normal Eye)

It is the condition in which parallel rays of light from infinity are focused on the retina with *accommodation at rest*, that is, second focal point of the eye is at retina (**Fig. 3.13**).

At **birth**, the average axial length is **18 mm**; so, the eye of newborn is **hypermetropic.** By the age of **3 years**, the axial length becomes **23 mm** and **hypermetropia reduces** gradually. From **3 to 14 years** of age, the axial length becomes **24 mm** and **emmetropia** is achieved.

This process is known as **emmetropization**.

Hypermetropic newborn may remain hyper-metropic, can reach emmetropia, or can become myopic.

■ Ametropia (Refractive Error)

It is the condition when parallel rays of light from infinity do not come to a focus on the retina with accommodation at rest, that is, second focal point of the eye is not located on retina. Causes of ametropia are as follows:

- Abnormal length of eyeball termed as "axial ametropia."
- Abnormal curvature of cornea or lens is termed as curvature ametropia.
- Abnormal position of lens is termed as positional ametropia.

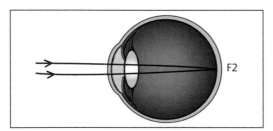

Fig. 3.13 Refraction in an emmetropic eye.

- Abnormal refractive index of media is termed as index ametropia.

The three types of ametropia or refractive errors are:

- Myopia.
- Hypermetropia (hyperopia).
- Astigmatism.

Myopia (Short Sightedness)

It is the condition in which parallel rays of light from infinity come to a focus in front of the retina with accommodation at rest. So, in myopia, there is difficulty to see at far distances, that is, the eye is near sighted (**Fig. 3.14**). It could be classified based on etiology and clinical presentation.

Etiological Types

Based on the cause of myopia, it can be:

- Axial myopia: It is due to *elongation* of the eyeball (normal axial length = 24 mm).

1 mm increase in axial length (anteroposterior length) leads to approximately 3D of myopia.

- Curvature myopia: It is due to increased curvature (less radius of curvature) of cornea/lens, as in:
  - ◇ Keratoconus.
  - ◇ Keratoglobus.
  - ◇ Lenticonus.

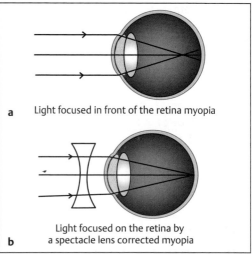

a Light focused in front of the retina myopia

Light focused on the retina by
b a spectacle lens corrected myopia

Fig. 3.14 (a) Light focused in front of the retina. **(b)** Light focused on the retina by a spectacle lens.

1 mm decrease in radius of curvature of cornea produces 6D of myopia.

- Index myopia: It is found in old age due to nuclear sclerosis. *In nuclear sclerosis*, RI of nucleus increases. Thus, *index myopia* (lenticular) is produced which improves near vision in existing presbyopia. This is termed as "second sight."
- Positional (displacement) myopia: *Anterior displacement of lens* causes myopia.

Clinical Types

Clinically, myopia can be classified into congenital, simple, and pathological myopia.

Congenital Myopia

Age of onset: It is present since birth and is rare.

Refractive error: Child is born with an abnormally long eyeball and may have—10 D myopia soon after birth.

Progression is rare.

Fundus: Myopic crescent may be present; choroidal vessel may be evident due to lack of pigmentation. Myopic crescent is a moon shaped feature that develops at the temporal border of the disc. It is primarily caused by atrophic changes from stretching due to elongation of the eyeball.

Simple Myopia (Developmental myopia)

It is the commonest form.

Age of onset: During childhood and adolescence (between 5–15 years of age).

Refractive error: It is mild to moderate and seldom exceeds 5 to 6 D.

Progression: It keeps on increasing during years of growth and does not progress after 21 years of age. It is also called as physiological myopia.

Fundus: No degenerative changes are seen although peripheral retinal degeneration may be seen later.

Pathological Myopia

Age: It appears in early childhood usually between 5 to 10 years of age and is more common in females. It is strongly hereditary.

Refractive error: It rapidly increases during period of active growth and may reach up to −15 D to −25 D, that is, high myopia.

Progression: It is essentially a degenerative and progressive condition.

Etiology: The condition is strongly hereditary and is more common in females than in males. The condition is essentially a disturbance of growth and results from rapid axial growth of eyeball. The degenerative changes in fundus do not appear until later in life.

Other factors which influence the progress of myopia are endocrine disturbances, nutritional disturbances, illness, or debility.

Fundus: Fundus shows chorioretinal degeneration, myopic crescent, and vitreous degeneration (**Fig. 3.15**).

Grades

Low myopia	–	≤ 2 D
Moderate myopia	–	2–6 D
High myopia	–	> 6 D

Symptoms

The signs and symptoms depend upon the grade of myopia (low or high) and these are:

- Poor vision for distance: Holding the book too close to the eyes while reading is the usual complaint of child's parents. It may be the only symptom in **low myopia**.

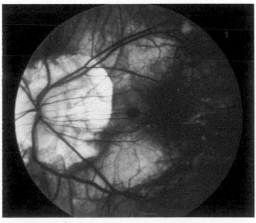

Fig. 3.15 High myopia.

- Eyestrain and headache *(asthenopic symptoms)* after near work. **In high myopia,** amplitude of accommodation is small, so convergence does not get an accommodative influence. Patient experiences discomfort after near work (**ocular asthenopia**).
- Exophoria: The imbalance between efforts of accommodation and convergence cause *exophoria*. In myopia, divergent squint is more common. Accommodation is of little value in myopia as any effort to accommodate would only accelerate his visual problem.
- Black spots floating before eyes due to vitreous degeneration.
- Occasionally flashes of light are noticed.
- Photophobia (i.e., eyes are sensitive to light) due to large pupils. Parents of child complain that the child squeezes his or her eyes to make a narrow slit. All myopes squeeze their palpebral aperture to reduce photophobia and improve their visual acuity if not corrected fully.

Signs

- Eyes are *prominent* due to increased axial length. The elongation of eyeball mainly affects the posterior pole.
- Anterior chamber: deep.
- Pupils: large.
- Apparent convergent squint due to large, negative-angle kappa. In myopes, there may be an impression of convergent squint although divergent squint is common in myopia.
- Fundus examination.

In **simple myopia,** fundus is usually normal and temporal myopic crescent may be seen.

In **pathological myopia** (very high myopia), ophthalmoscopy may reveal (**Fig. 3.16**):
- *Optic disc:*
  ◇ Large with mild pallor.
  ◇ Large physiological cup.
  ◇ Temporal crescent is present; sometimes, annular crescent may be

present encircling the disc. Supertraction crescent on nasal side of disc (due to pulling of retina over the disc margin) may be seen.
- *Macula:*
  ◇ **Foster Fuchs spot** (*a red central spot*) may be seen at fovea due to choroidal hemorrhage.
- *Peripheral retina:* Cystoid degeneration and lattice degeneration may be seen at the periphery.
- Chorioretinal atrophic patches may be present due to degenerative changes in retina and choroid.
- Degenerative changes in vitreous include liquefaction (causing vitreous floaters) and syneresis (causing posterior vitreous detachment). When posterior vitreous detachment (**PVD**) occurs at disc, it appears as a circular reflex called **Weiss reflex.**
- *Posterior staphyloma* (ectasia of sclera at posterior pole) may be present, which is recognized by change in course of vessels (**Flowchart 3.2**).

Treatment

Myopia may be treated by:
- Spectacles.
- Contact lens.
- Surgery.

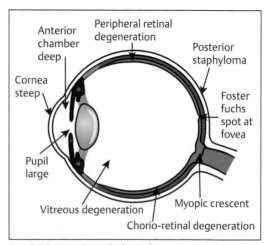

Fig. 3.16 Signs in pathological myopia.

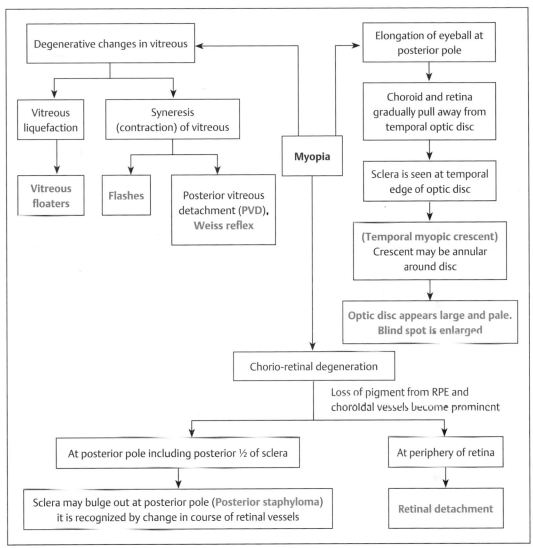

Flowchart 3.2 Changes seen in pathological myopia.

Spectacles

- *Concave lenses* are used in spectacles. Spectacles should be used constantly.
- Myopia must *never be overcorrected.*

Low and moderate myopia (up to 6D) are *fully corrected for distance.* If discomfort is experienced in near work, weaker lenses may be ordered for near work.

High myopia (>6D) is *always slightly under-corrected for distance* as strong concave lenses diminish the size of retinal images and make them very bright, which are not tolerated by the patient. For near work, still weaker lenses are prescribed.

- *If myopia is uncorrected:* Child loses interest in surroundings owing to blurred vision and tends to become unduly introspective.
- *In unilateral myopia:* Correction with spectacles induces aniseikonia (difference in size of images of both eyes).
- Periphery of thick concave lenses causes distortion of image.

Contact Lenses

These can be used instead of spectacles. Advantages of using contact lenses over spectacles include:

- Eliminate peripheral distortion caused by thick concave lenses.
- Provide wider field.
- Results in large image size compared with glasses.
- Causes no problem of aniseikonia.

Surgery

It is performed **after** 21 years of age when refractive error has stabilized.

- Surgical correction of myopia may involve:
  - ◊ Corneal surgery.
  - ◊ Lens surgery.

Corneal surgery

Aim: To flatten the cornea.

Methods: • Radial keratotomy (RK).
- Intracorneal rings (ICR).
- Photo refractive keratectomy (PRK).
- Excimer LASIK.
- Femtosecond LASIK.

Lens surgery

Aim: To reduce overall refractive power of the eye.

Methods: • Clear lens extraction for >15 D Myopia.
- Phakic IOL or ICL for high myopia– it involves placement of an anterior chamber/posterior chamber lens in a phakic eye anterior to natural crystalline lens.

Complications

Following are the complications of pathological myopia:

- Posterior staphyloma.
- Degenerative changes in vitreous and retina.
- Retinal detachment.
- Complicated cataract.
- Glaucoma.
- Choroidal hemorrhage.
- Vitreous hemorrhage.
- Strabismus fixus convergence.

Hypermetropia (Long Sightedness or Hyperopia)

It is an error of refraction in which parallel rays of light from infinity come to a focus behind the retina with accommodation at rest. Thus, posterior focal point is behind the retina (**Fig. 3.17**). Hypermetropia could be classified based on causation and clinical presentation.

Etiological Types

- Axial hypermetropia: It is due to *shortening of axial* (anteroposterior) *length* of eyeball. *1 mm shortening of axial length results in 3D of hypermetropia.* It is the commonest form.
- Curvature hypermetropia: It is due to *flat curvature* of the cornea or lens. Astigmatism is usually accompanied with curvature hypermetropia.
- Index hypermetropia: It is due to *decreased RI of the lens* as in cortical cataract. (In cortical cataract, RI of lens cortex increases relative to lens nucleus, so that overall refractive power of lens decreases).
- Positional (or displacement) hypermetropia: It is due to the posterior displacement of lens.

Accommodation has a considerable influence on hypermetropia.

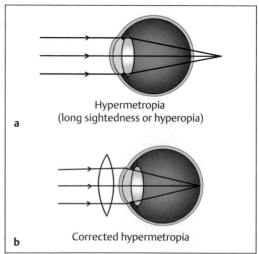

a Hypermetropia (long sightedness or hyperopia)

b Corrected hypermetropia

Fig. 3.17 (a) Hypermetropia (long sightedness or hyperopia). **(b)** Corrected hypermetropia.

Solid lines show course of rays with eye at rest, and *dotted lines* show the curvature of anterior surface of lens and course of rays with active accommodation (**Fig. 3.18**).

Clinical Types

Normally, ciliary muscle has a considerable amount of tone. A part of hypermetropia is corrected by this *physiological tone* of ciliary muscle which is called latent hypermetropia. Thus, latent hypermetropia can only be revealed under complete cycloplegia. The *remaining portion* of total hypermetropia is called the **manifest hypermetropia**, that is, it is the portion of hypermetropia not corrected by physiological tone of ciliary muscle. The part of manifest hypermetropia which can be *corrected by accommodation* is termed **facultative hypermetropia**.

The part of manifest hypermetropia which *cannot be overcome by accommodation* is termed **absolute hypermetropia**. This is the part which may lead to amblyopia.

Thus, total hypermetropia = latent + facultative + absolute hypermetropia
└──── Manifest ────┘

Pathological hypermetropia is seen in:
- Aphakia (absence of lens).

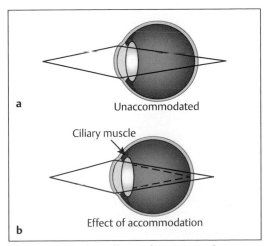

a Unaccommodated

Ciliary muscle

b Effect of accommodation

Fig. 3.18 (a, b) Effect of accommodation on hypermetropia.

- Occulomotor (3rd cranial nerve [CN]) palsy: Ciliary muscle tone decreases in occulomotor (3rd CN) palsy causing paralysis of accommodation. It results in hypermetropia.
- Consecutive hypermetropia (due to surgical over correction of myopia).

Grades

Low hypermetropia	-	≤ 2.0 D
Moderate hypermetropia	-	+ 2.0 D to + 5.00 D
High hypermetropia	-	> + 5.00 D

Symptoms

- Asthenopic symptoms—Strain on ciliary muscle due to sustained accommodative effort produces *asthenopic symptoms* (**eyestrain**) which include eye ache, burning, watering, frontal headache, and eye fatigue.

The asthenopic symptoms are noticed chiefly after prolonged near work and increase toward evening. Symptoms of eye strain may be absent if near work is avoided.
- Esophoria (latent convergent squint): Increased accommodative convergence due to continuous accommodation results in esophoria which further increases eye strain.
- Blurring of vision (near > distance) occurs when hypermetropia is *not fully corrected by voluntary accommodative effort*. It is associated with asthenopic symptoms due to sustained accommodative efforts. Inadvertent rubbing of eyes (due to eye strain) with dirty fingers may result in recurrent stye, chalazia, or blepharitis.

Symptoms vary with the age of patient and the degree of hypermetropia. The accommodational reserve is good in younger patients and decreases among older ones.
- *Mild* hypermetropia in *young* individuals: It is easily compensated by accommodation. Thus, mild hypermetropia may not cause any symptom in young individuals because of good accommodational reserve.

- *Mild* hypermetropia in *older* patients: Symptoms may appear because of decrease in accommodation in older patients.
- When *high* hypermetropia is present, especially in *adults* or *older* patients, it cannot be compensated by accommodation. Thus, there is marked blurring of vision for near and distance.

Signs

- *Eyeballs* are usually small with small cornea.
- *Anterior chamber* is shallow than usual. Such an eye is predisposed to angle-closure glaucoma.
- *Fundus: Disc* is small and hyperemic and margins may be seen blurred. So, it may be confused with papillitis, a condition known as **pseudopapillitis**:
  - ◊ *Blood vessels* may be unduly tortuous.
  - ◊ *Retina* shows glistening appearance (a bright reflex), resembling a watered silk appearance.

Complications of Untreated Hypermetropia

If hypermetropia is left untreated, it can lead to complications such as:

- Convergent strabismus (due to excessive use of accommodation).
- Amblyopia (lazy eye).
- Recurrent styes and blepharitis (infections due to rubbing of eyes resulting from eye strain).

Treatment

Hypermetropia may be treated by:

- Spectacles.
- Contact lenses.
- Surgery.

Spectacles

- If there is no symptom or tendency to develop convergent squint, no spectacles are prescribed.
- Hypermetropia with asthenopia is corrected by convex lenses. As hypermetropia in children tends to decrease with advancing age, therefore, annual checkup is must for a possible change in glasses. **Glasses must be used constantly**.
- In **young** patients **with active accommodation**, undercorrection is advised.
- In **older patients,** accommodation is poor; all manifest hypermetropia becomes absolute and full correction is advised.
- Refraction is conducted under cycloplegia:
  - ◊ In children <6 years, refraction under atropine (1% eye ointment twice a day × 3 days) is done.
  - ◊ In older children and adults, refraction with cyclopentolate 1% or homatropine 2% is performed.

Contact Lenses

Contact lenses are prescribed in unilateral hypermetropia (anisometropia) to avoid diplopia or amblyopia.

Surgery

- *Holmium laser thermokeratoplasty.*
- *Hypermetropic LASIK* to correct mild to moderate (+ 1 D to + 4 D) hypermetropia.
- *Phakic ICLs* for high hypermetropia (+ 4 D to + 10 D).
- *Conductive keratoplasty.*

Astigmatism

It is a condition in which *refraction varies in different meridians of eye; therefore*, a point object is not focused as a point.

Etiology

It may be:

- *Corneal astigmatism* due to abnormalities in curvature of cornea.
- *Lenticular astigmatism* due to:
  - ◊ Abnormalities in curvature of lens.
  - ◊ Tilting of lens as in subluxation of lens.
  - ◊ Unequal refractive index in different sectors of lens (index astigmatism).

In astigmatism, there are two principal meridians: Meridian of greatest curvature and meridian of least curvature.

Types

There are two types of astigmatism: regular and irregular astigmatism.

Regular Astigmatism

When these two principal meridians of greatest and least curvature of cornea *are at right angle (90°) to each other*, the condition is called *regular astigmatism*. The more curved meridian will have greater refractive power than the less curved. The two principal meridians may be horizontal and vertical at 90° to each other (*horizontal–vertical astigmatism*) or oblique (not horizontal and vertical) although still at 90° to each other (*oblique* astigmatism).

Bioblique Astigmatism

The two principal meridians are not at right angle to each other but are crossed obliquely. Normally, owing to the pressure of eyelids on the globe, *vertical curvature > horizontal curvature (normal rule)*.

With the Rule Astigmatism

When **vertical curvature > Horizontal curvature**, it is termed as astigmatism **'with the rule'**.

Vertical curvature > horizontal curvature

↓

Vertical rays will come to a focus sooner than horizontal

↓

Correction of this astigmatism will require Concave cylinder at 180° or Convex cylinder at 90°

(*Cylindrical lens has power only at right angle to axis*)

Against the Rule Astigmatism

When **horizontal curvature > vertical curvature**, it is termed as astigmatism "**against the rule.**" It occurs after cataract surgery through superior incision, in which vertical meridian flattens due to scarring.

Horizontal curvature > vertical curvature

↓

Horizontal rays will come to a focus sooner than vertical

↓

Correction of this astigmatism will require Concave cylinder at 90° or Convex cylinder at 180°

Irregular Astigmatism

When surface of cornea is irregular, rays of light are refracted irregularly, leading to multiple foci in various positions, and completely blurred image is produced on retina. This condition is called irregular astigmatism. It is *due to* corneal opacities or scarring and *cannot be corrected*. It is also seen in keratoconus and lenticonus (**Flowchart 3.3**).

Optics In Astigmatism

A more curved meridian has greater refractive power and will focus the rays sooner. Let us suppose vertical curvature > horizontal curvature. So, vertical rays come to a focus sooner than horizontal and, instead of a focal point, rays will have two foci. The configuration of rays refracted through the astigmatic (toric) surface is called **Sturm's conoid**. The distance between two foci is called **focal interval of sturm**. The focal interval is the degree or measure of astigmatism (**Fig. 3.19**). **Table 3.5** explains the various types of astigmatism.

Symptoms

These depend upon the type and the degree of astigmatism. Symptoms include:
- Defect in visual activity. Distance vision is often found to be good in mixed astigmatism as circle of least diffusion falls upon or near retina.
- Distortion of objects.
- Asthenopic symptoms:
  ◇ Burning.
  ◇ Eye ache.

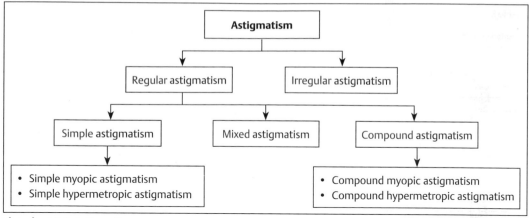

Flowchart 3.3 Astigmatism.

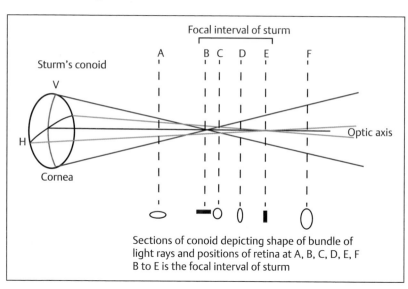

Fig. 3.19 Sturm's conoid.

◊ Headache.

◊ Eye fatigue.

In smaller degree of astigmatism, defect in visual activity is minimal but asthenopia or eye strain is marked due to efforts of accommodation (to produce a circle of least diffusion upon retina); however, in higher degree of astigmatism, asthenopic symptoms are absent because no attempts are made to ameliorate the blurred vision.

Signs

- *Head tilt,* especially in oblique astigmatism, in an attempt to bring the axes nearer to vertical and horizontal meridians.

- *Half closure of lids* as in myopes in an attempt to achieve the greater clarity of stenopaeic vision.
- Oval or tilted optic disc.

Determination of Astigmatic Power and Axis

It can be done with:

- Retinoscopy: It reveals power in two different axes.
- Keratometry: It measures corneal curvature in two different meridians.
- Jackson's cross cylinders: To verify the power of cylinder in the optical correction.
- Astigmatic fan test: To confirm the power and axis of the cylindrical lenses.

Table 3.5 Types of astigmatism

Position of object	Focal point of rays	Type of astigmatism
	At position **A**: Vertical rays are converging more than horizontal rays. So, shape of bundle of light rays, i.e., section will be horizontal oval or oblate ellipse.	If retina is situated at **A**: Rays from both meridian focus behind the retina, i.e., hypermetropia in both meridian. The condition is compound **hypermetropic astigmatism**.
	At position **B**: Vertical rays come to a focus while horizontal rays are still converging. So, bundle of light rays, i.e., section of conoid will be a horizontal straight line.	If a retina is positioned at **B**: Vertical meridian will be emmetropic while horizontal meridian will be hypermetropic. This condition is called simple **hypermetropic astigmatism**.
	At position **C**: Divergence of vertical rays and convergence of horizontal rays are equal. So, rays from both meridia meet forming a circle, known as **circle of least diffusion**.	If the retina is situated at **C**: Vertical meridian will be myopic. Horizontal meridian will be hypermetropic. The condition is called **mixed astigmatism**.
	At position **D**: Divergence of vertical rays > convergence of horizontal rays. So, bundle of rays will be vertical oval.	If retina is situated at **D**: Vertical meridian will be myopic. Horizontal meridian will be hypermetropic. The condition is called **mixed astigmatism**.
	At position **E**: Vertical rays diverging and horizontal rays come to a focus. So, shape of bundle of light rays will be a vertical straight line.	If retina is positioned at **E**: Vertical meridian will be myopic. Horizontal meridian comes to a focus. The condition is called simple **myopic astigmatism**.
	At position **F**: Divergence of vertical rays is more than that of horizontal rays. So, bundle of light rays will be vertical oval or prolate ellipse.	If retina is positioned at **F**: Both meridians will be myopic. This condition is called **compound myopic astigmatism**.

Treatment

Spectacles

- In small astigmatism (<0.5D) without symptoms, there is *no need of spectacles.*
- In astigmatism with asthenopic symptoms, *full optical correction* with cylindrical lenses (in simple astigmatism) or combination of spherical and cylindrical lenses (in mixed or compound astigmatism) is recommended. **Spectacles are advised for constant use**.

Toric Contact Lenses

Gas permeable contact lenses are rigid and retain their spherical shape on the eye. The irregular shape of the cornea of an astigmatic eye is rectified by the soft contact lenses for astigmatism. These are called Toric contact lenses. Regular lenses rectify the myopia/hypermetropia but toric contact lenses can rectify astigmatism as well.

Surgery

- Astigmatic LASIK.
- Toric phakic IOLs.
- Arcuate keratectomy.
- Photoastigmatic keratectomy with excimer laser.

Anisometropia

Isometropia is the condition of *equal refractive errors* in the two eyes.

Anisometropia is the condition in which there is *considerable difference in the refractive state of two eyes.*

A minor difference is common and seldom gives any symptom. *A difference of 0.25 D in two eyes causes 0.5% difference in the size of two retinal images*, that is, 1 D difference in refractive errors causes 2% difference in the size of two images.

Anisometropia up to 2.5 D creates aniseikonia (unequal size of image) of which approximately 5% is well-tolerated.

Anisometropia of >4 D is usually symptomatic and not tolerated.

Anisometropia may be congenital or acquired.

Types

Anisometropia may be:
- **Simple** anisometropia: One eye is emmetropic while the other has a refractive error.
- **Compound** anisometropia: Both eyes are ametropic and have same type of refractive errors but different in magnitude, for example, myopia of −1 D and −3 D in two eyes.
- **Mixed** anisometropia: Both eyes are ametropic but one is myopic and the other is hypermetropic. It is also called antimetropia.

Anisometropia and Binocular Vision

- In small degree of anisometropia, *binocular vision is usually maintained.*
- In anisometropia of >2.5D, fusion is not possible and binocular vision *is disrupted.* Vision is then **uniocular**. The eye with high-refractive error is suppressed and anisometropic amblyopia (partial loss of vision) results.
- When one eye is emmetropic or hypermetropic and other eye is myopic, emmetropic or hypermetropic eye is used for distance and myopic eye for near work. Both eyes have good visual activity (alternating vision). Before the glasses are prescribed, make sure that two eyes are functioning simultaneously. This can be assessed by the **FRIEND test**.

FIN—is written in green letters.

RED—is written in red letters.

Patient sits at a distance of 6 m wearing a diplopia goggle with red glass in front of right eye:
- If he or she reads FRIEND, he or she has binocular vision.
- If he or she reads RED or FIN persistently, he or she has uniocular vision.
- If he or she reads FIN at one time and RED at the other, he or she has alternating vision.

Treatment

- **Spectacles:** Anisometropia up to 2.5 D is well-tolerated with spectacles. In high-degree of anisometropia, aniseikonia occurs with spectacles. So, spectacles are not readily acceptable because of difficulty in fusion of images. If full correction is not tolerated, each eye is under corrected. If eye has become amblyopic, patching of emmetropic eye is done and amblyopic eye is used with spectacles.

- **Contact lenses** eliminate aniseikonia.
- **Surgery:** LASIK in anisometropic patients.

Correction of Refractive Errors (IM24.15)

Refractive errors can be corrected with:
- Spectacles.
- Contact lenses.
- Refractive surgery.

Spectacles

Important aspects of spectacles are as follows:
- Material of lenses.
- Type of lenses.
- Fitting of lenses.
- Frames.

Material of Lenses

- Glass lenses: They are usually made of *crown glass* having RI of **1.52.** For high myopes, *high-index lenses* (RI = 1.53–1.74) are used to minimize the thickness. Therefore, they are thin and light weight.
- Resilens *or* CR-39 plastic lenses are light-weight and made of allyl diglycol carbonate. They are often resistant to scratching.
- Polycarbonate lenses have high RI and are unbreakable. They are scratch and impact resistant, so ideal for children and sportsmen.

Types of Lenses

- Aspheric lenses: These have curves that flatten away from center; therefore, they do not cause spherical aberration and provide better peripheral vision.
- Bifocal lenses: These are used in presbyopic patients with refractive error for distance. The upper part contains correction for distant vision and lower part for reading or close work; between these two parts, there is a distinctive line.
- Trifocal lenses: In these lenses, a strip for intermediate distance is interposed between distant and near corrections.
- Multi focal (varifocal/progressive) lenses: These lenses provide continuous gradation from distant to near vision, having no distracting lines in between.

All these lenses can be tinted, coated, or photochromatic. Tinted glasses are advised for albinism and high myopia to reduce the amount of light entering the eye. Antireflection coating reduces glare. Photochromatic lenses change their color from light to dark on exposure to sunlight. They contain ultraviolet-activated, color-changing silver halide molecule. Exposure to short-wavelength light (UV light) causes conversion of Ag^+ into elemental Ag and the lenses darken in sunlight. The reaction is reversible, so lenses lighten when illumination decreases.

Fitting of Lenses

In *distant corrections*, lenses are fitted in the frames, so that their optical centers coincide with visual axes to avoid prismatic effects. In *reading*, eyes are directly downward and inward. So, presbyopic lenses are slightly decentered inwards. Ideally, lenses should be worn at 15 mm in front of cornea which corresponds to anterior principal focus of eye. At this distance, images formed on retina are of same size as in emmetropia.

Contact Lenses

Contact lenses are visual devices worn in apposition with cornea (**Table 3.6**). Contact lenses are used for:
- Corrective purpose.
- Cosmetic purpose.
- Therapeutic purpose.

Table 3.6 Advantages of contact lenses over spectacles

Feature	With contact lens	With spectacles
Prismatic effects on peripheral viewing	Eliminate prismatic effects as contact lenses move with the eyes	Present in spectacles lens
Field of clear vision	Greatly increased	Less than contact lenses
Binocular vision due to aniseikonia in high anisometropia	Binocular vision is retained due to less magnification of retinal image	Binocular vision is not possible
Irregular corneal astigmatism seen in keratoconus	Corrects	Not possible to correct
Cosmetically	Superior	Less acceptable
In rain and fog	Better optical aid	Poor optical aid

Table 3.7 Properties of contact lenses

Property	Hard CL	RGP CL	Soft CL
Material	PMMA	PMMA + silicone + PVP	HEMA
Oxygen permeability	Poor	Moderate	High
Adaptability	Required	Required	Not required
Deposits	Few	Few	Considerable
Use in astigmatism	Possible	Possible	Seldom corrects astigmatism of > 1D
Infective complications	Less	Less likely	May be contaminated by microorganisms
Size	Corneal CL smaller than corneal diameter	Corneal CL smaller than corneal diameter	Semiscleral CL 1–2 mm larger than corneal diameter
Durability	May undergo scratching	Do not scratch or tear	Tend to tear

Abbreviations: CL, contact lens; HEMA: hydroxyethyl methacrylate; PMMA, polymethyl methacrylate; PVP, polyvinyl pyrrolidone; RGP, rigid gas permeable.

Types

Contact lenses (CL) are of three types:
- Hard lenses.
- Rigid gas permeable (RGP) lenses.
- Soft lenses.

Hard contact lenses are made of PolyMethylMethAcrylate (**PMMA**).

RGP lenses are made of PMMA copolymerized with silicone and polyvinyl pyrrolidone (PVP).

Soft contact lenses are made up of HydroxyEthylMethAcrylate (**HEMA**) which is able to absorb fluid.

Differences in the properties of various types of contact lenses is listed in **Table 3.7**.

Special Types of CL

- For astigmatism: Toric CL.
- For presbyopia: Bifocal, trifocal, or multifocal CL.
- *Disposable CL*: Due to deposits with soft CL in the long-term, they are now used as disposable lenses. These are used for a specific period of time, then disposed of and replaced with new pair of lenses. These lenses can be daily, weekly, or monthly disposable.
- *Extended wear* (*continuous wear CL*) has increased water content and oxygen permeability than ordinary soft CL. These carry high-risk of infection.

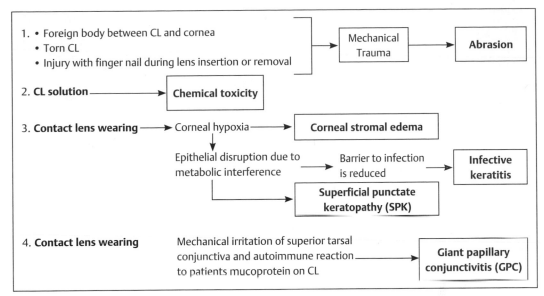

1. • Foreign body between CL and cornea
   • Torn CL
   • Injury with finger nail during lens insertion or removal → Mechanical Trauma → **Abrasion**

2. **CL solution** → **Chemical toxicity**

3. **Contact lens wearing** → Corneal hypoxia → **Corneal stromal edema**
   ↓
   Epithelial disruption due to metabolic interference → Barrier to infection is reduced → **Infective keratitis**
   → **Superficial punctate keratopathy (SPK)**

4. **Contact lens wearing** — Mechanical irritation of superior tarsal conjunctiva and autoimmune reaction to patients mucoprotein on CL → **Giant papillary conjunctivitis (GPC)**

Abbreviation: CL, contact lens.

Side Effects

These may be due to injury, CL solution, or improper fitting. *Most of the complications due to CL occur because of corneal hypoxia.*

- *Pseudomonas aeruginosa* is the pathogen most frequently involved.
- Fungi and Acanthamoeba may also infect the lenses.
- Incidence of microbial keratitis is more with extended wear CL than daily wear CL or RGP CL.

Contraindications

- Chronic dacryocystitis.
- Dry eye syndrome.
- Chronic blepharitis.
- Corneal degeneration.
- Chronic conjunctivitis.

■ Refractive Surgery (OP1.4, OP9.3)

Refractive surgeries are performed preferably after 21 years of age.

Pattern of treatment for correction of myopia, hyperopia, and astigmatism differs.

Myopia requires **greater tissue removal in center** of cornea than in periphery, resulting in flattening of central cornea.

Hyperopia requires **tissue removal from periphery**. For hyperopic ablation, the center is left untreated.

Astigmatism requires **greater treatment along one meridian than another,** creating a toric cut.

Details of refractive surgery will be discussed in Chapter 26 on "Eye surgery."

Ocular Therapeutics

Introduction 60
Routes of Administration 60
Antimicrobial Agents 62
Antiviral Agents 67
Antifungal Agents 69
Anti-Inflammatory Drugs 72
Antiallergic Drugs 73
Drugs Acting on Intraocular Muscles 74
Anti-Vascular Endothelial Growth Factor (Anti-VEGF) Agents 75
Viscoelastic Substances 75
Immunosuppressive Agents 76
Irrigating Solutions 78
Ocular Preservatives 78
Reactions to Medicines 79
Dyes Used in Ophthalmology 79

■ Introduction (PH1.58)

The drugs available for the treatment of ocular diseases include:

- Antibacterials.
- Antiviral agents.
- Antifungal agents.
- Anti-inflammatory drugs.
- Antiallergic drugs.
- Mydriatics and cycloplegics.
- Antiglaucoma drugs.
- Drugs used for dry eye.
- Anti-VEGF agents.
- Pharmacological agents used in intraocular surgery.

■ Routes of Administration

The therapeutic substances can be delivered by four routes (**Flowchart 4.1**).

■ Instillation

Topically instilled drugs are used in the form of *drops, ointment, gel, and suspension*. Ointment impairs the vision, hence must be applied at night.

Absorption and Bioavailability of Drug

The drug instilled into the conjunctival sac is absorbed largely through the cornea. The corneal layers have different selective permeability. The epithelium is more permeable to fat/lipid soluble substances, while the stroma is permeable to all water-soluble substances. The drug absorption is regulated by:

- Duration of drug contact in the eye, which is enhanced by the use of viscous carriers such as hydroxypropylmethylcellulose (HPMC), polyvinyl alcohol, and hyaluronic acid.
- Pressing the lower punctum by thumb to delay its nasal absorption.

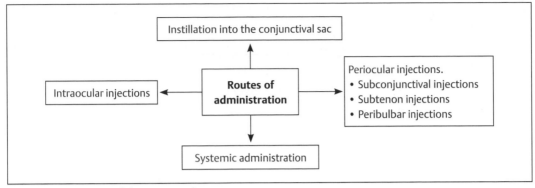

Flowchart 4.1 Routes of therapeutic substance.

Sustained release of the drug may be achieved by ocuserts placed in upper/lower fornix or by drug-impregnated contact lenses. The corneal epithelium forms the main barrier against drugs entering the eye. It is disrupted by local anesthetic or abrasion.

■ Periocular Injections

Subconjunctival Injections

Both antibiotics and steroids can be administered into the eye by subconjunctival injections. Antibiotics which do not penetrate the cornea, owing to their large molecular size, enter the eye through this route, as sclera allows the free transit of molecules of considerable size.

Subtenon Injections

Subtenon injections are employed for sustained release of steroids. These injections are used in the treatment of intermediate (pars planitis) and posterior inflammations. Depot preparation of corticosteroids (triamcinolone acetonide) is useful for the management of chronic intraocular inflammation without systemic side effects.

Peribulbar Injections

This route is used for administration of anesthetics, steroids, or antibiotics in the management of posterior uveitis. This route is preferred over retrobulbar injections for injecting anesthetics or

steroids in muscle cone, as retrobulbar injections may cause perforation of globe or damage to optic nerve.

■ Systemic Administration

Systemic therapy (oral or parenteral) is required in the inflammations/infections of posterior retina, optic nerve, or orbit that cannot be controlled by local applications alone. This route has certain limitations because of the impermeability of blood aqueous barrier. Lipid-soluble drugs (chloramphenicol, sulphonamides, etc.) can penetrate the barrier and enter the eye easily. The blood–aqueous barrier prevents the large-sized molecules (such as penicillin) or water-soluble drugs.

■ Intraocular Injections

In desperate cases, the drugs are injected either into the anterior chamber (intracameral injection) or in the vitreous (intravitreal injection). Intracameral injections of antibiotics are used in acute endophthalmitis. Intravitreal injections of antibiotics and antifungals are indicated in bacterial or fungal endophthalmitis, respectively. The effective concentrations of antibiotics in intravitreal injections last longer than in intracameral injections. Vitreous implants have been used for the treatment of cytomegalovirus (CMV) retinitis.

Bacterial Cell Wall

Gram +ve cell walls are thick and made of peptidoglycan (70–80%); the lipid content in the wall is very low and contains teichoic acid. It can be completely dissolved by lysozymes due to digestion of peptidoglycan layer except in Staph. aureus in which the cell wall is resistant to the action of lysozymes. These primarily produce exotoxins. It is more susceptible to antibiotics.

Gram −ve cell walls contain a thin peptidoglycan (10–20%) layer (without teichoic acids) that is surrounded by a thick plasma membrane adjacent to the **cytoplasmic membrane**. The lipid content in the wall is 20 to 30%. These primarily produce endotoxins. Periplasmic space is present in these bacteria. It is more resistant to antibiotics because their outer membrane comprises a complex lipopolysaccharide (LPS) whose lipid portion acts as an endotoxin.

Unlike mammalian and bacterial cells, **fungal cell membranes** comprise large amounts of **ergosterol** (Fig. 4.1).

■ Antimicrobial Agents

Antimicrobial drugs are synthetic as well as naturally obtained drugs that act against microorganisms.

Antibiotics are the substances obtained from the microorganisms which selectively kill other microorganisms at a very low concentration.

■ Classification

Antibiotics may be classified in a variety of ways:

On the Basis of Type of Action

Antibiotics may be bacteriostatic or bactericidal (**Table 4.1**).

On the Basis of Spectrum of Activity

Antibiotics may be narrow-spectrum or broad-spectrum. Narrow-spectrum antibiotics inhibit either gram +ve or gram −ve bacteria, for example, penicillin, streptomycin, erythromycin, and aminoglycosides. Broad-spectrum antibiotics inhibit both gram +ve and gram −ve as well as rickettsiae, chlamydia, spirochetes, and protozoa, for example, tetracyclines and chloramphenicol.

On the Basis of Mechanism of Action

Fig. 4.2 depicts the drugs having varying mechanisms of action.

1. Drugs inhibiting cell wall synthesis, these are **bactericidal drugs** and include:
   • Penicillin.
   • Cephalosporins.
   • Vancomycin.
   • Bacitracin.
2. Drugs affecting cell membrane function:
   • Polymyxins.
   • Amphotericin B.
   • Nystatin.
   • Natamycin.
3. Drugs acting on ribosome 50-S, these are **bacteriostatic drugs** and inhibit protein synthesis. These include:
   • Chloramphenicol.
   • Erythromycin.
   • Clindamycin.

Table 4.1 Types of antibiotics on the basis of action

Bacteriostatic drugs	Bactericidal drugs
• Tetracyclines • Chloramphenicol • Erythromycin • Clindamycin • Sulphonamides	• Penicillins • Cephalosporins • Vancomycin • Aminoglycosides • Fluoroquinolones

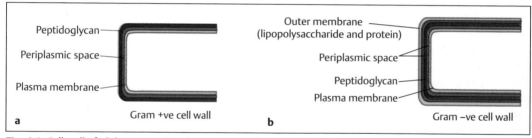

Fig. 4.1 Cell wall of: **(a)** gram positive bacteria and **(b)** gram negative bacteria.

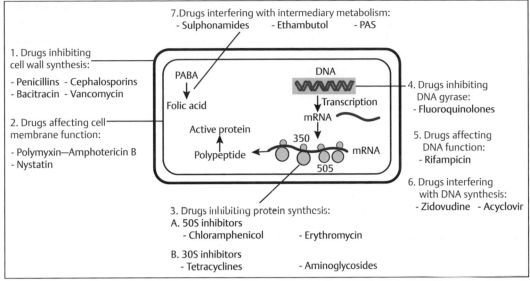

Fig. 4.2 Drugs with their mechanisms of action. Abbreviations: DNA, Deoxyribonucleic acid; mRNA, messenger ribonucleic acid; PABA, Para-aminobenzoic acid; PAS, Para-aminosalicylic acid.

4. Drugs acting on ribosome 30-S, these are **bactericidal drugs** and include:
   - Aminoglycosides.
   - Tetracyclines.
5. Drugs acting on nucleic acids, these are **bactericidal drugs**, inhibit DNA gyrase and include **fluoroquinolones**.
6. Drugs interfering with DNA synthesis:
   - Acyclovir.
   - Zidovudine.
7. Drugs interfering with intermediary metabolism:
   - Sulphonamides.
   - Ethambutol.
   - PAS.

Penicillins

Penicillins have narrow antibacterial spectrum and are effective against cocci and gram +ve organisms. In gram +ve bacteria, the cell wall is almost entirely made of peptidoglycan and extensively cross-linked. In gram −ve bacteria, it consists of alternating layers of lipoprotein and peptidoglycan. This may be the reason for higher susceptibility of gram +ve bacteria to penicillin.

Routes of Administration

- *Topical*: Penicillin G (benzyl penicillin) may be administered locally in the form of drops (100000 units/mL) instilled frequently specifically in gonococcal infections.
- *Subconjunctival injections*: Penicillin G as subconjunctival injections (0.5 million units).
- *Systemic.*

Common penicillins include the following:

Cloxacillin is penicillinase-resistant and is not affected by staphylococcal penicillinase. Therefore, it is used for treating staphylococcal infections which are resistant to other penicillins. Dose: 250 to 500 mg every six 6 hours. It is given orally/IM/IV.

Ampicillin is a broad-spectrum antibiotic. It is *acid-resistant* and *penicillinase sensitive*. Hence, it is administered orally and used for the organisms which do not produce penicillinase. Diarrhea is frequent after oral administration.

Dose: 250 to 500 mg every 6 hours. It is given orally/IM/ IV.

Amoxicillin is a broad-spectrum penicillin. Oral absorption is better. Hence, administered orally. Food does not interfere with its absorption. Dose: 250 to 500 mg every 8 hours.

Carbenicillin: The special feature of Carbenicillin is its *activity against Pseudomonas aeruginosa* and *proteus* which are not inhibited by penicillin G, ampicillin, or amoxicillin. It is not acid resistant, hence it is inactive orally.

Cephalosporins

Cephalosporins act in the same way as penicillins, that is, by inhibition of bacterial cell wall synthesis.

Cephalosporins are classified into four generations, depending on the antibacterial spectrum as well as potency (**Table 4.2**).

Routes of Administration

- **Topical:** Fortified cephazolin: Add 2.5 mL sterile water in 500 mg inj cerfazolin (dry powder). The reconstituted cefazolin 500 mg in 2.5 mL is added to 7.5 mL of preservative-free artificial tears to make 10 mL of solution. Thus, fortified cefazolin drops are prepared 5% (50 mg/mL). It is stable for 24 hours at room temperature or 96 hours if kept in a refrigerator. Cefazolin is most commonly used for Gram +ve organisms.

Problems with fortified antibiotics is its cost, short shelf life, need for refrigeration, and decreased sterility.

Vancomycin (Glycopeptide)

It is a *bactericidal* to gram + ve cocci and methicillin-resistant staphylococcus aureus (MRSA). It acts by inhibiting bacterial cell wall synthesis.

Routes of Administration

- **Topical:** Fortified vancomycin: Add 2.5 mL sterile water in 250 mg inj. vancomycin (dry powder). The reconstituted vancomycin 500 mg in 2.5 mL is added to 7.5 mL of artificial tears to make 10 mL of solution. Thus, fortified vancomycin drops are prepared. Refrigerate and use within 4 days.
- **Systemic:** It is not absorbed orally and administered intravenously (500 mg every 6 hours).
- **Intravitreal injection:** 1 mg in 0.1 mL of vancomycin is administered intravitreally. It is a drug of choice in endophthalmitis along with amikacin or ceftazidime.

Aminoglycosides

- All are *bactericidal* and *not absorbed orally.*
- They are active against **aerobic Gram –ve** bacilli. They do not inhibit anaerobes *because transport of aminoglycosides into the bacterial cell requires oxygen.*
- They exhibit **synergism** when combined with β-lactam antibiotics. *Therefore, cephazolin (β-lactam antibiotic) and fortified genticyn/tobramycin eye drops are effective in corneal ulcer cases.*
- All exhibit **ototoxicity** and **nephrotoxicity**.

Table 4.2 Classification of cephalosporins

Cephalosporins	Drugs	Spectrum
First generation	Cefazolin (P), Cephalexin, and cefadroxil (O)	Narrow spectrum. They are highly effective against Gram +ve cocci.
Second generation	Cefuroxime (P) and Cefaclor (O)	Intermediate spectrum. They are more active against Gram –ve but do not inhibit pseudomonas.
Third generation	Cefotaxime, Ceftriaxone, and Ceftazidime (P) Cefixime and Cefpodoxime proxetil (O)	Wide spectrum They are more active against Gram –ve but some inhibit pseudomonas.

Abbreviations: O, oral; P, parenteral.

Aminoglycosides include:

- Streptomycin.
- Gentamicin.
- Kanamycin.
- Tobramycin.
- Amikacin.
- Sisomicin.
- Netilmicin.
- Neomycin.
- Framycetin.

Inhibitors of bacterial wall synthesis (penicillin, cephalosporin,s and vancomycin) enhance entry of aminoglycosides and exhibit synergism.

Routes of Administration

- **Topical:** Fortified gentamicin/tobramycin: Add injection gentamicin/tobramycin 80 g in 2 mL (40 mg/mL) in commercially available 0.3% gentamicin/tobramycin drops (5 mL).

  Thus, fortified gentamicin/tobramycin 1.3% (13.6 mg/mL) drops are prepared. Refrigerate and use within 14 days.

  Gentamicin (0.3%) and tobramycin (0.3%)–drops are used topically.

  Neomycin (0.5%) and framycetin (0.5%)–drops or ointments are used topically.

- **Subconjunctival injection:** Gentamicin (20–40 mg), and tobramycin can be used subconjunctivally.

- **Intravitreal injection:** Amikacin is administered intravitreally (0.4 mg) along with vancomycin in the treatment of endophthalmitis.

Polypeptides

All are powerful **bactericidal** agents, but not used systemically due to toxicity. These include polymyxin B and bacitracin.

Bacitracin

Mechanism of action—It inhibits cell wall synthesis.

Route of administration—Its use is restricted to **topical application** generally in combination with neomycin and polymyxin B.

Polymyxin B

Mechanism of action—It has high-affinity for phospholipids and causes leakage from bacterial cell membrane. It is effective against gram –ve bacteria.

Route of administration—It is used **topically** in combination with neomycin, bacitracin, and gramicidin.

Chloramphenicol

It is a **broad-spectrum** antibiotic.

Mechanism of actions: It is **bacteriostatic** drug and inhibits bacterial protein synthesis.

Spectrum: It is similar to that of tetracyclines, that is, it is effective against gram +ve and gram –ve bacteria, spirochaetes, chlamydiae, rickettsiae, and mycoplasma. Like tetracyclines, it is ineffective against mycobacteria, pseudomonas, proteus, viruses, and fungi.

Routes of Administration

- **Topical:** It is used *topically* as drops (0.5%) or ointment (1%). It is least toxic to corneal epithelium.
- **Systemic:** It is lipid-soluble, so ocular penetration is better on systemic administration. Orally, it is administered in the dose of 250 to 500 mg every 6 hours.

Adverse effects:

- Bone marrow depression. Topical administration may rarely lead to blood dyscrasias.
- Gray baby syndrome.

Macrolides

These include:

- Erythromycin.
- Azithromycin.

Erythromycin

Erythromycin is bacteriostatic and inhibits protein synthesis.

Spectrum—It is a narrow-spectrum antibiotic effective mostly against gram +ve and a few gram –ve bacteria.

Route of administration—It is administered orally (250–500 mg every 6 hours).

Azithromycin

It is less active against gram + ve cocci but highly effective against gram −ve organisms, *Chlamydia trachomatis*, and *Toxoplasma gondii*.

Dose: 500 to 1500 mg (20–30 mg/kg) as a single dose.

Uses: It is used in the treatment of trachoma and toxoplasmosis.

Tetracyclines

These include:
- Tetracycline.
- Chlortetracycline.
- Oxytetracycline.
- Doxycycline.

Mechanism of action: These are *bacteriostatic* drugs and inhibit protein synthesis.

Spectrum: These are *broad-spectrum* antibiotics. They are effective against both gram +ve and gram −ve organisms and spirochetes. *All rickettsiae and chlamydiae are highly sensitive.*

Routes of Administration

- **Topical:** Tetracycline is used as drops and ointment (1%) for superficial ocular infections.
- **Oral:** Doxycycline 200 mg for one day then 100 mg/day for 9 days is administered orally in staphylococcal lid infections and trachoma.

Adverse effects—Tetracyclines have chelating property. Calcium-tetracycline chelate gets deposited in growing bones and teeth. Hence, tetracyclines should not be used during pregnancy, lactation, and in children.

Fluoroquinolones

They are **bactericidal** and include:
- Ciprofloxacin.
- Norfloxacin.
- Ofloxacin.
- Lomefloxacin.
- Pefloxacin.
- Levofloxacin.
- Gatifloxacin.
- Moxifloxacin.

Mechanism of action: They inhibit the bacterial DNA-gyrase enzyme and DNA synthesis.

Spectrum: These contribute toward their activity against gram +ve bacteria. Ciprofloxacin has a broad-spectrum activity, with the most susceptible ones are the aerobic gram −ve bacilli, while gram +ve bacteria are inhibited at relatively higher concentrations. It has good intraocular penetration. These drugs get deposited in the growing cartilage and hence contraindicated in children.

Route of administration: It could be topical and oral (**Table 4.3**).

Table 4.3 Routes of administration of fluoroquinolones

Fluoroquinolones	Administration
Ciprofloxacin	**Topical** (0.3%) drops or ointment. **Systemic**—orally (500 mg every 12 hours) IV 200 mg every 12 hours
Norfloxacin	**Topical** (0.3%) drops or ointment. **Systemic**—orally (400 mg every 12 hours)
Ofloxacin	**Topical** (0.3%) drops or ointment. **Systemic**—orally (200–400 mg every 12 hours)
Gatifloxacin	**Topical** (0.3%) drops or ointment.
Moxifloxacin	**Topical** (0.5%) drops or ointment. It is *self-preserved* 0.5% ophthalmic solution and has better intraocular penetration than other fluoroquinolones.

Sulphonamides

These are **bacteriostatic** but in high concentration they may be bactericidal.

Spectrum: They are effective against many gram +ve and gram −ve bacteria, chlamydiae, actinomyces, nocardia, and toxoplasma. Anaerobic bacteria are not sensitive to sulphonamides.

Route of Administration

- **Topical:** 10 to 30% sulphacetamide is used in the treatment of trachoma.
- **Systemic:** They can also be administered orally. They are lipid-soluble and pass blood–aqueous barrier easily. Therefore, their concentration in aqueous is high.

Adverse effects:
- Stevens–Johnson syndrome.
- Crystalluria.

■ Antiviral Agents

Viruses contain only one type of nucleic acid (DNA or RNA). So, viruses are either DNA viruses or RNA viruses.

DNA viruses:
- Adenovirus.
- Herpes simplex virus (HSV).
- H zoster virus (VZV).
- Epstein–Barr (EB) virus.

RNA viruses HIV (human immunodeficiency virus)—a retrovirus.

Antiviral agents are selectively active against either RNA or DNA viruses. Viruses can replicate only inside the host cells and utilize the host enzyme systems. Therefore, targeting the virus selectively is very difficult. Hence, antiviral drugs often produce severe toxic effects.

Antiviral agents are of two types:
- AntiHerpes agents (drugs used against herpetic infection)–
  ◇ **Purine derivatives.**
    - Acyclovir.
    - Ganciclovir.
    - Valacyclovir.
    - Famciclovir.
    - Vidarabine (adenine arabinoside/ Ara-A).
  ◇ **Pyrimidine derivatives.**
    - Idoxuridine (IDU or 5-Iodo 2-deoxyuridine).
    - Trifluorothymidine (TFT/F3T).
  There purine or pyrimidine analogues are incorporated to form abnormal viral DNA.
- Antiretroviral agents (drugs used against HIV infection), for example, foscarnet and zidovudine.

■ AntiHerpes Agents

Pyrimidine Derivatives

Idoxuridine (IDU)

It is a thymidine analogue that acts against *DNA viruses*. It substitutes thymidine in DNA synthesis and inhibits virus replication. It is a *virustatic drug*.

Preparation and use—It is used **topically** as 0.1% eye drops and 0.5% eye ointment for herpes simplex keratitis. The drops are instilled every 1 to 2 hours during day and ointment at night. It does not cure stromal keratitis or prevent recurrence.

Adverse effects:
- Superficial punctate keratitis.
- Follicular conjunctivitis.
- Punctal occlusion.

Trifluorothymidine (TFT/F3T)

It is also a pyrimidine analogue and has the same mechanism of action as IDU. It is soluble and is more effective than IDU.

Preparation and use—It is used as 1% eye drops instilled five times a day for 2 weeks in herpes simplex virus infections.

Adverse effect—It induces less epithelial toxicity than IDU.

Purine Derivative

Acyclovir

It is a selective virustatic drug. It is *selectively active against herpes group of viruses*: HSV-1, HSV-2, and varicella-zoster virus (VZV).

Order of sensitivity—HSV-1 > HSV-2 > VZV ≈ E.B. virus.

Cytomegalovirus (CMV) is practically not affected. So, it is used for the treatment of:
- Genital herpes (HSV-2).
- Mucocutaneous herpes (HSV-1).
- H. simplex keratitis (HSV-1).
- H zoster.
- Chicken pox.

Mechanism of action—Acyclovir is converted to its active form, acyclovir triphosphate, which inhibits DNA synthesis and viral replication. It is activated by herpes virus thymidine kinase to inhibit DNA polymerase; *thus, selectively active against herpes group of viruses.* (**Flowchart 4.2**)

Note: As acyclovir is activated by viral thymidine kinase in virus-infected cells, acyclovir has low-toxicity for host cells.

Advantages over IDU, TFT, and Ara-A:
- It penetrates intact corneal epithelium and stroma and produces therapeutic concentrations in aqueous.
- It demonstrates *less epithelial toxicity* then IDU, TFT, and Ara-A.

Route of Administration
- **Topical**.
- **Oral**.

Used as: 3% ointment and tablets.

Frequency of application and administration: Topically, 3% ointment is applied five times a day.

For acute **H. simplex infection**—400 mg 5 times a day × 5 to 7 days orally;

For **H. zoster ophthalmicus**—800 mg 5 times a day × 7 to10 days.

As intraocular penetration after oral and IV administration is good; so, it can be administered for treatment of keratouveitis and acute retinal necrosis.

Ganciclovir

It is an analogue of acyclovir.

Spectrum
- Herpes simplex.
- Herpes zoster.
- EB virus.
- CMV.

(**Flowchart 4.3**)

Route of Administration

IV—Initial dose: 5 mg/kg BD (10 mg/kg/day) × 2 weeks IV followed by maintenance dose of 5 mg/kg/day for long term.

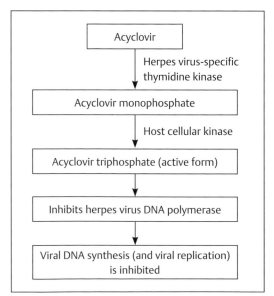

Flowchart 4.2 Algorithm explaining the mechanism of action of acyclovir.

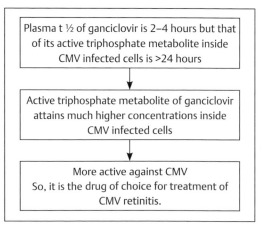

Flowchart 4.3 Ganciclovir in CMV retinitis. Abbreviation: CMV, cytomegalovirus.

Intravitreal implant containing 5 to 6 mg ganciclovir can be inserted into vitreous for CMV retinitis.

Toxicity: It may cause bone marrow depression.

Valacyclovir

It is 1-valyl ester of acyclovir, a pro drug of acyclovir.

Route of administration: It is given orally.

Dose: 1000 mg TDS × 7 to 10 days.

Famciclovir

Route of administration: It is used orally.

Spectrum: H. simplex and H. zoster but does not inhibits acyclovir-resistant strains.

Dose: 500 mg TDS × 7 to 10 days.

Vidarabine or Adenine Arabinoside (Vira-A or Ara-A)

It is a virustatic antiviral.

Mechanism of action: It acts by interfering in the synthesis of DNA.

Route of administration: Topical.

Used as: 3% ointment.

Frequency of application: Five times a day.

Spectrum: It is effective against DNA viruses, hence used in HSV epithelial keratitis but **ineffective in stromal disease.**

Toxicity: Same as with IDU.

■ Antiretroviral Agents

Foscarnet

Mechanism of action: It inhibits viral DNA polymerase and reverse transcriptase.

Spectrum: It is active against the following.
- H. simplex (including strains resistant to acyclovir).
- CMV (including strains resistant to ganciclovir).
- HIV.

So, it is used in the treatment of CMV retinitis in AIDS.

Route of administration: IV.

Toxicity: Nephrotoxic.

Zidovudine

It is a thymidine analogue.

Mechanism of action: It selectively inhibits viral reverse transcriptase (RNA-dependent DNA polymerase) in preference to cellular DNA polymerase which is essential for viral replication. Zidovudine thus prevents infection of new cells by HIV (**Flowchart 4.4**).

Spectrum: Only retroviruses (HIV).

Route of administration: Oral.

Toxicity: It causes anemia and neutropenia.

Use: Used in treatment of HIV-infected patients.

■ Antifungal Agents

Fungi can be classified into:
- **Filamentous fungi:** These are multicellular and produce tubular projections called hyphae. These may be aseptate (*Mucor and Rhizopus*) or septate (*Aspergillus, Fusarium,* and *Cephalosporium*).
- **Yeasts:** These are unicellular fungi and reproduce by budding, for example, *Candida* and *Cryptococcus*.
- **Dimorphic fungi:** These demonstrate both yeast phase in tissues and mycelial phase on culture media and saprophytic surfaces, for example, *histoplasma, blastomyces,* and *coccidioides*.

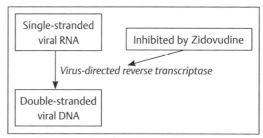

Flowchart 4.4 Mechanism of action of zidovudine.

Antifungal agents can be classified as shown in **Flowchart 4.5**.

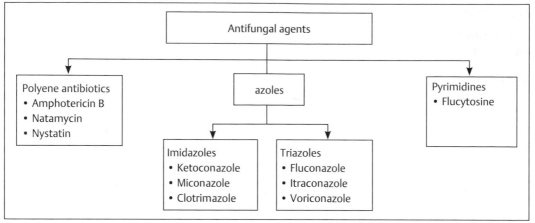

Flowchart 4.5 Classification of antifungal agents.

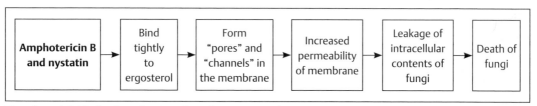

Flowchart 4.6 Mechanism of action of amphotericin B and nystatin.

Table 4.4 Route of administration of polyene antibiotics		
Antifungal drug	**Spectrum and use**	**Route of administration**
Amphotericin B It is insoluble in water, so poorly absorbed from gut	Effective against both yeast and filamentous fungi. *Used in:* • Keratomycosis • Endophthalmitis	**Topically** as 0.1 to 0.25% drops or a 2.5% ointment. **Intravitreally** (5–10 μg). **Intravenously** in 5 percent dextrose (0.05 mg/kg up to a total daily dose of 3 to 4 g).
Nystatin	It is effective against Candida albicans.	It is not absorbed orally. It is used **topically**.
Natamycin *(Pimaricin)* It is mainly fungicidal	It is effective against filamentous fungi and candida albicans.	It does not penetrate the cornea and is used **topically** as 5% ophthalmic suspension.

■ Polyene Antibiotics

Polyenes are effective against both filamentous and yeast forms.

Mechanism of action: Fungal cell membrane contains a sterol which resembles cholesterol and is called **'ergosterol' (Flowchart 4.6)**.

Natamycin blocks fungal growth by binding specifically to ergosterol, but without permeabilizing the membrane.

Amphotericin B is most toxic of all the antifungal agents. It may cause nephrotoxicity, bone marrow toxicity (anemia) or central nervous system (CNS) toxicity (convulsions and headache).

Use and routes of administration of various polyene antibiotics are explained in **Table 4.4**.

■ Azoles

Azoles may be either imidazoles or triazoles.

Imidazoles

Mechanism of action is explained in **Flowchart 4.7**.

Characteristic features of various imidazoles are listed in **Table 4.5**.

Clotrimazole

It is an imidazole derivative and alters the permeability of fungal cell wall, thus inhibiting the growth of fungal cells. It is effective against candida. It is used as topical cream and solution.

Econazole

It is similar in action to clotrimazole and is effective only in superficial infections. It is used topically as 1% ointment.

Triazoles

Characteristic features of various Triazoles are listed in **Table 4.6**.

Flucytosine (5-FC)

It is a synthetic pyrimidine antimetabolite and is fungistatic. After uptake into fungal cells (not human cells), it inhibits thymidylate synthesis. Thymidylic acid is a component of DNA and thus inhibits DNA synthesis.

It is often administered in combination with amphotericin B. Amphotericin B increases cell permeability, allowing more 5–FC to penetrate the cell, and is synergistic.

Toxicity of 5: FC consists of bone marrow depression, G.I. disturbances (enteritis and diarrhea), and elevation in hepatic enzymes.

Therapy with 5: FC is generally limited to the first 2 weeks of amphotericin B to avoid bone marrow depression.

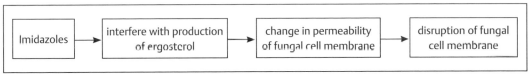

Flowchart 4.7 Mechanism of action of imidazoles.

Table 4.5 Differentiating features of miconazole and ketoconazole

Features	Miconazole	Ketoconazole
Effective against	Yeast and filamentous fungi	Candida (yeast)
Route of administration	Topical	Both topical and oral routes.
Preparation and dose	Used as 1% drops or 2% ointment every 6 hours	Topically used as 1% drops orally 200 to 800 mg/day

Table 4.6 Differentiating features of fluconazole, itraconazole, and voriconazole

Features	Fluconazole	Itraconazole	Voriconazole
Effective against	Candida and cryptococcus	Aspergillus	Used to treat invasive fungal infections (Candida and aspergillus)
Route of administration	Oral, topical, and intravitreal	Oral and topical	Topical and intravitreal
Preparation and dose	Oral absorption is good and given in the doses of 100 to 200 mg every 6 hours Topically, it is used as 0.2% drops. Intravitreally 0.1 mg	Orally, in the dose of 100–400 mg/day Topically, it is used as 1% eye drops	Topically, it is used as 1 to 2% eye drops Intravitreally, 100 µg

■ Anti-Inflammatory Drugs

Anti-inflammatory drugs are corticosteroids and non-steroidal anti-inflammatory drugs (NSAIDs).

■ Corticosteroids

Corticosteroids are anti-inflammatory, antiallergic, and immunosuppressive.

So, these are very effective in inflammatory and immune-mediated ocular diseases. They do not cure the disease as such but temporarily block the exudation in acute inflammations. The disease resumes its natural course once the steroids are withdrawn. Therefore, corticosteroids must not be withdrawn abruptly and the dose is gradually tapered.

Corticosteroids act by:
- Reducing the capillary permeability, therefore decreasing exudation.
- Suppressing the formation of arachidonic acid and other inflammatory mediators.
- Stabilizing lysosomal membranes and reducing the prostaglandins.
- Inhibiting fibroblast formation during tissue repair and delaying wound healing.
- Suppression of cell-mediated hypersensitivity reaction and modification of immune responses.

Corticosteroids are classified as per **Table 4.7**.

Ocular Indications of Corticosteroids

Corticosteroids are used in a large number of inflammatory ocular disease as (**Table 4.8**):
- Topical instillation.
- Systemic therapy.
- Injections.

Routes of Administration

Corticosteroids may be administered locally (topical and subconjunctival injections) or systemically (oral or parenteral) (**Table 4.9**).

Side Effects

Corticosteroids can cause side effects due to topical as well as systemic therapy. The side effects of corticosteroids are related to dose and duration of therapy as well as individual susceptibility.

Ocular Side Effects

Prolonged therapy may cause:
- Conjunctival necrosis.
- Delayed corneal wound healing.
- Worsening of corneal ulcers.
- Reactivation of herpetic keratitis.
- Keratomycosis.
- Posterior subcapsular cataract.

Table 4.7 Classification of corticosteroids (on the basis of duration of action)

Short-acting	Intermediate-acting	Long-acting
For example: • Cortisone • hydrocortisone	For example: • Prednisolone • methylprednisolone • triamcinolone	For example: • Dexamethasone • betamethasone

Table 4.8 Uses of corticosteriods (on the basis of routes of administration)

Corticosteroids	Uses
• As topical instillation (as eye drops or ointment)	• Allergic conjunctivitis • Scleritis • Iridocyclitis • Keratitis (Steroids are contraindicated in herpes simplex keratitis and ocular injuries).
• As systemic therapy	Retinitis, optic neuritis, and choroiditis in posterior segment require systemic steroid therapy.
• As injections	These may be given as subconjunctival, subtenon, or intravitreal injections.

Table 4.9 Routes of administration of corticosteroids

Corticosteroid	Route of administration (dose)
• Dexamethasone and betamethasone	Topical as 0.1% drops and ointment at night Subconjunctival and intravitreally (1 mg) Oral and parenteral (5 mg/day)
• Prednisolone acetate	Topical as 1% drops Orally, 1–2 mg/kg/day (50–150 mg/day)
• Methylprednisolone	Subconjunctival injection (20 mg/0.5 mL) Parenteral (30 mg/kg). High doses are given intravenously in "pulses"
• Triamcinolone acetonide	Periocular or posterior subtenon injection (40 mg) Intravitreal injection
• Medrysone	Topical as 1% drops
• Rimexolone	Topical as 1% drops
• Fluorometholone acetate	Topical as 0.1% drops
• Loteprednol	Topical as 0.5% drops

- Primary open-angle glaucoma (POAG).
- Central serous chorioretinopathy.
- Decreased resistance to infection.

Systemic Side Effects

Prolonged therapy may cause:
- Immunosuppression.
- Hyperglycemia (aggravate diabetes).
- Hypertension.
- Osteoporosis.
- Gastrointestinal ulceration.

Medrysone, rimexolone, fluorometholone, and loteprednol are less likely to cause a rise in intraocular pressure (IOP).

■ NSAIDs

These drugs inhibit the prostaglandin synthesis by blocking the enzyme cyclo-oxygenase. They are used in less severe or more chronic inflammations.

Route of administration: NSAIDs are used systemically as well as topically. *Topical NSAIDs must be used 3 to 4 times a day for 4 to 8 weeks.*

The commonly used NSAIDs are as follows:

Indomethacin: It is used orally as well as topically. It is given **orally** in the dose of 25 mg thrice a day to prevent cystoid macular edema (CME) and **topically** as 0.5 to 1% drops preoperatively to prevent intraoperative miosis and manage postoperative inflammation.

Diclofenac: The **oral** dose is 50 mg twice daily; **topically,** it is used as 0.1% drops postoperatively to treat uveitis and prevent CME.

Flurbiprofen: It is used **topically** as 0.03% drops preoperatively to prevent intraoperative miosis. It has good corneal penetration.

Ketorolac: It is used in the treatment of allergic conjunctivitis as 0.5% drops.

Bromfenac: It is used as 0.09% drops to treat inflammation and pain in the eye after eye surgery.

Nepafenac: It has the best corneal and intraocular penetration and used as 0.1% drops. It is a NSAID used to relieve eye pain, irritation, and redness following eye surgery.

■ Antiallergic Drugs

Antiallergic agents are classified as *mast cell stabilizers, antihistamines, and dual action agents.*

■ Mast Cell Stabilizers

These act by the following mechanism:
Mast cell stabilizers → Stabilize membrane of mast cells → Inhibition of mast cell degranulation Prevention of histamine release

Commonly used mast cell stabilizers are:
- Cromolyn sodium—It is topically used as 2 to 4% drops every 6 hours.
- Lodoxamide tromethamine—It is topically used as 0.1% drops instilled thrice a day.

These are used in allergic conjunctivitis.

■ Antihistamines

Topical antihistamines bind to receptors in the conjunctiva and show a competitive antagonism to histamine.

Antihistamines reduce the symptom of itching and are commonly combined with vaso-constrictors to relieve congestion. Commonly used antihistamines are:
- Chlorpheniramine is instilled topically four times a day.
- Emedastine (0.05%), a receptor antagonist, is also used topically four times a day.

Both of these are also used to treat allergic conjunctivitis.

■ Dual Action Agents

These agents have a dual action, that is, they prevent mast cell degranulation as well as prevent histamine binding to receptors. These include:
- Olopatadine (0.1%) drops instilled every 12 hours.
- Azelastine (0.5%) drops used once or twice a day.
- Ketotifen (0.025%) drops instilled thrice a day.
- Epinastine (0.05%) drops instilled twice a day.

All these are used to treat allergic conjunctivitis.

■ Drugs Acting on Intraocular Muscles

Intraocular muscles include pupillary muscles and ciliary muscle.

■ Pupillary Muscle

- **Sphincter pupillae** (Parasympathetic innervation)—It causes constriction of pupil (miosis).
- **Dilator pupillae** (Sympathetic innervation)—It causes dilatation of pupil (mydriasis).

■ Ciliary Muscle

- Ciliary muscle has parasympathetic innervation and cause accommodation.
- Drugs causing paralysis of accommodation or ciliary muscle are called **cycloplegics**. Side effects of cycloplegics are blurred vision, photophobia, and acute angle-closure glaucoma in hypermetropes with shallow chamber (due to mydriasis).
- Drugs causing mydriasis may be **parasympatholytic** or **sympathomimetics**.
- **Parasympatholytic drugs** cause dilatation and cycloplegia as they also paralyze accommodation, for example, atropine, homatropine, cyclopentolate, and tropicamide.
- **Sympathomimetic drugs** cause dilatation of pupil, for example, adrenaline (epinephrine) and phenylephrine.

Parasympatholytic Drugs

Atropine—It is used as 1% drops or ointment as atropine sulfate.

Application—The ointment is applied twice a day for 3 days before examination.

Duration of action—It has long duration of action and lasts for 7 to 10 days.

Uses:
- For refraction and fundus examination in children (<5 years of age).
- For penalization of better eye in amblyopia therapy.
- For relaxation of ciliary body in iridocyclitis.

Side effects—Systemic absorption of atropine may cause:
- Flushing of face.
- Fever in children.
- Paralytic ileus.
- Contact dermatitis.

Paralytic ileus in children causes distension of abdomen, hence ointment is preferred over drops in children.

Homatropine (2%) drops are less potent and its effect lasts for 48 to 72 hours. It is used for refraction and in the treatment of uveitis.

Cyclopentolate (1%) drops are used for refraction and fundus examination. Its effect lasts for up to 24 hours.

Tropicamide (0.5, 1%) drops are short-acting as its effect lasts for 4 to 6 hours.

Sympathomimetic Drugs

Adrenaline (0.1–1 mg/mL)—It is used in irrigating solution during intraocular surgery to dilate the pupil.

Phenylephrine (5 to 10%)—It is a selective agonist and causes mydriasis and vasoconstriction. It can cause a rise of blood pressure in few individuals.

■ Anti-Vascular Endothelial Growth Factor (Anti-VEGF) Agents

Retinal ischemia due to various retinal diseases leads to neovascularization of retina. The angiogenic factors are released in response to ischemia which induce angiogenesis. The main factor regulating angiogenesis is **VEGF**. To control neovascularization anti-VEGF agents have been developed. These include **bevacizumab** (*avastin*), **ranibizumab** (*lucentis*), and **pegaptanib** (*macugen*) (**Table 4.10**). These are administered by intravitreal injections.

■ Indications

- Wet, age-related macular degeneration.
- Diabetic retinopathy.
- Choroidal neovascular membrane (CNVM).
- Retinal venous occlusion.
- CME.
- Retinopathy of prematurity.
- Neovascular glaucoma (NVG).

■ Side Effects

- Raised IOP.
- Cataract.
- Retinal detachment.
- Endophthalmitis.

■ Viscoelastic Substances

An ideal viscoelastic must be viscous, inert, nontoxic, nonantigenic, and crystal-clear fluid. The viscoelastics are best for capsulorrhexis and intraocular lens (IOL) implantation. Pseudoplasticity of a viscoelastic is the ability to change under pressure from gel to liquid—Lower the surface tension, better is the coating.

■ Classification

Cohesive viscoelastic—In these viscoelastics, *molecules adhere to each other. These create and preserve the space* (i.e., prevent the collapse, deepen the anterior chamber, and distend the lens capsule). These are *easy to remove*.

Table 4.10 Differentiating features of various anti-VEGF agents			
Anti-VEGF agent	**Mechanism of action**	**Available as**	**Dose**
Bevacizumab (Avastin) It is a humanized monoclonal antibody against VEGF-A	It blocks VEGF-A by binding to its all isoforms.	4 mL vial containing 100 mg of drug.	1.25 mg/0.05 mL
Ranibizumab (Lucentis)	It binds and inactivates all isoforms of VEGF-A. It penetrates the ILM to gain access to the subretinal space.	As a single use glass vial.	0.5 mg/0.05 mL
Pegaptanib (Macugen)	It selectively binds and inhibits VEGF-165 isoforms of VEGF-A.	As a single dose prefilled syringe.	0.3 mg/90 µL
Abbreviation: ILM, internal limiting membrane.			

Dispersive viscoelastic–These viscoelastics coat the ocular surfaces and so are used to protect the corneal endothelium intraoperatively. These remain in position during irrigation.

Table 4.11 lists various viscoelastics.

■ Side Effects

Viscoelastic may cause postoperative rise of IOP, therefore it must be removed after completion of surgery by irrigation and aspiration.

■■ Immunosuppressive Agents

Immunosuppressant drugs are the drugs that suppress or reduce the body's immune responses. They are of use in organ transplantation and autoimmune diseases.

Use of immunosuppressant drugs in ophthalmology:
- Rheumatoid arthritis.

- Poly arteritis nodosa.
- Bechet's disease.
- VKH syndrome.
- Sympathetic ophthalmitis.
- Recalcitrant cases of intermediate uveitis.

■ Classification

Classification of immune suppressive agents is mentioned in **Flowchart 4.8**.

Antimetabolites

Azathioprine

It is a purine nucleoside analogue.

Mechanism of action–It interferes with DNA replication and RNA transcription.

Indications:
- Chronic uveitis.
- Sarcoidosis.
- Bechet's disease.

Table 4.11 Features of different viscoelastics		
Composition of viscoelastic	**Characteristics**	**Use**
HPMC 3%	It is viscous and elastic	In extracapsular cataract surgery (SICS and phacoemulsification).
Hypromellose 2%	It is like HPMC	In cataract surgery.
Sodium hyaluronate 1%	• Cohesive viscoelastic • High-molecular weight • High pseudoelastic • High-surface tension • Easily removed	It is an excellent spacer and maintains anterior chamber during cataract surgery, so it protects ocular tissue and facilitates IOL implantation.
Sodium hyaluronate 3% and chondroitin sodium sulfate 4%	• Dispersive viscoelastic • High-coating availability	It provides excellent tissue protection, hence used in compromised corneal endothelial function to protect it in phacoemulsification.
Abbreviations: HPMC, hydroxypropyl methylcellulose; IOL, intraocular lens; SICS, small incision cataract surgery.		

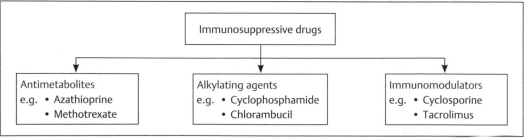

Flowchart 4.8 Classification of immunosuppressive agents.

Side effects:

- Bone marrow suppression (hence, total blood cell count should be performed regularly and the drug is stopped if TLC is less than 3000/mm³).
- Hepatotoxicity (hence, liver function tests should be carried out).

Methotrexate

It is a folic acid analogue.

Mechanism of action—It is a competitive inhibitor of many enzymes that use folates. It competitively inhibits dihydrofolate reductase, an enzyme that participates in tetrahydrofolates synthesis. Folic acid is essential for purine and pyrimidine base biosynthesis. Therefore, inhibition of their synthesis inhibits the synthesis of DNA and RNA.

Indications—In some autoimmune diseases, vasculitis, and orbital pseudotumor.

Side effects:

- Nausea and anorexia.
- Bone marrow suppression (hence, total blood cell count should be performed regularly).
- Hepatotoxicity (hence, liver function tests should be carried out).

Alkylating Agents

Cyclophosphamide

Mechanism of action—The main effect of cyclophosphamide is due to its metabolite phosphoramide mustard which forms DNA cross-linking. This is irreversible and leads to cell death.

Indications—In autoimmune disorders causing inflammation of uvea and sclera.

Side effects:

- Nausea and vomiting
- Bone marrow suppression.
- Cardiotoxicity.
- Hemorrhagic cystitis which is associated with hematuria and dysuria.
- Infertility in males and females.

Chlorambucil

Mechanism of action—It interferes with DNA replication.

Indications—In various autoimmune and inflammatory conditions.

Side effects:

- Bone marrow suppression.
- Gastrointestinal distress (nausea, vomiting, and diarrhea).
- Hepatotoxicity.
- Infertility.
- Opportunistic infections.

Immunomodulators

Cyclosporine

Mechanism of action—It inhibits the activity of T-cells and their immune response.

Indications— It is used topically as well as systemically. Topically, it is used in dry eye diseases. Systemically, it is used in uveitis, scleritis, etc.

Side effects:

- Nephrotoxicity (therefore, blood pressure monitoring and serum creatinine must be performed regularly).
- Enlargement of gums.
- Vomiting and diarrhea.
- Opportunistic infections.
- Hirsutism.
- Hepatotoxicity.

Tacrolimus

Indications—It is used topically as well as systemically. Topically, it is used as ointment (0.01%) in vernal keratoconjunctivitis and atopic keratoconjunctivitis.

Side effects:

- Its nephrotoxic effect is less than cyclosporine. Serum creatinine must be carried out regularly.

Mechanism of action—Tacrolimus binds to a protein (FK-binding protein 12) and inhibits Ca^{2+}—calmodulin-activated "phosphatase calcineurin." The response of helper T-cell to antigenic stimulation fails. Normally, calcineurin dephosphorylates a "nuclear factor of activated T-cell," which translocates to the nucleus and triggers transcription of cytokine genes, resulting in production of IL-2 and other cytokines. IL-2 is the major cytokine for T cell proliferation and differentiation, carrying forward the immune response.

Others

Few drugs inhibit the fibroblastic proliferation to prevent postoperative scarring in different ocular surgeries.

5-Fluorouracil (5-FU)

It is a pyrimidine antagonist and interferes with nucleic acid synthesis.

Use—It inhibits fibroblastic proliferation to prevent postoperative scarring and is used after trabeculectomy (glaucoma filtering surgery) when there is risk of failure of surgery due to excessive postoperative scarring.

Administration—It can be administered by subconjunctival injections (5 mg/mL) administered daily or on alternate days up to a total dose of 50 mg.

Complications—Corneal epithelial erosions and wound leak.

Mitomycin C (MMC)

It is an alkylating agent and inhibits RNA and protein synthesis. It is obtained from Streptomyces caespitosus.

Use—Topical drops 0.2 to 0.4 mg/mL of MMC are used after pterygium or glaucoma surgery to reduce scarring after glaucoma surgery or recurrence of pterygium.

Complications—It may induce scleral ulceration and iridocyclitis.

■ Irrigating Solutions

Intraocular irrigating solutions are used during all intraocular surgical procedures. The irrigating solutions for intraocular use during surgeries include:

- Ringer lactate (RL) solution.
- Balanced salt solution (BSS).
- Balanced salt solution plus (BSS plus).

The intraocular irrigating solutions subserve the following functions:

- These maintain IOP during surgery (**Table 4.12**).
- These maintain endothelial cell metabolism. Concentration of sodium lactate is much higher than aqueous in RL. So, its prolonged perfusion can cause endothelial cell breakdown. BSS is less protective to corneal endothelial cells. BSS plus is iso-osmotic with intraocular tissues and maintains the corneal endothelial function.

■ Ocular Preservatives

A variety of different preservatives have been used in multidose ophthalmic preparations. These inhibit the growth of microbial contaminants,

Table 4.12 Features of different irrigating solutions

Features	Ringer lactate	Balanced salt solution	Balanced salt solution plus
Composition	It is a mixture of NaCl, KCl, and CaCl₂ sodium lactate.	It is a mixture of NaCl, KCl CaCl₂, MgCl₂ Sodium acetate Sodium citrate	NaCl, KCl CaCl₂, MgCl₂ Sodiumbicarbonate Glutathione (oxidized) Dibasic sodium phosphate Dextrose
pH	6.5	7.4	7.4
Osmolality	273	300	305

Abbreviations: BSS, balanced salt solution; RL, Ringer lactate.

prevent biodegradation, and maintain drug potency.

Classification

Preservatives have been classified into two categories, namely, detergent preservatives and oxidizing preservatives.

Mechanism of Action

Mechanism of action of ocular preservatives is depicted in **Flowchart 4.9**.

Adverse Effects

The repeated use of ophthalmic drops has been linked to irritation, dryness, and surface epithelial cell loss. The severity of these effects is related to:

- The duration for which the medications are used.
- The types and concentrations of preservatives used.
- Total number of all eye drops used by the patient throughout the day.

Reactions to Medicines

Systemic toxic reactions may occur after local instillation of drugs. On the other hand, ocular side effects may occur after systemic administration of the drug.

Systemic Reactions to Eye Drops After Instillation

To decrease the systemic reactions due to instilled eye drops, pressure is given near medial canthus of closed eye lids for approximately 2 to 3 minutes after instillation. It prevents the entry into nasolacrimal ducts and systemic absorption of the drug. **Tables 4.13 and 4.14** list the systemic effects of instilled eye drops and ocular effects due to systemic drugs, respectively.

Dyes Used in Ophthalmology

Dyes are used in ophthalmology both as diagnostic and therapeutic aids. The ophthalmic dyes are used for anterior and posterior segments'

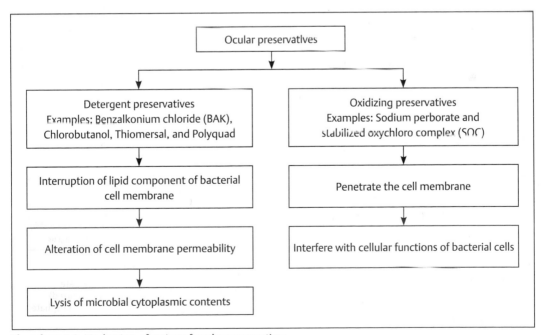

Flowchart 4.9 Mechanism of action of ocular preservatives.

Table 4.13 Summary of the systemic reactions of eye drops instilled

Drug instilled	Systemic side effects
Phenylephrine (10%)	• Increase in blood pressure • Cardiac arrhythmias • Cerebrovascular accidents
Cyclopentolate	• Behavioral changes • Hallucinations • Ataxia
Atropine (1%)	• Dry mouth • Raised body temperature • Red and hot skin • Abdominal distension (with eye drops)
Pilocarpine	• Sweating • Bradycardia • Decreased blood pressure • Increased GI activity
Timolol	• Bronchospasm in asthmatic patients • Cardiac arrhythmias in patients with heart block

Abbreviation: GI, gastrointestinal.

Table 4.14 Ocular side effects due to systemic drugs

Systemic drug	Ocular side effects
Corticosteroids	• Posterior subcapsular cataract • Glaucoma • Papilloedema (due to benign intracranial hypertension)
Ethambutol	• Optic neuritis
Chloroquine—It is related to the total cumulative dose. The risk of toxicity increases when the cumulative dose exceeds 300 gm (i.e., 250 mg/day × 3 years)	• Vortex keratopathy • Maculopathy (**"Bull's eye"** macular lesion) • Myopathy (failure of accommodation)
Phenothiazines (chlorpromazine)	• Pigmentary retinopathy • Conjunctival pigmentation (light brown) • Yellowish–brown granules on the anterior lens capsule within the pupillary area
Amiodarone (antiarrhythmia drug)	• Keratopathy • Anterior subcapsular lenticular opacity • Optic neuropathy
Sulphonamides	• Severe dry eyes

indications. The diagnostic dyes identify and track ocular structure at the cellular level. Dyes may be designated vital when they are used to stain living tissues or cells.

Dyes used in ophthalmology include:
• Fluorescein sodium.
• Indocyanine green.
• Rose Bengal.
• Trypan blue.
• Verteporfin.

Fluorescein is used extensively as a diagnostic tool in the field of ophthalmology. Rose Bengal is used to stain damaged conjunctival and corneal cells and thereby identify damage to the eye.

Fluorescein Sodium

It is a water-soluble dye. In powdered form, it is orange–red in color and yellow–green colored in solution.

Excitation peak of dye: **490 nm** (blue part of spectrum).

Emission peak of dye: **530 nm** (green part of spectrum).

Preparations and Uses

Topically, fluorescein sodium strips are used for the following conditions:
- Detection of corneal abrasion.
- Tear film breakup time.
- Applantation tonometry.
- Fitting assessment of rigid contact lens.
- Detection of the site of perforation (**Seidel's test**). The Seidel's test is used to assess the presence of anterior chamber leakage in the cornea. It is used as a screening test for corneal perforation. It is named after the German ophthalmologist **Erich Seidel**.

10% and 25% are used for intravenous use in the following conditions:
- Fundus fluorescein angiography (**FFA**).
- Iris angiography.
- Intraocular dynamic studies (**fluorometry**).

70 to 80% of fluorescein binds to serum albumin (bound fluorescein). Choriocapillaris contain fenestrations, so free fluorescein escape into extravascular space. **Fluorescein angiography** is an excellent method *for studying retinal circulation.* It is not helpful in delineating choroidal circulation, as fluorescein leaks from choriocapillaris, producing choroidal fluorescence.

Dose

5 mL of 10% OR 3 mL of 25% aqueous solution of fluorescein sodium.

Side Effects of Intravenous Dye

- Laryngeal or pulmonary edema.
- Severe hypotension and shock.
- Hypersensitivity.

Contamination

Fluorescein eye drops can be invaded by *pseudomonas aeruginosa.* Hence, very great care must be taken in the use of fluorescein drops, since these are frequently used on damaged tissue that is prone to infection. Therefore, strips are preferred over the solution.

Phenylmercuric acetate or nitrate (0.002%) is the best bactericide for preserving fluorescein drops and this is effective against pseudomonas.

Indocyanine Green (ICG)

- It is a high protein binding dye.
- **Excitation peak** of dye: **805 nm** (IR spectrum).
- **Emission peak** of dye: **835 nm** (IR spectrum).

Dose

ICG sodium salt is normally available in powder form and 25 to 40 mg ICG powder is dissolved in 2 mL of aqueous solvent (40 mg in 2 mL).

Contraindications

As dye contains 5% iodine, it should not be given to the patients allergic to any iodine compound and seafood.

Adverse Effects

These are less common than fluorescein and can cause anaphylactic shock, hypotension, dyspnea, and urticaria.

Uses

ICG angiography—*98% of ICG molecules bind with serum albumin.* So, dye remains within choriocapillaris as fenestrations of choriocapillaris are impermeable to albumin. It provides better resolution of choroidal vasculature; hence, it is used *for studying the choroidal lesions.*

Rose Bengal

Unlike fluorescein and lissamine green, it cannot be termed as a "vital" dye. Rose Bengal stains *mucus as well as devitalized* (dead and damaged)

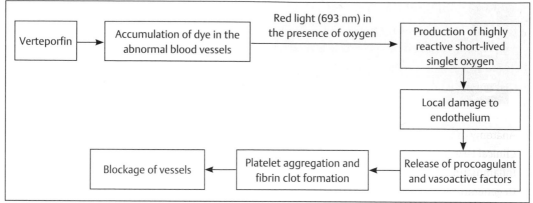

Flowchart 4.10 Mechanism of action of verteporfin.

cells red as in superficial punctate keratitis and filamentary keratitis. It is useful in diagnosis of keratoconjunctivitis sicca (**KCS**).

Rose Bengal dye is very irritating, so instill 2% xylocaine (local anesthetic) eye drop before using rose Bengal.

■ Trypan Blue

It is an azo dye used to stain the anterior capsule in the presence of mature cataract and aid in capsulorrhexis during cataract surgery. Endothelium is protected by using air bubble and the dye is washed off immediately with BSS and viscoelastic.

Preparation: It is available as 1mL ampoule and 2 mL vial. Each contains 0.6 mg/mL trypan blue.

■ Verteporfin

Verteporfin (trade name visudyne) is used as a photosensitizer for photodynamic therapy to eliminate the abnormal blood vessels. **Flowchart 4.10** explains the mechanism of action of verteporfin.

Uses

It is used in photodynamic therapy (PDT) for treatment of CNVM due to wet, age-related macular degeneration.

> **Medical therapy for glaucoma and dry eyes is discussed in their respective chapters.**

The Conjunctiva

Anatomy of Conjunctiva...83
Clinical Features of Conjunctival Disorders 85
Inflammation of Conjunctiva (Conjunctivitis) 89
Degenerative Changes in Conjunctiva 114

■ Anatomy of Conjunctiva

Conjunctiva is a thin, translucent mucous membrane. It lines the inner surface of eyelids and then reflects onto the surface of globe as far as the limbus (corneoscleral junction). Conjunctiva is divided into three parts, namely, palpebral conjunctiva, bulbar conjunctiva, and forniceal conjunctiva.

■ Palpebral Conjunctiva

It extends from the mucocutaneous junction of the lid margins and lines the inside of the eyelids. It is subdivided into:

- *Marginal conjunctiva*: It extends from the anterior lid margin to approximately 2 mm on the back of the lid (up to sulcus subtarsalis or subtarsal sulcus). It is a transitional zone between the skin of the lid and the conjunctiva proper and made up of stratified epithelium.
- *Tarsal conjunctiva*: It is highly vascular and adherent to tarsal plates. In the upper eyelid, it is fully adherent to whole tarsal plate, while adherence is less marked in the lower eyelid.
- *Orbital conjunctiva*: It is loose and lies between the border of the tarsal plate and fornix.

■ Bulbar Conjunctiva

It lines the anterior part of sclera and becomes continuous with corneal epithelium at the limbus.

It is separated from anterior sclera by episcleral tissue and Tenon's capsule. It is loosely attached to the underlying Tenon's capsule and freely movable over sclera except around cornea (limbal conjunctiva) where the attachment is firm. Limbal conjunctiva, a part of bulbar conjunctiva, covers the limbal region and is continuous with the corneal epithelium.

■ Forniceal Conjunctiva

It unites the palpebral and bulbar portions of conjunctiva. It is loose and thrown into folds. Plica semilunaris is a vertical semilunar fold present nasally and separates bulbar conjunctiva from caruncle at medial canthus, which is an ovoid mass covered by stratified squamous epithelium and contains hair follicles, sweat glands, and sebaceous glands (**Fig. 5.1**).

■ Histology

Conjunctiva consists of two layers, namely, epithelium and stroma. Epithelium is nonkeratinized and two to five layers thick. It is two-layered over palpebral conjunctiva and the layers gradually increase from fornix to limbus. It contains mucus glands, **"goblet cells"**, which secrete mucin for tear film. Stroma consists of richly vascularized connective tissue and consists of:

- *Superficial adenoid layer*: It contains lymphocytes, mast cells, and histiocytes. *It does not develop until 2 to 3 months after birth.* Hence, *conjunctival inflammation in*

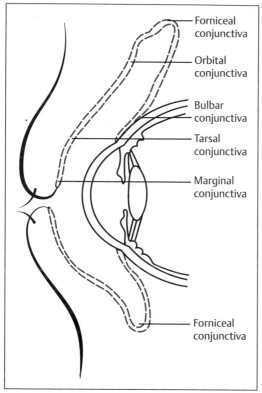

Fig. 5.1 Parts of conjunctiva.

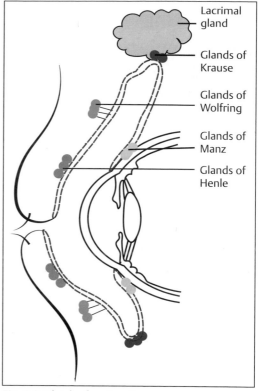

Fig. 5.2 Glands of conjunctiva.

the newborn does not produce a follicular reaction.

- *Deep fibrous layer*: It consists of collagen and elastic fibers and merges with tarsal plates.

Glands

Conjunctiva consists of two types of glands, namely, mucin secreting glands and accessory lacrimal glands (**Fig. 5.2**).

Mucin Secretors

These secrete mucin and include:

- *Goblet cells*–These are unicellular mucus glands located within epithelium of bulbar conjunctiva and fornix. These are most dense in inferonasal part of conjunctiva, so it is the best site for diagnostic biopsy.
- *Crypts of Henle*–These are present in tarsal conjunctiva.

- *Glands of Manz*– these are found in a circumferential ring of limbal conjunctiva.

Destructive disorders of conjunctiva damage the mucin secretors, leading to mucin deficiency which results in dry eye.

Accessory Lacrimal Glands

These are located in stroma and include:

- *Glands of Krause*–These are present in fornix.
- *Glands of Wolfring*–These are present along the upper border of superior tarsus and the lower border of inferior tarsus.

Nerve Supply

It is derived from **trigeminal nerve**. Long ciliary nerves supplying the cornea also supply the limbal conjunctiva. Branches from lacrimal nerve, infratrochlear (branch of nasociliary nerve), supratrochlear, and supraorbital (branches from frontal nerve) supply the rest of conjunctiva.

Blood Supply

It is derived from peripheral tarsal arcade, marginal tarsal arcade, and anterior ciliary arteries (**Fig. 5.3**). Marginal arcade, which lies 2 mm away from the margin of the eyelids, supplies the marginal conjunctiva. Peripheral arcade lies near the peripheral border of tarsal plate. Its perforating branches pierce the Müllers muscle to reach the conjunctiva and gives off ascending and descending branches. Descending branches supply the tarsal conjunctiva and also anastomose with vessels from the marginal arcade. Ascending branches pass into the superior fornix and continue around the fornices to the bulbar conjunctiva as the posterior conjunctival arteries which supply the bulbar conjunctiva.

Anterior ciliary arteries run along the tendon of rectus muscle and gives off anterior conjunctival arteries. Anterior ciliary arteries send branches to the limbal conjunctiva. Anterior conjunctival arteries anastomose with terminal branches of the posterior conjunctival artery, forming a *pericorneal plexus*. Thus, the superficial and deep systems of vessels are closely connected in the limbal area.

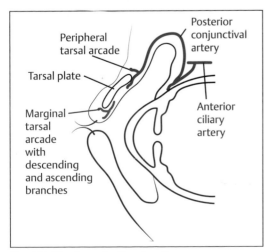

Fig. 5.3 Blood supply of conjunctiva.

Lymphatic Drainage

- Lymphatics from lateral side drain into preauricular lymph nodes.
- Lymphatics from medial side drain into submandibular lymph nodes.

Conjunctival Flora of Normal Eye

Eyelids and conjunctiva harbor a significant number of microorganisms. Organisms normally present in conjunctival sac are nonpathogenic. Frequent blinking mechanically washes away the bacteria by the tears. Bandaging arrests movements of lids and increases conjunctival sac temperature, leading to increase in bacterial content of conjunctiva. Also, low temperature of conjunctival sac, lysozyme (a bacteriostatic enzyme), and IgA in tears inhibit bacterial growth.

Organisms normally present in conjunctival sac include:

- Staphylococcus epidermidis.
- Neisseria catarrhalis.
- Corynebacterium xerosis.
- Propionibacterium acnes.

The organisms which are pathogenic and rarely found in normal eyes include:

- Streptococci.
- Neisseria gonorrhoeae.
- Moraxella.
- *Escherichia coli.*
- B. proteus.
- Haemophilus aegyptius.

The most dangerous pathogens in ocular infections include:

- Neisseria gonorrhoeae.
- Streptococcus pneumoniae.
- Pseudomonas pyocyanea.

Clinical Features of Conjunctival Disorders (OP3.1,3.2)

Common symptoms of conjunctival disorders include:

- Redness.
- Lacrimation.

- Itching.
- Stickiness.
- Burning.
- Foreign body sensation or grittiness.
- Bright light is resented (but if photophobia is present, it suggests associated corneal involvement or iritis).

Signs include discharge, conjunctival reaction, and associated keratopathy and lymphadenopathy.

■ Discharge

Eye discharge involves a combination of exudates filtered from dilated blood vessels, mucus, tears, and variable amount of epithelial debris. The eyes produce mucus throughout the day but tears flush them out with each blink before it hardens in the eye. During sleep, blinking is absent and the eye discharge collects and crusts in the corners of the eyes. Therefore, some discharge in eyes upon waking is normal, but excessive discharge differing in consistency, color, and quantity could indicate an eye infection or a disease.

Types of Discharge

There are four types of discharges in the eye which are as follows:
- *Watery discharge:* It is composed of serous exudates and tear and is seen in viral conjunctivitis and acute allergic conjunctivitis.
- *Mucoid discharge*: It is seen in vernal conjunctivitis and dry eye.
- *Purulent discharge:* It is seen in acute bacterial infections.
- *Mucopurulent discharge:* Such discharge gives rise to gluing up of eyelids in the morning. It is seen in mild bacterial infections and chlamydial infections.

■ Conjunctival Reaction

Conjunctival inflammatory reactions could be in the form of:
- Hyperemia of conjunctiva.
- Chemosis.
- Subconjunctival hemorrhage.
- Follicular reaction.
- Papillary reactions.

- Membranes.
- Xerosis.
- Subconjunctival scarring.

Hyperemia of Conjunctiva (Conjunctival injection)

It is the passive dilatation of conjunctival blood vessels and may be:
- More intense in fornices away from limbus– it indicates *conjunctivitis* (all types).
- Circum corneal or perilimbal congestion (**ciliary congestion**)– it indicates *involvement of cornea, iris, or sclera.*

Conjunctival congestion may be acute, transient, or chronic. Acute and recurrent occur due to concretions in palpebral conjunctiva or "in-growing" lashes. Transient congestion occurs due to foreign body. Chronic congestions occur due to dry, dusty climate, allergic conditions, and excessive ingestion of alcohol.

Topical instillation of decongestant drops (phenylephrine or naphazoline) blanch the blood vessels, providing temporary relief.

Chemosis (edema of conjunctiva)

It occurs due to exudation from abnormally permeable capillaries. It is particularly prominent in loosely attached bulbar and forniceal conjunctiva. The conjunctiva becomes swollen and gelatinous in appearance. Chemosis could be due to local or systemic causes.

Local causes include acute inflammation like:
- Severe infective conjunctivitis.
- Orbital cellulitis.
- Panophthalmitis.
- Inflammation of accessory structures of eye such as stye, insect bite on lid, dacryocystitis, and periostitis.

Owing to obstruction of blood and/or lymph drainage, it may occur with:
- Orbital tumors.
- Thyroid exophthalmos.
- Cavernous exophthalmos.
- Carotico-cavernous fistula (**Fig. 5.3**).

Systemic causes include the following:

- Hypersensitivity reaction.
- Angioneurotic edema.
- Urticaria.
- Decreased plasma osmotic pressure.
- Nephrotic syndrome.
- Congestive heart failure.
- Superior vena cava syndrome.
- Hypoproteinemia.

Subconjunctival Hemorrhage

It occurs due to rupture of small vessels. **Fig. 5.4** describes the causes of subconjunctival hemorrhage..

Treatment

Subconjunctival hemorrhage is symptomless and gets absorbed by itself within 2 to 3 weeks; however, the following points need to be kept in consideration:

- Cold compression in initial stages.
- Aspirin and nonsteroidal anti-inflammatory drugs (NSAIDs) should be avoided.
- Artificial tears–if mild ocular irritation is present.

Follicular Reaction

Follicles are lymph follicles with vascularization. These are prominent in the inferior forniceal conjunctiva. **Table 5.1** describes the follicular reaction in case of eye conjunctival disorders.

Papillary Reaction

Papillae are hyperplasia of the vascular system invaded by inflammatory cells. They form a mosaic-like pattern of elevated red dots.

A papillary reaction is more nonspecific being of less diagnostic importance than a follicular reaction (**Table 5.2**).

Membranes

Membranes are made up of fibrinous exudate that may or may not be firmly adherent to the epithelium of conjunctiva. These may be pseudomembranes or true membranes.

Pseudo Membranes

These are formed when the coagulated exudates adhere to the inflamed conjunctival epithelium. Therefore, it can be easily peeled off, leaving

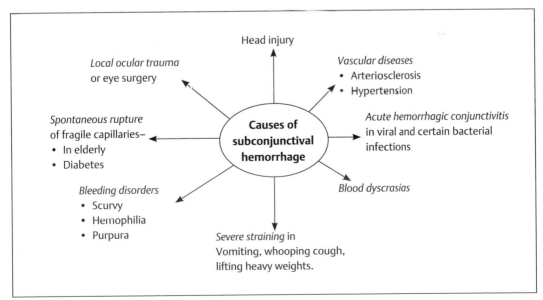

Fig. 5.4 Causes of subconjunctival hemorrhage.

Table 5.1 Follicular reaction			
Appearance	**Site**	**Histology**	**Causes**
Follicles are: • yellowish–white multiple, discrete round elevations. • 1–2 mm in diameter, encircled by tiny blood vessels	Follicles are most prominent in inferior forniceal conjunctiva but more numerous on upper palpebral conjunctiva in trachoma	Follicles are due to localized aggregation of lymphocytes in subepithelial adenoid layer of stroma. Follicles do not develop until about 2–3 months after birth.	Causes of follicular reaction include: • Viral conjunctivitis • Chlamydial conjunctivitis • Hypersensitivity to topical medications

Table 5.2 Papillary reaction		
Appearance	**Site**	**Causes**
Glomerulus-like appearance of capillaries growing into epithelium.	Most frequent in upper palpebral conjunctiva. Papillae can only develop in palpebral conjunctiva and limbal bulbar conjunctiva where it is attached to deeper fibrous layer.	• Bacterial conjunctivitis • Allergic conjunctivitis • Contact lens wear • Superior limbic keratoconjunctivitis

the underlying epithelium intact. These occur in severe adenoviral conjunctivitis and gonococcal conjunctivitis.

True Membranes

These are formed due to permeation of inflammatory exudates into the superficial layers of conjunctival epithelium. Therefore, attempts to remove the membrane tear the epithelium and results in bleeding. These occur in bacterial conjunctivitis due to the *Corynebacterium diphtheriae*.

Xerosis

It is a dry and lusterless condition of the conjunctiva.

Etiology

It is due to the deficiency of mucin which may occur as a sequel to a local disease of the conjunctiva, involving all its layers, or may be associated with general disease.

1. *Xerosis due to local conjunctival diseases*– it is a cicatricial degeneration of the conjunctiva due to:
   • Trachoma.
   • Burns.
   • Pemphigoid conjunctivitis.

• Diphtheritic membranous conjunctivitis.
• Prolonged exposure due to ectropion or proptosis.

The chief changes involve conjunctival epithelium and glands. The mucus secretion ceases and the epithelium becomes epidermoid like that of skin. This impaired secretory activity of conjunctiva results in xerosis in spite of normal or increased lacrimal secretion, as the watery tears then fail to moisten the conjunctiva.

2. *Xerosis due to systemic diseases*– it occurs due to vitamin A deficiency in the diet.

Subconjunctival Scarring

Subconjunctival scarring is significant tissue shrinkage with distortion of the fornices and/or the lids.

Etiology

These can be due to:
• Trauma: surgical, thermal, radiational, mechanical, chemical, trichiasis, or entropion.
• Autoimmune:
  ◇ Ocular cicatricial pemphigoid (OCP).

◇ Stevens–Johnson syndrome (erythema multiforme major).

◇ Graft versus host disease.

• Infection: trachoma.

• Allergy:

◇ Vernal keratoconjunctivitis.

◇ Atopic keratoconjunctivitis.

■ Lymphadenopathy

The preauricular lymph nodes are typically affected.

The most common causes are:

• Viral infection.

• Chlamydial infection.

• Bacterial conjunctivitis (particularly gonococcal).

• Parinaud oculoglandular syndrome.

■ Inflammation of Conjunctiva (Conjunctivitis (OP3.3))

Conjunctivitis is an inflammation of the conjunctiva. It may be of two types: infective and noninfective conjunctivitis.

Infective conjunctivitis may be:

• Bacterial.

• Viral.

• Chlamydial.

Noninfective conjunctivitis may be:

• Allergic conjunctivitis.

• Vernal keratoconjunctivitis.

• Atopic keratoconjunctivitis.

• Giant papillary conjunctivitis.

• Phlyctenular conjunctivitis.

• Toxic conjunctivitis.

• Oculocutaneous syndromes.

Conjunctivitis may be acute or chronic. Conjunctivitis that persists for > 4 weeks is considered chronic. Chronic conjunctivitis can be caused by a variety of microorganisms, environments, and environmental factors. Chronic conjunctivitis may occur due to:

• Inadequately treated acute conjunctivitis.

• Chronic bacterial conjunctivitis.

• Specific granulomatous conjunctivitis.

• Trachoma due to chlamydia trachomatis.

■ Infective Conjunctivitis

Bacterial Conjunctivitis

Bacterial conjunctivitis is caused by staphylococcus, streptococcus pneumoniae, hemophilus, corynebacterium diphtheriae, neisseria, moraxella, and Gram –ve bacilli. It is characterized by conjunctival hyperemia, lid edema, and mucopurulent discharge in one eye. The second eye becomes involved 1 to 2 days later. **Flowchart 5.1** describes the pathophysiology of bacterial conjunctivitis.

Depending on the onset, it may be acute, hyperacute, or chronic (**Table 5.3**).

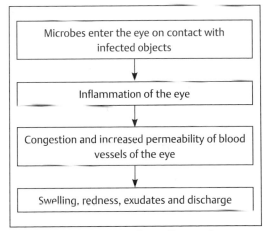

Flowchart 5.1 Pathophysiology of bacterial conjunctivitis.

Table 5.3 Types of bacterial conjunctivitis	
Acute	• Acute catarrhal or mucopurulent conjunctivitis • Acute purulent conjunctivitis • Acute membranous conjunctivitis • Acute pseudo-membranous conjunctivitis
Hyper acute	• Gonorrheal conjunctivitis
Chronic	• Chronic bacterial conjunctivitis • Chronic angular conjunctivitis

Acute Mucopurulent and Purulent Conjunctivitis (Fig. 5.5)

Etiology

The most common causative bacteria are:

- Staphylococcus aureus (a Gram + ve cocci)– its pathogenicity is proportionate to its coagulase activity.
- Koch–Weeks bacillus (Haemophilus aegyptius)– it is a Gram –ve bacilli.
- Pneumococcus.
- Streptococcus.

Clinical Presentation

The clinical presentation depends on the virulence and pathogenicity of the organism and the host immune response. Symptoms include:

- Redness of the eye.
- Mucopurulent discharge.
- Sticking together of lid margins, particularly in the morning, due to accumulation of discharge at night.
- Discomfort.
- Mild photophobia,
- Foreign body sensation,
- Colored halos due to prismatic action of discharge across the cornea.

Clinical signs include:

- Conjunctival congestion which is less marked in circum corneal zone.
- Flakes of mucopurulent discharge at fornices, canthi, and lid margins.
- Chemosis.
- Cilia are usually matted together.
- Yellow crust.
- Fine papillae.
- Ecchymosis.

Complications

If untreated, the disease may be complicated by:

- Marginal corneal ulcer.
- Superficial keratitis.
- Blepharitis or dacryocystitis.

Treatment

- Eyes should not be bandaged because band-aging the eye will raise the temperature of

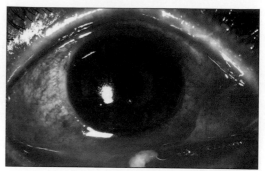

Fig. 5.5 Acute bacterial conjunctivitis (mucopurulent). Source: History. In: Singh K, Smiddy W, Lee A, ed. Ophthalmology review: A case-study approach. 2nd edition. Thieme; 2018.

conjunctival fornix, which will flare up the infection.

- Dark glasses must be used to avoid photophobia.
- Irrigation of conjunctival sac is carried out to remove the discharge, although frequent irrigation will wash out the lysozyme in the tears.
- Topical broad-spectrum antibiotics such as chloramphenicol, ciprofloxacin, gati-floxacin, and moxifloxacin are instilled 4 to 6 times a day.
- Antibiotic eye ointment is used at night.
- No steroids should be applied as the infection may flare up.

Acute Pseudomembranous and Membranous Conjunctivitis

It is the inflammation of conjunctiva characterized by the formation of pseudo membrane or fibrinous membrane covering the conjunctival surface in certain infections (**Fig. 5.6**).

Etiology

Membrane formation may take place in infections due to:

- Corynebacterium diphtheriae.
- Beta hemolytic streptococci.
- Streptococcus pneumoniae.
- Neisseria gonorrhoeae.
- Haemophilus aegyptius.

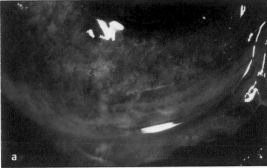 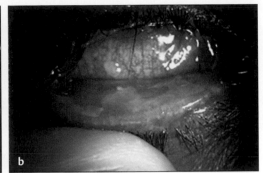

Fig. 5.6 (a) Pseudomembranous conjunctivitis. Source: History. In: Singh K, Smiddy W, Lee A, ed. Ophthalmology review: A case-study approach. 2nd edition. Thieme; 2018. **(b)** Membranous conjunctivitis.

- Staphylococcus aureus.
- *E. coli.*
- Viral infections.

Diphtheritic infection due to corynebacterium diphtheriae occurs chiefly in children, resulting in membrane formation. Membranous conjunctivitis of diphtheritic origin is often severe. Streptococcal conjunctivitis occurs in association with measles, whooping cough, and influenza. Chemical and thermal burns may also cause membrane formation.

Clinical Presentation

Mild cases are characterized by swelling of the lids, mucopurulent or sanguinous discharge, and white pseudo membrane on palpebral conjunctiva.

Severe cases are characterized by brawny lids and marked chemosis of conjunctiva. There is infiltration of conjunctiva with semisolid exudates impairing mobility and compressing the vessels. A true membrane is present which covers the whole palpebral conjunctiva. It is seldom found on the bulbar conjunctiva. The *membrane separates less easily and separation may lead to bleeding.* This form is referred to as membranous conjunctivitis. Regional (preauricular) lymph nodes are usually enlarged.

After the stage of infiltration, cornea and underlying conjunctiva tend to necrotize. The necrosed part sloughs out and may lead to corneal ulceration. Adhesions form between the palpebral and bulbar parts of conjunctiva (**symblepharon**).

Treatment

In children who are not immunized, every cause is treated as diphtheritic infection. It consists of:
- Freshly made topical (10,000 units/mL) penicillin drops from injectable solution are instilled on an hourly basis.
- Systemic administration of penicillin (crystalline penicillin 5 lacs units) on a 12-hour basis.
- Antidiphtheritic serum (4000–10,000 units repeated on a 12-hour basis).
- If cornea is involved, then cycloplegics (atropine 1%) are administered.
- In nondiphtheritic conjunctivitis, systemic and topical antibiotics are prescribed.

Complications

If the membrane is removed inadvertently, it may precipitate symblepharon. So, removal of membrane is not required.

Gonorrhoeal (Hyperacute) Conjunctivitis

Etiology

The severe form of acute purulent conjunctivitis is due to *Neisseria gonorrhoeae* (Gram –ve diplococci). This form of conjunctivitis is also termed hyperacute conjunctivitis. The disease is venereal in origin and the infection is transmitted from the genitals to the eye. Gonorrhoeal conjunctivitis occurs in two forms:
- In *newborns*, it occurs as ophthalmia neonatorum.

- In *adults*, it occurs as severe purulent conjunctivitis.

Clinical Presentation

The disease is acute and males are predominantly affected. The disease is characterized by severe purulent conjunctivitis with a tendency of corneal involvement.

Symptoms:
- Pain and redness in the eye.
- Photophobia.
- Blurring of vision.
- Gritty sensation in the eye.

Signs:
- Eye ball–painful and tender.
- Lids–tense and swollen.
- Conjunctiva–chemosed and bright-red velvety.
- Discharge–purulent, copious, and thick discharge.
- Lymph nodes–preauricular lymph nodes are enlarged.

Diagnosis

In gonococcal conjunctivitis, urethritis is almost present. Coincidence of urethritis with severe purulent conjunctivitis is the important point in diagnosis.

Complications

As Neisseria gonorrhoeae (gonococcus) can invade intact corneal epithelium, so *corneal complications are the rule*. The whole cornea becomes hazy with a gray area of necrosis in the center. Marginal ulcers usually develop due to retention of pus in the angle formed by chemotic conjunctiva. The ulcer produced progresses resulting in perforation. Iridocyclitis may develop independently of perforation.

Systemic complications include:
- Gonorrheal arthritis.
- Endocarditis.
- Septicemia.

Treatment

Systemic therapy: Gonococcal infection is usually treated with a third-generation cephalosporin such as ceftriaxone; quinolones are alternatives.
- *Gonococcal conjunctivitis* without septicemia in adults is treated with a single dose of ceftriaxone 1 g IM.
- Conjunctivitis with corneal involvement is treated with ceftriaxone 1 g IM or IV on a 12-hour basis for 5 days.
- Oral norfloxacin or ciprofloxacin are also effective.

Topical therapy:
- Irrigation of the eyes with warm saline.
- Intensive therapy with antibiotic eye drops such as *quinolones* (e.g., ofloxacin and ciprofloxacin eye drops) and *aminoglycosides* (tobramycin or gentamicin eye drops).
- Antibiotic ointment (e.g., erythromycin or bacitracin) is applied at night. Ointments and gels provide a higher concentration for longer periods than drops but they are not used during day time because of blurred vision.
- Cycloplegics (atropine 1 percent) must be applied if the cornea and uvea are involved.
- Patient and the sexual partner should be referred for evaluation of other sexually transmitted diseases.
- If venereal disease is present in teenagers, also treat with single dose of azithromycin (1 gm) because over 30% of these patients will be afflicted with concurrent chlamydial diseases.

Chronic Bacterial Conjunctivitis

Conjunctivitis longer than three weeks duration is defined as chronic bacterial conjunctivitis. It may result from several organisms.

Etiology

It is most commonly caused by Staphylococcus species, although other bacteria are occasionally involved. This type of conjunctivitis may often be associated with chronic dacryocystitis, rhinitis, and blepharitis.

Clinical Presentation

Staphylococcus aureus colonizes the eyelid margin from which it can cause direct infection of conjunctiva or may elaborate exotoxins to cause conjunctival inflammation. Recurrent styes and chalazia of the lid margin are concurrently seen from chronic inflammation of the meibomian glands. Meibomian glands secrete an oily component of the tear film. When inflamed, these glands produce chronic inflammation of eyelid margins and conjunctiva (**Fig. 5.7**). Symptoms include the following:

- Burning.
- Grittiness.
- Redness.
- Itching.
- Discharge is slight but there is abnormal amount of secretion from the meibomian glands.

Signs

It is marked by congestion of posterior conjunctival vessels when the lower lid is pulled down. The upper and lower palpebral conjunctiva may be congested with papillary hypertrophy.

Treatment

It consists of:

- Elimination of cause.
- Topical antibiotics to eliminate the infection.

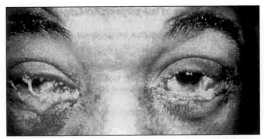

Fig. 5.7 Gonorrheal conjunctivitis. Source: Laboratory. In: Gallin P, ed. Pediatric ophthalmology: A clinical guide. 1st edition. Thieme; 2000.

- Astringent eye drops for symptomatic relief.

Chronic Angular Conjunctivitis

Angular conjunctivitis is a type of chronic conjunctivitis characterized by mild grade inflammation confined to the conjunctiva and lid margins near the angles (hence the name) associated with maceration of the surrounding skin.

Causative Organism

It is typically caused by *Moraxella–Axenfeld*, a Gram −ve diplobacilli. The bacilli are placed end to end, so the disease is also called diplobacillary conjunctivitis. The organism produces a proteolytic enzyme which macerates the epithelium of the lid margin.

The diplobacilli is often present in the nasal discharge in cases of angular conjunctivitis.

Mode of Infection

Infection is transmitted from nasal cavity to the eyes by contaminated fingers or handkerchief.

Pathology

The proteolytic enzyme produced by *Moraxella–Axenfeld* collects at the angles by the action of tears and thus macerates the epithelium of conjunctiva, lid margin, and the skin of the surrounding angles of eye. The maceration is followed by mild grade chronic inflammation. The skin may show eczematous changes.

Clinical Presentation

Symptoms include irritation in the eye, itching, and burning sensation in the eye, collection of dirty-white foamy discharge at the angles, and redness in the angles of eye.

Signs:
- Hyperemia of bulbar conjunctiva near the canthi.
- Hyperemia of lid margin near the angles.
- Excoriation of the skin around the angles.
- Presence of foamy mucopurulent discharge at the angles.

Complications

- If the condition is untreated, it becomes chronic and may give rise to *blepharitis*.
- A shallow, marginal, and catarrhal *corneal ulceration* may occur.

Treatment

- Tetracycline or oxytetracycline ointment (1%) two to three times a day for 2 weeks will eradicate the infection.
- Topical eye drops containing zinc inhibit the proteolytic ferment and thus help in reducing the maceration.

Viral Conjunctivitis

Viral conjunctivitis is extremely common and highly contagious. Most of the cases resolve spontaneously within days to weeks. The diagnosis is made clinically, hence laboratory investigations and viral cultures are rarely conducted. Viral conjunctivitis (**Fig. 5.8**) is caused by adenoviruses, herpes simplex, and less frequently by varicella-zoster virus, picornaviruses, pox, and papilloma viruses.

Transmission

The infection is transmitted by:
- Hand-to-eye contact.

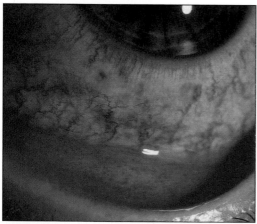

Fig. 5.8 Viral conjunctivitis. Source: Bulbar conjunctiva. In: Roth H, ed. Contact lens complications: Etiology, pathogenesis, prevention, therapy. 1st edition. Thieme; 2003.

- Contact with upper respiratory tract droplets.
- Infected swimming pools.
- Infected ocular instruments like tonometers.

Clinical Presentation

Acute viral conjunctivitis may present in three clinical forms: Acute serous conjunctivitis, acute hemorrhagic conjunctivitis, and acute follicular conjunctivitis. The follicular conjunctival reaction is more common in viral infections due to adenoviruses and herpes viruses. It can be acute or chronic. Acute follicular conjunctivitis may also occur in chlamydial inclusion conjunctivitis.

Patient complains of the following symptoms:
- Feeling of discomfort and foreign body sensation.
- Mild photophobia.
- Redness.
- Watering of the eyes.
- Mild mucoid discharge.
- A history of fever, pharyngitis, cough or rhinorrhea may be part of the viral prodrome.

Typical signs of viral conjunctivitis are as follows:
- Conjunctival hyperemia.
- Copious, clear, serous, and watery discharge.
- Lid edema.
- Follicular conjunctival reaction.
- Tender preauricular lymph node.
- Chemosis.

Adenoviral Infections

These infections are highly contagious and occur in epidemics. The onset of infection is abrupt. Patients with adenoviral conjunctivitis are contagious to others for 3 weeks. Subtypes of adenoviral conjunctivitis include:
- Epidemic keratoconjunctivitis (EKC).
- Pharyngoconjunctival fever (PCF).

Epidemic Keratoconjunctivitis (EKC)

Etiology

EKC is caused by adenovirus of serotypes 3, 7, 8, and 19 (**Fig. 5.9**).

Clinical Presentation

EKC is characterized by a sudden onset of signs and symptoms (**Fig. 5.10**).

Symptoms:
- Red eye.
- Photophobia.
- Irritation.
- Foreign body sensation.
- Excessive watery discharge.

Signs:
- Follicular conjunctival reaction.
- Discrete subepithelial corneal infiltrates which appear approximately 2 weeks after the onset of conjunctivitis.

These are associated with photophobia. These gradually diminish and finally disappear, but may persist for weeks to months or even years.
- Preauricular lymphadenopathy.

Occasionally, pseudo membranes develop on palpebral conjunctiva.

Treatment

EKC is a highly contagious disease and its transmission usually occurs from eye to finger to eye. Tonometers and eye drops are the other

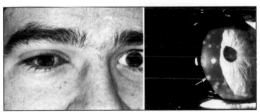

Fig. 5.9 Epidemic keratoconjunctivitis. Source: Epidemic keratoconjunctivitis. Viral conjunctivitis. In: Lang G, ed. Ophthalmology. A pocket textbook atlas. 3rd edition. Thieme; 2015.

routes of transmission. It is nonspecific and symptomatic with:
- Broad-spectrum antibiotic drops to prevent secondary bacterial infection.
- Lubricants.
- Acyclovir is not effective against adenovirus infections.

Prophylaxis

Patient should be advised to wash their hands frequently, use separate towels, and avoid close contact with other people. To prevent the spread of epidemic, sterilization of all instruments touching the patient's eye must be done.

Pharyngoconjunctival Fever (PCF)

Etiology

It is caused by adenovirus of serotypes 3, 4, and 7. It primarily affects children in epidemic form.

Clinical Presentation

It is characterized by:
- **Pharyngitis.**
- **Conjunctivitis** (acute follicular).
- **Fever.**
- **Preauricular lymphadenopathy** (large and tender preauricular lymph nodes).
- Signs are less severe than in EKC and corneal involvement is rare but may occur as superficial punctate keratitis.

Treatment

There is no specific treatment. Topical antibiotics are used to prevent the secondary bacterial infections.

> *Newcastle Conjunctivitis*
> It is rare and occurs among poultry workers. It is caused by the **Newcastle virus** which is derived from contact with diseased fowls. It is clinically indistinguishable from PCF.

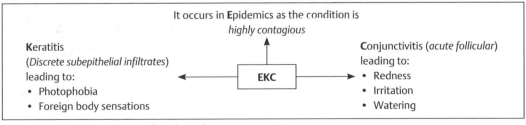

It occurs in **Epidemics** as the condition is *highly contagious*

Keratitis
(*Discrete subepithelial infiltrates*)
leading to:
- Photophobia
- Foreign body sensations

← EKC →

Conjunctivitis (*acute follicular*)
leading to:
- Redness
- Irritation
- Watering

Fig. 5.10 Clinical presentation of epidemic keratoconjunctivitis.

Herpes Simplex Conjunctivitis

Etiology

It is caused by herpes simplex virus (HSV) type I in young children who are infected by contamination from the carriers of virus. In neonates, infection is due to maternal genital infection with HSV type II which is acquired by direct contamination of the eye from the birth canal.

Clinical Presentation

It is characterized by:
- Acute follicular conjunctivitis.
- Vesicular lesions on the lids and dendritic keratitis, with reduced corneal sensations are highly suggestive of herpetic infection (**Fig. 5.11**).
- Preauricular lymph nodes are usually involved.

Treatment

It consists of:
- Topical lubricating eye drops.
- Topical antiviral therapy with acyclovir (3%) eye ointment five times a day.

Acute Hemorrhagic Conjunctivitis

Etiology

It is caused by picornaviruses (coxsackie virus and enterovirus 70). It is also known as Apollo conjunctivitis due to the epidemic that occurred at the time when the Apollo spacecraft was launched. It is highly contagious and is transmitted by hand-to-eye contact.

Clinical Presentation

Symptoms:
- Redness.
- Lacrimation.
- Photophobia.
- Pain.
- Lid swelling.

Signs:
- Swollen lids.
- Conjunctival follicles (**Fig. 5.12**).
- Subconjunctival hemorrhages (**Fig. 5.13**).
- Chemosis.
- Preauricular lymphadenopathy.

Cornea is usually unaffected but superficial punctate keratopathy can be seen sometimes in the cornea.

Treatment

The infection usually resolves without sequelae. There is no specific treatment but broad-spectrum antibiotics are used to prevent secondary bacterial infections.

Molluscum Contagiosum Conjunctivitis

Molluscum contagiosum is a cutaneous or conjunctival pox viral infection that causes a raised, waxy, and umblicated lesion on the eye

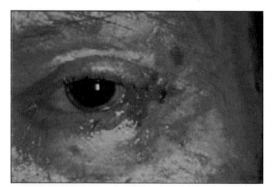

Fig. 5.11 Herpes simplex conjunctivitis. Source: Medical disorders. In: Probst L, Doane J, ed. Refractive surgery: A color synopsis. 1st edition. Thieme; 2000.

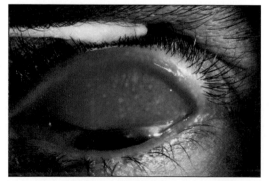

Fig. 5.12 Follicular conjunctivitis. Source: General notes on the causes, symptoms, and diagnosis of conjunctivitis. In: Lang G, ed. Ophthalmology. A pocket textbook Atlas. 3rd edition. Thieme; 2015.

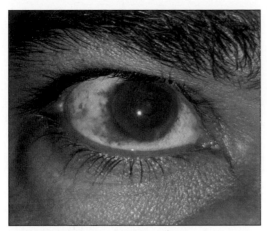

Fig. 5.13 Subconjunctival hemorrhage.

lids near the lid margin and face. Virus particles that are shed into the tear film from eyelid lesions may cause a reaction of conjunctiva and cornea, resulting in chronic follicular conjunctivitis and epithelial keratitis with subepithelial corneal infiltration. Usually, there is no enlargement of lymph nodes. Typical umblicated eyelid lesions help in establishing the diagnosis. Treatment is carried out by surgical excision of the eyelid nodule. The conjunctivitis and keratitis typically resolve after removal of skin lesion. The skin lesions can also be treated by cryotherapy or cauterization.

Chronic follicular conjunctivitis occurs in:
• Drug users (pilocarpine)
• Trachoma
• Molluscum contagiosum

Chlamydial Conjunctivitis

Chlamydia are obligate, intracellular, and Gram –ve bacteria. Chlamydia species consists of three subgroups: *C. trachomatis, C. pneumoniae, and C. psittaci.* Humans are the reservoir of C. trachomatis and C. pneumoniae; C. psittaci causes zoonosis.

Based on serological typing, *C. trachomatis* can be divided into:
• Serotypes A, B, Ba, and C which induce trachoma.
• Serotypes D to K cause inclusion conjunctivitis, urethritis, and epididymitis

in males, and cervicitis and salpingitis in females.
• Serotype L 1, 2, and 3 cause lymphogranuloma venereum.

Although C. trachomatis is the infectious agent for both trachoma and inclusion conjunctivitis, the clinical presentation and epidemiologic characteristics of the two diseases are very different.

Transmission

• Serotypes A, B, Ba, and C of C. trachomatis are transmitted generally with contact of conjunctival exudates directly or via flies.
• Subtypes D-K as well as the L varieties are transmitted sexually and therefore cause venereal disease, in which ocular involvement represents secondary infection.

Chlamydial conjunctivitis consists of three clinical syndromes:
• Adult inclusion conjunctivitis.
• Neonatal chlamydial conjunctivitis.
• Trachoma.

Adult Inclusion Conjunctivitis

Etiology

It is caused by C. trachomatis serotypes D to K.

Transmission

Adult chlamydial inclusion conjunctivitis is sexually transmitted from genital infection. The primary infection produces mild urethritis in males and cervicitis in females. Ocular infection commonly occurs from the genitals by the fingers or through the water of the swimming pool. Thus, the disease may occur in local epidemics (**swimming pool conjunctivitis**).

Clinical Features

It has an acute onset with an incubation period of about a week. The disease may be unilateral or bilateral.

Symptoms:
• Ocular irritation.
• Redness.
• Watering.
• Photophobia.

Signs:
- Watery or mucopurulent discharge.
- Conjunctival hyperemia with follicular conjunctival reaction which is always more prominent in inferior fornix.
- Superficial punctate keratitis with occasional micropannus is common (**Fig. 5.14**).
- *Preauricular lymph nodes* are tender and enlarged.

Diagnosis

The diagnosis is made by:
- Giemsa staining of conjunctival scrapings for basophilic intracytoplasmic bodies in epithelial cells (**called Halberstaedter-von Provazek inclusion bodies**).
- Direct immunofluorescent antibody tests.
- Enzyme-linked immunosorbent assay (ELISA) and PCR tests of ocular specimens.
- Mc Coy cell culture is highly specific.

In addition, whenever possible, cervical or urethral specimens should be obtained.

Treatment

All patients with chlamydial conjunctivitis must be referred to a genitourinary specialist.

Systemic therapy–Because of frequent concomitant systemic infections, systemic therapy involves one of the following:
- Only a single 1 gm dose of oral azithromycin is generally the treatment of choice.

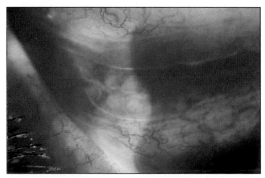

Fig. 5.14 Adult inclusion conjunctivitis (Follicles in lower fornix). Source: Clinical aspects. In: Hoang-Xuan T, Baudouin C, Creuzot-Garcher C, ed. Inflammatory diseases of the conjuctiva. 1st edition. Thieme; 2001.

- Doxycycline 100 mg twice daily for 2 weeks (oral tetracyclines are contraindicated in pregnancy, breast feeding, and in children under 12 years of age).
- Erythromycin, Ofloxacin are alternatives.

Therapy of both patient and his/her sexual partner is necessary.

Topical therapy–Topical erythromycin (0.5%) or tetracycline (1%) ointment are used to achieve rapid relief, but are insufficient alone.

Neonatal Chlamydial Conjunctivitis

It manifests from 5 to 14 days after the birth and is a cause of ophthalmia neonatorum. It is a venereal infection derived from the birth canal of the mother.

Typical signs are:
- Eyelid edema.
- Chemosis.
- Mucopurulent discharge.
- Superficial keratitis with peripheral pannus formation.
- Conjunctival membrane or pseudo membrane without follicular reaction.

In contrast to infections in the adults, there are no follicles in neonatal chlamydial conjunctivitis due to the absence of a subconjunctival adenoid layer in children.

Trachoma (OP3.4)

Trachoma is a cause of preventable blindness. Trachoma is also called *granular conjunctivitis or Egyptian ophthalmia*. The incidence of trachoma is highest in unhealthy, dirty, crowded, and poor hygienic conditions. It is contagious in its acute stage and transmitted by contact of conjunctival secretions through fingers, flies, or towels.

Etiology

It is caused by chlamydial trachomatis serotypes A, B, Ba, and C. The organism is an obligate intracellular parasite and forms colonies in the conjunctival epithelial cells called Halberstaedter-von Provazek inclusion bodies. Chlamydia trachomatis cannot replicate extracellularly and hence depends on host cells.

Pathology

The essential lesion is the trachomatous follicle. Histologically, there is lymphocytic infiltration in the adenoid layer of conjunctiva. The aggregation of lymphocytes form follicles. The follicles appear as round swellings that are paler than the surrounding conjunctiva. The follicles are invaded by multinucleated macrophages (Leber's cells) which engulf the cytoplasmic nuclear debris. The fibroblast grows and the trachomatous follicles show necrosis and cicatricial changes. The cicatricial bands are characteristic of trachomatous follicles and never formed in other forms of follicular conjunctivitis.

Clinical Features

The infection involves both the conjunctiva and cornea in the majority of cases. The primary infection is epithelial. The bacteria have an incubation period of 5 to12 days. Features of trachoma are divided into:
- Active inflammatory stage.
- Chronic cicatricial stage.

Active Inflammatory Stage (Active Trachoma)
Symptoms:
- Redness.
- Foreign body sensation.
- Watering.
- Itching.
- Photophobia.

Active trachoma will often be irritating and have a watery discharge. Bacterial secondary infection may occur and cause a purulent discharge.

Signs:
- Congestion.
- Mixed papillary and follicular conjunctivitis.

The *essential lesion* is in the form of **trachomatous follicles** which are characteristic lesions of trachoma. In most cases, they appear on upper palpebral conjunctiva and sometimes on lower palpebral conjunctiva as well. Follicles may also appear at the junction of cornea and sclera (limbal follicles). The trachomatous follicles are bigger in size and undergo necrotic and cicatricial changes (*nontrachomatous follicles resolve without cicatrization*).

Chronic Cicatricial Stage

The structural changes of trachoma include scarring in the eyelid (tarsal conjunctiva), resulting in distortion of the eyelid and trichiasis. Trichiasis results in corneal opacity and blindness. The linear scar present in sulcus subtarsalis is called **Arlt's line** (named after Carl Ferdinand von Arlt).

The cornea may be involved with conjunctiva and manifests initially as superficial keratitis, typically in the upper part of cornea. At a later stage, lymphoid infiltration with vascularization of the upper limbus may be evident as **trachomatous pannus**.

In progressive pannus, the cellular infiltration lies beyond the vessels which are nonanastomosing and parallel to each other. In regressive pannus, the infiltration recedes, so the vessels extend a short distance beyond the area of cellular infiltration. The corneal ulcers are common at the advancing edge of the pannus. In the beginning, the pannus lies between the epithelium and the Bowman's membrane, and the pannus may resolve completely, if treated, at this stage. When the pannus destroys the Bowman's membrane and invades the stroma, the resolution of pannus leaves a permanent opacity. The limbal follicles resolve and may leave small depressions (**Herbert's pits**). *These pits are highly pathognomonic of trachoma* (**Fig. 5.15**).

WHO recommended a simplified grading system for trachoma (**Table 5.4**).

Sequelae
- *Corneal ulceration.*
- *Trachomatous ptosis* (dropping of upper lids may develop following dense infiltration and cicatrization).
- *Entropion* (lid margin rolls inward due to contraction of newly formed scar tissue).
- *Trichiasis* (lashes turn inside and rub against the cornea due to entropion).

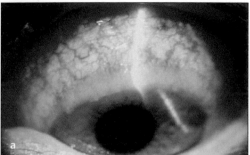

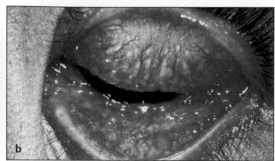

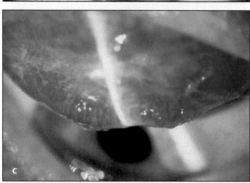

Fig. 5.15 (a) Superior limbal follicles in florid trachoma. Source: Chlamydial conjunctivitis. In: Hoang-Xuan T, Baudouin C, Creuzot-Garcher C, ed. Inflammatory diseases of the conjuctiva. 1st edition. Thieme; 2001. **(b)** Trachoma (stage II–III). Source: Trachoma. In: Lang G, ed. Ophthalmology. A pocket textbook atlas. 3rd edition. Thieme; 2015. **(c)** Superior limbal follicles in florid trachoma. Source: Chlamydial conjunctivitis. In: Hoang-Xuan T, Baudouin C, Creuzot-Garcher C, ed. Inflammatory diseases of the conjuctiva. 1st edition. Thieme; 2001.

Table 5.4 World Health Organization (WHO) grading of trachoma

Grading	Features	Significance
TF (**T**rachomatous inflammation - **F**ollicular)	Presence of ≥ 5 follicles of > 0.5 mm in upper tarsal conjunctiva.	The patient, if treated properly at this stage, should recover with no/minimal scarring.
TI (**T**rachomatous inflammation **I**ntense)	Tarsal conjunctiva is diffusely involved. Follicles and papillae are numerous. The inflammatory thickening of upper tarsal conjunctiva obscures > 50% of the normal deep tarsal vessels.	This stage indicates severe infection with high-risk of complications. The disease needs urgent treatment.
TS (**T**rachomatous **S**carring)	Tarsal conjunctiva shows cicatrization. Scars are easily visible as white fibrous bands in tarsal conjunctiva.	It implies that the infection is old but inactive at present.
TT (**T**rachomatous **T**richiasis)	Presence of at least one eyelash rubbing the eyeball.	Corrective surgery is required.
CO (**C**orneal **O**pacity)	Presence of corneal opacity in pupillary area which blur the details of the part of pupillary margin.	It signifies the dense corneal scarring which blurs a part of the pupillary margin, when seen through the opacity, and also causes significant visual impairment.

Note: In this system, TF and TI represent active trachoma.

- *Tylosis* (thickening of tarsal plate).
- *Dry eye* (caused by destruction of goblet cells and ductules of lacrimal gland).
- *Corneal opacity* may cause visual impairment and blindness.

Diagnosis

In most cases, diagnosis is made on clinical features and depend on the presence of, at least, two of the following signs:

- More follicles in upper than lower palpebral conjunctiva.
- Superficial keratitis in early stages in upper part of cornea.
- Pannus in upper part of cornea.
- Limbal follicles or Herbert's pits.
- Linear conjunctival scarring of upper tarsus.
- Histological demonstration of inclusion bodies in conjunctival scrapings.
- Culture of C. trachomatis (inclusion conjunctivitis can be excluded by culture of organism).
- Nucleic acid amplification test such as PCR (polymerase chain reaction).

Treatment

WHO has developed the "SAFE" strategy for trachoma management which is an acronym for:

S– **S**urgery for trichiasis.

A– **A**ntibiotics for active disease.

F– **F**acial hygiene.

E– **E**nvironmental improvement.

1. **Antibiotics:**
   WHO recommends antibiotics for trachoma control: oral azithromycin and tetracycline eye ointment.
   - *Systemic therapy*
     ◊ A single dose of oral azithromycin (20 mg/kg up to 1 gm) is the treatment of choice.
     ◊ Erythromycin 250 to 500 mg 4 times a day for 14 days.

     or
     ◊ Doxycycline 100 mg twice daily for 10 days. (Oral tetracyclines cannot be given to children <8 years of age and during pregnancy or breast feeding).
     ◊ Sulphonamides are effective orally but have a high risk of allergic reactions such as Stevens–Johnson syndrome and erythema multiforme.

   - *Topical therapy*
     Topical treatment with tetracycline (1%) eye ointment is less effective than oral treatment.
2. **Facial hygiene** is a critical preventive measure which reduces both the risk and severity of active trachoma in children.
3. **Environmental improvement** activities are as follows:
   - Promotion of improved water supply.
   - Improved household sanitation.
   - Fly control that transmits trachoma.
4. **Surgery:** the management of entropion and trichiasis requires surgical intervention.

Ophthalmia Neonatorum (Neonatal Conjunctivitis)

It is the form of conjunctivitis developing within the first month of life (**Fig. 5.16**). It may be infectious or noninfectious (**Table 5.5**). In infectious conjunctivitis, the organism is transmitted from the genital tract of an infected mother during birth.

Clinical Presentation

- *Chemical conjunctivitis* is due to silver nitrate used as prophylaxis against infection. In the past, a drop of silver nitrate solution (1%) was instilled into each eye if maternal infection was suspected (Crede's method) but nowadays it is rare, as prophylaxis with 1% silver nitrate solution is no longer in common use. In most countries, antibiotics eye drops or ointment are used instead.

  There is a history of instillation of prophylactic chemical preparation.

  Timing of onset– it is usually seen in first few hours of its application and lasts 2 to 4 days.

  *Discharge–*It is characteristically watery.
- Ophthalmia neonatorum due to neisseria gonorrhoeae (gonococci):

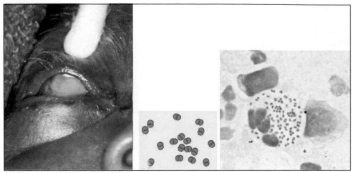

Fig. 5.16 Gonococcal conjunctivitis (ophthalmia neonatorum). Source: Neonatal conjunctivitis. In: Lang G, ed. Ophthalmology. A pocket textbook atlas. 3rd edition. Thieme; 2015.

Table 5.5 Causes of ophthalmia neonatorum

Ophthalmia neonatorum	Causes
Noninfectious	• Chemical irritants such as silver nitrate (AgNO₃)– chemical conjunctivitis. • Neonatal conjunctivitis due to reactions with chemicals in eye drops.
Infectious	• Neisseria gonorrheae. • Chlamydia trachomatis. • Other agents causing ophthalmia neonatorum include: ◇ Herpes simplex virus (typically HSV 2). ◇ Staphylococcus aureus. ◇ Streptococcus haemolyticus. ◇ Streptococcus pneumoniae.

Timing of onset–It typically manifests in the first 5 days after birth.

Discharge–It is associated with marked bilateral purulent discharge.

Features:
- Severe eyelid edema.
- Marked chemosis.
- Purulent conjunctivitis.
- Intense conjunctival congestion.

There is risk of corneal ulceration with rapid progression as gonococcus can invade intact epithelium. It can result in perforation and its sequelae. When vision is not completely destroyed but seriously impaired, nystagmus develops because central macular fixation is impaired, which takes place during the first 3 weeks of life.
- Ophthalmia neonatorum due to chlamydia trachomatis:

Timing of onset–It manifests usually from 1 to 3 weeks after birth.

Discharge–It is mucopurulent.

Features–It is a venereal infection derived from the urogenital tract of the mother. The inflammation is less severe.

Chemosis may be present. There are no follicles due to the absence of conjunctival adenoid layer in children. If it is left untreated, a baby infected with chlamydia may develop pneumonitis at a later stage.
- Ophthalmia neonatorum due to **herpes simplex virus** (**typically, HSV 2**):

Timing of onset–It manifests from 1 to 2 weeks after birth.

Discharge–It is characteristically watery.

Features:
- Eyelid and periocular vesicles.
- Dendritic or geographical corneal ulcer.

Investigations

These are tailored to the clinical picture and are as follows:
- Parental prenatal testing for sexually transmitted infection.

- Conjunctival scrapings for PCR in chlamydial and HSV infections.
- Conjunctival smears for Gram and Giemsa staining. Gram –ve intracellular diplococci with polymorphonuclear leucocytes indicate infection with N. gonorrhoeae, whereas polymorphonuclear leucocytes and lymphocytes without bacteria suggest infection with C. trachomatis.
- Conjunctival swabs for culture in N. gonorrhoeae infection.

Differential Diagnosis

As the tears are not secreted early in life, so in case of any discharge from baby's eyes during first month rule out the following:

- Congenital nasolacrimal duct (NLD) obstruction.
- Acute dacryocystitis.
- Congenital glaucoma.

Prophylaxis

As the disease is preventable, prophylaxis is routinely performed and it requires antenatal, natal, and postnatal care.

- Antenatal measures—Include treatment of genital infections in mother.
- Natal measures—Deliveries should be conducted under hygienic conditions taking all aseptic measures. The newborn baby's closed lids should be thoroughly cleansed and dried.
- Postnatal measures—These include use of tetracycline (1%) or erythromycin (0.5%) ointment into the eyes of babies immediately after birth if the mother is suspected to be infected with gonococci or chlamydia.

Treatment

Conjunctival cytology samples and culture sensitivity swabs should be taken before starting treatment.

- Chemical ophthalmia neonatorum is a self-limiting condition and does not require any treatment apart from artificial tears.
- Gonococcal ophthalmia neonatorum needs prompt treatment to prevent complications.

Topical therapy should include:

- Irrigation of eyes with saline till the discharge is eliminated.
- *Bacitracin* eye ointment four times a day. Many authorities advocate use of penicillin but topical penicillin therapy is not reliable because of resistant strains. However, in penicillin-sensitive cases, penicillin drops (5000–10,000 units/mL) should be instilled till the infection is controlled.
- Atropine (1%) ointment is applied in case of corneal involvement.

Systemic therapy:

- Gonococcal conjunctivitis treated systemically with IV or IM ceftriaxone 25 to 50 mg/kg once a day for 7 days is also effective if there is suspicion of penicillinase-producing strain.
  ◊ Injection or
  ◊ Cefotaxime IV or IM.
- Chlamydial neonatal inclusion conjunctivitis responds well to:
  ◊ Systemic (oral) erythromycin for 2 to 3 weeks or azithromycin for 3 days.
  ◊ Topical treatment with tetracycline (1%) or erythromycin (0.5%) eye ointment can be used in addition.
- Herpes simplex neonatal conjunctivitis should be treated with IV acyclovir for 14 days to prevent systemic infection. Topical acyclovir (3%) five times a day may be considered in addition.
- Other bacterial neonatal conjunctivitis (other than gonococcus or chlamydia) is treated with broad-spectrum antibiotic drops and ointments such as chloramphenicol or erythromycin for 2 weeks.

Gentamycin, tobramycin, or fluoroquinolone drops four times a day can be used for Gram –ve organisms.

Granulomatous Conjunctivitis

It is the unilateral, chronic inflammatory granuloma of the conjunctiva. Granulomatous conjunctivitis in association with preauricular lymphadenopathy is known as Parinaud oculo-glandular syndrome.

The common granulomatous conjunctival inflammations leading to granulomatous conjunctivitis are:
- Tuberculosis.
- Sarcoidosis.
- Syphilis.
- Leprosy.
- Tularemia.
- Ophthalmia nodosa.

Parinaud's Oculoglandular Syndrome (POS)

It is characterized by follicular conjunctivitis with ipsilateral preauricular lymphadenopathy. Common causes of POS are listed in **Table 5.6**.

Cat-scratch disease (caused by Bartonella henselae) is the most common cause of POS, which is usually associated with a scratch by a cat or kitten 2 weeks or less before the onset of symptoms.

Clinical Features

Symptoms:
- Redness.
- Foreign body sensation.
- Mucopurulent discharge.

Signs:
- Follicular conjunctivitis.
- Preauricular lymphadenopathy.
- Malaise.
- Fever.
- Skin rash.

Table 5.6 Common causes of POS	
Cause of POS	**Bacteria responsible**
Cat-scratch disease	Bartonella henselae
Tularemia	Francisella tularensis
Syphilis	Treponema pallidum
Tuberculosis	Mycobacterium tuberculosis
Lymphogranuloma venereum	C. trachomatis serotypes L1, 2, 3

Abbreviation: POS, Parinaud's oculoglandular syndrome.

Investigations

- Conjunctival scrapings for staining (Gram, Giemsa, and Acid-fast staining) and culture.
- Complete blood count.
- FTA-ABS.
- Chest X-ray.
- Mantoux test.
- Serological tests for tularemia and cat scratch disease.

Treatment

At present, no definitive treatment is available but NSAIDs and specific treatment for underlying cause may be helpful.

Ophthalmia Nodosa (Caterpillar Hair Conjunctivitis)

It is a granulomatous inflammation of the conjunctiva which is characterized by formation of a nodule on the bulbar conjunctiva.

Etiology

It is due to irritation caused by the retained hair of caterpillars. The disease is, therefore, common in summers.

Histopathological examination

It reveals hair surrounded by giant cells and lymphocytes.

Treatment

It consists of excision biopsy of the nodule.

■ Noninfective Conjunctivitis

Allergic Conjunctivitis

Hypersensitivity is a set of undesirable reactions produced by the body's immune system, including allergies and autoimmunity, in response to the foreign substance (allergens). It consists of four types: I, II, III, and IV. Type I, II, and III are antibody-mediated and type IV is cell-mediated. Allergic conjunctivitis is a type I (immediate) hypersensitivity reaction. In type I hypersensitivity, B-cells are stimulated to produce IgE antibodies specific to an antigen (**Fig. 5.17**).

During sensitization, IgE antibodies bind to the receptors on the surface of tissue mast cells and blood basophils. These mast cells coated by IgE antibodies are called "sensitized" (**Flowchart 5.2**). Mast cells are particularly abundant in the conjunctival stroma, especially at the limbus.

Distinguishing Features

Allergic conjunctivitis shows the following distinguishing features from the infective conjunctivitis:

- Itching—It is a prominent symptom.
- Hyperaemia—It is less marked.
- Discharge—The discharge is watery, not purulent, and often contains eosinophils.
- Allergic conjunctivitis shows a tendency toward recurrences.

The hallmark of allergic conjunctivitis is itching. A patient having red itchy eyes with no palpable preauricular lymph nodes is most probably afflicted with allergy.

Symptoms

- Itching.
- Watering.
- Foreign body sensation.
- Redness.
- Lid swelling.

Treatment

The pharmacological agents may include:

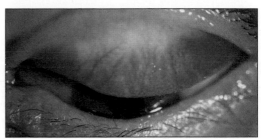

Fig. 5.17 Seasonal allergic conjunctivitis. Source: Clinical entities. In: Hoang-Xuan T, Baudouin C, Creuzot-Garcher C, ed. Inflammatory diseases of the conjuctiva. 1st edition. Thieme; 2001.

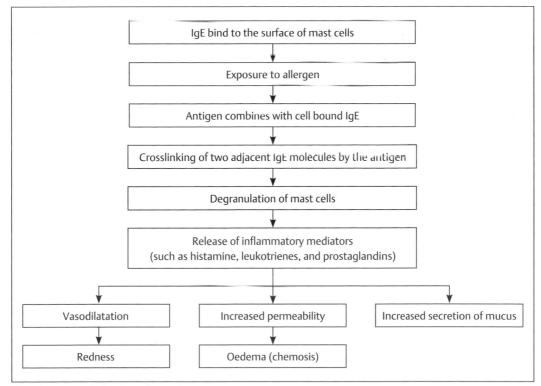

Flowchart 5.2 Mechanism of sensitivity reaction.

Topical vasoconstrictors

These provide short-term relief to vascular congestion and redness. These include:

- Naphazoline.
- Phenylephrine.
- Oxymetazoline.

Generally, the common problem with vasoconstrictors is that they *may cause rebound conjunctival congestion*, inflammation, and dryness. *These pharmacological agents are ineffective against severe ocular allergies.*

Antihistamines

Systemic and/or topical antihistamines may be given to relieve acute symptoms due to interaction of histamine at ocular H_1 and H_2 receptors.

Systemic antihistamines (chlorpheniramine, astemizole, cetrizine, and loratadine) often relieve ocular allergic symptoms but patients may experience systemic side effects such as drowsiness and dry mouth.

Topical antihistamines include:

- *Emedastine.*
- *Epinastine.*
- *Levocabastine.*

Mast cells stabilizers

Mast cell stabilizers do not relieve existing symptoms and are to be used on a prophylactic basis to prevent mast cell degranulation with subsequent exposure to the allergen. Therefore, they need to be used long-term in conjunction with various other classes of medication. Common mast cell stabilizers include *sodium cromoglycate* and *lodoxamide.*

Dual action drugs

These agents have both antihistamine and mast cell stabilizing activities. These include *olopatadine, azelastine,* and *ketotifen.*

NSAIDs

These act on the cyclo-oxygenase metabolic pathway and include *ketorolac* tromethamine and *diclofenac* sodium. They can provide symptomatic relief.

Corticosteroids

These inhibit the arachidonic acid released from phospholipids by inhibiting phospholipase A_2. Corticosteroids effectively block both cyclo-oxygenase and lipoxygenase pathways in contrast to NSAIDs which act only on the cyclo-oxygenase pathway (**Flowchart 5.3**).

Corticosteroids include:

- Prednisolone.
- Dexamethasone.
- Hydrocortisone.
- Fluorometholone.
- Loteprednol.
- Rimexolone.
- Medrysone.

Relatively weak steroids such as rimexolone, medrysone, loteprednol, and fluorometholone tend to have fewer ocular side effects. In contrast, agents such as prednisolone acetate are more potent and have a higher incidence of side effects (raised intraocular pressure [IOP] and posterior subcapsular cataract).

A general rule of thumb: *topical steroids should be prescribed only for a short period of time and for severe cases that do not respond to conventional therapy.*

Immune modulators

Cyclosporin may be indicated if steroids are ineffective or poorly tolerated.

Prophylaxis

- Prevent exposure to the allergen.
- Frequent use of cold compresses.
- Artificial tears.
- Sunglasses.

Various Types of Allergic Conjunctivitis

Type I (immediate) hypersensitivity reaction is the most common allergic response of the eye. There is evidence of an element of type IV (delayed) hypersensitivity in, at least, some forms. Ocular example of type IV hypersensitivity includes phlyctenular keratoconjunctivitis.

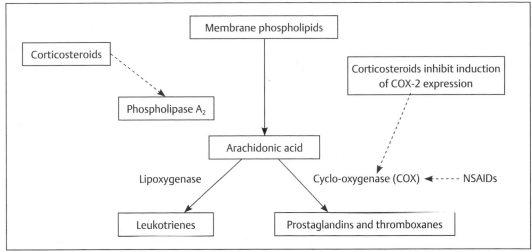

Flowchart 5.3   Mechanisms of action of corticosteroids and NSAIDs.

Allergic conjunctivitis may be divided into:
- Seasonal allergic conjunctivitis (SAC).
- Perennial allergic conjunctivitis (PAC).
- Vernal keratoconjunctivitis (VKC).
- Atopic keratoconjunctivitis (AKC).
- Giant papillary conjunctivitis (GPC).
- Phlyctenular keratoconjunctivitis.
- Contact allergic (toxic) conjunctivitis.

Seasonal and Perennial Allergic Conjunctivitis (SAC and PAC)

Allergens
Since the conjunctiva is a mucosal surface similar to the nasal mucosa, the same allergens that trigger allergic rhinitis may be involved in the pathogenesis of allergic conjunctivitis. Common airborne antigens include dust, molds, pollen, grass, and weeds.

The main distinction between SAC and PAC, as implied by the names, is the timing of symptoms.

Individuals with SAC typically have symptoms of acute allergic conjunctivitis for a different period of time, that is,
- In spring– the predominant airborne allergen in this period is tree pollen.
- In summer– the predominant airborne allergen in this period is grass pollen.

- In autumn– the predominant airborne allergen in this period is weed pollen.

Typically, persons with SAC are symptom-free during the winter months because of decreased airborne transmission of these allergens.

Individuals with PAC have symptoms throughout the year, generally worse in autumn.

Common household allergens such as dust, mite, and pet dander are usually the causes of PAC.

Clinical features
Symptoms:
- Ocular itching.
- Redness.
- Burning.
- Watering.
- Sneezing and nasal discharge.

Signs:
- Conjunctival congestion.
- Chemosis.
- Eyelid edema.

Edema is generally believed to be the direct result of increased vascular permeability caused by the release of histamine from conjunctival mast cells.

Treatment

The following classes of medication may be effective:

- Artificial tears for mild symptoms.
- Mast cells stabilizers, for example, sodium cromoglycate.
- Topical antihistamines, for example, *emedastine, epinastine, and levocabastine.*
- Dual action drugs, for example, olopatadine.
- NSAIDs.

Topical steroids are effective but rarely necessary.

Vernal Keratoconjunctivitis (VKC) or Spring Catarrh (OP3.5)

VKC is chronic, recurrent, and bilateral inflammation of the conjunctiva in which both IgE and cell-mediated immune mechanisms (Type I and Type IV hypersensitivity reactions) play the roles. It is more common in tropical climate, less common in temperate zones, and almost nonexistent in cold climate. Predisposing factors include:

Sex—It primarily affects boys.

Age—It affects children between 5 to 15 years. More than 90% cases show remission by the late teens.

Types– the disease is usually seen in two forms:
- Palpebral.
- Limbal.

Both forms may coexist in a patient.

Clinical Features
Symptoms:
- Severe itching.
- Foreign body sensation.
- Thick stringy mucoid discharge.
- Lacrimation.
- Photophobia.
- Burning.
- Increased blinking.

Signs:

Palpebral **VKC**—It primarily involves the upper tarsal conjunctiva. It is characterized by the presence of giant papillae. Giant papillae are large, polygonal with flat top, and are often described as "**cobblestone papillae.**" The papillae consist chiefly of dense fibrous tissue with thickened epithelium over them. It imparts a bluish–white or milky color to the papillae. Mucous deposits between the giant papillae. In severe cases, large papillae may cause mechanical ptosis. The papillae may also appear in the lower palpebral conjunctiva (**Fig. 5.18a**).

Limbal **VKC**—The limbal or bulbar VKC is frequently seen in black races. It is characterized by papillae at the limbus which have a gelatinous appearance. They are commonly associated with multiple white spots (**Horner–Trantas dots**) which are accumulations of degenerated epithelial cells and eosinophils (**Fig. 5.18b**).

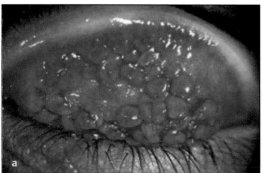 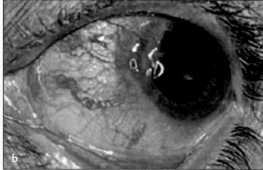

Fig. 5.18 (a) Vernal conjunctivitis (palpebral), **(b)** Vernal conjunctivitis (limbal). Source: Superior limbic keratoconjunctivitis. In: Agarwal A, Jacob S, ed. Color atlas of ophthalmology. The quick-reference manual for diagnosis and treatment. 2nd edition. Thieme; 2009.

Both types of vernal conjunctivitis are complicated by the following five types of *corneal lesions*:

- **Superficial punctate keratitis** occurs in the upper part of cornea.
- As the areas of superficial punctate keratitis coalesce, they may result in **epithelial erosions** and a **shield ulcer** which is typically shallow. It is pathognomonic of VKC.
- Subepithelial scarring.
- Another type of corneal involvement is **pseudogerontoxon** which is a degenerative lesion in the peripheral cornea adjacent to a previously inflamed segment of the limbus. It resembles a local area of arcus senilis with a cupid's bow appearance.
- **Vernal corneal plaques,** resulting from the coating of epithelial erosions with mucous and calcium phosphate. Keratoconus is more common in VKC.

Treatment

It is purely symptomatic and depends on the intensity and the severity of the disease. It includes:

- Cold compression.
- Sunglasses.
- The patient must be advised to stop eye rubbing as rubbing further induces mast cell degranulation and release of histamine. It sets up a vicious cycle.
- *Topical combined antihistamine and vasoconstrictor* may offer relief in mild VKC.
- Antihistamine reduces itching and vasoconstrictor reduces the redness and chemosis.
- *Mast cell stabilizers* (sodium cromoglycate) are administered twice daily in mild to moderate VKC. They reduce the need for steroids but are seldom effective in isolation. They are safe for long-term use.
- *Olopatadine* has combined mast cell stabilizing and antihistaminic actions and is prescribed twice daily.
- *Mucolytic agents* such as acetylcysteine dissolves mucous filaments and deposits and may provide relief in VKC.
- *Topical steroids*:
  - ◊ These are the most effective drugs and often required in moderate to severe VKC.

- ◊ Steroids must be reserved for severe cases that do not respond to conventional therapy.
- ◊ They should be prescribed at the lowest effective concentration and for a short duration due to potential side effects. Relatively weak steroids (fluorometholone, loteprednol, or rimexolone) must be used as these have lower potency with fewer ocular side effects.

Instillation of steroids should be tapered gradually

- To avoid steroid-induced complications, a pulse (intermittent) therapy is generally recommended, such as 1% prednisolone acetate is prescribed every two hours for 5 to 7 days followed by a rapid taper over 10 days. This may be repeated if symptoms recur.
- The indiscriminate use of steroids, particularly self-medication by the patient, must be discouraged.
- Antibiotics must be used in conjunction with steroids to prevent bacterial infection.
- 2% cyclosporine may be indicated if steroids are ineffective or poorly tolerated.
- A *supratarsal steroid injection* (triamcinolone acetonide 40 mg/mL) may be considered in severe palpebral disease or for noncompliant patients.

Atopic Keratoconjunctivitis (AKC)

AKC is a bilateral inflammation of the conjunctiva and eyelids, which has a strong association with atopic dermatitis and asthma. It is seen in adulthood (30–50 years). It is a type I hypersensitivity response. AKC tends to be more chronic and severe than VKC (**Fig. 5.19**).

Clinical Features

Symptoms: These are similar to those of VKC but are more severe.

Signs: AKC may affect eyelid skin and lid margins, conjunctiva, cornea, and lens.

- **Eyelids**—The skin of the eyelids may exhibit eczematoid dermatitis with dry,

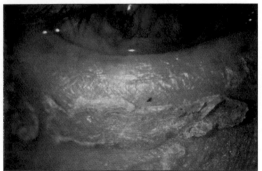

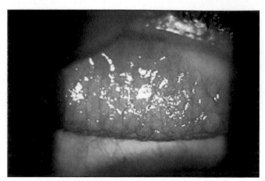

Fig. 5.19 Atopic keratoconjunctivitis (AKC). Source: Clinical entities. In: Hoang-Xuan T, Baudouin C, Creuzot-Garcher C, ed. Inflammatory diseases of the conjuctiva. 1st edition. Thieme; 2001.

Fig. 5.20 Giant papillary conjunctivitis.

scaly, and inflamed skin. Lid margins may show meibomian gland dysfunction and keratinization. Staphylococcal colonization of eyelid margins is very common and may result in blepharitis.

- **Conjunctiva**—The conjunctiva may show chemosis and typically a papillary reaction, which is more prominent in the inferior tarsal conjunctiva, in contrast to that seen in vernal keratoconjunctivitis. Hyperplasia of limbal regions may result in a gelatinous thickening, similar to the limbal variant of VKC. Fibrosis or scarring of the conjunctiva may result in symblepharon formation.
- **Cornea**—Corneal involvement ranges from punctate epithelial keratopathy early in the course of the disease to neovascularization, stromal scarring, and possibly ulceration. Keratoconus is common, as with VKC, and may be secondary to chronic ocular rubbing.
- **Lens**– lenticular changes in AKC include anterior or posterior subcapsular cataract formation. There may be an association with chronic use of topical corticosteroids.

Treatment

Treatment of patients with AKC is similar to that of VKC, that is, topical mast cell stabilizers and topical corticosteroids provide significant relief of symptoms. Topical steroids used in a pulsed

fashion may help in controlling symptoms and mast cell stabilizers have to be used for several weeks. Systemic cyclosporine may be indicated if the disease is severe and steroids are ineffective.

Giant Papillary Conjunctivitis (GPC)

GPC is an immune-mediated inflammatory disorder affecting the superior tarsal conjunctiva. As the name implies, the primary finding is the presence of "giant" papillae, which are typically greater than 0.3 mm in diameter (**Fig. 5.20**). The underlying mechanism is a hypersensitivity reaction of type I and type IV.

Etiology

It is believed that GPC represents an immunological reaction to a variety of foreign bodies, which may cause prolonged mechanical irritation to the superior tarsal conjunctiva. These include:

- Contact lenses (hard and soft) are the most common irritant.
- Ocular prostheses.
- Extruded scleral buckles.
- Exposed sutures following previous surgical intervention.

Clinical Features

Symptoms:
- Itching.
- Watering.
- Foreign body sensation.

- Photophobia.
- Redness.
- Blurring.
- Increased mucus production.

Signs:
- Superior tarsal hyperemia.
- Macro papillae (0.3–1.0 mm) and giant papillae (>1 mm in diameter) on superior tarsal conjunctiva.
- Another clinical sign of GPC may be chronic limbal vascularization due to hypoxia associated with prolonged and persistent use of contact lenses.

Treatment
It consists of:
- Removal of stimulus.
  ◊ Discontinuation of contact lens or ocular prosthetics.
  ◊ Removal of exposed sutures or scleral buckle.
- Effective cleaning of contact lens or prosthesis.
- Topical treatment.
  ◊ Mast cell stabilizers.
  ◊ Artificial tears.
  ◊ Antihistaminic and decongestant drops.
- Topical steroids can be used for the acute phase and for a short while.
- Subtarsal injection of long-acting steroid in severe cases (provided the patient is not a steroid responder).

Contact Allergic (toxic) Conjunctivitis

Etiology
Certain chemicals and toxins cause an allergic or toxic effect. The causative agent may be:
- *Ocular medications*—Atropine, gentamicin, neomycin, tobramycin, antivirals, epine-phrine, pilocarpine, brimonidine and prostaglandin analogues, etc.
- *Preservatives*—Benzalkonium chloride, thiomersal, etc.
- *Chemicals*—Chemicals in cosmetics applied around the eyes and hair spray.

Clinical Features
All these chemicals and toxins can produce follicular hypertrophy, predominantly on the inferior tarsal conjunctiva and fornix. Usually the patient presents with a puffy swollen eyelid. The corneal staining with fluorescein may show punctuate epithelial keratopathy of inferior cornea.

Treatment
- Removal or discontinuation of the precipitant.
- Use of preservative-free drugs.
- Topical lubricant eye drops.
- Sometimes a mild topical steroid ointment may be required.

Phlyctenular Conjunctivitis

It is an allergic response of conjunctival and corneal epithelium to some endogenous allergens to which they have become sensitized.

Etiology
It is a delayed hypersensitivity (type IV) reaction to endogenous microbial protein which may be either tubercular or staphylococcal protein. These children suffer from mild, long-standing infections of tonsils.

Predisposing Factors
- *Age*—It is common between 5 and 15 years of age.
- *Undernourishment*—The disease is common in malnourished and debilitated children.
- *Season*—Its incidence is high in spring and summer.

Clinical Features
Symptoms:
- Discomfort in the eye.
- Irritation.
- Reflex watering.

The disease may be complicated by mucopurulent conjunctivitis due to secondary infection.

Signs:

In phlyctenular conjunctivitis, the characteristic lesion is phlycten or phlyctens (blebs) which are single or multiple, small, round, yellow or gray, elevated nodules found at or near the limbus. Exudation and infiltration of leucocytes into deeper layers of conjunctiva leads to nodule formation in which central cells are polymorphonuclear and peripheral cells are lymphocytes. Neighboring blood vessels dilate and proliferate.

The phlyctens are rare on the palpebral conjunctiva. Vessels around the phlyctens on bulbar conjunctiva are congested (*simple phlyctenular conjunctivitis*).

Overlying epithelium on large phlycten undergoes necrosis and ulceration, leading to severe pustular conjunctivitis (*necrotizing phlyctenular conjunctivitis*). The conjunctival phlyctens heal without the formation of a scar. Phlyctens may be multiple, arranged in the ring form (*miliary phlyctenular conjunctivitis*), and form a ring ulcer on necrosis and ulceration.

When phlycten occurs on the cornea (corneal phlycten), it often causes pain and photophobia. Vascularization is seen around the phlycten. When ulceration occurs in the corneal phlycten, it forms a fascicular ulcer with prominent vascularization and undergoes fibrovascular corneal scarring with thinning.

Clinical Types
- Phlyctenular conjunctivitis (conjunctiva alone is involved).
- Phlyctenular keratoconjunctivitis (both conjunctiva and cornea are involved).
- Phlyctenular keratitis (cornea alone is involved).

Differential Diagnosis
Phlyctenular conjunctivitis must be differentiated from:
- Episcleritis.
- Conjunctival foreign body granuloma.
- Inflamed pinguecula.
- Filtering bleb after glaucoma surgery.

Investigations
These are indicated in multiple or recurrent phlyctens. These include:

- TLC, DLC, ESR, Mantoux test, X-ray chest to exclude tubercular infection.
- Stool examination for ova, parasite, and cyst to rule out parasitic infestation.
- ENT consultation to rule out tonsillitis and adenoiditis.

Treatment
- Encourage use of dark glasses.
- Topical steroid drops or ointment.
- Antibiotic drops should be added for associated secondary infection.
- Cycloplegics are added when cornea is involved.
- Treatment of causative factor, for example, treatment of tuberculosis, tonsils, adenoids, or parasitic infestation.

Conjunctivitis in Blistering Mucocutaneous Diseases

Mucocutaneous blistering diseases comprise ocular cicatricial pemphigoid (OCP), Stevens–Johnson syndrome, Reiter's syndrome, and Behçet's syndrome.

Ocular Cicatricial Pemphigoid

It generally affects the patients above 50 years of age. It is characterized by bilateral conjunctivitis of insidious onset with remissions and exacerbations.

Clinical Features

Symptoms:
- Foreign body sensation.
- Redness.
- Watering.
- Photophobia.

Signs:
Ocular features—There is progressive cicatrization leading to:
- Shrinkage of conjunctiva.
- Formation of inferior symblepharon.
- Shallowing of the inferior fornix.
- Severe dry eye due to destruction of goblet cells and accessory glands with occlusion of main lacrimal ductules.

- Superficial punctate keratopathy.
- Entropion.
- Trichiasis.
- Peripheral corneal vascularization.
- Keratinization and conjunctivalization of corneal surface due to epithelial stem cell failure.
- Consequent opacification of the cornea.

Systemic features—Mucosal involvement is very common and most frequently oral. Blisters may be found in nose, mouth, palate, pharynx, esophagus, anus, vagina, and urethra. Skin lesions are less common.

Treatment

Systemic
- Systemic immunosuppressive therapy.
- Systemic steroids.

Local
- Artificial tears.
- Topical steroids may be used.
- Retinoic acid may reduce keratinization.
- Contact lenses may be used to protect cornea.

Reconstructive surgery
It should be considered when the active disease is controlled. It includes:
- Mucous membrane grafts.
- Limbal stems and transfer for corneal re-epithelialization.
- Keratoprosthesis for end-stage corneal disease.

Stevens–Johnson Syndrome

Stevens–Johnson syndrome is uncommon but potentially lethal. It may be associated with severe eye problems. It causes painful blisters and lesions on the skin and mucous membranes and is most commonly caused by drug reactions.

Etiology

It is a type II hypersensitivity reaction usually due to:
- Drugs—Sulphonamides, antibiotics, NSAIDs, and anticonvulsants.

- Infections due to—Mycoplasma pneumoniae and herpes simplex virus.

Clinical Features

Ocular features
- Eyelid:
  ◊ Cicatricial entropion.
  ◊ Trichiasis.
  ◊ Keratinization of lid margins.
- Conjunctiva:
  ◊ Pseudo-membranous conjunctivitis.
  ◊ Conjunctival cicatrization.
  ◊ Shortening of fornices.
  ◊ Symblepharon formation.
- Cornea:
  ◊ Keratinization.
  ◊ Vascularization.
  ◊ Scarring.

Cornea is involved as a result of the primary inflammation as well as cicatricial entropion and aberrant lashes.
- Severe dry eye as a result of fibrosis of lacrimal gland ductules and loss of goblet cells.

Systemic features

Mucosal involvement—Blisters may involve the mucous membranes of mouth and the eyes.

Skin lesions—These are vesicular, erythematous, and epidermal necrosis.

Treatment

Ocular treatment
- Topical preservative-free lubricants.
- Antibiotics to prevent secondary bacterial infections.
- Lysis of developing symblepharon with a glass rod coated with antibiotic or plain paraffin ointment in the fornices.
- Punctal occlusion.
- Topical transretinoic acid may reverse keratinization.
- Bandage contact lens to protect cornea from trichiasis.
- Mucous membrane graft.

- Transplantation of limbal stem cells.
- Keratoprosthesis in end-stage disease.

Systemic treatment
- Discontinuation of drug and treatment of suspected infection.
- Immunosuppressive therapy.
- Systemic antibiotics as prophylaxis against systemic infection.

■ Degenerative Changes in Conjunctiva

■ Concretions

These occur as elevated, minute, hard, yellow spots in the palpebral conjunctiva. The term concretion is a misnomer as they never become calcareous.

Etiology

These are due to the accumulation of epithelial cells and inspissated mucus in depressions known as Henle glands. They are common in elderly persons suffering from trachoma or chronic conjunctivitis.

Clinical Features

Foreign body sensation is the main symptom. On rubbing, a corneal abrasion may develop.

Treatment

It includes removal of concretions with a sharp needle after topical anesthesia.

■ Pinguecula

It is a degeneration of the bulbar conjunctiva in the interpalpebral zone (**Fig. 5.21**). It is usually found among elderly people.

Etiology

It occurs among those exposed to dusty and windy climate, strong sunlight, and ultraviolet (UV) exposure. It is considered as a precursor of pterygium.

Pathology

Histopathology of pinguecula reveals *elastotic degeneration* of collagen fibers of conjunctival stroma, and deposition of amorphous hyaline material. However, the epithelium appears normal.

Clinical Features

It is usually bilateral, symptom-free, and characterized by triangular, yellowish–white patch near the limbus, commonly the nasal limbus. In congested conjunctiva, it stands out as an avascular patch.

Complications

- Inflammations.
- Conversion into pterygium.

Treatment

Most cases of pinguecula do not require any treatment. If desired, excision can be performed. Artificial tears or lubricants can be prescribed for ocular irritation.

Prophylaxis

Avoid exposure to sunlight, dust, smoke, etc.

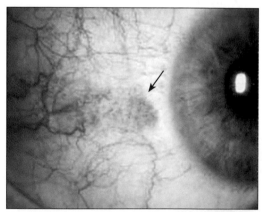

Fig. 5.21 Pinguecula (*arrow*). Source: Pinguecula. In: Lang G, ed. Ophthalmology. A pocket textbook atlas. 2nd edition. Thieme; 2006.

Pterygium (OP3.6, OP4.5)

It is a degenerative condition of subconjunctival tissue which grows onto the cornea as fibrovascular tissue (**Fig. 5.22**).

Location

It occurs in palpebral fissure area, usually on the nasal side.

Etiology

It is common in hot climates and is associated with chronic dryness and UV light exposure, such as parts of Australia, Middle East, south Africa, and Texas. Outdoor work in situations with high-light reflectivity, including sand and water, enhances pterygium development. Currently, pterygium is believed to be caused by damage to limbal stem cells by UV light and overproduction of growth factor, resulting in proliferation of fibrovascular tissue. A pterygium frequently follows a pinguecula.

Pathology

Pathologic changes include:
- Elastotic degeneration of collagen.
- Proliferation of fibrovascular tissue beneath the conjunctival epithelium.
- Destruction of Bowman's membrane and superficial corneal stroma.

Types of Pterygium

Progressive pterygium—It is thick and vascular and encroaches upon cornea with infiltrates (Fuch's

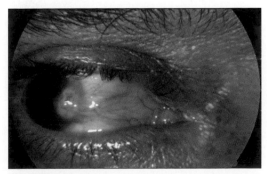

Fig. 5.22 Pterygium.

spots). It is loosely adherent to sclera across its entire length.

Regressive pterygium—When pterygium stops growing, infiltration and vascularization disappears (but pterygium never disappears) and it becomes thin and pale.

Clinical Features

In the early stages, it is often asymptomatic, except for mild irritation, redness, and cosmetic disfigurement. Progression may cause diminution of vision due to astigmatism and serious visual impairment when it involves pupillary area. **Table 5.7** lists the various grades of pterygium.

Parts

Pterygium appears as a triangular fold of conjunctiva encroaching the cornea with:
- Head (apex of the pterygium, typically raised and highly vascular).
- Body (flashy elevated portion congested with tortuous vessels).
- Neck—It is the limbal part connecting the main body with head.

Differential Diagnosis

Pterygium must be differentiated from pseudopterygium, which is a conjunctival adhesion to cornea (**Table 5.8**).

Treatment

Surgical excision is the only treatment but recurrence is the main problem.

Indications
- Cosmetic reasons,
- Progression toward visual axis, that is, grade II and III pterygium.
- Restriction of ocular motility.
- Excessive astigmatism due to it.

Procedures
- Surgical excision with bare sclera (D'Ombren's operation).
- Transplantation of pterygium in the lower fornix (Mc Reynolds operation).

Table 5.7 Grades of pterygium

Grade of pterygium	Extension on cornea
Grade 1	Extends <2 mm onto the cornea. A deposit of iron may be seen in corneal epithelium anterior to advancing head of pterygium and is called Stocker's line.
Grade 2	Involve up to 4 mm of cornea and may induce astigmatism.
Grade 3	Invade >4 mm of cornea and involve visual axis. Extensive lesions may be associated with subconjunctival fibrosis resulting in mild restriction in ocular motility.

Table 5.8 Differentiating features of true and pseudopterygium

True pterygium	Pseudopterygium
• It is adherent to underlying structures throughout.	• It is fixed only at its apex to cornea.
• Location—It is always in palpebral aperture.	• It may be present at any site.
• Probe cannot be passed under it.	• Probe can be passed under it.
• Progressive or stationary.	• Almost always stationary.
• Etiology—Degenerative process.	• It is secondary to previous trauma or inflammation such as peripheral corneal ulceration.

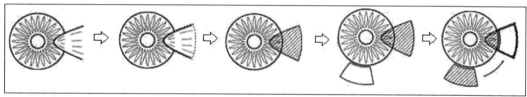

Fig. 5.23 Pterygium excision with free conjunctival autograft.

The above operations are not performed now. Currently, procedures used are:

- Pterygium excision with free conjunctival autograft.
- Pterygium excision with amniotic membrane transplantation.

Free *conjunctival autograft* should not be taken from upper region, because it may adversely affect the future glaucoma surgery, but should be obtained from lower conjunctiva. Recurrence is reduced with this technique and presently it is preferred technique (**Fig. 5.23**). *Amniotic membrane transplant* is used when there is extensive damage sustained in conjunctiva. For deep extensive lesions, peripheral lamellar keratoplasty may be required.

Adjunctive treatment to minimize recurrence

To reduce recurrence of pterygium, postoperative mitomycin C has been tried but late scleral necrosis may occur.

The Cornea

Anatomy and Physiology of Cornea 117

Pathological Changes in Cornea 120

Symptoms of Corneal Diseases 124

Evaluation of Corneal Diseases 124

Inflammation of Cornea 127

Corneal Degenerations 154

Corneal Dystrophies 156

Ectatic Conditions of Cornea 161

■ Anatomy and Physiology of Cornea

Cornea is **avascular and transparent**. Its horizontal and vertical diameters are 12 mm and 11.5 mm, respectively (**Fig. 6.1**). Its thickness at the center and periphery is 0.5 mm and 0.7 mm, respectively. Radius of curvature of anterior surface of cornea (in central region) is 7.8 mm, while that of posterior surface is 6.5 mm. Its refractive index is 1.376 (≈1.38). Cornea provides 3/4th of the total refractive power of the eye. Refractive power of anterior convex surface of cornea is +48.8 D; refractive power of posterior concave surface is −5.8 D, so the total refractive power of cornea is 43.0 D. The junction of cornea with sclera is called **limbus**. The corneal curvature is greater than the rest of the globe. Cornea is *devoid of lymphatic channels.*

■ Histology

Histologically, cornea consists of five layers (**Fig. 6.2**):

1. Epithelium (anterior most).
2. Bowman's membrane.
3. Stroma or substantia propria.
4. Descemet's membrane.
5. Endothelium (posterior most).

Epithelium

It may be regarded as continuation of conjunctiva over cornea. Embryologically, it is derived from surface ectoderm at 5 to 6 weeks of gestation. Characteristic features of epithelium are as follows:

- It is stratified and *4 to 6 cell layers thick.*
- The epithelial cells contain microvilli with glycocalyx layer which facilitate adsorption of mucinous portion of tear film and

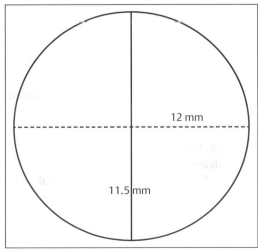

Fig. 6.1 Diameters of cornea.

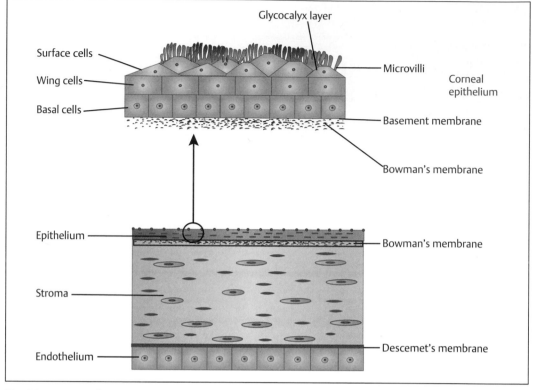

Fig. 6.2 Anatomy of cornea.

hydrophilic spreading of tear film with each eyelid blink. *Loss of glycocalyx from injury or disease results in loss of stability of tear film.*

- Superficial cells undergo desquamation and are replaced by deeper cells of corneal epithelium. *Basal cells are the only corneal epithelial cells capable of mitosis. Because of excellent ability to regenerate, epithelium does not scar as a result of inflammation.*
- Tight junctions between its cells provide *barrier function and* restrict entry of tears into intercellular spaces. *Thus, healthy epithelial surface repels dyes such as fluorescein or Rose Bengal.*
- *Epithelial regeneration*: Epithelial stem cells (undifferentiated pluripotent cells) are principally localized to limbal basal epithelium and serve as an important source

of new corneal epithelium. Junctional barrier prevents conjunctival tissue from growing on the cornea. So, *dysfunction or deficiency of limbal stem cells results in the following* chronic epithelial defects:

◊ Overgrowth of conjunctival epithelium onto the corneal surface.

◊ Vascularization.

These problems can be *treated by limbal cell transplantation.*

Bowman's Membrane

It is an acellular structure which, once destroyed, does not regenerate.

Stroma (Substantia Propria)

Stroma forms 90% of total corneal thickness. It may be regarded as forward continuation of sclera. It is composed of collagen fibrils, forming lamellae which are loosely adherent to each other and regularly arranged in many layers. The layers crisscross at approximately right angles to each other. Corneal lamellae become continuous with scleral lamellae at limbus. *The layered structure of stroma results in corneal splitting, as in superficial keratectomy.* Ground substance occupies the space in between lamellae and is composed of glycosaminoglycans (mucopolysaccharides). Corneal cells and **keratocytes** are found between lamellae which are collagen-producing fibroblasts. *Corneal stroma is markedly hydrophilic due to osmotic force of stromal glycosaminoglycans (GAG).*

Descemet's Membrane

It is a thin elastic membrane secreted by endothelium throughout life. It is composed of collagen fibrils and separates corneal stroma from endothelium. Unlike Bowman's membrane, it can regenerate (regenerated by endothelial cells). It is quite resistant to inflammatory process of cornea. Therefore, **descematocele** can maintain integrity of eye for long after all other layers of cornea are destroyed. It fuses with trabecular meshwork. The fusion site is known as *Schwalbe's line* which defines the end of Descemet's membrane and start of the trabecular meshwork.

Endothelium

It is derived from neural crest cells. It consists of single layer of flat hexagonal cells and appears as honey comb mosaic (**Fig. 6.3**). It contains a high-density of Na⁺–K⁺ ATPase pump. It secretes Descemet's membrane throughout life. It cannot regenerate but adjacent cells slide to fill in a damaged area. Endothelial cell density decreases with advancing age and declines from 3,000–4,000 cells/mm² to 2,500 cells/mm² in adults. At a cell density of approximately 500 cells/mm², corneal edema develops. It is examined by a specular microscope.

The primary physiological role of endothelium is fluid regulation in corneal stroma. This function is most important as it keeps the cornea clear.

■ Blood Supply of Cornea

Normal cornea is an avascular tissue which gets its nourishment from:

- Capillaries at limbus which are derived from episcleral branches of the anterior ciliary arteries.
- Aqueous by diffusion.
- Oxygen dissolved in tear film.

■ Nerve Supply of Cornea

Cornea is supplied by the ophthalmic division of the trigeminal nerve (v_1) through *long ciliary nerves* (**Fig. 6.4**).

Course

Long ciliary nerves pierce sclera posterior to limbus and form annular plexus (pericorneal plexus). Branches from annular plexus travel radially to enter the corneal stroma and lose their myelin sheaths. They divide into anterior group, which forms subepithelial plexus, and posterior group, which forms stromal plexus. Branches from subepithelial plexus pierce Bowman's membrane to form intraepithelial plexus. *Due to rich nerve supply, cornea is extremely sensitive structure.* In eyes with corneal abrasions or bullous keratopathy, direct stimulation of these nerve axons causes pain, reflex lacrimation, and photophobia.

■ Metabolism of Cornea

Energy is needed for normal functions of a tissue. In cornea, energy is needed for maintenance of its

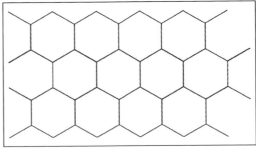

Fig. 6.3 Honey comb mosaic appearance of endothelium of cornea.

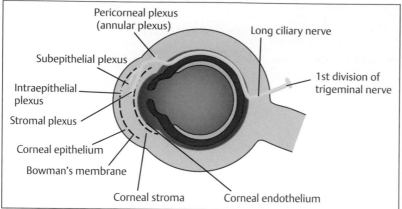

Fig. 6.4 Nerve supply of cornea.

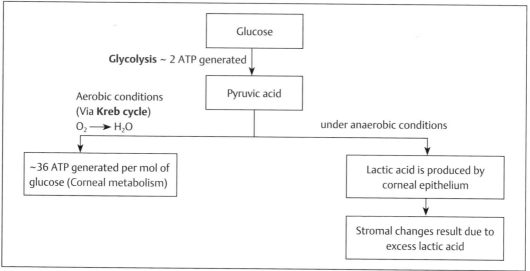

Flowchart 6.1 Metabolism of cornea. Abbreviation: ATP, adenosine triphosphate.

transparency and dehydration. Energy in the form of adenosine triphosphate (ATP) is generated by breakdown of *glucose* and utilization of *oxygen* (**Flowchart 6.1**).

Source of glucose for cornea is aqueous (90%), tears and limbal capillaries (10%).

Source of oxygen for cornea—Most of the O_2 in cornea is consumed by epithelium and endothelium. *Epithelium* gets much of its O_2 from limbal capillaries or precorneal tear film. *Endothelium* gets most of its O_2 from aqueous humor, and the cornea is **mainly aerobic**.

If access of O_2 to epithelium is abolished by tight contact lenses or replacement of air in goggles with N_2, cornea swells and become cloudy due to production of lactic acid by corneal epithelium under anaerobic conditions.

Pathological Changes in Cornea

The pathological changes in cornea can be categorized in (**Table 6.1**) as follows:

- Loss of transparency (corneal edema and corneal opacity).
- Vascularization of cornea.

Table 6.1 Difference between normal and pathological cornea

Normal cornea	Pathological cornea
Transparent	Loss of transparency due to corneal edema and corneal opacity
Avascular	Vascularization of cornea
Absence of pigments	Corneal pigmentation

- Pigmentation of cornea.
- Corneal filaments.
- Prominent corneal nerves.
- Infiltrates.

■ Transparency of Cornea (OP4.3, 4.5)

Normal cornea is a transparent structure. Corneal transparency occurs due to *regular arrangement of collagen fibrils* (corneal lamellae) in stroma, *avascularity* of cornea and *relative state of dehydration*. Water content of normal cornea is approximately 78%. It is maintained at a steady level by a balance between various factors. Disturbance of any of these factors leads to corneal edema.

Corneal Edema (OP4.3, 4.5)

It is the accumulation of fluid in the cornea. Corneal edema may be epithelial or stromal and can affect the entire cornea.

Factors Leading to Corneal Edema

Following factors are responsible for the development of corneal edema:
- Stromal GAG: Osmotic force of stromal GAG plays a role in hydration. *Accumulation of GAG in the cornea (as in Mucopolysaccharidoses)* leads to corneal edema.
- Intraocular pressure (IOP): *Raised* IOP (≥ 50 mm Hg) often results in corneal edema due to easy passage of aqueous through corneal stroma but its escape is retarded by epithelium and accumulation of fluid in basal cells of epithelium results in epithelial edema.

- Integrity of endothelium and epithelium: *Damage to epithelium or endothelium* due to any cause results in corneal swelling and loss of transparency. However, *damage to endothelium* is far more serious which can occur during intraocular surgery/postuveitis.
- Corneal endothelial Na^+–K^+ ATPase pump and intracellular carbonic anhydrase pathway in endothelium: Activity in both these pathways produces a net flux from stroma to aqueous. *Inhibition of endothelial Na^+–K^+ ATPase pump, as in Fuch's endothelial dystrophy*, leads to corneal edema.

If edema lasts for a long period, epithelium is raised into large vesicles or bullae (vesicular or bullous keratopathy). Bullae periodically burst and symptoms like ocular pain and irritation occur.

Clinical Features

Corneal edema presents with symptoms like impairment of vision, photophobia, watering, ocular discomfort, pain due to periodic rupture of bullae, and halos around light.

On slit lamp examination, corneal thickness is increased with haze. Epithelial edema is visible on retroillumination with slit lamp.

Management

It includes:
- Treatment of primary causes such as lowering of IOP, and control of ocular inflammation.
- Protection of endothelium during intraocular surgery by use of viscoelastics.
- Hypertonic agents:
  ◊ 5% sodium chloride eye drops × QID.
  ◊ 6% sodium chloride eye ointment at bed time.
  ◊ Anhydrous glycerine.
- Bandage (therapeutic) contact lens to minimize discomfort of bullous keratopathy.
- Penetrating keratoplasty (corneal transplant) is done in long-standing corneal edema which is nonresponsive to medical treatment.

Prognosis

It depends on the status of corneal endothelium. If endothelium is healthy, edema usually resolves completely. Corneas with reduced endothelial cell counts may not be able to recover.

Corneal Opacity (OP4.5)

Corneal opacity occurs in the epithelial breech that involves Bowman's membrane (**Fig. 6.5**). It may be congenital due to developmental anomalies or birth trauma. The common causes include infection, injury or corneal abrasion. Corneal opacification (loss of transparency) may follow the noninflammatory diseases or inflammation. The term "scar" is reserved for the opacity following inflammation. Scar tissue is white and opaque, and varies in density.

Based on the density of scarring, corneal opacity may be nebular, macular or leucomatous (**Table 6.2**).

Nebular corneal opacity may be so faint that it could be missed on routine examination. A corneal opacity in pupillary area causes blurring of vision.

- If iris becomes adherent to the back of leucoma in perforated corneal ulcer, it is called adherent leucoma.
- In a sloughing corneal ulcer, where the whole cornea sloughs, prolapse of iris occurs. Exudates which cover the prolapsed iris become organized and form a layer of fibrous tissue over which corneal epithelium rapidly grows, resulting in the formation of pseudocornea. More commonly, iris and cicatricial tissue are too weak to support the IOP. Cicatrix (scar) becomes ectatic. Ectasia of pseudocornea with incarceration of iris tissue is known as anterior staphyloma.

> **Bowman's membrane does not regenerate.** So, some opacity always remains when Bowman's membrane has been destroyed.

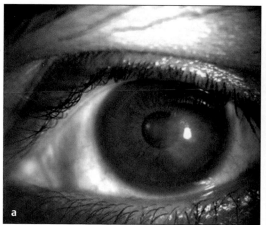 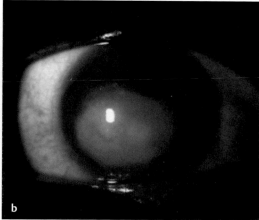

Fig. 6.5 Corneal opacity. **(a)** Macular grade. **(b)** Leucoma grade.

Table 6.2 Types of corneal opacities			
	Nebular corneal opacity (nebula)	**Macular corneal opacity (macula)**	**Leucomatous corneal opacity (leucoma)**
Density	Less dense +	Moderately dense ++	Very dense +++
Involves	Bowman's membrane and superficial stroma	Less than half the thickness of corneal stroma	More than half the thickness of corneal stroma
Structure seen through opacity	Details of iris can be seen through opacity	Details of iris cannot be seen through opacity	Obscures view of iris and pupil

Treatment

The ideal procedure either involves

- Excimer laser PTK (phototherapeutic keratectomy), or
- Corneal transplantation (keratoplasty).

■ Vascularization of Cornea (OP4.5)

Normal cornea is avascular. Vascularization of cornea is always pathological. Vascularization, which is considered as a defence mechanism (immunological defence) against disease, interferes with corneal transparency. It may be superficial or deep.

Superficial Vascularization

It arises from conjunctival superficial vascular plexus. The vessels are wavy and lie in the epithelial layer. Continuity of vessels can be traced with conjunctival vessels at the limbus. It is seen in the following:

- Trachoma.
- Phlyctenular keratoconjunctivitis.
- Superficial corneal ulcers.
- Rosacea keratitis.
- Contact lens wearers.

Pannus

When superficial vascularization is associated with cellular infiltration, it is termed as **pannus**. It may either be progressive when infiltration is ahead of vessels, or regressive, when infiltration is behind the vessels, that is, infiltration recedes. Pannus may be located superiorly, inferiorly, or generalized. Superior pannus occurs in trachoma and contact lens wearers. Inferior pannus is associated with exposure keratopathy and rosacea. Generalized pannus may be seen in chemical burns, Stevens–Johnson syndrome, and Mooren's ulcer.

Deep Vascularization

It arises from anterior ciliary vessels. The vessels run a fairly straight course and lie in the corneal stroma. The continuity of vessels cannot be traced beyond the limbus. It is seen in the following:

- Chemical burns.

- Deep corneal ulcers.
- Disciform keratitis.
- Sclerosing keratitis.
- Interstitial keratitis (IK).

Once the cornea has been vascularized, the vessels remain throughout life, but these blood vessels may become empty ("ghost vessels") when stimulus is eliminated.

Treatment

Vascularization can be prevented by timely and adequate treatment of predisposing conditions. Treatment is usually unsatisfactory. The following treatment regimens may be effective:

- *Topical corticosteroid* causes vasoconstriction and decrease in permeability of vessels.
- *Beta irradiation.*
- *Peritomy* is the surgical treatment of superficial vascularization in intractable cases.

■ Pigmentation of Cornea (OP4.5)

Pigments deposited may be iron, silver, gold, copper, melanin, etc.

Deposition of Iron

In **hyphema** (blood in anterior chamber), hemosiderin becomes embedded in the corneal stroma. Rise of IOP promotes blood staining of cornea. *Blood staining of cornea simulates dislocation of lens in the anterior chamber.*

In **keratoconus**, deposition of iron hemosiderin surrounds the base of the cone in the corneal epithelium (**Fleischer's ring**).

In **pterygium**, iron is deposited as a golden brown line in front of its head (**Stocker's line**) in the corneal epithelium.

In **filtering bleb**, iron is deposited anterior to the filtering bleb (**Ferry's line**) in the corneal epithelium.

In **old age**, deposition of iron is seen as a brown horizontal line (**Hudson–Stahli line**) in the corneal epithelium. It is located at the junction of the upper 2/3rd and 1/3rd along the line of lid closure.

Deposition of Silver

Prolonged topical use of silver nitrate causes impregnation of salt in the stroma and Descemet's membrane, resulting in brownish discoloration of Descemet's membrane (**Argyrosis**).

Deposition of Copper

When a copper foreign body is retained in the eye, deposition of copper occurs around the periphery of the cornea in the region of Descemet's membrane and deeper stroma. A gray–green or golden–brown pigmentation of the peripheral corneal stroma is produced (**Chalcosis**).

In Wilson's disease (hepatolenticular degeneration), deposition of copper in the periphery of Descemet's membrane is seen as a golden-brown or green ring just inside the limbus when examined on slit lamp (**Kayser–Fleischer ring, Fig. 6.6**).

If viewed in cobalt blue light, the ring appears almost black. The condition is reversible with time, if the disease is treated with penicillamine.

Deposition of Melanin

In pigment dispersion syndrome, uveal pigment (melanin) is deposited on the corneal endothelium in the form of a vertical spindle (**Krukenberg's spindle**). The spindle may be associated with pigment dispersion glaucoma.

Deposition of Gold

Gold is deposited in the epithelium in patients with **chrysiasis.**

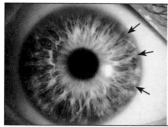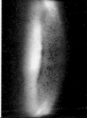

Fig. 6.6 Kayser Fleischer ring (deposition of copper). Source: Wilson disease (hepatolenticular degeneration). In: Biousse V, Newman N, ed. Neuro-ophthalmology illustrated. 3rd Edition. Thieme; 2019.

■ Corneal Filaments

These are the epithelial threads attached to cornea at one end, and the other unattached end is often club-shaped. These hang over the cornea and move freely with each blink, thereby producing irritation and foreign body sensation.

■ Prominent Corneal Nerves

These may be associated with—Local ocular disorders, for example,

- Keratoconus.
- Acanthamoebic keratitis.
- Fuch's endothelial dystrophy.
- Congenital glaucoma.

Systemic diseases, for example,

- Neurofibromatosis.
- Refsum syndrome.

■ Infiltrates

These originate from the limbal vascular arcades and are indicative of active inflammation. These are located usually within the anterior stroma and appear as focal, granular, gray–white opacities. These are composed of leucocytes and cellular debris.

■ Symptoms of Corneal Diseases

Symptoms of corneal diseases include pain or slight irritation, visual impairment, lacrimation (excessive tear production), photophobia, halos, redness, and foreign body sensation. Specific symptoms pertaining to different pathologies of cornea are listed in **Table 6.3**.

■ Evaluation of Corneal Diseases

Corneal examination can be done with the following:

- Slit lamp.
- Placido's disc.
- Pachymeter.
- Corneal staining.
- Specular microscopy.
- Confocal microscopy.
- Corneal aesthesiometer.

Table 6.3 Corneal pathology and symptoms

Corneal pathology	Symptoms
• Corneal abrasions or bullous keratopathy, resulting in direct stimulation of bare nerve endings	• Lacrimation. • Pain. • Photophobia associated with reflex blepharospasm because of corneal irritation. The reflex blepharospasm is not completely abolished in dark but is greatly diminished by anaesthetization.
• Loss of central corneal transparency due to: ◊ Stromal edema ◊ Corneal opacity	Visual impairment.
• Epithelial edema resulting in diffraction of light	Halos around light with blue end of spectrum nearest to light source.
• Corneal foreign body or corneal filaments	Foreign body sensation.

Cornea is examined for the following:

1. Size
   - Normal size: Horizontal diameter 12 mm and vertical diameter 11.5 mm.
   - Megalocornea (increased size): It may be congenital and due to buphthalmos.
   - Microcornea (decreased size): It may occur isolated or as a part of microphthalmos (small eye).

2. Shape:
   - Normal cornea: It is like a part of a sphere.
   - Flat cornea (cornea plana): It may occur congenitally or in phthisis bulbi.
   - Conical cornea: In keratoconus.
   - Globular cornea: In Keratoglobus.

3. Surface: Corneal surface and curvature can be evaluated by slit lamp, Placido's disc, Placido keratoscope, corneal topography, and keratometer.

Placido's keratoscopic disc: Kerato means cornea and scopic means visualization. The corneal surface is visualized by a disc painted with alternating black and white circles and contains a hole in the center. Light is kept behind the patient and the examiner looks at corneal image of circles through the hole.

Uniform and sharp image of circles is seen in normal cornea, while irregularities in rings are seen if corneal surface is uneven as in keratoconus, keratoglobus, and corneal astigmatism.

Corneal topography: It is computerized video keratography. It provides an objective record of the condition of anterior corneal surface (optical and anatomical condition) in the form of color-coded maps.

Green color represents normal curvature.

Blue color represents flat curvature.

Red color represents steep curvature.

It is important in preoperative evaluation for refractive surgery, for example, in patient with keratoconus, refractive surgery is deferred.

Orbscan is an improved technology which uses scanning slit technology with Placido disc. It provides information regarding curvature of anterior and posterior surfaces of cornea, and depth of anterior chamber. Curvature of anterior surface of cornea can also be measured by a *keratometer.*

4. Transparency: Cornea is optically transparent, and it becomes hazy in corneal edema, ulcers, opacity, vascularization, dystrophies and degenerations, and corneal deposits. The examination for corneal edema and corneal opacity is carried out with the help of a slit lamp. The corneal opacity is examined for its density (nebular, macular, or leucomatous), sensations, location, and its size.

If keratitis (ulcerative or nonulcerative) is suspected, corneal staining is performed.

5. Corneal Staining: Staining of cornea with vital dyes (*Fluorescein or Rose Bengal,* **Table 6.4**) is important in evaluating corneal epithelial lesions. It should be performed before corneal sensation is tested and also prior to measurement of IOP.

Alcian blue dye stains mucus selectively, so it stains excess mucus, as in keratoconjunctivitis sicca **(KCS)**.

> In a geographical herpetic ulcer, peripheral devitalized cells are stained with Rose Bengal dye, while the base of the ulcer (epithelial defect) is stained with Fluorescein dye.

6. Corneal Vascularization: The normal cornea is avascular. If corneal vascularization is present, note the following points:
- Whether the vessels are superficial or deep.
- Whether the distribution is localized, circumferential, or peripheral.

7. Corneal Thickness (Pachymetry): Corneal thickness indirectly reflects endothelial function. It is measured by with the help of the pachymeter.

Average corneal thickness at center, that is, central corneal thickness (CCT) is about 0.5 mm (490–560 μm). CCT of ≥0.6 mm is suggestive of endothelial disease. At periphery corneal thickness is ≈ 0.7 mm.

CCT can alter measurement of IOP: Patients with increased CCT record **high IOP**, while patients with decreased CCT record **low IOP**.

8. Corneal Sensitivity: Cornea is richly supplied by nerves. Corneal sensitivity can be tested by:

- Touching cornea with wisp of cotton wool— Normally, there is brisk blink reflex as a response.
- Corneal aesthesiometer provides a more qualitative measurement of corneal sensations. In aesthesiometer, a single horse hair of varying length is used. The longest length which induces blinking is a measure of the threshold of corneal sensitivity. Normally, the cornea is most sensitive in the center.

Corneal sensations are diminished in the following:
- Herpetic keratitis.
- Neuroparalytic keratitis.
- Absolute glaucoma.
- Cerebellopontine angle tumor.
- Leprosy.
- Trigeminal block for neuralgia.

9. Endothelial Function: Corneal endothelium can be examined by specular microscopy or confocal microscopy on a slit lamp.

Specular microscopy: Specular microscope photographs the endothelial cells and enables the study of their morphology (their number [count], size and shape).

Average cell count is 2,500 cells/mm². In adults, it declines with age from 3,500 cells/mm² in children to 2,000 cells/mm² in old age. There is a certain amount of endothelial cell loss after intraocular surgery. Intraocular surgery is deferred in endothelial cell count cases of <1,000 cells/mm².

Table 6.4 Difference between Fluorescein and Rose Bengal dyes	
Fluorescein dye 2%	**Rose Bengal dye 1%**
• It remains *extracellular* and *does not stain mucus.* It stains tear film and shows up epithelial corneal defects. • It *delineates* areas denuded of epithelium (abrasions, ulcer) which *stains brilliant green* when examined under a cobalt blue filter.	• It *stains mucus as well as devitalized* (dead and damaged) *cells red* as in superficial punctate keratitis and filamentary keratitis. • It is useful in diagnosis of **KCS.** • Rose Bengal dye is very irritating, so instill 2% xylocaine (local anesthetic) eye drop before using Rose Bengal.

Abbreviation: KCS, keratoconjunctivitis sicca.

Normally, endothelial cells are hexagonal. Variability in the shape of cells is called **pleomorphism**. *In the presence of 50% nonhexagonal cells, intraocular surgery is contraindicated.* Variation in cell size is called **polymegathism**.

Confocal microscopy: It is performed by a confocal microscope. In cases with corneal edema, endothelium is not adequately visualized by specular microscopy due to edema. *Confocal microscopy may be of value in cases with corneal edema.*

Confocal microscope allows direct visualization of corneal cells. It acquires multiple images of cornea from epithelium to endothelium. Magnified images provide detailed information regarding cell count, shape, and size.

Confocal microscopes are of two types: Confocal slit-scanning microscope and confocal laser-scanning microscope.

■ Inflammation of Cornea

Inflammation of cornea is known as **Keratitis**.

■ Source of Inflammation

Inflammation of cornea may arise from:

- Exogenous source: Cornea is involved by way of exogenous organisms.
- Endogenous source: Inflammation due to endogenous source is typically immunological in nature. *As cornea is* avascular, the immunological changes are common near limbal blood vessels close to the corneal margin and called **marginal keratitis**.
- Contiguous spread (owing to direct anatomical continuity).
- Diseases of conjunctiva spread to corneal epithelium, for example, trachoma and vernal keratoconjunctivitis.
- Diseases of sclera spread to corneal stroma, for example, sclerosing keratitis.
- Diseases of uveal tract spread to corneal endothelium, for example, herpetic uveitis with endotheliitis.

■ Classification

Keratitis can be classified as follows:

- Based on depth:
  - ◊ Superficial keratitis: It is the inflammation involving epithelium and Bowman's membrane.
  - ◊ Deep keratitis: It is the inflammation deep to Bowman's membrane.
- Based on location:
  - ◊ Central.
  - ◊ Peripheral.
- Based on epithelial defect:
  - ◊ Ulcerative.
  - ◊ Nonulcerative.
- Based on etiology:
  - ◊ Infectious.
  - ◊ Noninfectious.

Infectious Keratitis (OP4.1, 4.2)

It is the corneal inflammation caused by bacterial, viral, fungal, or parasitic (protozoal or helminthic) organisms. It can be classified as:

- Depending on depth:
  - ◊ Superficial.
  - ◊ Deep.
- Depending on pus formation:
  - ◊ Purulent (suppurative).
  - ◊ Nonpurulent (Nonsuppurative).
- Depending on epithelial defect:
  - ◊ Ulcerative wherein corneal epithelium shows discontinuity. Loss of epithelium with inflammation in surrounding cornea is called corneal ulcer.
  - ◊ Nonulcerative wherein epithelium is intact (corneal abscess).

Inflammation in cornea is visible as a grayish haze. If it is accompanied by accumulation of leucocytes and cellular debris, this hazy area is called an *infiltration* and appears as gray–white or off–white opacities. *Infiltrates are indicative of active inflammation.*

Noninfectious Keratitis

It is the corneal inflammation with no known infectious cause. It may be:
- Allergic/immune-mediated:
  1. *Localized immune-mediated keratitis:*
     ◊ Phlyctenular.
     ◊ Vernal.
     ◊ Mooren's ulcer.
     ◊ Marginal.
     ◊ Atopic.
  2. *Keratitis in systemic immunological disorders:*
     ◊ Associated with collagen disorders.
     ◊ Dermatological disorders: Rosacea.
       – Erythema multiforme.
       – Mucous membrane pemphigoid.
- Nonimmune-mediated:
  ◊ Neurotrophic in Vth cranial nerve (CN) palsy and diabetes.
  ◊ Neuroparalytic in VIIth CN palsy.
  ◊ Traumatic:
    – Chemical injury.
    – Thermal injury.
    – Radiation.
  ◊ Mechanical:
    – Entropion with trichiasis.
    – Lagophthalmos.
    – Exophthalmos.
  ◊ Nutritional in keratomalacia.
  ◊ In KCS.
  ◊ Others:
    – Thygeson's superficial punctate keratitis (SPK).
    – Superior limbic keratoconjunctivitis.

■ Infectious Keratitis

Bacterial Keratitis

The conjunctival sac is never free from organisms. Most of the organisms, normally, present on the ocular surface are:
- Staphylococcus albus or epidermidis.
- Propionibacterium acnes.
- Neisseria catarrhalis.
- Diphtheroids.
- Corynebacterium xerosis, etc.

All these organisms are nonpathogenic commensals. Streptococci, *E. coli*, B proteus, Neisseria gonorrhoeae, Hemophilus aegyptius, Moraxella, etc., are pathogenic and rarely found in normal eyes.

Defence Mechanisms

The following mechanisms help in defending against the microbial invasion of the corneal surface:

1. **Blinking** regularly sweeps away debris trapped in the mucin layer of tears.
2. **Tight junctions between** corneal and conjunctival epithelial cells.
3. **Tears** which contain:
   - Lactoferin (secreted by lacrimal gland): It inhibits complement activation.
   - Lysozyme, which promotes microbial aggregation and causes lysis of bacterial cell membrane.
   - IgA: It causes bacterial agglutination and inhibits bacterial adherence to corneal and conjunctival surface.
   - β-lysin: It causes bacteriolysis.
4. **Mast cells of conjunctiva:** Stimulation of mast cells cause degranulation of mast cells. It results in vascular dilation and increased vascular permeability. Thus, transudate is produced which is antimicrobial.
5. **Resident normal microbes** produces bacteriocins (high-molecular weight proteins), which inhibit growth of pathogens.

Predisposing Factors

Compromising one or more of the defense mechanisms represent a risk factor in the development of bacterial keratitis. These mechanisms are:

Trauma: Accidental, agricultural or surgical (refractive surgery).

Topical steroids (cause impairment of local immune defense).

Trigeminal nerve paralysis causes corneal anesthesia and exfoliation of epithelial cells.

A—Vitamin **A** deficiency.

B—**B**ullous keratopathy (corneal epithelial problem).

C—**C**hronic blepharitis.

Contact lens wear, particularly extended wear soft lenses, causing hypoxia and trauma to corneal epithelium.

D—**D**iabetes mellitus.

Dry eyes (Poor tear production results in reduction of antimicrobial tear component and epithelial desiccation and damage).

E—**E**ntropion with trichiasis (results in breakdown of protective corneal epithelium).

F—**F**acial nerve palsy (results in exposure keratopathy).

It does not appear that AIDS serves as an independent risk for development of infectious keratitis, but infectious keratitis in AIDS patients might follow a more aggressive course.

Causative Organisms

Bacteria that can penetrate normal (intact) corneal epithelium are Neisseria gonorrhoeae, Neisseria meningitidis, and Corynebacterium diphtheriae.

However, most other bacteria are capable of producing keratitis with damaged epithelium. Purulent keratitis is usually exogenous due to pyogenic bacteria. The most common pathogens are listed in **Flowchart 6.2**.

Pseudomonas aeruginosa is a frequent cause of contact lens-associated keratitis and found in moist environments.

Pathogenesis of Corneal Ulcer

For a bacterial keratitis to become established, bacterial adherence to cornea requires a defect in the continuity of the corneal epithelium (**Fig. 6.7**). Pathological changes occurring during development of corneal ulcer can be described

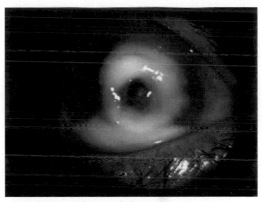

Fig. 6.7 Bacterial corneal ulcer.

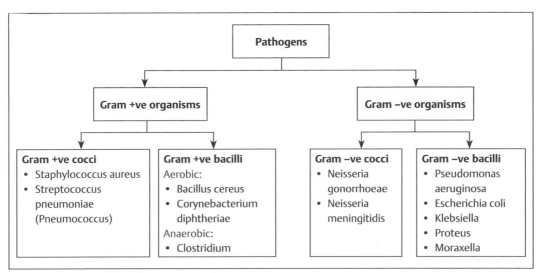

Flowchart 6.2 Types of pathogens causing keratitis.

in four stages, namely, infiltration, ulceration, regression and cicatrization (**Fig. 6.8**).

Stage of Infiltration

The bacterial adherence to the cornea on damaged epithelium is facilitated by binding of microbial adhesins and toxins to host cell receptors and glycocalyx coat. The corneal infection and inflammation stimulates immigration of polymorphonuclear leucocytes (polymorphs) via tear film and proliferating limbal blood vessels. The epithelium becomes edematous and is raised at the site of infiltration.

Stage of Ulceration

The stage of infiltration is followed by the necrosis and desquamation of corneal stroma, leading to ulceration. Polymorphs phagocytose bacteria and necrotic stroma. If bacteria overwhelms host defense, necrosis progresses unchecked and corneal perforation takes place.

Stage of Regression

If infection is brought under control, infiltration decreases in size. Superficial vascularization develops from the limbus which supplies antibodies. Immune response increases and epithelium heals over ulcer.

Stage of Cicatrization

Cicatrization, which occurs in vascularized ulcer, involves regeneration of collagen and formation of fibrous tissue. Newly formed fibers are not arranged regularly as in normal corneal lamellae. These refract light irregularly. Scar is, therefore, opaque.

If ulcer is superficial and involves epithelium only, ulcer heals without leaving any opacity behind. **If ulcer involves Bowman's membrane**, some degree of permanent opacification remains, as **Bowman's membrane never regenerates**.

Clinical Features

Clinical features depend on virulence of organism, duration of infection, and use of steroids.

Symptoms

- Pain and photophobia (due to exposure of nerve endings of 1st division of trigeminal [V] nerve).
- Redness.
- Blepharospasm.
- Lacrimation.
- Discharge.
- Blurred vision.

Signs

- Circum corneal (ciliary) congestion of conjunctiva.
- Epithelial defect is associated with gray–white infiltrate around the margin of ulcer. Corneal lamellae imbibe fluid, and margin of ulcer becomes edematous and overhangs above the surface with sloping edges (**saucer-shaped appearance of ulcer**).
- *Corneal ulcer takes a green stain with Fluorescein dye.*
- Lid erythema and edema.
- Anterior chamber inflammation is often present with cells and flare and may produce a hypopyon.

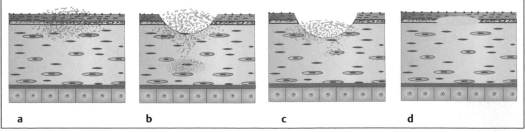

Fig. 6.8 Pathogenesis of corneal ulcer. **(a)** Stage of infiltration. **(b)** Stage of ulceration. **(c)** Stage of regression. **(d)** Stage of cicatrization.

Hypopyon Corneal Ulcer

Development of hypopyon: Some of the toxins produced by bacteria diffuse into the anterior chamber and irritate the vessels of iris and ciliary body **(keratouveitis)**. Polymorphs from vessels are poured into the anterior chamber and thereafter gravitate to the bottom of the anterior chamber to form **hypopyon**. *Hypopyon is sterile since* accumulation of polymorphs is due to toxins, and not to actual invasion by bacteria. Indeed, bacteria and leucocytes are incapable of passing through the intact Descemet's membrane. Such hypopyons are fluid and always move to the lowest part of the anterior chamber with change in the position of the patient's head. Once the ulcerative process is controlled, hypopyon is easily and rapidly absorbed.

Thus, in absence of a full-thickness corneal perforation, hypopyon often represents a sterile accumulation. Development of hypopyon depends on:

- *Virulence of infecting organism*: Pyogenic organisms producing hypopyon are Staphylococci, Streptococci, Gonococci (N-gonorrhoeae), Moraxella, and Pseudomonas.

Pseudomonas and Pneumococcus (Streptococcus pneumoniae) are most dangerous and are likely to be present if there is dacryocystitis (inflammation of lacrimal sac).

- *Resistance of tissues*: Hypopyon corneal ulcers are much more common in elderly individuals, debilitated persons, and alcoholics.

Hypopyon corneal ulcer caused by pneumococci is characteristic and is called **ulcus serpens** because of its tendency to **creep over cornea in a serpiginous fashion**. It starts as a gray–white or yellowish disc-like lesion near the central part of the cornea with shaggy undermined infiltrating edges. One edge of the ulcer, along which the ulcer spreads, shows more infiltration which often looks like a yellow crescent. The tissues breakdown and ulcer spreads (**Fig. 6.9**).

There is violent iritis, leading to hypopyon, which increases in size very rapidly. Massive hypopyon often causes rise in IOP (*secondary glaucoma*).

In severe cases, ulcer spreads rapidly. The entire cornea is affected by the ulcerative process and perforation of ulcer results if there is sudden coughing or sneezing.

Pseudomonas corneal ulcer

Pseudomonas produces destructive enzymes (such as protease, lipase, elastase, and exotoxin) which melt corneal stroma and results in a necrotic soupy ulceration with **greenish-yellow mucopurulent discharge** adherent to the ulcer. The corneal epithelium away from the primary ulcer typically develops a diffuse, semi-opaque **"ground glass" appearance**. The ulcer is associated with marked anterior chamber reaction and hypopyon formation. Rapidly spreading ulcer often extends peripherally, deeply involving the entire cornea and resulting in sloughing corneal ulcer and **perforation**. *If cornea sloughs*, iris is prolapsed and covered by exudates which become organized, resulting in **formation of pseudocornea (Fig. 6.10).**

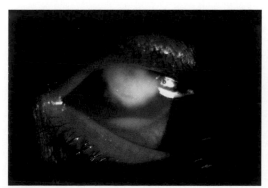

Fig. 6.9 Hypopyon corneal ulcer.

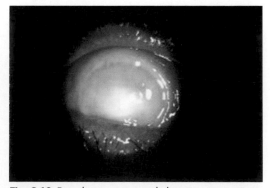

Fig. 6.10 Pseudomonas corneal ulcer.

Management of Corneal Ulcer

It includes identification of organism and treatment. For identifying the causative organisms, corneal scrapings are taken from the margins and base of ulcer for Gram's and Giemsa staining (**Table 6.5**) and culture and sensitivity (**Table 6.6**).

Treatment

Fundamental principles for treating corneal ulcer are protection, cleanliness, and specific treatment of infection. Treatment should be initiated before the results of culture and antibiotic sensitivity are available. Treatment includes the use of antibiotics and cycloplegics.

Antibiotics

Commonly used antibiotics are:
- *Aminoglycosides, for example,* Gentamicin, Tobramycin, and Amikacin.
- *Fluoroquinolones, for example,* Ciprofloxacin, Gatifloxacin, Ofloxacin, Moxifloxacin, and Levofloxacin.
- *Cephalosporins, for example,* Cefazolin.
- *Penicillins, for example,* Penicillin G, Methicillin, and Piperacillin.
- *Vancomycin.*

Routes of administration could be topical, subconjunctival, or systemic. *Topical administration* is the route of choice because it provides rapid, high-levels of drugs in the cornea and anterior chamber. The infection is controlled by the broad-spectrum antibiotic, while in severe infection, the fortified antibiotic drops are preferred. Fortified drops are not commercially available and are freshly prepared from their injectable preparations.

Treatment Regimen for Topical Antibiotics

Initial therapy should be initiated with a broad-spectrum regimen. Broad-spectrum coverage can be achieved with
- Fluoroquinolone antibiotic alone **or**
- Combination of aminoglycoside + cephalosporin.

Since increasing resistance to fluoroquinolones has been reported, therapy with fluoroquinolones is not a standard practice. *Initial therapy should be a combination of two* fortified antibiotics:

An aminoglycoside (gentamicin or tobramycin) for Gram –ve organisms

+

A cephalosporin (cefazolin is most commonly used for Gram +ve organisms)

Table 6.5 Staining of corneal scrapings

Stain	Organism identified
• Gram's and Giemsa: Gram's staining differentiate into Gram +ve and Gram –ve species	Bacteria, fungi
• Potassium hydroxide (KOH) fixation	Fungi
• Calcofluor white (it is a fluorescent dye with an affinity for amoebic cysts and fungi)	Fungi and acanthamoeba

Table 6.6 Corneal scrapings for culture and sensitivity

Culture media	Organism isolated
• Blood agar	It promotes growth of: • Aerobic bacteria **except** Neisseria, Haemophilus and Moraxella • Saprophytic fungi
• Chocolate agar	It is used to isolate neisseria, hemophilus, and moraxella
• Sabouraud's dextrose agar	Promotes growth of fungi
• E. coli plated non-nutrient agar	For acanthamoeba

Amikacin is useful against Gram –ve organisms resistant to gentamicin and tobramycin. The *instillation frequency* of topical antibiotics is as follows:

- Every 1 hour day and night for 48 hours.
- Every 2 hours during daytime for a further 48 hours.
- 4–6 hourly for another week.

Treatment is continued until epithelium has healed. When combination of two antibiotics is prescribed, drops are given in an alternating fashion every half an hour.

Initial therapy with aminoglycoside and cephalosporin can be changed for effective treatment, if needed, after microbiological investigation (culture and sensitivity) reports. For example, fluoroquinolone treatment is significantly more effective in the treatment of Neisseria infection than an aminoglycoside combined with a cephalosporin.

Treatment Regimen for Oral Antibiotics

These are not usually necessary. Systemic antibiotics provide relatively low-level of antibiotic in the cornea because of avascularity. Therefore, these are advised only when keratitis is complicated by scleritis (as in peripheral ulcers with scleral extension) or there is risk of perforation or endophthalmitis.

N. gonorrhoeae should be treated systemically with IM ceftriaxone or IV penicillin G along with topical fluoroquinolone.

N. meningitidis should be treated with i.v. penicillin G along with topical fluoroquinolone.

Treatment Regimen for Subconjunctival Antibiotics

Subconjunctival injections are indicated if there is poor compliance with topical treatment (**Table 6.7**).

Cycloplegics

Atropine 1% as drops or ointment is preferred. Other cycloplegics are homatropine 2% eye drops and cyclopentolate 1% eye drops. These are instilled two to three times a day. Cycloplegics relieves ciliary spasm and reduces pain. These also prevent posterior synechiae formation as anterior uveitis generally accompanies corneal ulceration.

Treatment of Perforated Corneal Ulcer

If perforation has occurred, the treatment depends upon its size and location. Small perforation in pupillary area is managed with rest, antibiotics, atropine, and pressure bandage. Small perforation over iris results in adhesion of iris to cornea, forming adherent leucoma. In case of perforation, anterior chamber must be restored as quickly as possible. It can be done by use of tissue adhesive (cyanoacrylate glue). It is applied to the area of perforation after careful debridement. Drying of the adhesive may take 5 to 10 minutes. A surgical procedure such as therapeutic penetrating keratoplasty or conjunctival flap can be undertaken thereafter. Persistent anterior stromal scar can be removed by excimer laser phototherapeutic keratectomy.

Topical Corticosteroids in Corneal Ulcer

Steroids are best avoided, since they may retard epithelialization and inhibit repair by fibrosis. If inflammation is severe and persists, it is safest to use steroids when there is evidence of successful antibiotic treatment and cultures become sterile.

Additional therapeutic measures taken for healing of ulcer are as follows:

- Treatment of cause
  - ◊ Dacryocystitis should be treated with dacryocystorhinostomy (**DCR**).
  - ◊ If IOP is raised, it is reduced by antiglaucoma therapy.
  - ◊ Peritomy (excision of 2 mm strip of limbal conjunctiva) is performed for corneal vascularization.

Table 6.7 Dosage of subconjunctival injections for the treatment of corneal ulcers

Drug	Subconjunctival dose
Gentamicin/tobramycin	40 mg
Amikacin	50 mg
Cefazolin	125 mg
Note: Subconjunctival injections are given at 24 hourly intervals for 5 days.	

- Removal of necrotic tissue by repeated scraping of the floor of ulcer.
- Cauterization of ulcer with pure (100%) carbolic acid or 10% trichloroacetic acid.
- Conjunctival flaps might be especially useful in peripheral infectious ulceration.

If infection is brought under control, cicatrization occurs in corneal ulcer. The residual scar may cause irregular astigmatism or may be visually debilitating (**Table 6.8**).

Treatment of Nonhealing Corneal Ulcer

If ulcer does not respond to therapeutic measures and continues to progress, a thorough search must be made for the cause, which could be either local or systemic. Local causes include lagophthalmos, trichiasis, raised IOP, dacryocystitis and

Table 6.8 Outcome of treatment in bacterial keratitis

Outcome of bacterial keratitis	Treatment
• If irregular astigmatism occurs	• It is treated with rigid contact lens.
• If scar is anterior stromal	• It is removed by excimer laser phototherapeutic keratectomy.
• If scar is deep	• It requires lamellar or penetrating keratoplasty.

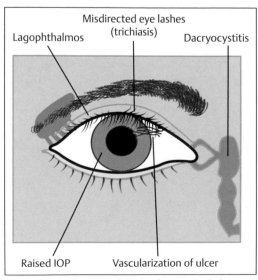

Fig. 6.11 Local causes of nonhealing corneal ulcers.

vascularization of ulcer, while systemic causes include diabetes mellitus and systemic steroid administration (**Fig. 6.11**).

Complications

Following are the complications of corneal ulcers:

1. **Ectatic cicatrix** (secondary keratectasia): Deep ulcer may lead to marked thinning of cornea which may bulge under normal IOP. The corneal scar (cicatrix) becomes consolidated with permanent bulging as secondary keratectasia.

2. **Secondary glaucoma:** Corneal ulcer causes absorption of toxins in the anterior chamber, leading to the formation of toxic iridocyclitis. This further causes blockage of an angle of the anterior chamber with fibrinous exudates leading to secondary glaucoma.

3. **Descemetocele**: Some ulcers become adequately deep (due to virulent organisms) to involve the whole thickness of cornea except *Descemet's membrane*. Descemet's membrane being elastic offers resistance to inflammation and is unable to support IOP and herniates. The herniation of Descemet's membrane through the ulcer is known as descemetocele.

4. **Perforation of corneal ulcer** (perforated corneal ulcer, **Fig. 6.12**).

Descemetocele is a sign of impending perforation which may convert into perforation on

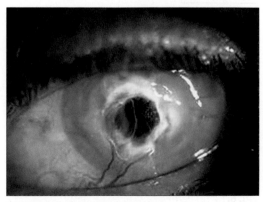

Fig. 6.12 Perforated corneal ulcer.

coughing, sneezing, straining at stool, or spasm of orbicularis muscle. Pain is alleviated after perforation. Perforation of ulcer is accompanied by sudden escape of aqueous and fall in IOP. The iris lens diaphragm moves forward and cicatrization of corneal ulcer results (**Fig. 6.13**).

Factors responsible for preventing perforation are as follows:

- Forced expiration (blowing the nose, coughing, etc.) must be avoided.
- IOP is reduced by oral acetazolamide and/ or i.v. mannnitol and topical IOP-lowering eye drops.

Sequelae and complications of perforation: The effect of perforation largely depends on its size and position. These include the following:

- **Endophthalmitis** or **panophthalmitis**: Due to perforation of ulcer, organisms gain access to the interior of the eye, leading to the development of endophthalmitis or panophthalmitis.
- **Intraocular/expulsive hemorrhage**: Sudden perforation of large ulcer causes sudden lowering of IOP, hence there is dilatation of intraocular blood vessels. This leads to the development of intraocular/ expulsive hemorrhage (profuse bleeding along with extrusion of contents of globe).
- **Anterior synechiae**: If perforation is small and opposite the iris, anterior synechiae develop, leading to leucoma adherens.

- **Iris prolapse**: If perforation is large and opposite the iris, iris prolapse occurs. There is deposition of exudates on the iris surface which becomes organized. Iris and cicatricial tissue are too weak to support IOP, hence anterior ectasia of cicatrix with incarceration of iris, which is called **anterior staphyloma**, develops.
- **Anterior capsular cataract**: If perforation is opposite the pupil (central perforation), the lens comes in contact with the ulcer-causing anterior capsular cataract. **If perforation is not plugged by iris but exudates fill the gap,** the repeated ruptures of exudates fill the gap, causing the opening to become permanent and leading to the formation of **corneal fistula**.

Fungal Keratitis (Mycotic Keratitis)

For clinical purpose, fungi are of the following two types:

- Filamentous fungi.
- Nonfilamentous fungi **(yeasts)**.

Risk Factors

The following risk factors are involved in the development of fungal keratitis:

- *Trauma* with vegetable matter or animal tail.
- *Systemic immunosuppression* by use of corticosteroids or immunosuppressives.
- Diabetes.

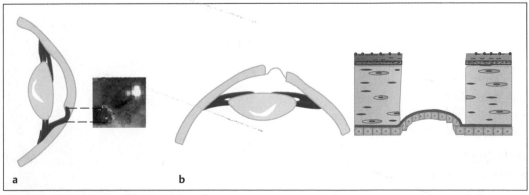

Fig. 6.13 (a) Perforation. **(b)** Descemetocele.

- *Hydrophilic contact lens* wear.
- *Corneal surgery* (fungal infection at lamellar interface has been described following LASIK).

Etiology

Fungal keratitis is rare in temperate countries but common in tropical countries, warm and humid climates, rural areas, and immuno-compromised individuals. It is most prevalent in agricultural areas and typically preceded by ocular trauma with vegetable matter. It is commonly due to infections with Aspergillus, Fusarium, and Candida albicans.

Clinical Features

The onset is gradual and slowly progressive. Symptoms are relatively minimal, much milder than clinical signs, and include foreign body sensation, photophobia, blurred vision, and discharge.

Clinical signs of filamentous fungi are:
- Organism adherence results in *gray–white, elevated infiltrate.* Epithelium over *infiltrate may be elevated* above the remainder of the corneal surface.
- Invasion into corneal lamellae and extension along corneal lamellae results in *feathery borders* and *satellite lesions.*
- Penetration of intact Descemet's membrane by filamentous fungi results in thick and immobile *hypopyon* with upper convex border (**Fig. 6.14**). Infection in anterior chamber is difficult to eradicate.
- Sometimes, a white immune ring (**Wessely ring**) may be seen around the ulcer due to deposition of immune complexes.

In case of nonfilamentous fungi (candida), keratitis is characterized by a yellow–white stromal infiltrate, associated with dense suppuration, which appears as a collar-button abscess without feathery edge.

Diagnosis

History of trauma with vegetable matter, wood, animal tail, or chronic use of steroid is present.

Investigations helpful for coming to a diagnosis include:
- Scrapings from the floor of ulcer are stained with 10% KOH.
- Scrapings are also plated on Sabouraud dextrose agar for culture and sensitivity. Cycloheximide should not be included in the medium since it inhibits fungal growth.

Treatment

As *most antifungals are only fungistatic,* topical treatment should be continued for several weeks. Removal of epithelium over the lesion enhances penetration of antifungal agents.

Topical treatment includes the following considerations:
- Infection due to *filamentous fungi* is treated with natamycin 5%, amphotericin B 0.15%, or miconazole 1% drops. Voriconazole eye drops are more effective against Aspergillus. The drops are instilled initially every 1 hour and tapered gradually.
- *Candida infection (yeast)* is usually treated with amphotericin B. Nystatin eye ointment applied five times a day is only effective against candida.

If infection fails to respond to single agent therapy, amphotericin B and natamycin can be used alternatively on an hourly basis.

Systemic antifungal drugs (**itraconazole or voriconazole**) may be required in endophthalmitis.

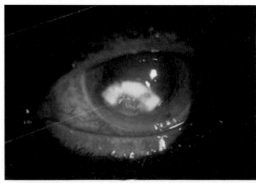

Fig. 6.14 Fungal keratitis with satellite lesions and hypopyon.

If medical treatment fails, surgical intervention may be required. **Penetrating keratoplasty** should be performed sooner to minimize the risk of endophthalmitis or infectious scleritis. Clear margins should be included in excised cornea. Corticosteroid use is not recommended in management of fungal keratitis.

Viral Keratitis

Viruses are obligate, intracellular parasites. Viruses that cause corneal disease include:

- Herpes simplex virus (**HSV**).
- Varicella zoster virus (**VZV**).
- Epstein–Barr virus (**EBV**).
- Adenovirus.
- Cytomegalovirus (**CMV**): It is a more common entity in association with AIDS.

Herpes Simplex Keratitis

HSV is a DNA virus and is of two types: HSV-1 and HSV-2. HSV-1 causes infection above waist and affects face, lips and eyes, while HSV-2 is associated with genital infection (genital herpes). HSV infection can be categorized into neonatal, primary, and recurrent infections.

Neonatal Infection

It is the infection of newborns by maternal genital herpes.

Fetus passes through the birth canal, so *neonatal HSV infection occurs by way of Type-2 virus (Fetus)*. It may affect the central nervous system (CNS) or can remain localized to the eye. Neonatal ocular HSV infection can present as conjunctivitis, keratitis, iridocyclitis, iris atrophy, cataract, chorioretinitis, or optic neuritis (**Fig. 6.15**).

Primary Infection (i.e., no previous virus exposure)

Neonates are usually protected by maternal antibodies against HSV infection during the first 6 months of life. So, primary infection by HSV-1 is uncommon during the first 6 months of life. Transmission occurs by droplet transmission via contaminated adult saliva. So, children under 3 years of age are more prone to get HSV infection, owing to close contact, that is, it typically occurs between 6 months to 5 years of age.

Primary infection remains *often subclinical* and may cause mild fever, malaise, upper respiratory tract symptoms, and local lymphadenopathy. Oral mucosa is more commonly involved than eye in primary infection.

Children may develop **follicular kerato conjunctivitis. Epithelial punctate keratitis** may be found in nearly 50% of the cases. Primary

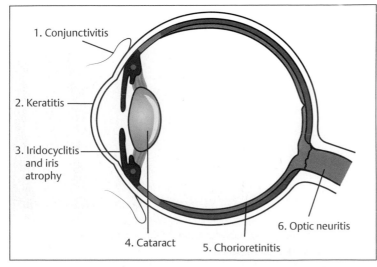

Fig. 6.15 Presentation of neonatal ocular HSV. Abbreviation: HSV, herpes simplex virus.

1. Conjunctivitis
2. Keratitis
3. Iridocyclitis and iris atrophy
4. Cataract
5. Chorioretinitis
6. Optic neuritis

herpetic infection is usually *benign and self-limited.* An attack does not produce lasting immunity and recurrences are frequent, particularly associated with upper respiratory tract infection (URTI). A person once infected frequently becomes a carrier.

Recurrent Infection (i.e., reactivation in presence of cellular and humoral immunity)

After primary infection with HSV-1, the virus reaches the sensory ganglion, where it may lie dormant for many years. Risk factors for recurrence are fever, stress, trauma, malnourishment, measles, and use of corticosteroids and other immunosuppressive.

The above stimuli (risk factors) may cause a clinical reactivation and replication of the virus. The virus travels down the sensory ganglion (e.g., trigeminal ganglion) and result in recurrent ocular HSV disease. Fortunately, ocular HSV disease tends to be a form of unilateral disease.

Clinical Features

Clinical features depend upon the part affected. Recurrent ocular HSV infection can affect lids, conjunctiva and cornea (epithelium, stroma and endothelium).

Note: Epithelial lesions are caused by replicating live virus. Stromal and endothelial lesions involve both live virus activity and immune reaction to viral antigen.

I. *Involvement of* lids causes lid vesicles and blepharitis.

II. *Involvement of* conjunctiva manifests as severe follicular conjunctivitis.

III. *Involvement of* corneal epithelium by way of HSV results in **epithelial keratitis**.

Symptoms include mild discomfort, foreign body sensation, redness, watering, blurred vision, and photophobia.

Following are the clinical signs of involvement of corneal epithelium due to recurrent HSV infection:

- Characteristic epithelial lesion of recurrent HSV infection is **dendritic ulcer** (**Fig. 6.16**).

Virus replication results in opaque epithelial cells on the cornea, arranged in a row or group. Central desquamation of these results in linear branching ulcer (dendritic ulcer). *The ends of the ulcer have characteristic terminal knobs which are pathognomonic. The central ulcerated area stains with Fluorescein dye,* while the *peripheral cells* at the margin containing live virus *stain with Rose Bengal dye.* Indiscriminate use of topical steroids results in progressive enlargement of dendritic ulcer to an amoeboid or geographical configuration known as **geographical ulcer**.

- Corneal sensation *is reduced.* The ulcer may resolve spontaneously or with treatment over 1 to 2 weeks. A nonhealing epithelial defect after live virus disappears with prolonged topical treatment is referred to as **"metaherpetic" ulcer**. It is caused by basement member damage, resulting in failure of reepithelialization. It is not caused by reactivation of virus (viral replication). *Margins of these ulcers do not stain with Rose Bengal.*

IV. *Involvement of* corneal stroma: Stromal lesion might be an immunological reaction, be infectious, or may involve combined mechanism. Stromal lesions in herpetic disease include disciform

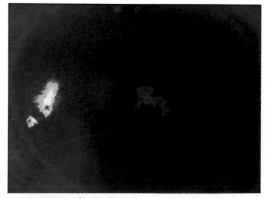

Fig. 6.16 Dendritic ulcer. Source: Uveitis. In: Glass L, ed. Ophthalmology Q&A Board Review. 1st Edition. Thieme; 2019.

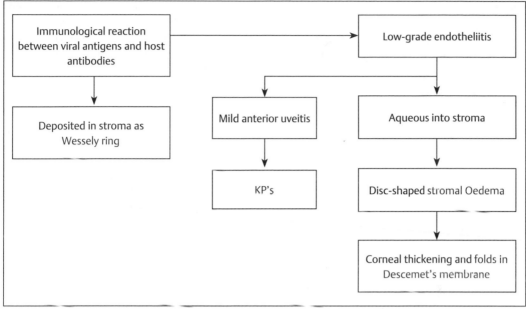

Flowchart 6.3 Signs of disciform keratitis.

keratitis and stromal necrotizing keratitis. **Disciform keratitis:** It is a *hypersensitivity reaction* to HSV antigen in the cornea. Symptoms include blurred vision and halos around lights. Following are the clinical signs of disciform keratitis due to recurrent HSV infection (**Flowchart 6.3**):

- Disc-shaped *stromal edema*, often with overlying epithelial edema, is a dominant feature.
- Folds in Descemet's membrane.
- Mild anterior uveitis with keratic precipitates (KPs).
- A ring of stromal haze may be present surrounding the stromal edema called the **Wessely ring.** It signifies deposition of viral antigen and host antibody complexes.
- Corneal sensations are reduced. There is no stromal neovascularization or necrosis.

Stromal necrotizing keratitis: It is caused by *active viral invasion*. The infiltration of cornea by polymorphs, lymphocytes, macrophages, and plasma cells mediate tissue destruction and stromal necrosis.

Typical lesion has a cheesy, yellow–white necrotic appearance. There may be associated anterior uveitis with KPs. Scarring, vascularization, and lipid deposition are common.

- In advanced disease, corneal stromal melting results in descematocele formation and perforation.
- If peripheral cornea is involved, inflammation and necrosis spread to sclera, resulting in *sclerokeratitis.*

V. Involvement of corneal endothelium (endotheliitis) results in corneal edema, anterior uveitis, which in turn leads to hypopyon and synechiae formation, and trabeculitis resulting in elevated IOP.

Complications

Complications of herpetic eye disease include:

- Secondary infection.
- Secondary glaucoma.
- Cataract (secondary to inflammation or prolonged use of steroids).
- Iris atrophy (secondary to keratouveitis).

Diagnosis

Diagnosis of ocular HSV disease is based on a constellation of:

- Assessment of *corneal sensations*.
- *Staining characteristics* with Fluorescein and Rose Bengal dye.
- Enzyme-linked immunosorbent assay *(ELISA)* test identifying viral antigens.
- Polymerase chain reaction *(PCR)* which detects HSV viral DNA in tissues, aqueous, and tears.

Treatment

Treatment of HSV ocular disease depends on the nature of ocular involvement. Ocular HSV disease is treated by antiviral agents. These are purine or pyrimidine analogues that are incorporated to form abnormal viral DNA.

> To define the role of oral antiviral agents and topical corticosteroids in the treatment and prevention of recurrent HSV ocular disease, a study termed **H**erpetic **E**ye **D**isease **S**tudy (HEDS) was conducted. According to HEDS:
> 1. **Oral acyclovir**: Provides no extra benefit over topical steroids and topical antiviral agents in treatment of stromal keratitis. It provides benefit in HSV iridocyclitis. So, concurrent administration of oral acyclovir is recommended in HSV iridocyclitis. It does not seem to prevent recurrent stromal keratitis or iridocyclitis.
> 2. **Topical steroids**: In absence of accompanying HSV epithelial keratitis, topical steroids along with topical antiviral agents reduce progression of stromal inflammation and shorten the duration of stromal keratitis (i.e., stromal keratitis improves more rapidly).

- Treatment of **epithelial keratitis** *without stromal involvement* includes the following considerations:

    1. Debridement of the edges of dendritic ulcer with cotton-tipped applicator to reduce infected (virus-laden) epithelial cells.
    2. Antiviral agents:
        ◊ TFT (Trifluorothymidine) 1% drops every 2 hours

        or

◊ Vidarabine (Ara - A) 3% ointment 5 times daily.

TFT and acyclovir both are active against HSV-1 and HSV-2.

Early IDU (Idoxuridine) 0.1% drops and 0.5% ointment were used, but due to the relative toxic effect on epithelium (punctate keratopathy), it is seldom used now. The most frequently used drug is Acyclovir 3% ointment. Recently, Ganciclovir 0.15% gel 5 times daily is effectively used. Antiviral agents are used until the epithelial ulcer has healed.

3. Lubricants are also given.
4. Cycloplegics, if required.
5. Topical antibiotics to prevent secondary bacterial infections.
6. Topical steroids are contraindicated in epithelial HSV keratitis because of the presence of active viral replication in HSV epithelial keratitis.

> *Advantages of acyclovir* over IDU, TFT, and Vidarabine.
> 1. It has less epithelial toxicity.
> 2. It penetrates intact corneal epithelium and stroma, achieving therapeutic levels in aqueous humour.
> 3. It acts preferentially on virus-laden epithelial cells and has low-toxicity for host cells.

- *Treatment of metaherpetic ulcers (postinfectious ulcer):* If ulcer is truly metaherpetic, that is, persistent epithelial defect after live virus disappears with topical treatment; antiviral agent serves no purpose and most likely will only inhibit epithelial regeneration. Treatment is directed toward encouraging epithelial healing and includes:
    ◊ Lubrication of eye with preservative free drops.
    ◊ Therapeutic (bandage) soft contact lens.
    ◊ Temporary tarsorrhaphy (if above measures fail) (OP4.7).
    ◊ Conjunctival flap.
- *Treatment of **stromal keratitis:*** It is treated with topical steroids and topical antiviral

agents. Important points of consideration are:

◇ Topical Prednisolone (1% drops) is used 4 to 5 times daily and gradually tapered. It reduces inflammation.

◇ Acyclovir 3% ointment is recommended five times daily. It penetrates intact corneal epithelium and stroma and can therefore be used to treat stromal herpetic keratitis.

Oral acyclovir provides no extra benefit over topical steroids and topical antiviral agents in treatment of stromal keratitis.

- Treatment of patients with **HSV irido-cyclitis**: HSV endotheliitis, trabeculitis, and iridocyclitis are treated with topical steroids (Prednisolone 1% drops tapered gradually) plus topical antiviral agent (Acyclovir 3% ointment five times daily) and oral Acyclovir (400 mg five times daily for 7–10 days).

- To reduce rate of **recurrent herpetic eye disease**: Low-dose oral Acyclovir 400 mg BD for 6 to 12 months reduces the rate of recurrent HSV ocular disease but this effect reduces or even disappears when the drug is discontinued. So, long-term prophylactic treatment should be considered in patients with frequent recurrences and at the risk of visual loss, particularly involving an only eye.

- Patients with **stromal scarring** and **opacity** can be treated by penetrating keratoplasty (PKP). Recurrence of active herpetic infection in corneal grafts is often a problem. Since long-term oral antiviral treatment can reduce recurrence rate, oral Acyclovir 400 mg BD should be given to patients undergoing PKP for herpetic eye disease to improve the survival of corneal grafts.

Varicella-Zoster Virus Keratitis (VZV Keratitis)

Varicella-zoster virus causes **varicella** (chicken-pox) *on initial infection* and **zoster** or shingles *on recurrence* (herpes zoster). Thus, herpes zoster is caused by same virus that causes chicken pox. After initial varicella (chicken pox) infection in childhood or youth, the virus remains latent in a sensory ganglion (like herpes simplex virus). It can reactivate to cause shingles (herpes zoster) after depressed cellular immunity. Depressed cellular immunity can occur with age, AIDS, immunosuppressives, blood dyscrasias, neoplasms, and radiotherapy. Thus, herpes zoster represents a form of recurrent disease.

The virus travels via sensory nerve to skin dermatome or eye where peripheral inflammation develops. *Trigeminal nerve infection is second in frequency as a site of recurrence after the thoracic region.*

Herpes zoster ophthalmicus (HZO) is a consequence of Gasserian ganglion (trigeminal nerve) involvement. Involvement of ophthalmic (1st) division occurs far more commonly than involvement of 2nd or 3rd divisions of trigeminal nerve. Of the 1st division, frontal nerve is the most commonly involved branch. The virus travels via branches of ophthalmic division of trigeminal nerve to the skin, eye, and adenexae (**Fig. 6.17**).

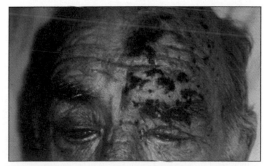

Fig. 6.17 Herpes zoster ophthalmicus. Source: The diagnosis of binocular diplopia. In: Biousse V, Newman N, ed. Neuro-ophthalmology illustrated. 3rd Edition. Thieme; 2019.

Pathology

There is prominent *vasculitis with granulomatous or lymphocytic infiltration.* Tissue damage caused by zoster infection is due to both inflammation and vasculitis-induced ischemia.

Clinical Features

Prodromal stage of HZO precedes the appearance of rashes (eruptive stage) and lasts 3 to 5 days. The disease starts with fever, malaise, and headache followed by neuralgic pain along the distribution of the 1st division of the trigeminal nerve.

Eruptive stage follows the prodromal stage and lasts for approximately 3 weeks. The vesicles appear on one side of the forehead of the scalp along the distribution of the ophthalmic division of the trigeminal nerve and does not cross the midline. The pain sometimes diminishes after the appearance of vesicles but may persist for months or years.

The skin of lid and affected area becomes red and edematous. The vesicles suppurate before they crust and leave behind pitted scars. Anesthesia of skin follows as the eruptions subside.

Postherpetic neuralgia is the pain that persists for months to years after the skin lesions (rashes) have healed.

Contact with nonimmune or immunosuppressed individuals should be avoided until the crusting is complete.

Ocular involvement: Ocular complications arise as the eruptions subside. The eye is frequently affected if the vesicles appear on the tip and the side of the nose due to *involvement of the nasociliary branch of the trigeminal nerve* (**Hutchinson sign**). The eye involvement may rarely occur when disease affects maxillary nerve (2nd division of trigeminal nerve) (**Table 6.9**).

Table 6.9 Ocular manifestations in HZO	
Structure involved	**Ocular manifestation**
• *Involvement of **lid***	• Lid scarring may result in cicatricial entropion or ptosis.
• *Involvement of **conjunctiva***	• Conjunctivitis is common. It can be follicular or necrotizing.
• *Involvement of **sclera***	• Scleritis may become chronic and frequently recurrent, leading to staphyloma.
• *Involvement of **cornea***	• Corneal involvement in acute phase can manifest as: ◊ Punctate epithelial keratitis. ◊ Dendritic lesions (*in contrast to HSV dendrites, these have tapered ends without terminal bulbs*). ◊ Nummular keratitis. ◊ Disciform keratitis. ◊ Sclerokeratitis. ◊ Kerato uveitis. • Chronic corneal lesions that follow HZO are: ◊ Mucous plaque keratitis. ◊ Neurotrophic keratitis. ◊ Exposure keratitis.
• *Involvement of **uvea***	• Anterior uveitis is frequently associated with sector iris atrophy.
• *Involvement of **trabecular meshwork***	• *Trabeculitis* may cause secondary glaucoma.
• ***Occlusive vasculitis***	• It may cause ARN and anterior segment ischemia.
• *Involvement of **optic nerves***	• Optic neuritis is rare and a late complication.
• *Involvement of **motor nerves***	• HZO affecting 3rd, 4th, and 6th CN results in extraocular muscle palsy, while facial N (7th CN) involvement results in facial palsy (**Bell's palsy**).

Abbreviations: ARN, acute retinal necrosis; CN, cranial nerve; HSV, herpes simplex virus; HZO, herpes zoster ophthalmicus.

Treatment

A. Treatment of **acute systemic** herpes zoster.

1. Systemic antiviral agents: Oral Acyclovir – 800 mg five times daily × 7 to 10 days and initiated within 72 hours of the onset of symptoms.

It accelerates healing of skin lesions. It reduces period of viral shedding, severity of acute pain, incidence of episcleritis, keratitis, and iritis. Other antivirals are oral Famciclovir 500 mg TDS × 7 to 10 days **and** oral Valaciclovir 1000 mg TDS × 7 to 10 days.

2. Systemic steroids are used in combination with antiviral agents. These are not only recommended to reduce acute pain but also used in the treatment of inflammatory complications of HZO such as severe scleritis, uveitis or orbital inflammation.

Dose: 60 mg/day and then reduced gradually.

B. Treatment of **postherpetic neuralgia**.

Nonsteroidal anti-inflammatory drugs (NSAIDS) are ineffective in postherpetic neuralgia. Initially, it is treated with:

Topical Lidocaine 5% gel (local anesthetic) or topical Capsaicin cream (depletes substance P). If it is ineffective, then the following drugs are given:

- Amitriptyline (a tricyclic antidepressant)— 12.5 to 25 mg at night and increased gradually to 75 mg/day, or
- Carbamazepine 400 mg daily to reduce pain.

C. **Local ocular treatment** of HZO.

For cutaneous lesions, antibiotic–corticosteroid skin ointment is applied on skin and lids. **Calamine lotion is better avoided** as it promotes crust formation. In the eye itself:

- Topical antivirals are not effective.
- Topical antibiotics are instilled to prevent secondary bacterial infection in acute stage of disease.

- Topical steroids and antiviral eye ointment are given if there is scleritis, sclerokeratitis, or iridocyclitis to reduce inflammation. Steroids are tapered gradually.
- Major complication of HZO, neurotrophic ulceration, is treated with bandage contact lens, tarsorrhaphy (OP4.7), and cyanoacrylate glue/penetrating keratoplasty (in case of corneal perforation).

Parasitic Keratitis

Acanthamoeba Keratitis

It is caused by Acanthamoeba (a protozoan) found in soil and water environments such as ponds, swimming pools, contact lens solutions, and tap water.

Source of infection

- Contact lens solutions are the usual source of infection. Once contact lens is contaminated, risk of infection is established, since the organism can adhere to and penetrate an intact epithelium.
- Swimming or bathing in contaminated water may be the source in noncontact lens wearers.

Acanthamoeba exists in dormant cystic form and active trophozoite form. Trophozoite produces a variety of enzymes and binds to corneal epithelium, resulting in thinning and necrosis of corneal epithelium. Early infection can be confined to the epithelium, but in advanced cases, the organism can enter the stroma and anterior chamber.

Clinical Features

Symptoms of acanthamoeba keratitis include severe ocular pain, blurred vision, photophobia, and lacrimation.

Clinical signs of acanthamoeba keratitis include the following:

- Early infection is confined to the epithelium which shows irregular surface as well as infiltrates and pseudodendrites mimicking

H simplex keratitis. The epithelium is intact initially and later breaks down.

- Deep linear stromal infiltrates might be seen around corneal nerves (radial keratoneuritis) and are pathognomonic.
- The infiltrates coalesce to form a ring abscess in stroma and resemble stromal herpetic disease. Scleritis may develop. In spite of severe inflammation, corneal vascularization is typically absent.
- Corneal melting may occur at the periphery of the area of infiltrates. Satellite lesions can appear. Anterior chamber inflammation can cause anterior uveitis and hypopyon.

Differential Diagnosis

This condition should be differentiated from herpetic keratitis and fungal keratitis. Patients with acanthamoeba keratitis are younger than patients with bacterial keratitis or fungal keratitis, and have a longer duration of symptoms before being treated. In terms of clinical signs, acanthamoeba keratitis is more likely to have disease confined to the epithelium and ring infiltrate.

Diagnosis

- *Staining of corneal scrapings* with calcofluor white stain. It is a fluorescent dye with an affinity for amoebic cysts which demonstrates the walls of the cysts but requires a fluorescent microscope.
- Polymerase chain reaction (PCR) to detect acanthamoebic DNA.

Nonsuppurative keratitis in a contact lens wearer is a high-index of suspicion, and treatment should be as for acanthamoeba infection.

Treatment

It includes the following considerations: Debridement to remove infected epithelium for early disease. Topical antiamoebics which include:

- **Cationic antiseptics** (inhibit membrane function) include Chlorhexidine and PHMB (polyhexamethylene biguanide).

- **Azoles** (destabilize cell walls) include Clotrimazole, Fluconazole, Ketoconazole, and Miconazole.
- **Aminoglycosides** (disrupt plasmalemma of organism) include Neomycin and Paromomycin.
- **Aromatic diamidines** (inhibit DNA synthesis) include Propamidine isethionate, Hexamidine, and Pentamidine.

Topical ameobicides are given as dual therapy (diamidines + cationic antiseptics) with:

- Propamidine isethionate + PHMB drops

or

Hexamidine + Chlorhexidine

Topical neomycin and miconazole are quite effective. The diseases may require a prolonged treatment for several months. Since cysts are difficult to eradicate, stromal relapses are common, as treatment is tapered.

- Topical steroids should be avoided, if possible.
- Persistent corneal inflammation occurs due to necrotic protozoa (acanthamoeba antigen) rather than viable organism and may result in scarring and impaired vision. PKP is needed for residual scarring.

■ Noninfectious Keratitis

Interstitial Keratitis (IK)

It is an inflammation of the corneal stroma without primary involvement of epithelium or endothelium.

Etiology

It is most often associated with congenital syphilis but may also be seen in acquired syphilis, tuberculosis, leprosy, and viral infections (**Table 6.10**). **Cogan's syndrome** (IK and deafness) is a rare cause affecting both eye and ear.

IK due to congenital syphilis occurs via *transplacental route,* usually *bilateral,* and affects children between the ages of *5 and 25 years.*

In IK, the uveal tract is almost always affected. The disease is fundamentally uveitis and keratitis is secondary. **Keratitis is the result of immune-mediated reaction.** *Treponema pallidum is not seen in cornea even during the acute phase.*

Course of the Disease

It is divided into three stages: Progressive, florid, and regressive stages.

Progressive Stage

The cellular infiltration in deeper layers of cornea (just anterior to Descemet's membrane) occurs after anterior uveitis with ciliary congestion. The stromal cloudiness involves the whole cornea, giving it a ground glass appearance in 2 to 4 weeks. Anterior uveitis may be obscured by corneal clouding.

Florid Stage

In this stage, deep vascularization of stroma occurs. The vascular growth begins at the limbus and grows in a brush-like manner. Since these vessels are covered by hazy cornea, vessels look dull reddish pink, resulting in a characteristic **salmon patch**. There is superficial vascularization but it never extends far over the cornea. Conjunctiva may heap up at the limbus.

Regressive Stage

In this stage, stromal vessel become nonperfused and remain as fine opaque lines (empty or ghost vessels), which indicates the previous occurrence of the disease. The cornea clears slowly from periphery toward center. If cornea does not clear within 18 months, visual prognosis is poor.

Clinical Features

Symptoms include pain, blurring of vision, photophobia, and watering of eyes.

Following are the clinical signs of IK:
- Signs in *progressive stage:* Keratic precipitates, ciliary congestion, and ground glass appearance of cornea with stromal edema.
- Sign in *florid stage*: Deep vascularization with salmon patch.
- Sign in *regressive stage*: Ghost vessels. Since infiltration of cornea is almost limited to deeper layers, ulceration of corneal surface is rare.

Diagnosis

It depends on:
- Other evidences of congenital syphilis include:
  ◊ Frontal eminence.
  ◊ Flat nasal bridge.
  ◊ Hutchinson's teeth (notching of two upper central incisors in permanent dentition).
  ◊ Vestibular deafness.
  ◊ Rhagades at the angles of the mouth.
- **Hutchinson's triad** includes IK, Hutchinson's teeth, and vestibular deafness. Coagan's syndrome include non syphillitic IK and deafness.
- **Serological tests**: All patients with IK should have treponemal serology including rapid reagin test, FTA–ABS (fluorescent treponemal antibody absorption) test, **and** venereal disease research laboratory (VDRL) test.

Table 6.10 Differentiating features of syphilitic and tubercular IK

	Syphilitic IK	Tubercular IK
Laterality	Usually bilateral	Usually unilateral
Involvement	Involves whole cornea	Frequently sectorial involving lower sector of cornea
Treatment (Systemic)	Antisyphilitic	Antitubercular
	(Topical treatment is same in both)	

Abbreviation: IK, interstitial keratitis.

Treatment

Active IK is dealt with the help of:

- Systemic treatment with penicillin and systemic steroids tapered gradually.
- Topical treatment with topical steroids (as IK is a hypersensitivity reaction), and cycloplegics for uveitis.
- Lubricating eye drops.
- PKP in cases with dense corneal opacity.

Immunologically Mediated Keratitis

Immunologically mediated keratitis includes the following:

- Keratitis secondary to conjunctival diseases, for example, phlyctenular keratitis and vernal keratitis.
- Marginal ulcer (catarrhal ulcer).
- Mooren's ulcer.
- Keratitis associated with collagen vascular disorders such as rheumatoid arthritis, systemic lupus erythematosus (SLE), polyarteritis nodosa, and Wegener's granulomatosis.

Phlyctenular Keratitis

Cornea is often involved in phlyctenular kerato-conjunctivitis, which is essentially a conjunctival disease.

Phlyctens are commonly found at the limbus but may occur within the corneal margin (*corneal phlycten*).

Etiology

It is thought to be delayed hypersensitivity (Type IV and cell-mediated) to an endogenous microbial antigen, mostly staphylococcal or tubercular.

Clinical Features

Symptoms include photophobia, lacrimation, blepharospasm, and pain. *Corneal phlyctens* cause much pain and photophobia.

Clinical signs of phlyctenular keratitis include:
- Phlycten appears as a gray nodule at the limbus, which is associated with superficial vascularization.

- A limbal phlycten may extend onto the cornea and appear as slightly raised above the corneal surface. The overlying epithelium breaks down and a triangular yellowish ulcer is formed with prominent vascularization known as **fascicular ulcer**.

As the disease is essentially conjunctival, so the epithelium and superficial layer of cornea are involved. The ulcer remains superficial and seldom perforates. A healed corneal phlycten leaves a triangular scar associated with superficial vascularization and thinning.

Treatment

Treatment includes use of topical steroids, topical antibiotics, and cycloplegics, in case of corneal involvement.

It is also essential to treat associated staphylococcal blepharitis.

Vernal Keratitis

Cornea can be involved in up to 50% of cases with vernal keratoconjunctivitis. It is more frequent in palpebral type of disease. Several types of corneal lesions may be produced such as:

- Punctate epithelial keratitis which begins as discrete micro erosions in the superior cornea (punctate epithelial erosions).
- Epithelial macro erosion due to continued epithelial loss.
- **Shield ulcer** (vernal ulcer): A vernal ulcer is noninfectious, horizontally oval, shallow, nonvascularized, and indolent ulcer of the superior cornea. It is associated with sub-epithelial scarring and mild corneal opacity. Chronic inflammation in the absence of ulcer may develop peripheral superficial vascularization, especially superior.

Treatment

- Punctate epithelial keratitis responds to usual treatment of vernal kerato-conjunctivitis.
- For persistent epithelial defects with ulceration, amniotic membrane graft with lamellar keratoplasty is carried out to enhance reepithelialization.

Marginal Ulcer (Catarrhal Ulcer)

Marginal ulcer is a *superficial* ulcer situated *near the limbus and* frequently seen *in old people.*

Etiology

It is thought to be caused by immune reaction to exotoxins produced by *Staphylococcus aureus.* These ulcers may also be caused by *Moraxella* and *Haemophilus.* They are often associated with Staphylococcal blepharitis in which an immune reaction occurs in the toxins produced by staphylococcus. This antigen–antibody complex is deposited in the peripheral cornea with secondary lymphocytic infiltration.

Clinical Features

Symptoms include mild irritation, lacrimation, photophobia, and pain. The subepithelial marginal infiltrates, *separated from limbus by a clear zone of cornea*, are typically located at the point of contact of eyelids with cornea (i.e., at 4, 7, 10, and 2 o'clock positions). The infiltrates coalesce with the circumferential spread which is accompanied by the breakdown of overlying epithelium. The ulcer formed is *shallow and frequently become vascularized.* Resolution occurs but *recurrences are common* and ulcer runs a chronic indolent course (**Fig. 6.18, Table 6.11**). Differentiating features between marginal keratitis and bacterial keratitis can be remembered by the mnemonic, PEDAL.

Lesions are culture negative, but S. aureus can frequently be isolated from lid margins.

Treatment

Treatment includes topical antibiotic + steroid drops. Treatment of coexisting blepharitis is done to prevent recurrences.

Mooren's Ulcer

It is a rare peripheral ulcerative keratitis also known as **chronic serpiginous ulcer** or **rodent ulcer**.

Etiology

Its exact etiology is unknown but autoimmune mechanism appears to be involved. It can be triggered in genetically susceptible individuals by trauma.

It may be unilateral or bilateral and affects males more commonly than females. Unilateral involvement affects older patients, is slowly progressive and responds better to treatment; bilateral involvement affects younger patients and is more aggressive.

Clinical Features

Symptoms include severe pain, lacrimation, photophobia, and blurred vision due to irregular astigmatism.

It begins as gray infiltrates near the margin of the cornea which breakdown, forming peripheral ulcer. The ulcer spreads circumferentially and toward the center of the cornea. Typically, advancing edge of ulcer undermines the corneal epithelium and superficial stroma. The base of the ulcer soon becomes vascularized. Healing takes place behind the active margin of the ulcer, but the healed area remains thin, vascularized and opaque. It rarely perforates. Spontaneous perforation is rare; however, minor trauma may lead to perforation.

Differential Diagnosis

It includes the conditions that are characterized by peripheral corneal ulceration and/or melting. Patients with bilateral Mooren's ulcer must be investigated for collagen vascular disorders.

Treatment

Treatment for Mooren's ulcer is difficult and disappointing as ischemia is the underlying cause.

Stepladder approach to manage this aggressive disease includes local, systemic, and surgical therapy.

- **Local treatment** includes: *Topical* treatment with corticosteroids, cyclosporine, and Acetylcysteine 10% (collagenase inhibitor). *Conjunctival resection* is done if inflammation is not controlled. It eliminates conjunctival sources of collagenase, proteoglycanase, and other inflammatory mediators.
- **Systemic treatment**: Systemic immuno-suppression with cyclophosphamide, cyclosporine, steroids, or methotrexate may be

Table 6.11 Comparison between marginal and bacterial keratitis (i.e., distinction between noninfectious and suppurative infiltrates)

	Marginal keratitis	Bacterial keratitis
Pain	Less	More
Epithelial defect	Small or absent (<1 mm)	Present (>1 mm)
Discharge	Watery	Purulent
Anterior chamber reaction (uveitis)	–	+
Location	Peripheral	Central

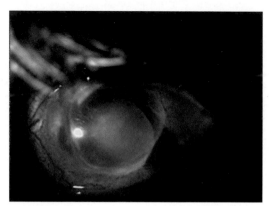

Fig. 6.18 Peripheral ulcerative keratitis (PUK).

initiated if the treatment with conjunctival resection fails.

- **Surgical treatment**: It includes lamellar keratoplasty and cyanoacrylate glue to treat small perforations.

> Lamellar keratoplasty with systemic immunosuppression may reduce the risk of recurrence; without systemic immunosuppression, recurrence rate is high.

Conditions causing peripheral corneal ulceration and thinning:
- Marginal ulcer.
- Mooren's ulcer.
- Systemic collagen vascular disorders:
  ◊ Rheumatoid arthritis.
  ◊ Polyarteritis nodosa.
  ◊ SLE.
  ◊ Wegener's granulomatosis.
- Oculo-dermatologic conditions:
  ◊ Rosacea keratitis.
- Corneal degenerations:
  ◊ Terrien's marginal degeneration.
  ◊ Pellucid marginal degeneration.

■ Miscellaneous Keratitis

Superficial Keratitis

It involves corneal epithelium, Bowman's membrane, and superficial corneal stroma. It is divided into:
- Superficial punctate keratitis (SPK).
- Superior limbic keratoconjunctivitis.
- Filamentary keratitis.
- Recurrent corneal erosions.
- Photophthalmia.

Superficial Punctate Keratitis (SPK)

It is characterized by multiple, punctate lesions in the superficial layers of the cornea (**Fig. 6.19**). It is caused by:
- *Viral infections*: Most common causes are: adenovirus, H-simplex, and H-zoster.
- *Chlamydial infections*: Trachoma and inclusion conjunctivitis.
- *Toxic:* It may be due to staphylococcal toxins in blepharoconjunctivitis.
- *Dry eye syndrome*: In KCS.
- *Idiopathic*: Thygeson's SPK.

Location

Location of lesions may serve as a clue to the etiology of SPK.

Superior location of SPK: The probable etiology may be vernal keratoconjunctivitis (VKC), superior limbic keratoconjunctivitis (SLK), and trachoma.

Inferior location: The probable etiology is Staphylococcal blepharitis, trichiasis, entropion, and lagophthalmos.

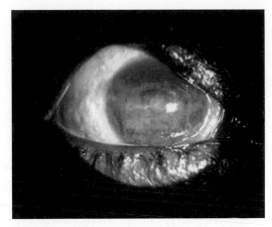

Fig. 6.19 Superficial punctate keratitis.

Interpalpebral location: The probable etiology is seborrheic blepharitis and KCS.

Clinical Features

Symptoms include mild ocular discomfort, photophobia, and lacrimation. It is characterized by punctate epithelial lesions which stain with Fluorescein dye. Subepithelial lesion may be present which do not stain with Fluorescein dye.

It is usually associated with conjunctivitis. One of the most characteristic features of Thygeson's SPK is lack of associated conjunctival inflammation (conjunctivitis). All other disease entities have associated conjunctivitis.

Treatment

It is treated with topical steroids with gradual tapering, lubricants, and treatment of cause.

Superior Limbic Keratoconjunctivitis (SLK)

As the name suggests, it is superior, limbic, corneal and conjunctival inflammation. It typically affects those belonging to the middle age group, with a greater affinity for females than males. It is usually bilateral. It is associated with abnormal thyroid dysfunction, usually hyperthyroidism. Its exact etiology is unknown. It appears to be the result of blink-related mechanical trauma which is supported by increased lid apposition of exophthalmic thyroid patients, who are known to have an increased incidence of SLK. SLK runs a chronic course with remissions and exacerbations. *Thyroid function tests* should be performed due to strong association with thyroid disease.

Clinical Features

Symptoms include foreign body sensation, burning, irritation, redness, watering, and photophobia.

Characteristic signs are seen in cornea and conjunctiva:
- Conjunctiva: Hyperemia of superior bulbar conjunctiva and opposing superior tarsal (palpebral) conjunctiva with papillary reaction is marked.
- Cornea shows filamentary keratitis of the superior cornea and limbus.
  ◊ SPK in the superior part of cornea which stains with Fluorescein and Rose Bengal.
  ◊ Superior corneal pannus.
- KCS in 25 to 50% of cases.

Treatment

Treatment is symptomatic as the condition is usually self-limiting and include the following:
- Topical lubricants to reduce friction between lid and bulbar conjunctiva. Lubricant must be preservative-free.
- Topical steroids to reduce inflammation.
- Topical Acetyl Cysteine drops (10%) for filamentary keratitis.
- Topical retinoic acid to prevent keratinization.
- Punctal occlusion as 25 to 50% patients with SLK also have KCS (dry eyes).
- Soft contact lenses which intervene between lid and superior bulbar conjunctiva and may be useful.
- Resection of superior limbal conjunctiva and Tenon's capsule.

Filamentary Keratitis

It is a superficial keratitis associated with formation of corneal filaments.

Etiology

KCS is the most common cause. Other causes include recurrent corneal erosions, H. simplex keratitis, prolonged eye patching, neurotropic keratitis, and SLK.

Clinical Features

Symptoms include irritation and foreign body sensation. Filaments consist of the core of mucous strands lined with epithelium. One end of the filament is attached to the corneal epithelium, while the other is unattached (free), moves with each blink, and causes foreign body sensation. They *stain well with Rose Bengal* (**Fig. 6.20**).

Treatment

Treatment includes the following:

- Mechanical removal of filaments.
- Hypertonic 5% saline drops to encourage adhesion of loose epithelium.
- A topical mucolytic agent such as Acetyl Cysteine (10%).
- Bandage contact lens.
- Treatment of underlying cause.
- Short-term topical steroids.

Recurrent Corneal Erosions

It is characterized by recurrent breakdown of epithelium. The basic cause is abnormalities in the underlying basement membrane microstructure. The condition may be associated with trauma, epithelial basement membrane or anterior stromal dystrophy, and diabetes.

Pathogenesis

Trauma or epithelial basement membrane dystrophy results in microscopic derangement in the epithelial basement membrane (such as thickening and discontinuity). It leads to abnormally weak attachment between basal cells of epithelium and basement membrane. Thus, epithelial layers are prone to separation and frequent erosions.

Minor injuries such as opening the eyes after sleep can cause shearing forces, resulting in tearing of epithelium.

Clinical Features

Symptoms often occur on wakening and include severe pain, blurring, photophobia, foreign body sensation, blepharospasm, and watering.

Characteristic Signs of recurrent corneal erosions include the following:

- Frank epithelial defects, particularly in the lower part of cornea.
- Signs of epithelial basement membrane dystrophy (intraepithelial microcysts and finger print lines) may be present in both eyes.

Typically, onset of corneal erosion occurs upon awakening in the morning, although it may occur at any time. Sleep causes relative anoxia, leading to edema of corneal epithelium. Vulnerable epithelium is easily rubbed off on sudden opening of eyelids upon awakening.

Treatment

Treatment includes the following:

- Lubricants: Eye drops during waking hours and gel or ointment at night.
- Therapeutic soft contact lenses (bandage contact lens).
- Topical antibiotics and cycloplegics.
- If erosions are severe or frequent, *excimer laser phototherapeutic keratectomy can be performed.*
- Anterior stromal micropunctures over and surrounding the erosions not involving the visual axis.

Photophthalmia

It is caused by exposure to ultraviolet (UV) rays in the range of 290 to 311 nm. UV damage to cornea is both wavelength- and intensity-dependent.

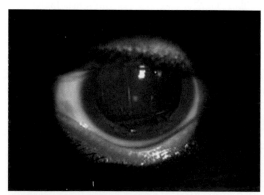

Fig. 6.20 Filamentary keratitis.

For short wavelength, a very small amount of UV energy may produce a corneal lesion. Nucleic acids of corneal epithelium maximally absorb these wavelengths. *Sources of UV rays* are welding flashes, germicidal lamps, and snow surface.

> Most damaging range of wavelength is 260 to 290 nm but absorbed by ozone layer. So, radiation of these wavelengths rarely penetrates the Earth's surface.

Pathology

After 4 to 6 hours of exposure to UV rays damaged epithelial cells desquamate and multiple erosions result, which produces characteristics punctate Fluorescein staining (superficial punctate keratitis).

Symptoms

Symptoms include burning pain, lacrimation, photophobia, and blepharospasm.

Prophylaxis consists of wearing dark glasses made of crooks glass which cuts off nearly all infrared and UV rays.

Treatment

Treatment includes cold compression, lubricant drops, and bandaging both eyes for a day.

■ Trophic Keratitis

Neurotrophic Keratitis

Sensory innervation is vital for the health of corneal epithelium and stroma. Neurotrophic keratitis occurs in an anesthetic cornea, that is, it *results from damage to the trigeminal nerve* which supplies the cornea. Following are the causes of neurotrophic keratitis:

1. Damage to trigeminal nerve: It may occur due to surgery for trigeminal neuralgia, injection of alcohol in gasserian ganglion for trigeminal neuralgia, and tumors: acoustic neuroma and neurofibroma.
2. Ocular disease such as the following:
   - Herpes simplex keratitis.
   - Herpes zoster keratitis.

3. Systemic diseases such as diabetes (peripheral neuropathy may result in decreased corneal sensation) and leprosy.

Pathogenesis of neurotrophic keratitis is explained in **Flowchart 6.4**.

Clinical Features

Symptoms include red eye, **absence of pain**, decreased aqueous tear production, mild foreign body sensation, and blurred vision.

Following are the clinical signs of neurotrophic keratitis:
- Presence of ciliary congestion.
- Decreased corneal sensation.
- Persistent epithelial defects. The ulcer is typically found in the interpalpebral area, and the cornea appears dull. It is followed by stromal edema and melting (**Flowchart 6.5**).

Treatment

- Decreased aqueous tear production in neurotrophic keratitis is treated with:
- Topical lubricant eye drops (**preservative-free**).
- Punctal occlusion abolishes drainage of tears.
- Tarsorrhaphy to prevent drying and reduce exposure. It is a good alternative and kept for at least 1 year (OP4.7).
- Amniotic membrane transplantation.

Exposure Keratitis

Lids resurface the cornea with the help of precorneal tear film at each blink and keep the cornea moist. Exposure keratitis is caused by improper wetting of corneal surface by precorneal tear film despite the presence of normal tear secretions.

Etiology

It is caused by the conditions that lead to exposure of cornea, that is, due to incomplete closure of lids. Causes of exposure keratitis (**lagophthalmos**) are:

1. Facial nerve palsy (**neuroparalytic keratitis**): VIIth nerve palsy may be idiopathic or can follow surgery for

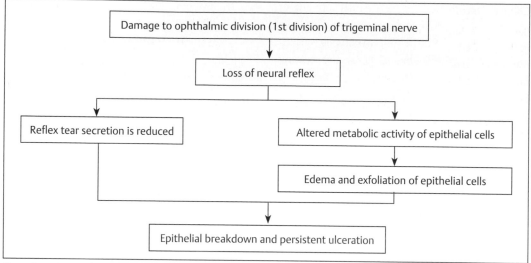

Flowchart 6.4 Pathogenesis of neurotrophic keratitis.

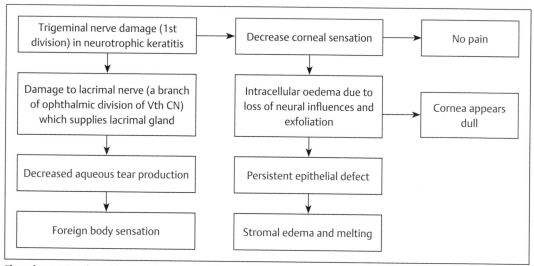

Flowchart 6.5 Clinical features in neurotrophic keratitis.

acoustic neuroma/parotid tumor. It results in the paralysis of orbicularis muscle and incomplete closure of lid.

2. Severe proptosis due to thyroid ophthalmopathy and orbital tumor.
3. Eyelid scarring associated with cicatricial pemphigoid, burns, and trauma.
4. Reduced muscle tone as in coma.

Occasionally corneal exposure during sleep may occur in normal healthy individuals if there is poor Bell's phenomenon.

Pathogenesis

Incomplete closure of lids results in desiccation of cornea. The epithelium is cast off, and invasion of cornea by infective organisms may occur.

Clinical Features

Because of lagophthalmos, cornea is exposed in lower part. So, initial desiccation occurs in the lower part of cornea, leading to inferior punctate epithelial keratitis *followed by* epithelial breakdown, stromal melting, infection, and even perforation (**Fig. 6.21**).

Treatment

- Tear substitutes (preservative-free lubricants) during day time.
- At night, application of eye ointment and closure of lids by tape or bandage.
- Treatment of the cause of exposure, but in the meantime, tarsorrhaphy may be required by suturing lids together (OP4.7).

> Combined neurotrophic (Vth CN damage) and neuroparalytic (VIIth CN palsy) keratitis is difficult to manage.

Nutritional Deficiency (Vitamin A Deficiency)

Ocular manifestations caused by vitamin A deficiency are referred to as **xerophthalmia.** **Cornea in vitamin A deficiency shows the following changes:**

1. Corneal xerosis: Earliest changes in cornea involve loss of corneal luster due to xerosis and bilateral punctate corneal epithelial erosions.

2. Keratomalacia: It reflects very severe vitamin A deficiency, often as early as the first year of life. Night blindness and conjunctival signs of vitamin A deficiency precede keratomalacia. The condition is usually bilateral. Bilateral melting of cornea is associated with conjunctival xerosis, and vitamin A deficiency is referred to as **keratomalacia.**

In keratomalacia, cornea becomes dull, insensitive, and hazy. The ulcer is formed with yellow infiltrates. Typically, it is devoid of usual inflammatory reaction and is a **characteristic** **feature.** The lesion rapidly involves full-thickness of cornea. Finally, whole tissues undergo necrosis and melt away (corneal melting by liquefactive necrosis).

Treatment

Systemic treatment involves oral or IM administration of vitamin A. Locally, intense lubrication and topical antibiotics are advised.

Atheromatous Corneal Ulcer

It occurs in old leucoma undergoing degenerative changes or it may start after a minor trauma. It is readily vulnerable to infection, as cornea is devitalized and insensitive. It is treated with the usual treatment, conjunctival flap, or keratoplasty. The amniotic membrane transplantation may be effective for the treatment of deep ulceration.

■ Keratitis Associated with Skin Diseases

Rosacea Keratitis

Acne rosacea is a skin disease characterized by erythema of cheeks and nose in butterfly configuration, progressing to telangiectasia, hypertrophy of sebaceous glands, papules and pustules. Rosacea keratitis is usually associated with seborrheic blepharitis. It is generally seen among elderly women.

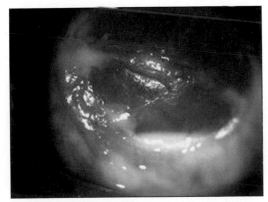

Fig. 6.21 Exposure keratitis.

Clinical Features

Symptoms include irritation, mild redness, and lacrimation.

Clinical signs of rosacea keratitis are:
- Seborrheic blepharitis and recurrent chalazia.
- Conjunctival vessels in the interpalpebral region are dilated.
- Yellowish-white infiltrates are seen in the cornea near the limbus which may ulcerate and then corneal vascularization takes place.
- Punctate epithelial keratopathy involving lower cornea.

Treatment

Local treatment: Topical *corticosteroids* as drops or ointment.

Systemic treatment: The essential treatment involves treating the skin condition with *systemic tetracycline* 250 mg 4 times daily for 3 weeks and then once daily for 6 months or *doxycycline* 100 mg twice daily for 3 weeks.

■ Corneal Degenerations (IM24.15)

There is marked distinction between degeneration and dystrophy. Degenerations are nonhereditary and usually unilateral, while dystrophies are hereditary and usually bilateral.

■ Etiology

Degenerations could arise due to age-related changes like arcus senilis, Vogt limbal girdles and Hassell–Henle bodies or pathological changes like lipid degenerations, amyloid degeneration, band keratopathy, Salzmann's nodular degeneration, Terrien's marginal degeneration, and spheroidal degeneration.

■ Classification

Corneal degenerations can be divided into:
- Primary degenerations.
- Secondary degenerations due to some compromising factors, for example, trauma, chemicals, systemic diseases, or inflammation.
- Infiltration associated with lipid and mucopolysaccharide metabolisms.

■ Arcus Senilis (Gerontoxon)

It is a lipid infiltration of peripheral corneal stroma. It begins in the superior and inferior perilimbal cornea as a crescent and gradually progresses circumferentially to form a circle. It is approximately 1 mm wide and does not affect vision. It is seen among the elderly population. It has a diffuse central border and a sharper peripheral border. It is separated from limbus by a clear zone which is known as the lucid interval of Vogt.

Arcus juvenilis (anterior embryotoxon): If the arcus appears in young persons (below 40 years of age), it is known as arcus juvenilis. It may be associated with familial lipidemia.

■ Vogt Limbal Girdle

It is an age-related change characterized by bilateral, chalky white crescentric lines in the interpalpebral area along both nasal and temporal limbus.

■ Hassell–Henle Bodies

These are the excrescences of hyaline material present in peripheral Descemet's membrane and are part of normal aging process.

■ Terrien's Marginal Degeneration

It is an idiopathic, noninflammatory thinning of peripheral cornea. It is usually bilateral, but may be unilateral. It is more frequently seen in males. It is most frequent in middle-aged to elder persons.

Signs: It starts with fine yellow–white punctate stromal opacities and superficial vascularization, usually superiorly. The lesion spread circumferentially and separated from the limbus by a clear zone. Progressive circumferential thinning results in peripheral gutter. Astigmatism develops from associated corneal flattening which may be irregular and results in visual deterioration. Usually, there is no pain or inflammation. Perforation may rarely occur following blunt trauma.

■ Band Shaped Keratopathy (Calcific Degeneration)

Band keratopathy is characterized by deposition of calcium salts in the subepithelial layers (Bowman's layer, epithelial basement membrane, and anterior stroma) of the cornea. Calcium is deposited as hydroxyapatite salt.

Etiology

1. Ocular causes: It occurs in eyes with chronic diseases, particularly chronic uveitis, glaucoma, chronic keratitis, Pthisis bulbi, and silicone oil in anterior chamber, that is, in aphakic eyes which have undergone vitrectomy with silicone oil.
2. Increased serum calcium or phosphate.
3. Systemic associations like sarcoidosis, hyperparathyroidism, vitamin D toxicity, and metastatic neoplasms to bone. All these conditions are associated with elevated serum calcium.

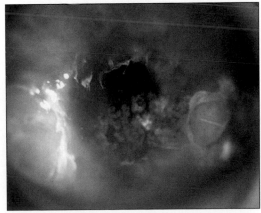

Fig. 6.22 Band-shaped keratopathy. Source: Band-shaped keratopathy. In: Gulani A, ed. The art of pterygium surgery: mastering techniques and optimizing results. 1st Edition. Thieme; 2019.

4. Juvenile rheumatoid arthritis (Still's disease): Chronic uveitis in Still's disease causes band-shaped keratopathy.
5. Chronic renal failure (CRF).

Clinical Features

Calcium is deposited as a horizontal band in the interpalpebral area of the cornea. Calcification starts near the corneal periphery which is separated from the limbus by a clear zone of cornea as in so many degenerative conditions, probably owing to better nutrition close to blood vessels. Calcium deposition gradually progresses toward the center to form a band-like chalky plaque (**Fig. 6.22**). The calcium plaque contains clear holes where Bowman's membrane is traversed by nerve endings and the surface of this opaque band appears stippled. Epithelium usually remains intact as deposition is beneath it.

Treatment

It is indicated if the vision decreases or persistent discomfort occurs. Central deposits may be removed by:

- *Chelation*—It involves removal of epithelium over deposits followed by application of 0.01 molar solution of **EDTA** (ethylene diamine tetra acetic acid), which is a chelator of calcium. It removes most of the deposited calcium. Pad and bandage for reepithelialization is taken care of.
- Treat any underlying systemic conditions or persistent uveitis to prevent recurrences.
- **PTK** with excimer laser to remove band keratopathy.
- Lamellar keratoplasty may be performed.

■ Spheroidal Degeneration (Climatic Droplet Keratopathy)

It is also called oil droplet keratopathy or actinic droplet keratopathy.

Etiology

It is thought to be a result of UV light exposure and occurs most often in men who work outdoor in the sun and in areas that have sunlight reflection off snow or sand.

Clinical Features

It is always bilateral and characterized by the presence of subepithelial, golden or yellow, fine droplets in the interpalpebral area of peripheral cornea and advance toward the center. Droplets appear oily although they are not of lipid origin. These globules are made up of a protein material with elastotic features. As the condition advances, droplets become larger and form large corneal nodules with elevated corneal epithelium.

Treatment

Majority of cases are asymptomatic. In cases with central lesions affecting vision, PTK with excimer laser or lamellar keratoplasty can be carried out.

■ Salzmann Nodular Degeneration

Etiology

It occurs in persons with previous chronic keratitis, particularly associated with trachoma, phlyctenular keratitis, vernal keratitis and IK.

It is characterized by bluish-white, avascular nodules in superficial stroma and Bowman's membrane that elevate the epithelium and may be associated with recurrent corneal erosions. The base of the nodule may be outlined by epithelial iron deposits.

Treatment

Most of the cases are asymptomatic and require no treatment. If nodules encroach the central cornea, affecting vision, PTK with excimer laser or lamellar keratoplasty can be done.

■ Corneal Dystrophies (OP4.5)

Corneal dystrophies are a group of opacifying disorders of cornea which are progressive, bilateral, symmetrical, hereditary, non inflammatory and nonvascularized. *All corneal dystrophies are*

autosomal dominant except macular dystrophy which has autosomal recessive inheritance.

■ Classification

On the basis of corneal layer primarily involved, corneal dystrophies are classified into (**Fig. 6.23**).
- Epithelial dystrophies:
  ◊ Epithelial basement membrane dystrophy.
  ◊ Meesmann dystrophy.
- Bowman layer dystrophies:
  ◊ Reis-Buckler dystrophy.
  ◊ Thiel-Behnke dystrophy.
- Stromal dystrophies:
  ◊ Lattice dystrophy.
  ◊ Granular dystrophy.
  ◊ Macular dystrophy.
  ◊ Gelatinous drop-like dystrophy.
- Endothelial dystrophies:
  ◊ Fuch's endothelial dystrophy.
  ◊ Posterior polymorphous dystrophy.
  ◊ Congenital hereditary endothelial dystrophy.

Epithelial Dystrophies

Epithelial dystrophies include:
- Epithelial basement membrane dystrophy (*Cogan's microcystic dystrophy* or *map-dot-fingerprint dystrophy*).
- Meesmann's dystrophy (juvenile epithelial dystrophy).

Epithelial Basement Membrane Dystrophy

Onset: In the second decade, the condition is asymptomatic. In a few patients, recurrent corneal erosions develop in the third decade.

Clinical features: It is characterized by bilateral, intraepithelial lesions which are best visualized by retroillumination. The pattern of lesions may be: dot-like opacities, epithelial microcysts, fingerprint-like lines or map-like gray patches. Simultaneous bilateral recurrent corneal erosions suggest epithelial basement membrane dystrophy.

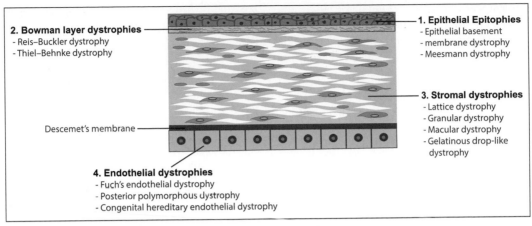

2. Bowman layer dystrophies
- Reis–Buckler dystrophy
- Thiel–Behnke dystrophy

1. Epithelial Epitophies
- Epithelial basement
- membrane dystrophy
- Meesmann dystrophy

3. Stromal dystrophies
- Lattice dystrophy
- Granular dystrophy
- Macular dystrophy
- Gelatinous drop-like
  dystrophy

Descemet's membrane

4. Endothelial dystrophies
- Fuch's endothelial dystrophy
- Posterior polymorphous dystrophy
- Congenital hereditary endothelial dystrophy

Fig. 6.23 Classification of corneal dystrophies.

Histology: It shows thickening of basement membrane and deposition of fibrillar material between basement membrane and Bowman's membrane.

Meesmann's Dystrophy (Juvenile Epithelial Dystrophy)

Onset: It is in the first 2 years of life, and has autosomal dominant inheritance.

Clinical features: It is characterized by multiple, tiny intraepithelial vesicles which are maximum centrally. The patient remains asymptomatic until middle age, then vesicles break through the anterior epithelial surface and cause intermittent irritation and decrease in visual acuity. Corneal sensations are reduced.

Bowman Layer Dystrophies

These include:

- **Reis–Buckler dystrophy** (corneal dystrophy of Bowman's layer type I or granular corneal dystrophy).
- **Thiel–Behnke dystrophy** (Honey comb dystrophy or corneal dystrophy of Bowman's membrane Type II).

Characteristics of both types of Bowman layer dystrophies:

Inheritance: Autosomal dominant.

Clinical features: These are characterized by gray–white, round opacities in the central cornea. Over time, these result in a reticular pattern in the Reis–Buckler dystrophy and assume a honeycomb pattern in the Thiel–Behnke dystrophy. Patients have recurrent corneal erosions which are painful initially. Later, the pain diminishes, as corneal sensitivity decreases. Vision is impaired due to fibrosis at Bowman's layer.

Histology: It shows destruction of Bowman's membrane and fibrous tissue, replacing Bowman's layer in both dystrophies.

Treatment: Symptomatic for **recurrent erosions**. Excimer laser keratectomy for visual disturbance. Lamellar keratoplasty is associated with relatively rapid recurrence of dystrophy on the graft and penetrating keratoplasty (PKP) may become necessary in both dystrophies.

Stromal Corneal Dystrophies

- These include: Granular corneal dystrophy.
- Macular corneal dystrophy.
- Lattice corneal dystrophy.
- Schnyder crystalline dystrophy.

Granular Dystrophy

Inheritance: Autosomal dominant.

Onset: In first decade of life.

Clinical features: Opacities are dense, white and granular in the anterior stroma of central cornea, sparing the peripheral cornea. The intervening cornea between the opacities also remains clear (**Fig. 6.24**).

Histopathology: The opacities are formed due to the hyaline degeneration of collagenous protein and stain with Masson trichrome.

Effect on vision: Glare is present but the vision is good. The opacities coalesce into various irregular shapes and vision is impaired.

Treatment: PKP is usually required by the fifth decade.

Macular Dystrophy

Inheritance: Autosomal recessive.

Onset: In the first decade of life (6–9 years).

Clinical features: Opacities assume a discrete granular form in the central cornea which spreads to the periphery. There is no clear space between the opacities.

Histopathology: The opacities are composed of glycosaminoglycans (GAG) and stain with alcian blue.

Effect on vision: Vision is affected at an early age.

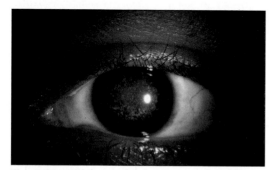

Fig. 6.24 Granular dystrophy. Source: Corneal disorders. In: Narang P, Trattler W, ed. Optimizing suboptimal results following cataract surgery. 1st Edition. Thieme; 2018.

Treatment: Penetrating keratoplasty is indicated but recurrence in graft may occur.

Lattice Dystrophy

Inheritance: Autosomal dominant.

Onset: During the second decade.

Clinical features: It is characterized by presence of branched, crisscross lines along with punctate opacities in between.

Histopathology: Histopathology reveals that it is a form of amyloidosis, that is, amyloid is deposited in the corneal stroma and stain with Congo red.

Effect on vision: The crisscross lines form an irregular lattice work and cause impairment of visual acuity.

Treatment: PKP is the treatment of choice when acuity decreases significantly.

Schnyder Crystalline Dystrophy

It is a disorder of corneal lipid metabolism associated with systemic hypercholesterolemia (raised serum cholesterol).

Inheritance: Autosomal dominant.

Features: It is caused by central subepithelial corneal crystals, often in a ring pattern, initially in the first decade of life. With advancing age, central corneal haze becomes evident.

Histology: Shows accumulation of cholesterol and phospholipids throughout stroma.

Treatment: Excimer laser keratectomy is advised.

Endothelial Corneal Dystrophies

- These include: Fuch's endothelial dystrophy.
- Posterior polymorphous dystrophy.

Fuch's Endothelial Dystrophy

It is bilateral and associated with increased incidence of primary open-angle glaucoma.

Inheritance: It is autosomal dominant.

Age: It occurs after 50 years.

Sex: It is more common in females.

Stagings: It is characterized by progressive loss of corneal endothelial cells, resulting in reduced vision, and the severity of disease varies as follows (**Flowchart 6.6**):

Stage 1: Earliest finding in Fuch's dystrophy is the presence of excrescences (irregular warts) of Descemet's membrane called guttae in the central corneal endothelium (**corneal guttata**) which involve the corneal periphery as well with time. The confluence of guttae produces a roughened surface with beaten metal appearance. Stroma and epithelium are uninvolved and patient's vision is normal at this stage.

Stage 2: Disruption of normal endothelial mosaic takes place with endothelial dysfunction. It results in stromal edema which is significant upon awakening and clears later in the day due to evaporation. Stromal edema results in Descemet membrane's folds with increase in corneal thickness.

Patient complains of blurred vision in morning that improves during the day, Glare and colored halos around lights in the morning.

Stage 3: Due to progressive endothelial decompensation, epithelial edema with bullae formation takes place (**bullous keratopathy**). The periodic rupture of bullae causes:
- Pain and discomfort due to exposure of naked nerve endings, and eye is prone to secondary infection.
- Profound reduction in vision.

Diagnosis—It is diagnosed by:
- Specular microscopy: It is done for endothelial cell count (**Fig. 6.25**).
- Corneal pachymetry: It is done to document increased corneal thickness.
- Confocal microscopy: It is done to image endothelium in the presence of corneal edema (corneal opacification precludes specular microscopy).

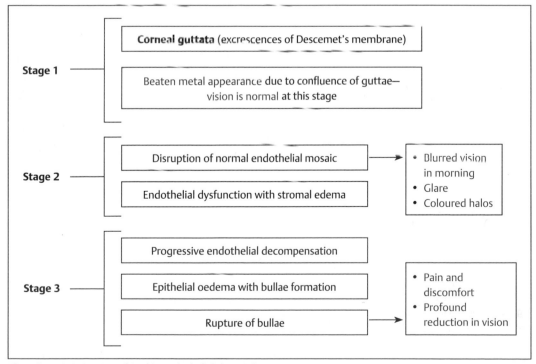

Flowchart 6.6 Staging of Fuch's endothelial dystrophy.

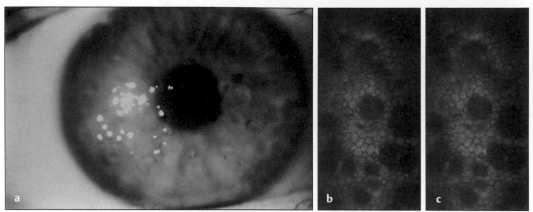

Fig. 6.25 Fuch's dystrophy. **(a)** On slit lamp. Source: History. In: Singh K, Smiddy W, Lee A, ed. Ophthalmology review: a case-study approach. 2nd Edition. Thieme; 2018. **(b)** Moderate type. **(c)** Advanced type with endotheliopathy (on specular biomicroscopy). Source: Specular microscopy and pachymetry. In: Narang P, Trattler W, ed. Optimizing suboptimal results following cataract surgery. 1st Edition. Thieme; 2018.

Differential diagnosis—It includes:

- Posterior polymorphous dystrophy.
- Congenital hereditary endothelial dystrophy.
- Aphakic/pseudophakic bullous keratopathy (**Fig. 6.26**).
- Hassell–Henle bodies.

Treatment

- Topical Sodium Chloride as drops (5%) and ointment (6%).
- Lubricating eye drops.
- Bandage contact lenses to relieve pain caused by rupture of bullae.
- PKP.
- If IOP is >20 mm Hg, reduce it. Lowering of IOP may reduce the force that drives the fluid into stroma.

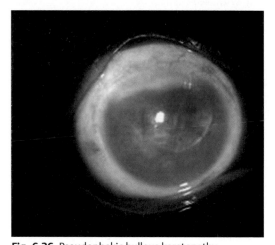

Fig. 6.26 Pseudophakic bullous keratopathy.

Cataract surgery and Fuch's endothelial dystrophy

Cataract surgery may accelerate endothelial cell loss. Extra precautions during intraocular surgery (such as intraoperative soft shell viscoelastics technique) should be taken to protect the endothelium from surgical trauma:

- In eye with corneal epithelial edema or corneal thickness >640 µm by pachymetery, consider triple procedure, that is, cataract surgery + IOL implantation + keratoplasty.
- If corneal thickness is <640 µm, good visual outcome is expected.

Posterior Polymorphous Dystrophy

Inheritance: Usually autosomal dominant.

Clinical features: It occurs early in life and is characterized by the presence of multilayered endothelium. The single cell layer of endothelium is transformed into a multilayered epithelium-like tissue. The posterior surface of cornea shows vesicular pattern, band-like lesions of diffuse opacities.

Treatment

It is usually asymptomatic and treatment is not required. Those with corneal opacification require PKP.

■ Ectatic Conditions of Cornea

Disorders of corneal shape include:
- Keratoconus.
- Keratoglobus.
- Pellucid marginal degeneration.

■ Keratoconus (Conical Cornea) (OP4.5)

It is a progressive steepening of cornea secondary to stromal thinning whereby it assumes a conical shape. The apex of cone always being slightly below the center of cornea. It occurs around puberty with slow progression. It is usually bilateral but the patients have asymmetrical involvement.

Etiology

It is unknown but seems to be multifactorial. It may be:
- Due to congenital weakness of the cornea.
- Secondary to trauma.
- Associated with Down syndrome.
- Due to repeated rubbing of the eyes.

Clinical Features

Symptoms include progressive bulging of cornea which induces myopic astigmatism and subsequently becomes irregular. It causes marked visual impairment and the patient may complain of frequent changes in spectacle power and decreased tolerance to contact lens wear.

Ocular manifestations of keratoconus are limited to cornea and include:
- Conical protrusion of cornea with apex of cone slightly below the center of cornea (**Fig. 6.27a**).
- Bulging of lower eyelid by cone of cornea on down gaze (**Munson's sign**).
- With direct ophthalmoscope at 1 m distance, a ring of shadow concentric with the margin of cone is seen in red reflex "oil droplet" reflex which alters its position on moving the ophthalmoscope (**Fig. 6.27b**).
- Retinoscopy shows irregular "scissor" reflex.
- A ring of iron deposition occurs in the epithelium at the base of cone (Fleischer ring). It is best seen with a cobalt-blue filter.
- Presence of vertical striae in deep stroma (Vogt striae) may be noticed. These deep stromal stress lines disappear with external pressure on the globe (**Fig. 6.27c**).
- Distortion of corneal reflex is best seen with Placido disc or corneal topography.
- When light beam is focused from the temporal side across the cornea, a conical reflection is seen on the nasal cornea (**Rizutti's sign**).

Sometimes, rupture in Descemet's membrane develops, which causes influx of aqueous into cornea (**acute hydrops**) and sudden stromal edema with opacification. It results in sudden impairment of visual acuity. Break usually heals within 6 to 10 weeks, corneal edema clears, and stromal scarring may develop.

Keratoconus can be graded by keratometry, as depicted in **Table 6.12**.

Associations

Systemic associations: Keratoconus may be associated with:
- Down's syndrome.
- Marfan's syndrome.
- Ehlers Danlos syndrome.
- Apert's syndrome.
- Atopy.

Ocular associations—These include:
- Vernal keratoconjunctivitis.
- Leber's congenital amaurosis.
- Retinopathy of prematurity.
- Fuch's dystrophy.
- Blue sclera.
- Aniridia.
- Ectopia lentis.

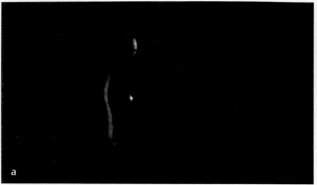

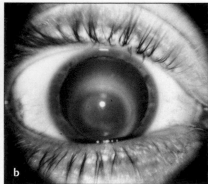

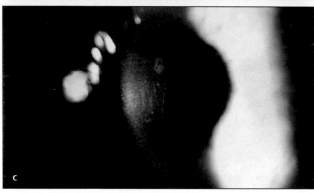

Fig. 6.27 (a) Conical protrusion of cornea. **(b)** Oil droplet red reflex. **(c)** Vogt's striae. Source: History. In: Singh K, Smiddy W, Lee A, ed. Ophthalmology review: A case-study approach. 2nd edition. Thieme; 2018.

Posterior keratoconus

In posterior keratoconus, the posterior corneal surface protrudes into the stroma. Frequently, scarring occurs in stroma, anterior to Descemet's bulge. It is congenital, nonprogressive, and usually unilateral.

Table 6.12 Grading of keratoconus

Grade of keratoconus	Keratometry reading
Mild	< 48 D
Moderate	48–54 D
Severe	> 54 D

Treatment

- Spectacles in early stages to correct refractive errors.
- Rigid gas permeable contact lenses to eliminate irregular corneal curvature. So, these are required to correct higher degree of astigmatism.
- Intracorneal rings in low to moderate keratoconus.
- **Corneal collagen cross linking** (**CCC**): It is a new technique to arrest progression of keratoconus. In this procedure, corneal epithelial is removed and *riboflavin 0.1% eye drops* are instilled over cornea till cornea is adequately saturated, which is exposed to UV radiation. Riboflavin triggers increased

cross-linking of corneal collagen fibrils by formation of intrafibrillary and interfibrillar covalent bonds and stabilizes the corneal stroma. Bandage soft contact lenses are prescribed to permit the epithelium to heal.

- **Corneal transplantation** (Keratoplasty): It is done if disease progresses despite all measures and in case of acute hydrops.

PKP or **deep lamellar keratoplasty** is currently becoming procedure of choice. It removes entire corneal stroma, sparing the host's Descemet membrane and endothelium. It reduces the risk of rejection and the donor cornea with low endothelial cell count can be used.

Table 6.13 Differentiating features between keratoglobus and buphthalmos

	Keratoglobus	Buphthalmos
Corneal transparency	Clear cornea	Hazy
IOP	Normal	Increased
Angle of anterior chamber	Normal	Angle anomaly present
Optic disc	No cupping	Cupping present

Abbreviation: IOP, intraocular pressure.

■ Keratoglobus

It is congenital, nonprogressive, and bilateral. It is inherited as an autosomal recessive trait. It is characterized by hemispherical (globular) corneal protrusion due to thinning of entire cornea (i.e., limbus-to-limbus corneal thinning). In contrast, keratoconus shows central stromal thinning. It may be associated with blue sclera and systemic connective tissue abnormalities. *Vogt striae and Fleischer's ring are absent.* It must be differentiated from buphthalmos (**Table 6.13**).

Corneal topography shows generalized steepening, and cornea is more prone to rupture on relatively mild trauma in keratoglobus. It is treated with scleral contact lenses because results of surgery are very poor.

■ Pellucid Marginal Degeneration

It is a progressive, bilateral peripheral corneal thinning typically affecting the inferior cornea (usually 4 to 8 o'clock positions).

The following clinical signs helps in diagnosing pellucid marginal degeneration:

- Area of thinning is 1 to 2 mm inside the inferior limbus and measures approximately 2 mm in width and 6 to 8 mm in horizontal extent (4–8 o'clock).
- Cornea above the crescent-shaped band of thinning protrudes with flattening in vertical meridian. Therefore, there is a marked against-the-rule astigmatism and reduced visual acuity.
- Epithelium is intact.
- Vogt striae (deep stromal stress lines) and Fleischer's ring do not occur.
- Acute hydrops is rare.
- **Corneal topography** shows a classical "butterfly" pattern.

Treatment

- Contact lenses are prescribed for correction of astigmatism. Spectacles usually fail due to increasing irregular astigmatism.
- Surgery includes:
  ◊ Large eccentric penetrating keratoplasty.
  ◊ Crescentric lamellar keratoplasty.
  ◊ Thermocauterization.

Anatomy 164

Inflammation of Sclera 165

Staphyloma 170

Blue Sclera 172

■ Anatomy

Sclera is an avascular, dense fibrous tissue. It forms the posterior 5/6th part of the outer coat of the eyeball. Developmentally, it is derived from the neural crest. Its primary function is to protect the eye and maintain the shape of the eyeball.

Anteriorly, it is continuous with cornea at the limbus. The anterior most sclera near the limbus is marked by an indentation (furrow) on the inner surface called scleral sulcus. Posteriorly, it ends at the optic nerve canal. Its outer surface is covered by Tenon's capsule which is separated from the sclera by an episcleral tissue. Its inner surface is separated from the choroid by the suprachoroidal space.

The **thickness of sclera** varies from one place to the other. It is thickest (1 mm) *near the optic nerve* and thinnest (0.3 mm) at the *insertion of extraocular muscles*. At *limbus*, the thickness of sclera is 0.83 mm.

Histologically, sclera can be divided into three parts from outward to inward (**Fig. 7.1**):
- Episcleral tissue.
- Scleral stroma (sclera proper).
- Lamina fusca.

■ Episcleral Tissue

It is a thin, loose layer of connective tissue overlying the sclera and situated below the Tenon's capsule. It is a densely vascularized layer. Apart from the vessels and nerves, it contains collagen, fibroblasts, and occasional melanocytes. Anteriorly, it is supplied by anterior ciliary arteries, while the posterior part of episcleral tissue is supplied by posterior ciliary artery.

■ Scleral Stroma (Sclera Proper)

It is composed of collagen bundles, elastic fibers, fibroblasts, and ground substances (proteoglycans and glycoproteins). The collagen fibers in sclera are of varying sizes and are irregularly arranged.

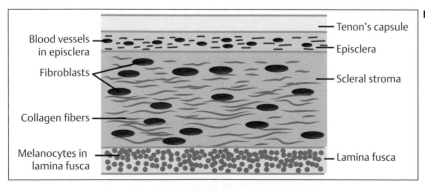

Fig. 7.1 Parts of sclera.

Blood vessels in episclera — Tenon's capsule — Episclera — Fibroblasts — Scleral stroma — Collagen fibers — Melanocytes in lamina fusca — Lamina fusca

Due to this irregularity of collagen fibers, the sclera is opaque (cornea is transparent due to uniform orientation of collagen fibers). The fibroblasts in sclera play an important role in the synthesis of collagen, proteoglycans, and glycoproteins.

■ Lamina Fusca

It is the inner most layer of sclera. The connective tissue of this layer is loosely arranged than the rest of the sclera and contains an abundance of melanocytes, mostly migrated from the choroid. It is separated from the choroid by a potential space known as *suprachoroidal space.*

The sclera is **perforated by** many nerves and vessels. Posteriorly, it is pierced by optic nerve and blends with dural and arachnoid coverings of optic nerve at its exit. The sclera is modified into a sieve-like membrane (*lamina cribrosa*) through which the optic nerve fibers pass. It is also penetrated by 8 to 20 short posterior ciliary arteries in a ring (*circle of Zinn*) which are accompanied by short ciliary nerves. Little anterior to these, two long posterior ciliary arteries and nerves also pierce the sclera to enter the eye ball. Posterior to the equator, it is perforated by four vortex veins which drain the veins of uveal tract. Anteriorly, the anterior ciliary arteries and veins penetrate the sclera 3 to 4 mm away from the limbus (**Fig. 7.2**).

■ Blood Supply

It is almost avascular and gets its nourishment from the episclera and choroid.

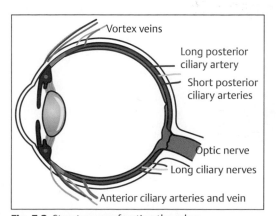

Fig. 7.2 Structures perforating the sclera.

■ Nerve Supply

Sclera is supplied by branches from long and short posterior ciliary nerves.

■ Inflammation of Sclera

The inflammation of sclera may be:
- Superficial or episcleritis.
- Deep or scleritis.

■ Episcleritis (OP5.1)

It is a benign, self-limiting but recurrent inflammatory disease affecting the episclera which lies between the Tenon's capsule and the sclera proper.

Age and sex– It commonly affects young females.

Etiology

Most of the time it is idiopathic. It may be associated with:
- Connective tissue diseases (rheumatoid arthritis, systemic lupus erythematosus [SLE], and relapsing polychondritis).
- Systemic vasculitic diseases (polyarteritis nodosa)
- Dermatologic disease (Rosacea)
- Metabolic disease (gout).
- Herpetic infection.
- Atopy.

It is often regarded as a hypersensitivity reaction to an endogenous toxin.

Pathophysiology

The inflammatory response is localized to the superficial episcleral vascular network. Histopathology shows a nongranulomatous inflammation with vascular dilatation and perivascular lymphocytic infiltration of subconjunctival and episcleral tissues.

Clinical Features

Symptoms:
- Redness.
- Ocular discomfort.
- Photophobia.
- Lacrimation.

Signs:

Episcleritis appears as two clinical types, namely, simple or diffuse episcleritis and nodular or focal episcleritis.

Simple or Diffuse Episcleritis

The large episcleral vessels run radially beneath the conjunctiva. Therefore, engorgement of these vessels in episcleritis results in *sectoral or diffuse redness* of one or both eyes. The *pain is unusual,* but if present, it is localized to the eye itself. It is the most common type and presents with sudden redness and generalized discomfort (**Fig. 7.3a**).

Nodular or Focal Episcleritis

It has a less acute onset and more prolonged course than simple episcleritis. It presents with a circumscribed nodule situated 2 or 3 mm from the limbus. *The nodule is hard, tender, immovable,* and often temporal in location. The *overlying conjunctiva moves freely* over it. It is traversed by deeper episcleral vessels which impart a bright red or salmon pink color to it. It is usually *transient* but has a tendency to *recur*. The *nodule never ulcerates* and leaves a slate-colored scar (**Fig. 7.3b**).

Occasionally, a fleeting but frequently repeated episcleritis (episcleritis periodica fugax) may be seen.

Differential Diagnosis

It must be differentiated from scleritis, conjunctivitis, and foreign body or granuloma.

- The episcleritis is differentiated from scleritis (**Table 7.1**) by:
- Phenylephrine **2.5%** eye drops blanch conjunctival vessels, allowing the differentiation of *conjunctivitis* and episcleritis.
- The nodular episcleritis may be confused with congestion due to *foreign body* or *granuloma* which must be ruled out as the causes for the episcleral nodule.

Investigations

The recurrent attacks of episcleritis may require systemic evaluation. The basic tests to order include:

- Rheumatoid factor.

Table 7.1 Differentiating features of episcleritis and scleritis

Episcleritis	Scleritis
• Instillation of phenylephrine **(10%)** blanches the conjunctival and episcleral vessels. Therefore, patient's eye redness improves after phenylephrine instillation. • Diffuse or sectoral bright red or pink bulbar injection.	• Instillation of phenylephrine **(10%)** does not blanch the deep scleral vessels. • In scleritis, there is violaceous hue.

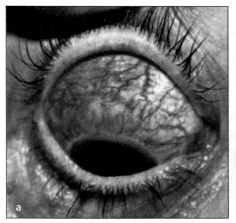 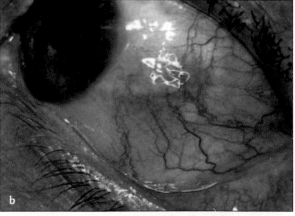

Fig. 7.3 (a) Diffuse episcleritis. Source: Episcleritis. In: Agarwal A, Jacob S, ed. Color Atlas of Ophthalmology. The Quick-Reference Manual for Diagnosis and Treatment. 2nd Edition. Thieme; 2009. **(b)** Nodular episcleritis. Source: Episcleritis. In: Agarwal A, Jacob S, ed. Color Atlas of Ophthalmology. The Quick-Reference Manual for Diagnosis and Treatment. 2nd Edition. Thieme; 2009.

- Anti-nuclear antibody.
- Serum uric acid.
- Chest X-ray.
- Total leukocyte count (TLC), differential leukocyte count (DLC), and erythrocyte sedimentation rate (ESR).
- Venereal disease research laboratory (VDRL)/fluorescent treponemal antibody absorption (FTA-ABS) test.
- Urine analysis.

Treatment

- Mild episcleritis is treated with lubricants.
- Moderate to severe episcleritis:
  ◇ Topical and systemic nonsteroidal anti-inflammatory drugs (NSAIDs) may be preferred as initial therapy.
  ◇ Topical steroid drops or ointment.
  ◇ Oral (NSAIDs) such as:

Flurbiprofen 100 mg t.i.d. for 10 days and indomethacin 25 mg t.i.d. are given for the cases where topical treatment is unsuccessful.

■ Scleritis (OP5.2)

Scleritis is the inflammation of sclera proper and is characterized by oedema and cellular infiltrate deep within the sclera tissue. It is usually a bilateral disease (50%). It is also less common than episcleritis and extends more deeply. *Pain is a hallmark symptom.* It usually occurs in elderly patients between the 4th and 6th decades. Females are more affected than males. **Flowchart 7.1** details the pathophysiology of scleritis.

Etiology

- Scleritis is commonly associated with systemic causes, usually an autoimmune disease such as:
  ◇ Rheumatoid arthritis.
  ◇ SLE.
  ◇ Relapsing polychondritis.
  ◇ Polyarteritis nodosa.
  ◇ Ankylosing spondylitis.
  ◇ Reiter's syndrome.

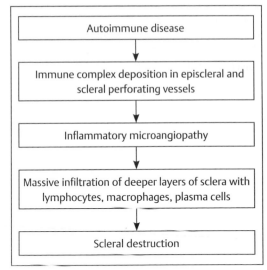

Flowchart 7.1 Pathophysiology of scleritis.

  ◇ Wegener granulomatosis.
  ◇ Giant cell arteritis.
- Metabolic disorders such as gout.
- Infections such as herpes zoster ophthalmicus.
- Granulomatous diseases such as sarcoidosis, syphilis, and tuberculosis.
- Postsurgical such as after cataract extraction and retinal detachment surgery.

Classification

Flowchart 7.2 explains the classification of scleritis.

The most common clinical forms are diffuse and nodular scleritis (non-necrotizing). Necrotizing scleritis with or without inflammation is much less frequent and frequently associated with systemic autoimmune disorders.

Clinical Features

Symptoms:
- Pain.
- Redness.
- Photophobia.
- Lacrimation.
- Diminution of vision.

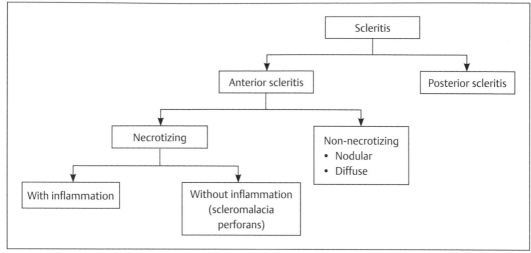

Flowchart 7.2 Classification of scleritis.

The pain often typically wakes the patients early in the morning. The pain is exacerbated by eye movements. Worsening of the pain during eye movement is due to the extraocular muscle insertions into the sclera. This pain may radiate to involve the ear, scalp, face, and jaw.

Signs:
The signs in scleritis vary depending on the location of the scleritis and the degree of involvement. The signs of different types of scleritis are explained below.

Anterior Scleritis

Anterior Non-necrotizing Scleritis

Diffuse Scleritis
The inflammatory reaction may involve the sector or the whole sclera with marked reactive scleral edema and characteristic violet–bluish hue of involved area (**Fig. 7.4**).

Nodular Scleritis
It is characterized by the appearance of one or more nodules. The nodule is *hard, purplish, elevated, immovable, and situated near the limbus.* Sometimes, the nodules encircle the cornea forming a ring (annular scleritis).

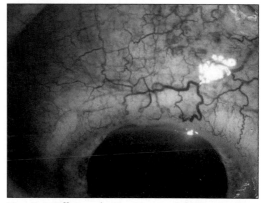

Fig. 7.4 Diffuse scleritis. Source: Scleritis. In: Lang G, ed. Ophthalmology. A Pocket Textbook Atlas. 3rd Edition. Thieme; 2015.

Anterior Necrotizing Scleritis

With Inflammation
The localized inflammatory reaction is associated with local infarction, owing to the occlusive vasculitis. The inflammation spreads to the adjoining areas and the necrotic patches coalesce, proceeding to scleral necrosis. The necrosed sclera becomes thin and the uveal tissue shines through it, leading to subsequent staphyloma formation. It is usually associated with anterior uveitis.

Without Inflammation (Scleromalacia Perforans)

It is a rare form of progressive scleral thinning without inflammation. The typical signs of inflammation (pain and redness) are absent. The sclera is white (without vascular congestion) and thin. Due to scleral thinning, the exposure of underlying uvea and staphyloma formation may occur. Despite the nomenclature, perforation of the globe is extremely rare, as integrity is maintained by a thin layer of fibrous tissue, but trivial trauma may lead to the perforation of the globe.

Posterior Scleritis

It is rare and involves the sclera posterior to the insertion of rectus muscles. It is potentially a blinding condition and the diagnosis is commonly delayed. The inflammation may involve the adjacent structures, giving rise to the following symptoms and signs. Posterior scleritis may involve:

- Extraocular muscles (myositis).
- Orbital tissues.
- Uveal tissue.

Involvement of extraocular muscles result in:

- Pain in eye movements.
- Restricted ocular movements resulting in diplopia.
- Tenderness to touch
- Redness around muscle insertion.

Involvement of orbital tissues result in:

- Proptosis.
- Disc edema.
- Macular edema.
- Diminution of vision.

Involvement of uveal tissue result in:

- Choroidal folds.
- Choroidal detachment.
- Uveal effusion syndrome.
- Exudative retinal detachment.

Complications

Table 7.2 lists the possible complications of scleritis.

Investigations

- B-scan ultrasonography.
- Orbital magnetic resonance imaging (MRI).
- Computed tomography (CT) scan.
- X-ray of chest (for tuberculosis and sarcoidosis) and spine (for ankylosing spondylitis)
- *Laboratory test*– Due to the association of scleritis with many systemic diseases, laboratory workup becomes extensive and includes:
  ◇ TLC.
  ◇ DLC.
  ◇ ESR.

Table 7.2 Complications of scleritis	
Structure involved	**Complications**
Cornea	Scleritis may extend to cornea, resulting in: • Sclerosing keratitis in which the peripheral cornea adjacent to the site of scleritis resembles sclera. It is triangular or tongue-shaped with the round apex toward the center of cornea. There is no corneal vascularization and ulceration. • Peripheral ulcerative keratitis which is characterized by progressive melting and ulceration due to stromal melting.
Sclera	• The scleral thinning may not withstand the IOP, resulting in ectasia (staphyloma). Secondary glaucoma is a common sequel to the ciliary staphyloma.
Uvea	• Uveitis • Intraocular pressure can be very difficult to control in the presence of active scleritis with inflammation resulting in glaucoma. • Hypotony may result due to inflammatory damage or ischemia of ciliary body.
Lens	• Cataract
Retina and optic nerve in posterior scleritis	• Macular edema • Disc edema • Retinal detachment

◊ C-reactive protein (CRP).
◊ Antinuclear antibodies (ANA).
◊ Anti-DNA antibodies.
◊ Rheumatoid factor.
◊ Antineutrophil cytoplasmic antibodies.
◊ Urine analysis.
◊ FTA-ABS and VDRL (for syphilis).
◊ Serum uric acid (for gout).
◊ Serum ACE enzyme (for sarcoidosis).

Treatment

* For **non-necrotizing scleritis**
  ◊ Oral NSAIDs (indomethacin and flurbiprofen) twice a day should be used alone only in non-necrotizing disease.
  ◊ Concurrent therapy with antacids or receptor blockers is advised to reduce gastrointestinal side effect of NSAIDs.
  ◊ Topical steroids are generally ineffective and reduce ocular inflammation but treatment is generally systemic.
  ◊ Systemic corticosteroids may be used in patients unresponsive to NSAIDs.
* For **necrotizing scleritis**
  ◊ Necrotizing scleritis needs oral steroids (prednisolone 1–1.5 mg/kg/day) tapered slowly.
  ◊ Intravenous methylprednisolone may be used for severe scleritis.
  ◊ Immunosuppressive agents (methotrexate or cyclophosphamide) may be required in nonresponsive cases to steroids.
  ◊ *Periocular steroid injections are contraindicated in necrotizing scleritis* because they may lead to scleral thinning and perforation.
  ◊ Scleral patch grafting may be required in case of marked thinning or risk of perforation.

If scleritis is infectious, causes are treated with appropriate topical and systemic antimicrobial agents.

If scleritis is caused by an underlying disease, treatment of that disease may be needed.

Patient must be informed about the potential serious adverse effects of steroids and immunosuppressive drugs.

■ Staphyloma

It is an ectasia of outer coats (cornea, sclera or both) in which the uveal tissue is incarcerated. The inflammatory or degenerative diseases of the outer tunic of the eyeball leads to weakening of the outer coat resulting in its localized bulging. Raised intraocular pressure (IOP) and trauma also contribute to the development of staphyloma.

■ Classification

Depending on the site involved, staphyloma can be classified into (**Fig. 7.5**):
* Anterior.
* Intercalary.
* Ciliary.
* Equatorial.
* Posterior.

Anterior Staphyloma

It occurs mainly due to perforation of a large sloughing corneal ulcer (**Flowchart 7.3**). It may be partial or total.

Intercalary Staphyloma

It is the localized bulging of the outer coat at the limbal area (from limbus up to 2 mm behind the limbus) lined by the root of the iris.

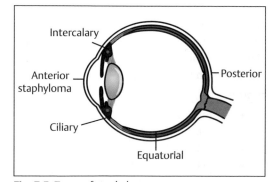

Fig. 7.5 Types of staphyloma.

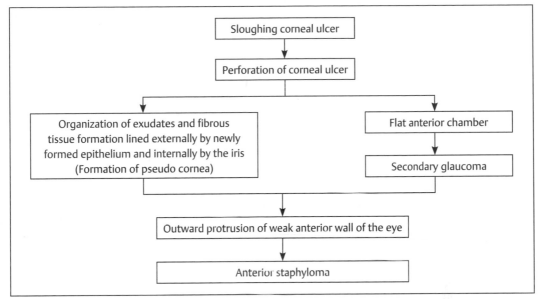

Flowchart 7.3 Formation of anterior staphyloma.

Causes

- Perforated injury of peripheral cornea.
- Perforated marginal corneal ulcer.
- Anterior scleritis.

Clinical Features

There is marked corneal astigmatism resulting in defective vision. In untreated cases, secondary angle closure glaucoma occurs, leading to progression of staphyloma.

Treatment

Localized staphylectomy under heavy doses of oral steroids.

Ciliary Staphyloma

It is located about 2 to 3 mm behind the limbus, affecting the ciliary zone. The ciliary body is incarcerated in the bulge of weak sclera. It is bluish in color with lobulated appearance (**Fig. 7.6**).

Causes

- Perforating injury resulting in thinning sclera.
- Scleritis.
- Absolute glaucoma.

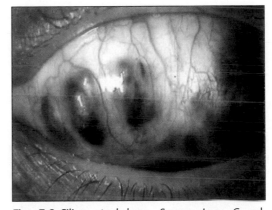

Fig. 7.6 Ciliary staphyloma. Source: Lang G, ed. Ophthalmology. A Pocket Textbook Atlas. 3rd Edition. Thieme; 2015.

Equatorial Staphyloma

It is the bulge of sclera in the equatorial region with incarceration of choroid. It is located 14 mm behind the limbus (corresponding to the position of equatorial region). The equatorial region is relatively weak, owing to the passage of vortex veins.

Causes

- Scleritis.
- Degeneration of sclera in high myopia.

Posterior Staphyloma

It is the bulge of weak sclera at the posterior pole of the eye and is lined by the choroid.

Causes

- Pathological myopia.
- Posterior scleritis.
- Perforating injuries.

Location

It is present as a crescentric shadow in the macular region (2–3 DD) on the temporal side of the optic disc.

Diagnosis

It is not visible externally and can be detected on fundus examination by ophthalmoscope and *B-scan ultrasonography* (**Fig. 7.7**). On ophthalmoscopy, the retinal vessels dip into the ectatic area and are seen to change their direction.

■ Treatment of Staphylomas

- Prompt treatment of inflammatory diseases to prevent the formation of staphylomas.

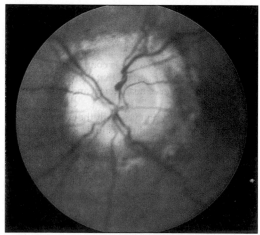

Fig. 7.7 Posterior staphyloma on fundus examination. Source: Scott I, Regillo C, Flynn H et al., ed. Vitreoretinal Disease: Diagnosis, Mnagement, and Clinical Pearls, 2nd Edition. Thieme; 2017.

- Control of raised IOP.
- Local excision and repair by corneal or scleral grafting.
- Enucleation with an implant may be performed in a blind disfiguring eye.

■ Blue Sclera

In babies, the scleral collagen fibers are thin and immature, resulting in thinning of underlying uveal tissue. Therefore, the sclera appears blue in babies (**Fig. 7.8**). This blue discoloration reduces with the age. It is an asymptomatic condition. It may also be associated with keratoconus and keratoglobus.

■ Causes

- Osteogenesis imperfecta (Type I and II).
- Marfan's syndrome.
- Ehlers–Danlos syndrome.
- High myopia
- Pseudoxanthoma elasticum.
- Buphthalmos.
- Healed scleritis.

Osteogenesis imperfecta is a hereditary condition due to abnormalities of the type I collagen gene. The thinness and transparency of the collagen fibers of the sclera allow visualization of the underlying uvea, leading to characteristic blue sclera. This condition is characterized by:

- Frequent bone fractures (fragilitas ossium).
- Blue sclera.
- Deafness.

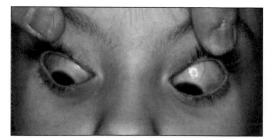

Fig. 7.8 Blue sclera. Source: Blue Sclera and Scleral Staphyloma. In: Agarwal A, Jacob S, ed. Color Atlas of Ophthalmology. The Quick-Reference Manual for Diagnosis and Treatment. 2nd Edition. Thieme; 2009.

Anatomy and Physiology 173
Inflammation (Uveitis) 177
Anterior Uveitis (Iridocyclitis) 180
Intermediate Uveitis (Pars Planitis) 190
Posterior Uveitis 191
Specific Types of Uveitis 193
Endophthalmitis 205
Panophthalmitis 207
Pigment Dispersion Syndrome 208
Degenerative Changes in Uveal Tract 208
Detachment of Choroid 211
Congenital Anomalies of Uveal Tract 212

■ Anatomy and Physiology

Uveal tract is the middle and highly vascular coat of eyeball. It consists of the following three parts: iris, ciliary body, and choroid.

Iris is the anterior most part of the uveal tract. **Ciliary body** extends from the scleral spur anteriorly up to ora serrata posteriorly, **Choroid** extends from the ora serrata anteriorly up to optic disc posteriorly. Ciliary body and choroid line the sclera. These anatomically distinct parts of the uveal tract are closely related; hence, the inflammatory processes affecting one part often involve the other part too.

■ Iris

It forms a free circular diaphragm in the coronal plane which contains an aperture in the center called *pupil* (diameter 2.5–4 mm). The iris is attached with the ciliary body. This attachment is called *root*. The root is the thinnest part; hence,

prone to tear on trauma. *Collarette* divides the anterior surface of iris into the pupillary and ciliary zones. *Crypts* (minute depressions) are mainly found in the ciliary zone (**Fig. 8.1**).

Microscopically, iris is composed of four layers (anterior to posterior, **Fig. 8.2**):

- *Anterior limiting layer*: It covers the anterior surface of the iris and is deficient in areas of crypts; this allows easy transfer of fluid between iris and anterior chamber.
- *Iris stroma*: It consists of loosely arranged collagenous network and also contains–
  ◊ Blood vessels which run in a radial direction.
  ◊ Nerves.
  ◊ Pigment cells.
  ◊ Two unstriped muscles: sphincter pupillae and dilator pupillae (**Fig. 8.3** and **Table 8.1**).
- *Anterior pigmented epithelium* consists of flattened cells.

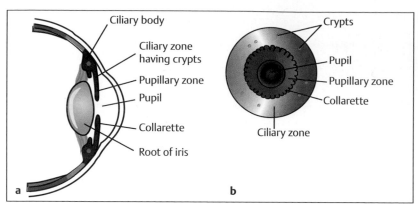

Fig. 8.1 (a, b) Anterior surface of iris.

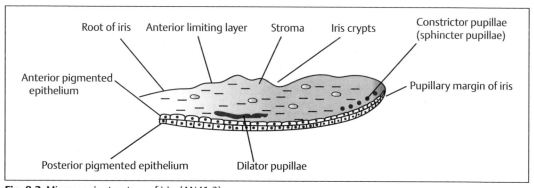

Fig. 8.2 Microscopic structure of iris. (AN41.3)

Table 8.1 Differentiating features of muscles of iris stroma (AN41.3)		
	Sphincter pupillae	**Dilator pupillae**
• Fibers	Fibers are circular around pupillary margin	Fibers are arranged radially near the root of iris.
• Nerve supply	Parasympathetic fibers via oculomotor (IIIrd) nerve	By cervical sympathetic nerves
• Function	Constriction of pupil (**miosis**)	Dilatation of pupil (**mydriasis**)

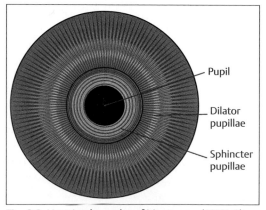

Fig. 8.3 Unstriped muscles of iris stroma. (AN41.3)

- *Posterior pigmented epithelium* consists of cuboidal cells. These two layers of pigmented epithelium, developmentally, are derived from retina and are continuous with each other at the pupillary margin.

The sensory nerve supply of the iris is derived from the trigeminal (Vth) nerve.

■ Ciliary Body

It is triangular in cross-section with the base forward. The iris is attached at the middle of the base, so the base forms part of the angle of the anterior and posterior chambers. The **outer**

surface of the ciliary body lies against the sclera. The **stroma** of the ciliary body is composed of collagen fibers as well as ciliary muscle, vessels and nerves. The **inner surface** of the ciliary body is divided into two regions:

Anterior part: It is called **pars plicata** and has approximately 40 villi which form ridges around the circumference called which are known as *ciliary processes.*

Posterior part: It is smooth and called **pars plana (Fig. 8.4).**

Ciliary Processes

The core of ciliary processes contains blood vessels embedded in loose connective tissue. These are the **site of aqueous production.** The inner surface is lined by epithelium which is two layered (**Fig. 8.5**):

Outer pigmented layer: It is a continuation of the retinal pigment epithelium; in forward direction, it is continuous with anterior pigmented epithelium of iris.

Inner nonpigmented layer: It represents forward continuation of sensory retina and is continuous with posterior pigmented epithelium of iris.

Ciliary Muscle (AN41.3)

It is an unstriped muscle and forms the chief mass of the ciliary body. Ciliary processes contain no part of the ciliary muscle. It is composed of three types of fibers with a common origin.

1. *Meridional (longitudinal) fibers:* These are inserted at the scleral spur and run anteroposteriorly on the inner aspect of sclera. These are involved in regulation of aqueous outflow.
2. *Radial (oblique) fibers:* These are inserted in the root of iris in close relation to the dilator muscle.
3. *Circular fibers:* These help in accommodation.

Nerve supply of ciliary muscle: It is supplied by the oculomotor nerve (through short ciliary nerves). Its *sensory nerve supply* is derived from the trigeminal (Vth) nerve.

Functions of Ciliary Body

The ciliary body serves the following functions:
- Formation of aqueous humor (by ciliary processes).
- Accommodation (through circular fibers of the ciliary muscle).

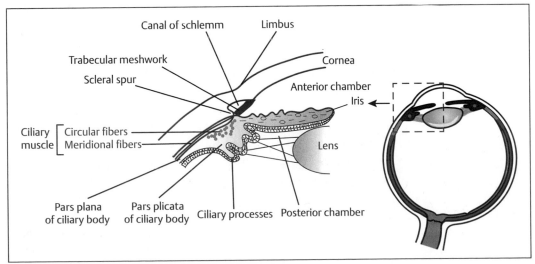

Fig. 8.4 Parts of ciliary body. (AN41.3)

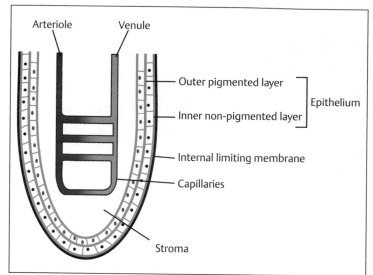

Fig. 8.5 Layers of ciliary processes.

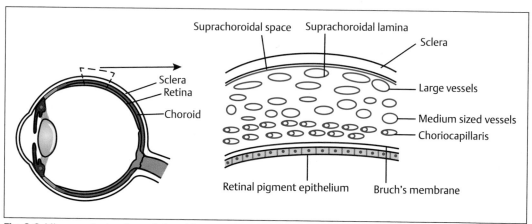

Fig. 8.6 Microscopic structure of choroid.

- Regulation of aqueous outflow (through insertion of the meridional fibers of ciliary muscle at the scleral spur).

■ Choroid

It is an extremely vascular part of the uveal tract. Outer surfaces (suprachoroidal lamina) lie in contact with sclera, with a potential space between the two structures, the **suprachoroidal space**, which contains long and short posterior ciliary arteries and nerves. The inner surface is in contact with *Bruch's membrane*, a thin elastic

membrane. The stroma of choroid is largely composed of blood vessels which increase in size from within outward . Thus, the innermost (immediately beneath Bruch's membrane) zone comprises ciliary plexus formed by fenestrated vessels called **choriocapillaris** which nourish the outer layer of retina (**Fig. 8.6**).

Nerve supply of choroid: The sensory fibers are derived from the trigeminal (V) nerve, and the vasomotor function is regulated by autonomic nerves (**Table 8.2**).

Table 8.2 Nerve supply of uveal tract

Sensory nerve supply:	Trigeminal (V) nerve
Motor nerve supply:	
• Sphincter pupillae and ciliary muscle	• **Oculomotor** (III) **nerve** (parasympathetic nerve fibers)
• Dilator pupillae	• **Cervical sympathetic nerves**
Vasomotor function	Regulated by **autonomic nerves**

■ Blood Supply of Uveal Tract

Arterial supply: Uveal tract is supplied by three groups of ciliary arteries:
- Short posterior ciliary arteries.
- Long posterior ciliary arteries.
- Anterior ciliary arteries.

The choroid is supplied by short posterior arteries, reinforced anteriorly by anastomosed recurrent branches from the major arterial circle of iris. Ciliary body and iris are supplied by long posterior ciliary arteries and anterior ciliary arteries via the major arterial circle.

Venous drainage: Uveal tract is drained by the following three groups of ciliary veins:
- Short posterior ciliary veins
- Vortex veins (venae vorticosae).
- Anterior ciliary veins.

Short posterior ciliary veins receive blood only from the sclera. **Vortex veins** (four in number) receive blood from the uveal tract with the exception of the outer part of ciliary muscle. These open into ophthalmic veins. **Anterior ciliary veins** receive blood from the outer part of ciliary muscle.

The high vascularity of the uveal tract makes it vulnerable for its frequent involvement in various infections as well as systemic vascular and immune diseases.

■ Inflammation (Uveitis) (OP6.1, 6.2, 6.3, 6.8)

The inflammation of the uveal tract is generally not confined to a single part of the uvea and tends to involve uvea as a whole. The inflammation of iris (**iritis**) is almost always associated with some amount of inflammation of the ciliary body (**cyclitis**) and vice versa.

■ Classification

Uveitis may be classified anatomically, clinically, etiologically, and pathologically as follows:
- Anatomical classification (**Fig. 8.7**):
  ◊ Anterior uveitis.
  ◊ Intermediate uveitis.
  ◊ Posterior uveitis.
  ◊ Panuveitis.
- Clinical classification:
  ◊ Acute uveitis.
  ◊ Chronic uveitis.
  ◊ Recurrent uveitis.
- Etiological classification:
  ◊ Infective uveitis.
  ◊ Secondary to systemic diseases.
  ◊ Neoplastic uveitis.
  ◊ Traumatic uveitis.
  ◊ Idiopathic uveitis.
- Pathological classification:
  ◊ Granulomatous.
  ◊ Nongranulomatous.

The "International Uveitis study group" has recommended to follow anatomical classification.

Anatomical Classification of Uveitis

Based on the anatomical site of involvement, uveitis can be:
- Anterior uveitis: It is the inflammation of the anterior uvea (iris and pars plicata of ciliary body). It is further subdivided into–
  ◊ *Iritis:* Inflammation predominantly involves iris.

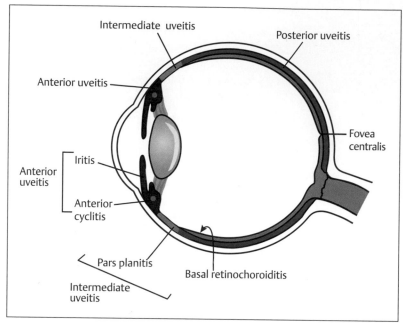

Intermediate uveitis

Posterior uveitis

Fig. 8.7 Anatomical classification of uveitis.

Anterior uveitis

Fovea centralis

Iritis

Anterior uveitis

Anterior cyclitis

Pars planitis

Basal retinochoroiditis

Intermediate uveitis

◊ **Anterior cyclitis:** Inflammation predominantly involves the anterior part of ciliary body (pars plicata)

◊ **Iridocyclitis:** Both iris and pars plicata of the ciliary body are equally involved in this condition.

- Intermediate uveitis is subdivided into:
  ◊ **Pars planitis:** There is predominant involvement of pars plana (the posterior part of ciliary body).
  ◊ **Basal retinochoroiditis:** There is predominant involvement of the extreme periphery of retina.

- Posterior uveitis: It is the inflammation of the uveal tract posterior to vitreous base. It can be subdivided into:
  ◊ **Choroiditis:** It is the primary involvement of choroid which may be focal, multifocal, or diffuse.
  ◊ **Chorioretinitis:** Choroiditis associated with retinitis is known as chorioretinitis.
  ◊ **Retinochoroiditis:** Here, retina is primarily involved with associated choroidal involvement.

- Panuveitis: It is the inflammation involving the entire uveal tract.

Clinical Classification of Uveitis

Uveitis is classified according to the mode of onset and duration:

- Acute: It is sudden in onset and symptomatic too. It persists for ≤6 weeks.
- Chronic: It has insidious onset and asymptomatic. It persists for months/years, or if inflammation recurs in less than 3 months after cessation of therapy.
- Recurrent: When there are repeated episodes of uveitis with period of inactivity (without treatment) between the episodes lasting at least 3 months, it is called recurrent uveitis.

Etiological Classification of Uveitis

- Infective uveitis: It may be due to:
  ◊ **Bacterial infections,** for example, tuberculosis, leprosy, gonorrhea and brucellosis.
  ◊ **Spirochaetal infections,** for example, syphilis, leptospirosis and Lyme disease.

◊ *Viral infections*, for example, herpes simplex, herpes zoster, cytomegalovirus (CMV) and acquired immune deficiency syndrome (AIDS).

◊ *Fungal infections*, for example, presumed ocular histoplasmosis syndrome (POHS), candidiasis and cryptococcosis.

◊ *Parasitic infections*, for example, toxoplasmosis, toxocariasis and onchocerciasis.

- Secondary to systemic diseases: Uveitis is found in association with the following diseases:

    ◊ *Auto immune disorders*
    - Ankylosing spondylitis.
    - Reiter's disease (or syndrome).
    - Psoriatic arthritis.
    - Juvenile chronic arthritis (JCA).
      Behcet's syndrome.
    - Rheumatoid arthritis.
    - Systemic lupus erythematosus (SLE).
    - Polyarteritis nodosa.
    - Vogt–Koyanagi–Harada (VKH) syndrome.

    ◊ *Sarcoidosis*

    ◊ *Metabolic disorder*: Diabetes mellitus.

    ◊ *Gastrointestinal disorders*
    - Whipple's disease.
    - Ulcerative colitis.
    - Crohn disease.

- Neoplastic uveitis: May be associated with
    ◊ Acute leukemia.
    ◊ Iris melanoma.
    ◊ Reticulum cell sarcoma of brain.
    ◊ Large cell lymphoma.
    ◊ Histiocytic cell sarcoma.

All these can present features of uveitis and are termed "**masquerade syndromes**."

- Traumatic—trauma to the eye may be:
    ◊ Blunt trauma: It may cause uveitis due to mechanical or irritative effect to intraocular blood.
    ◊ Penetrating injury.
    ◊ Surgical trauma.

- Idiopathic (uveitis of unknown etiology):
    ◊ Pars planitis.
    ◊ Sympathetic ophthalmitis.
    ◊ Glaucomatocyclitic crisis (Posner–Schlossman syndrome).
    ◊ Uveitis-glaucoma-hyphema (UGH) syndrome.
    ◊ Geographical choroidopathy.

- Miscellaneous:
    ◊ Lens-induced uveitis: It may be phacolytic or phacoanaphylactic.
    ◊ Fuch's heterochromic iridocyclitis.
    ◊ Uveitis associated with ocular ischemia: Ischemia alters permeability of vessels, leading to leakage of cells and proteins which, in turn, result in uveitis.

Pathological Classification of Uveitis

Pathologically, uveitis can be of two types: nongranulomatous and granulomatous (**Table 8.3**).

Nongranulomatous uveitis: In this type, the reaction is exudative *(or allergic)*. Exudation of protein-rich fluid results in *aqueous flare*. Outpouring of lymphocytes and polymorphs which adhere to corneal endothelium results in *fine keratic precipitates* (**KPs**). It tends to be of *acute onset* and *short duration*.

Granulomatous uveitis: It is usually due to invasion of eye by living organisms, but it can also be of immunological etiology. So, hypersensitivity reaction is common in granulomatous uveitis and exudative type of reaction is not encountered. This type of inflammation tends to be of *insidious onset* and *chronic course* with *minimal aqueous flare*. It is common in tuberculosis, leprosy, sarcoidosis, syphilis, etc. Granulomatous uveitis is characterized by dense nodular infiltration of the uveal tissue (**Flowchart 8.1**).

■ Investigations

The investigations are ordered after assessing the type of uveitis suspected on clinical examination. If there is single attack of mild, unilateral, acute anterior uveitis without specific

Table 8.3 Differences between nongranulomatous uveitis and granulomatous uveitis

	Nongranulomatous uveitis	Granulomatous uveitis
Onset	Acute	Insidious
Course	Short	Long
Symptoms		
• Pain	Marked	Minimal
• Photophobia	Marked	Slight
Signs		
• Ciliary congestion	Marked	Mild
• KPs	Fine and lymphocytic	'Large mutton fat' and macrophagic
• Aqueous Flare	Marked	Mild
• Iris nodules	Absent	Usually present
• Posterior synechiae	Thin	Thick and broad based

Abbreviation: KP, keratic precipitates.

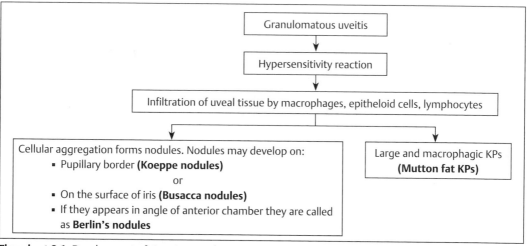

Flowchart 8.1 Development of signs in granulomatous uveitis.

features of underlying disease, investigations are not necessary. Indications for investigations are recurrent uveitis, bilateral uveitis, and posterior uveitis. **Table 8.4** lists the investigations performed for uveitis along with the rationale behind those investigations.

■ Anterior Uveitis (Iridocyclitis) (OP6.1, 6.2, 6.3, 6.8) (OP6.6)

Clinically, anterior uveitis (iridocyclitis) may present in two forms: acute and chronic, as explained in **Table 8.5**.

■ Clinical Features

Symptoms

The main symptoms of acute anterior uveitis are pain, photophobia, blurred vision, redness, and reflex lacrimation through fifth nerve stimulation supplying iris. Pain is of sudden onset, worse at night, and radiates along distribution of 1st (ophthalmic) division of 5th nerve to forehead, scalp and check. Causes of blurring of vision are depicted in **Fig. 8.8**.

Table 8.4 Rationale for various investigations

Investigations	Rationale

• Hematological
  ◇ **TLC** (Total leucocyte count)
  ◇ **DLC** (Differential leucocyte count)
  ◇ **ESR** (Erythrocyte Sedimentation Rate)
 	
  ◇ **Blood sugar**
	TLC and DLC give information about inflammatory response.
	ESR provides information regarding any chronic inflammatory condition.
	Blood sugar is done to rule out diabetes mellitus.

• Serological Tests
  ◇ **VDRL** (Veneral Disease Research Laboratory)
  ◇ **RPR** (Rapid Plasma Reagin)
  ◇ **FTA–ABS test:** It is highly sensitive and specific (Fluorescent Treponemal antibody absorption test)
  ◇ **Sabin–Feldman dye test:** It utilizes live organisms
  ◇ **Immunofluorescent–antibody test:** It utilizes dead organisms
  ◇ **ELISA** (Enzyme Linked Immuno Sorbent Assay)
	These tests are done to rule out syphilis.
	
	These tests are done for toxoplasmosis.

• Enzyme assay
  ◇ **Serum ACE** (Serum Angiotensin converting enzyme)
  ◇ **Serum lysozyme** – less specific than ACE
	These tests are done to rule out **sarcoidosis**.
	It is done for uveitis of immunological origin.

• **HLA [Human leucocyte Antigen] tissue typing** HLA type (antigen) **HLA – B27** **HLA – B51** **HLA – A29** **HLA – B7, HLA – DR2**	Associated disease • Ankylosing spondylitis and Reiter's syndrome. • Behcet syndrome. • Birdshot chorioretinopathy. • POHS (Presumed Ocular Histoplasmosis Syndrome).

• Radiological
  ◇ X-Ray chest
  ◇ X-Ray sacro-iliac joint
	• It is done to exclude tuberculosis and sarcoidosis.
	• It is done to exclude ankylosing spondylitis (It should be done in presence of low back pain and uveitis).

• Imaging
  ◇ **CT** and **MRI** of brain and thorax
  ◇ **OCT** (optical coherence tomography)
  ◇ **Angiography**
Fluorescein angiography (FA)
 	
Indocyanine green (ICG) angiography
	For sarcoidosis and for accompanying cysticercus infection in brain.
	To detect cystoid macular edema.
	Fluorescein dye leak out of choroidal vessels resulting in choroidal flush. So, deep lesions will be hidden by this choroidal flush. Thus, **FA is less appropriate in choroiditis**.
	
	ICG dye does not readily leak out of choroidal vessels. Hence, choroidal vessels are better visualized through retinal pigment epithelium. So, **ICG angiography is better suited for choroidal diseases.** ICG is able to detect non perfusion of choriocapillaris and provide information about inflammation affecting stroma of choroid.

• Skin Test
  ◇ **Mantoux test** (Tuberculin test)
  ◇ **Kveim test**
	For tubercular uveitis.
	For sarcoidosis.

• Biopsy
  ◇ **Aqueous samples**
  ◇ **Vitreous biopsy**
  ◇ **Lungs and lymph nodes biopsy**
	For polymerase chain reaction (**PCR**).
	For culture and PCR.
	For sarcoidosis.

Abbreviations: ACE, angiotensin-converting enzyme; ANA, antinuclear antibody; DLC, differential leucocyte count; ELISA, enzyme-linked immunosorbent assay; ESR, erythrocyte sedimentation rate; FA, fluorescein angiography; FTA-ABS test, fluorescent treponemal antibody absorption test; HLA, human leucocyte antigen; ICG, indocyanine green; JIA, juvenile idiopathic arthritis; OCT, optical coherence tomography; PCR, polymerase chain reaction; POHS, presumed ocular histoplasmosis syndrome; RPR, rapid plasma regain; TLC, total leucocyte count; VDRL, veneral disease research laboratory; USG, ultrasonography.

Table 8.5 Differentiating features of acute and chronic anterior uveitis

	Acute anterior uveitis	Chronic anterior uveitis
Occurrence	More common	Less common
Onset	Sudden	Insidious
Duration	3 months or less	Persistent inflammation lasting longer than 3 months
Symptoms	Severe So, patient seeks Medical attention	Asymptomatic or minimal symptoms So, diagnosed during routine examination of eye
Laterality	Usually unilateral	Simultaneous bilateral involvement is more common
Course and prognosis	With appropriate therapy completely resolve within 5–6 weeks with an excellent visual prognosis	Remissions and exacerbations of inflammatory activity are common. Prognosis is guarded
Complications	Are related to delayed or inadequate management	Complications such as cataract and glaucoma are common

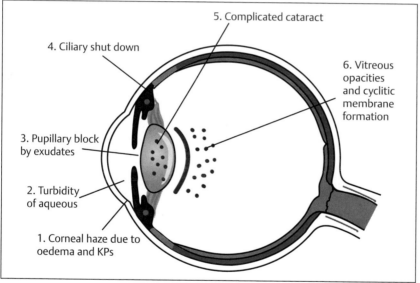

5. Complicated cataract

4. Ciliary shut down

6. Vitreous opacities and cyclitic membrane formation

3. Pupillary block by exudates

2. Turbidity of aqueous

1. Corneal haze due to oedema and KPs

Fig. 8.8 Causes of blurring of vision in acute anterior uveitis.

Signs

Anterior uveitis is characterized by signs, as depicted in **Fig. 8.9**.

1. **Circum corneal (ciliary) congestion:** It is deep and has a violaceous hue (**Fig. 8.10**).
2. **Corneal signs:**
   - *Endothelial dusting:* It is the deposition of small inflammatory cells on corneal endothelium in the early stages of uveitis. It gives rise to a dirty appearance.
   - KPs: These are the clusters of inflammatory cells on corneal endothelium. These appear only after a few days. They are seldom present in simple iritis but are characteristics of cyclitis and iridocyclitis (**Fig. 8.11**).

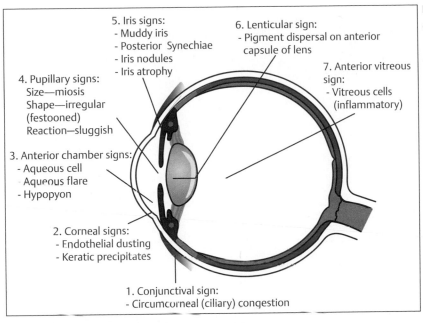

5. Iris signs:
- Muddy iris
- Posterior Synechiae
- Iris nodules
- Iris atrophy

6. Lenticular sign:
- Pigment dispersal on anterior capsule of lens

7. Anterior vitreous sign:
- Vitreous cells (inflammatory)

4. Pupillary signs:
Size—miosis
Shape—irregular (festooned)
Reaction—sluggish

3. Anterior chamber signs:
- Aqueous cell
- Aqueous flare
- Hypopyon

2. Corneal signs:
- Endothelial dusting
- Keratic precipitates

1. Conjunctival sign:
- Circumcorneal (ciliary) congestion

Fig. 8.9 Signs in anterior uveitis.

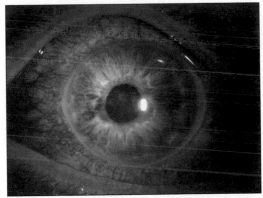

Fig. 8.10 Anterior uveitis with circum corneal (ciliary) congestion. Source: Anisocoria. In: Biousse V, Newman N, ed. Neuro-Opthalmology Illustrated. 3rd Edition. Thieme; 2019.

Keratic precipitates (KPs)
- *Distribution:* KPs are distributed commonly in mid and inferior zones of cornea. Large KPs found in granulomatous uveitis are sometimes distributed over a triangular area, with the apex pointing up on the inferior part of cornea (**Arlt triangle**). This is due to the effect of gravity and normal convection flow of aqueous.
- *Size:* Small and medium KPs are found in nongranulomatous uveitis and are white and round. Large KPs are usually mutton fat greasy and typically occur in granulomatous uveitis.

- *Old KPs:* In nongranulomatous uveitis, KPs shrink, fade, and become pigmented. Old mutton fat KPs take on a "ground glass" appearance (**hyalinized**).
- *KPs are composed of* epitheloid cells, lymphocytes, and polymorphs.

3. **Anterior chamber signs**:
   - *Aqueous cells:* Presence of circulating cells is a strong indication of an active inflammation of uvea.
   - *Aqueous flare:* It is due to leakage of proteins into aqueous and not necessarily a sign of active uveitis (**Fig. 8.12a**).
   - *Hypopyon* (OP6.4): It is a feature of intense inflammation where poured polymorphs settle down at the bottom of anterior chamber to form hypopyon with a horizontal level (**Fig. 8.12b**).

   Grading of aqueous flare and cells is performed with 2 mm long and 1 mm wide slit beam of slit lamp biomicroscope. Cells are graded by counting cells per field, while aqueous flare is graded by degree of obscuration of iris details (**Table 8.6**).

4. Four **iris signs:**
   - *Iris pattern* becomes blurred and indistinct as exudation in iris stroma

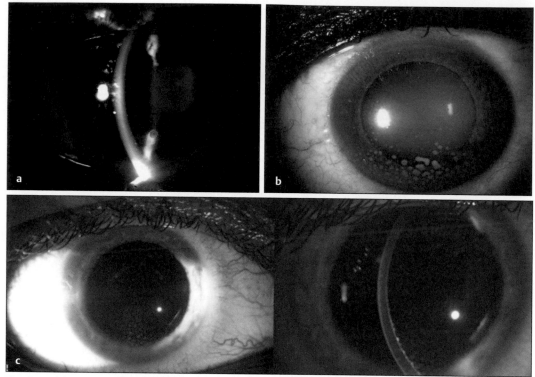

Fig. 8.11 (a) Keratic precipitates. **(b)** Mutton fat keratic precipitates. **(c)** Keratic precipitates in anterior uveitis. Source: Ocular Examination. In Biousse V, Newman N, ed. Neuro-Opthalmology Illustrated. 3rd Edition. Thieme; 2019.

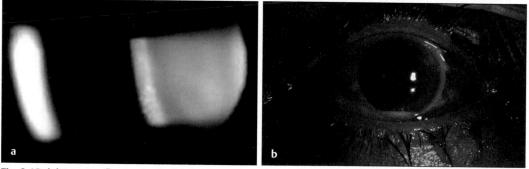

Fig. 8.12 (a) Aqueous flare and cells. **(b)** Hypopyon. Source: History In: Singh K, Smiddy W, Lee A, ed. Opthalmology Review: A Case-Study Approach. 2nd Edition. Thieme; 2018.

causes filling of crypts on the anterior surface of iris (**muddy iris**).

- *Iris nodules:* These are of two types: **Koeppe's nodules,** found at pupillary margin, and **Busacca nodules,** found on anterior surface of iris. *These nodules typically occur in granulomatous uveitis.*

- *Posterior synechiae:* These are the adhesions between anterior lens surface and posterior surface of iris. Posterior synechiae show predilection

Table 8.6 Grading of aqueous cells and flare

(a) Grading of aqueous cells		(b) Grading of aqueous flare	
Grade	Cells per field	Grade	Aqueous flare
0	0	0	Absent
+	5–10	+	Faint, barely detectable
++	10–20	++	Moderate (iris details clear)
+++	20–50	+++	Moderate (iris details hazy)
++++	>50	++++	Intense (fibrinous aqueous)

for lower part of pupil in early stages due to the gravitation of exudates. These must not be allowed to become organized. These may be segmental (adhesions at some points) or annular, that is, ring synechiae (extending for 360 degree). The condition is called **seclusio pupillae.**

- *Iris atrophy:* It is an important feature of Fuchs heterochromic iridocyclitis and uveitis due to herpes virus.

5. **Pupillary signs:**
   - *Size—***miosis:** Due to spasm of sphincter pupillae.
   - *Shape—***irregular shape:** When pupil with segmental posterior synechiae is dilated with mydriatic (atropine and homatropine), intervening portion of pupillary margin (between posterior synechiae) dilate and pupil assumes a festooned appearance (**festooned pupil, Fig. 8.13**).
   - *Reaction—***sluggish** pupillary reaction (due to edema of iris).

If exudation from iris and ciliary body is profuse, it may cover the surface of iris as well as the pupillary area. This type of uveitis is called *plastic iridocyclitis.* Exudates upon iris surface may become organized and contract, resulting in eversion of pupillary margin (*ectropion pupillae*). Exudates may block the pupil and get organized. The condition is called *occlusio pupillae.*

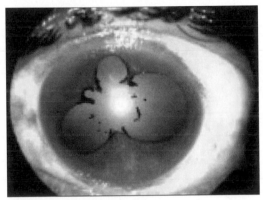

Fig. 8.13 Festooned pupil. Source: Antiinflammatories. In: Agarwal A, Jacob S, ed. Color Atlas of Opthalmology. The Quick-Reference Manual for Diagnosis and Traetment. 2nd Edition. Thieme; 2009.

6. **Lenticular sign:** Pigment dispersal on anterior capsule of lens.
7. **Anterior vitreous sign:** *Vitreous cells* (inflammatory cells in anterior vitreous).

In iritis, aqueous cells are more than vitreous cells.

In iridocyclitis, cells are equally distributed in aqueous and vitreous humor.

In cyclitis, exudates in vitreous are more. When they organize, they form *cyclitic membrane* behind the lens.

To understand the development of signs in anterior uveitis, it is necessary to remember the anatomy and pathological changes occurring in the iris (**Fig. 8.14** and **Flowchart 8.2**).

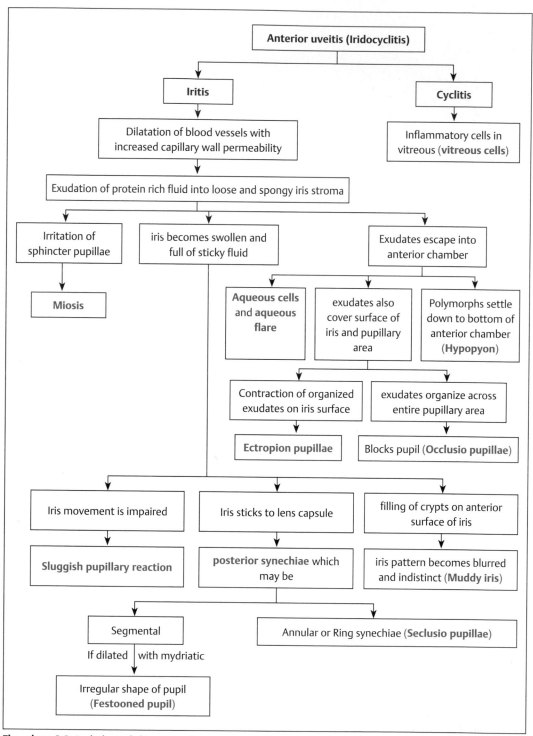

Flowchart 8.2 Pathological changes in iris.

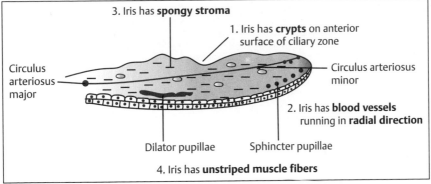

3. Iris has **spongy stroma**

1. Iris has **crypts** on anterior surface of ciliary zone

Circulus arteriosus major

Circulus arteriosus minor

2. Iris has **blood vessels** running in **radial direction**

Dilator pupillae   Sphincter pupillae

4. Iris has **unstriped muscle fibers**

Fig. 8.14 Anatomy of iris.

Anatomy of Iris

1. Iris has **crypts** on the anterior surface of ciliary zone.
2. Iris has **blood vessels** running in the radial direction.
3. Iris has **spongy stroma** consisting of loosely arranged collagenous network.
4. Iris has **unstriped muscle fibers**.

■ Investigations

- Hematological investigations (total leucocyte count [TLC], differential leucocyte count [DLC], erythrocyte sedimentation rate [ESR], blood sugar).
- Serological test (antinuclear antibody [ANA], rheumatoid factor, human leucocyte antigen [HLA] typing, venereal disease research laboratory [VDRL], fluorescent treponemal antibody absorption test [FTA-ABS], enzyme-linked immunosorbent assay [ELISA], etc.).
- Radiological investigations (X-ray chest and sacroiliac joints, CT scan).
- Skin test (Mantoux test and Kveim test).
- Urine examination to rule out urethritis.
- Anterior chamber paracentesis for polymerase chain reaction (PCR) to diagnose organisms and cellular analysis.

■ Differential Diagnosis (OP3.1)

Acute iridocyclitis must be differentiated from acute conjunctivitis and acute angle closure glaucoma (**Table 8.7**). *Dilatation of pupil is urgently required in acute anterior uveitis (iridocyclitis), but it may worsen acute angle closure glaucoma, so it is a must to differentiate between the two.*

■ Treatment

It includes general treatment of uveitis with cycloplegics and mydriatics, corticosteroids and immunosuppressives; specific treatment of underlying cause; and treatment of sequelae and complications.

General Treatment (OP6.9)

Cycloplegics and Mydriatics

Short-acting preparations are Tropicamide 0.5% or 1% drops and Cyclopentolate 1% drops, while long-acting preparations are Homatropine 2% drops and Atropine 1% drops or ointment (most powerful cycloplegic).

Mode of Action

These relieve the spasms of ciliary muscle and sphincter pupillae so, give comfort and rest to the eye. These prevent formation of posterior synechiae. It is best achieved by short-acting cycloplegics which keep the pupil mobile. Pupil should not be kept constantly dilated in chronic anterior uveitis, as posterior synechiae can still form in dilated position. These break down recently formed posterior synechiae. Once synechiae have formed, topical Atropine 1% drop or ointment is used.

Table 8.7 Differentiating features of acute conjunctivitis, acute anterior uveitis and acute angle closure glaucoma (OP6.1)

	Acute conjunctivitis	Acute anterior uveitis	Acute angle closure glaucoma
Symptoms			
• Discharge	Mucopurulent	Watery	Watery
• Colored halos	May be present	–	+
• Vision	Normal	Slightly impaired	Markedly impaired
• Pain	±	Moderate	Severe
Signs			
• Congestion (injection)	Superficial	Deep ciliary	Deep ciliary
• Cornea	Normal	KPs on endothelium	Epithelial edema
• Aqueous	Clear	Flare ++	Flare ±
• Pupil			
◇ Size	Normal	Small	Dilated
◇ Shape	Normal	Irregular	Vertical oval
◇ Reaction	brisk	Sluggish	Non reacting
• IOP	Normal	Often normal	Markedly raised
• Tenderness	–	+	+

Note: (+) denotes presence and (–) denotes absence

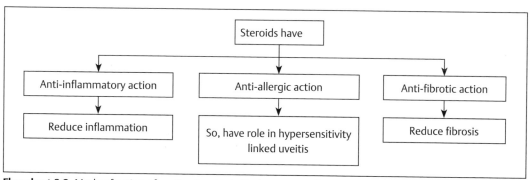

Flowchart 8.3 Mode of action of corticosteroids in the treatment of anterior uveitis.

In eyes that do not respond to mydriatic drops, a *subconjunctival (s/c) injection* of mydricaine 0.3 mL (a mixture of adrenaline + atropine + procaine) may be effective. *Subconjunctival mydricaine induces tachycardia and hypertension, so should be used cautiously in patients with cardiovascular disease.* To breakdown persistent posterior synechiae *"tissue plasminogen activator"* is injected into anterior chamber. It dissolves fibrinous exudates. When the pupil is well dilated, frequency of instillation is gradually reduced and then discontinued.

Corticosteroids

These are the mainstays in the treatment of uveitis. Potent steroid preparations include betamethasone, dexamethasone and prednisolone, while weak steroid preparations include fluorometholone and loteprednol. Mode of action of corticosteroids in the treatment of anterior uveitis is described in **Flowchart 8.3**.

Routes of Administration

Topical steroids: These are given in the form of eye drops and ointment. Frequency of instillation depends on the severity of inflammation. Initially, potent steroids are given. Weaker steroids are used as the inflammation subsides. Weaker preparations are reserved for mild uveitis in patients who are steroid responders.

Complications of topical steroids include elevation of intraocular pressure (IOP), cataract, corneal melting due to inhibition of collagen synthesis, and secondary infection with bacteria and fungi.

Periocular injections: Subconjunctival injections or anterior subtenon injections are given mainly in severe cases of anterior uveitis. Short-acting (1 day) preparations include betamethasone and dexamethasone. long-acting (several weeks) preparations include triamcinolone acetonide and methylprednisolone acetate.

Systemic administration: It is given orally and includes prednisolone which is given in initial dose of 1 to 2 mg/kg body weight/day (60–80 mg/day) as a single morning dose after breakfast. The dose is gradually tapered over several weeks to avoid reactivation. If steroids are given for <2 weeks, there is no need to reduce the dose gradually. There are certain side effects from the use of systemic therapy. Short-term therapy causes dyspepsia and peptic ulceration, and also mental changes. Prednisolone can cause mental problems, including psychosis, mania and clinical depression. Severe psychiatric illness was uncommon with dose less than 40 mg/day of prednisolone, but increased doses above 80 mg/day of prednisolone strongly supporting that these symptoms are dose-dependent. Long-term therapy causes cataract (posterior sub capsular), worsening of diabetes, cushingoid state, osteoporosis, electrolyte imbalance, and reactivation of infections such as TB. *Presence of a flare in absence of cells is not an indication for systemic steroid therapy.*

Immunosuppressive (Cytotoxic Agents)

These are given to patients who do not respond to systemic steroids. Drugs used for immuno-suppression are azathioprine, cyclophosphamide, chlorambucil, cyclosporin and methotrexate. All of these drugs are potentially toxic. Complications of immunosuppression are bone marrow depression, hepatotoxicity, gastro-intestinal ulceration, sterility, alopecia and nephrotoxicity (with cyclosporin). Monitoring with immunosuppressives is done by complete blood count, liver function tests (because of hepatotoxicity) and renal function tests (because of nephrotoxicity).

Specific Treatment of Underlying Cause

When exact etiology is identified, the underlying disease needs the specific treatment.

Treatment of Sequelae and Complications

Glaucoma (*Hypertensive iridocyclitis*): In this condition, IOP increases due to inflammation before the synechiae develops (inflammatory glaucoma). It requires the following:

- Control of inflammation by steroids and atropine.
- Lowering of IOP by systemic acetazolamide, 250 mg 4 times a day and 0.5% Timolol maleate eye drops.

> Pilocarpine and Latanoprost are contraindicated as uveitis may be exacerbated.

Secondary glaucoma: Secondary glaucoma develops after ring synechiae, so mental problems, including psychosis, mania and clinical depression. Severe psychiatric illness was uncommon with dose less than 40 mg/aim of treatment is to restore communication between posterior and anterior chambers which is achieved by:

- Laser iridotomy.
- Surgical iridectomy: It is not done during acute stage of iritis because opening will be filled with exudates, and the aim of operation will not be achieved.

Complicated cataract: The lens is removed surgically 2 to 3 months after a quiescent interval of acute iritis.

Band keratopathy: It is treated with excimer laser photoablation or phototherapeutic keratectomy (PTK)

Cystoid macular edema (CME): Intravitreal triamcinolone is given for it.

■ Complications

- Complicated cataract: It is characterized by polychromatic luster at the posterior pole of lens. Cataract progresses rapidly in the presence of posterior synechiae.
- Cyclitic membrane (retrolental membrane): It is due to organized exudates behind the lens in severe cases of plastic uveitis.
- Rise of IOP: In the active stage of iridocyclitis, sticky albuminous aqueous clogs the trabecular meshwork at the angle of anterior chamber. It results in reduced aqueous drainage and rise in IOP (**hypertensive iridocyclitis**). In the later stages, pupillary block due to seclusio pupillae or occlusio pupillae reduces the flow of aqueous from posterior chamber to anterior chamber. It results in iris bombe. The apposition of iris to cornea at periphery forms peripheral anterior synechiae, with subsequent obliteration of angle of anterior chamber. It causes rise in IOP (**secondary glaucoma**).
- Panuveitis and retinal complications: In cases of longstanding uveitis, choroid is involved, owing to the continuity and resulting in panuveitis which, in turn, may cause retinal complications such as exudative retinal detachment, cystoid macular edema and neuro retinitis.

In plastic uveitis, exudates and strands of fibrous tissue are formed in vitreous. Contraction of these fibrous strands, formed in vitreous and attached to retina, may result in tractional retinal detachment.

- Band-shaped keratopathy.
- Phthisis bulbi: Chronic and recurrent uveitis can lead to degenerative changes in ciliary body with reduced aqueous secretion.

It results in **ocular hypotony** (soft eye) with shrinkage of eyeball (Phthisis bulbi).

■ Intermediate Uveitis (Pars Planitis)

It is also known as *chronic posterior cyclitis*. It involves pars plana of ciliary body and periphery of choroid. It is an insidious, chronic, and relapsing disease. It particularly affects a child or a young adult. The condition is typically bilateral (80%) but involvement is frequently asymmetrical. Etiology is usually unknown.

It presents as floaters in the eye and leads to blurring of vision. Blurred vision is due to opacities in anterior vitreous. It is characterized by the presence of the following clinical signs:

- Cells in anterior vitreous.
- White snowball-like exudates near ora serrata, involving inferior pars plana. Coalescent exudates give the appearance of a "snow bank" (**snow banking, Fig. 8.15**).
- Mild peripheral periphlebitis and peri-vascular sheathing.
- Absent or minimal anterior uveitis with minimal aqueous flare and occasional KPs.
- Posterior synechiae are absent.

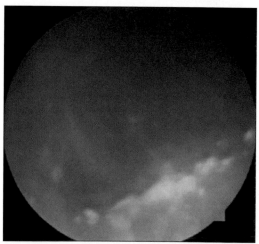

Fig. 8.15 Snow banking in pars planitis, Source: Intermediate Uveitis. In: Steidl S, Hartnett M, ed. Clinical Pathways In Vitreoretinal Disease. 1st Edition. Thieme; 2003.

■ Differential Diagnosis

Pars planitis must be differentiated from chronic conditions which produce vitritis or peripheral retinal changes, mimicking pars planitis, for example:

- Peripheral toxocariasis.
- Syphilis.
- Sarcoidosis.
- Multiple sclerosis.
- Whipple disease (vitritis without snowballs).

■ Treatment

The main **indication** of treatment is decreased visual acuity due to chronic macular edema. The treatment includes:

- Posterior subtenon injection of triam-cinolone should be given initially.
- In the event of resistance to injections (in unresponsive cases), systemic steroids are given.
- In severe steroid resistant cases, immuno-suppressive agents are considered.
- Vitrectomy: It is indicated in case of tractional retinal detachment, nonresolving vitreous hemorrhage, and severe vitreous opacification.

■ Complications

- Macular edema: If it becomes chronic, cystoid changes develop (cystoid macular edema).
- Cataract.
- Retrolental cyclitic membrane.
- In advanced cases, exudate becomes vas-cularized, resulting in contraction of fibro-vascular tissue and leading to tractional retinal detachment and vitreous hemor-rhage (**Fig. 8.16**).

■ Posterior Uveitis

Posterior uveitis is the inflammation of choroid (posterior uvea). The inflammation of choroid almost always involves retina, because outer layers of retina depend upon choroid for their nourishment. According to the site of primary involvement, posterior uveitis can be:

- Chorioretinitis: The primary focus is in choroid.
- Retinochoroiditis: The primary focus is in retina.

■ Classification

According to the number and location of areas involved, choroiditis can be focal, multifocal and diffuse.

Focal Choroiditis

It is characterized by a patch (or patches) of choroiditis localized in a particular area. It may be (**Fig. 8.17**):

- *Central:* If choroiditis involves posterior pole or macular region.
- *Juxtapapillary:* If patch of choroiditis is close to the optic disc.

Multifocal Choroiditis

It is the choroiditis with fewer and more discrete foci. When it is confined to anterior (peripheral) part of choroid, it is termed as anterior choroiditis (**Fig. 8.18**).

Disseminated or Diffuse Choroiditis

When multiple, small areas of inflammation are scattered all over the fundus behind the equator,

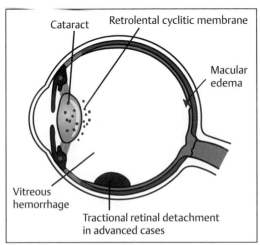

Fig. 8.16 Complications of intermediate uveitis.

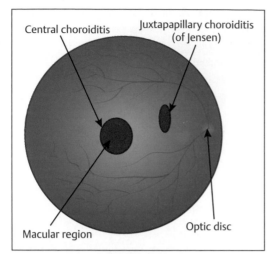

Fig. 8.17 Types of focal choroiditis.

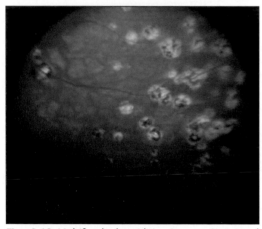

Fig. 8.18 Multifocal choroiditis. Source: Signs and Symptoms of Uveitis. In: Steidl S, Hartnett M, ed. Clinical Pathways In Vitreoretinal Disease. 1st Edition. Thieme; 2003.

it is called disseminated choroiditis. It is syphilitic or tuberculous in origin. The healed lesions appear as atrophic patches.

■ Clinical Forms

Clinically, it is similar to iridocyclitis, and may be granulomatous and nongranulomatous choroiditis. Nongranulomatous choroiditis (also known as exudative choroiditis) is characterized by acute leucocytic infiltration and marked exudation. Granulomatous choroiditis is usually associated with direct organismal infection and characterized by aggregation of chronic inflammatory cells (lymphocytes, plasma cells, etc.).

■ Clinical Features

Symptoms

The presenting symptoms vary according to the location of inflammatory lesion. Peripheral lesions present with floaters and minimal visual symptoms, while central lesions cause marked blurring of vision and may not notice the presence of floaters. Various visual symptoms related to central choroiditis are:

- Black spot in front of eye (positive scotoma).
- Retinal irritability leading to subjective sensation of flashes of light (photopsia).
- Inflamed area is slightly raised, causing alterations in the contour of retina. These alterations further lead to:
  ◊ Distortion of image and apparent change in size of objects (metamorphopsia).
  ◊ Straight lines appear wavy.
  ◊ Objects appear small (micropsia) due to separation of rods and cones, and sometimes larger (macropsia) due to crowding of rods and cones.

Signs

In active stage: Inflammatory cells and *vitreous opacities* are present. The patch of choroiditis is seen as a *yellowish area deep to retinal vessels*. Retinal signs include exudates in retina, edema of overlying retina and retinal vasculitis. In this, commonly retinal veins are involved (periphlebitis) with sheathing of vessels.

In healed stage: White areas are surrounded by black pigment clumps at the edges, and the affected area becomes more sharply defined, lying deep to retinal vessels (*in retinitis pigmentosa, retinal pigment lies anterior to retinal vessels*).

■ Treatment

Topical steroids are useful only for anterior uveitis, because therapeutic levels are not reached behind the lens. Treatment protocols include the following:

- Periocular injection: Periocular steroids should be considered as first-line therapy to control inflammation and CME. Posterior subtenon injection of long-acting preparations such as triamcinolone or methylprednisolone is given. *Complications* of posterior subtenon injection are:
  ◇ Globe penetration.
  ◇ Elevation of IOP.
  ◇ Optic nerve injury.
  ◇ Extraocular muscle (EOM) paresis.
- Intraocular steroids: Triamcinolone injection 4 mg in 0.1 mL is given in treatment of uveitis and CME unresponsive to other forms of therapy. It produces fast resolution of CME.

  Complications of intraocular steroids are:
  ◇ Rise of IOP.
  ◇ Cataract.
  ◇ Endophthalmitis.
  ◇ Retinal detachment.
- Systemic steroids: These are indicated when there is no improvement with periocular steroids or when posterior uveitis is sight threatening. Routes of administration are IV and oral administration. IV methylprednisolone in dose of 1 g/day through infusion bottle is given for 3 days, followed by oral prednisolone given in the dose of 1–2 mg/kg body wt/day and tapered gradually over several weeks.
- Specific treatment of underlying cause.

■ Complications

- Complicated cataract owing to impaired nutrition of lens.
- Papillitis.
- Retinal detachment.

■ Specific Types of Uveitis

■ Bacterial Uveitis

Tubercular Uveitis

It is a chronic granulomatous infection caused by mycobacterium tuberculosis. It can cause either a direct infection or a delayed hypersensitivity reaction in the uveal tissue. Tuberculosis can involve both anterior and posterior uvea.

Ocular Manifestations

Anterior uveitis: It is usually granulomatous but occasionally it may be nongranulomatous. Granulomatous type may occur in the miliary form (yellowish white nodule surrounded by multiple satellites) or conglomerate form (larger yellowish white tumor).

Posterior uveitis: Tuberculous choroiditis is caused by direct infection. It can manifest as:

- Multiple, miliary tubercles in choroid (choroidal tubercles).
- Disseminated choroiditis.
- Large, solitary choroidal granuloma (choroidal tuberculoma).

Diagnosis

Diagnosis is reached with the help of the following investigations:

- Mantoux test.
- Chest X-ray.
- ESR.
- PCR on samples obtained from ocular tissues.
- Histopathology of ocular tissues to demonstrate tubercular bacilli.
- Therapeutic isoniazid test: If there is a dramatic improvement in uveitis to 300 mg/day isoniazid for 3 weeks, the diagnosis of tuberculosis is highly likely.

Treatment

Usual treatment of anterior uveitis is recommended. Antitubercular treatment (ATT) is also given. This included a 4-drug regimen (isoniazid + rifampicin + ethambutol + pyrazinamide) for 2 months followed by isoniazid + rifampicin for 6 months. Concomitant systemic steroid therapy is also frequently necessary. *Ethambutol may cause optic neuropathy.* So, periodical eye examination is needed.

Leprotic Uveitis

Leprosy (Hansen's disease) is caused by Mycobacterium leprae. It predominantly involves skin, peripheral nerves, and anterior segment of the eye. Two types of leprosy are lepromatous (cutaneous) type and tuberculoid (neural) type (**Table 8.8**).

Ocular Manifestations

Involvement of anterior segment of the eye causes uveitis. Involvement of peripheral nerves leads to varied types of symptoms, for example:

- Involvement of facial nerve causes neuroparalytic lagophthalmos, leading to exposure keratopathy.
- Involvement of trigeminal nerve causes either loss of corneal sensations, leading to neurotrophic keratopathy or loss of iris sensations. *Hence, eye with chronic uveitis usually tolerates surgery for secondary cataracts.*
- Damage to sympathetic innervation of dilator pupillae causes unopposed action of sphincter pupillae, leading to miosis.

Other ocular features include conjunctivitis, episcleritis, keratitis, uveitis, miosis and iris atrophy. Leprosy involves predominantly anterior uvea. Lepromatous leprosy may result in **granulomatous anterior uveitis**. It is characterized by presence of small, glistening nodules

known as **iris pearls**—a *pathognomonic sign.* Iris pearls are composed of dead bacilli within histiocytes which are located at the pupillary margin and resemble a necklace. There is low-grade inflammation associated with formation of synechiae.

Treatment

It includes local treatment of anterior uveitis and also specific treatment for leprosy. **Dapsone** 50 to 100 mg/day for 1 to 2 years is the drug of choice for the treatment of leprosy. Dapsone is a systemic sulphone. Other drugs recommended by WHO are **clofazimine and rifampicin**. They are potent drugs effective against resistant cases.

■ Uveitis in Sarcoidosis

It is a systemic disease of unknown etiology characterized by formation of **noncaseating** granuloma in affected tissues. The clinical presentation may vary from single organ involvement to multisystem involvement. Commonly involved tissues are lungs, skin, joints, eyes, central nervous system (CNS), liver and spleen.

Ocular Manifestations

Uveitis is the most common ocular manifestation. It may involve the anterior or posterior segment.

Anterior segment involvement presents as (**Fig. 8.19**):

- Anterior uveitis:
  ◊ Acute iridocyclitis.
  ◊ Chronic iridocyclitis: It is granulomatous, usually bilateral, and more common than acute form.
- Other ocular features:
  ◊ Conjunctival nodules.
  ◊ Band-shaped keratopathy.

Table 8.8 Differentiating features of different types of leprosy

	Lepromatous type	**Tuberculoid type**
• Cellular immunity	Depressed	Good
• Ocular involvement	It is due to direct invasion of iris by bacilli	It is indirect due to involvement of peripheral nerves resulting in neuroparalytic and neurotrophic keratopathy
• Uveal involvement	More common	Rare

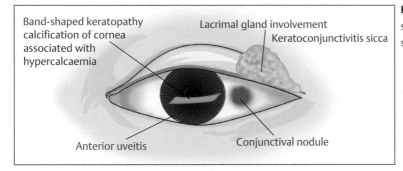

Band-shaped keratopathy calcification of cornea associated with hypercalcaemia

Lacrimal gland involvement

Keratoconjunctivitis sicca

Anterior uveitis

Conjunctival nodule

Fig. 8.19 Ocular lesions in sarcoidosis due to anterior segment involvement.

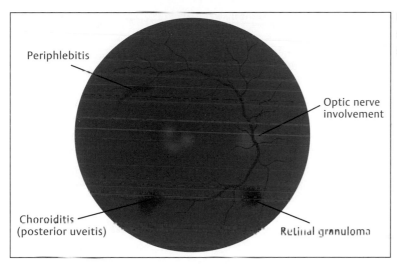

Periphlebitis

Optic nerve involvement

Choroiditis (posterior uveitis)

Retinal granuloma

Fig. 8.20 Ocular lesions in sarcoidosis due to posterior segment involvement.

◇ Keratoconjunctivitis sicca (due to lacrimal gland involvement)

Involvement of both lacrimal and salivary glands constitute **Mikulicz syndrome**.

Posterior segment manifestations are caused by involvement of:

- Choroid: Choroidal involvement may result in *posterior uveitis (chorioretinitis) and choroidal or retinal granuloma* (**Fig. 8.20**).
- Blood vessels– Involvement of blood vessels cause peripheral retinal periphlebitis which is characterized by:
  ◇ Perivenous sheathing.
  ◇ Peripheral retinal hemorrhages due to increased vascular permeability.
  ◇ Perivenous exudates known as "**candle wax drippings**."

Uveoparotid fever: Sarcoidosis may present as **uveoparotid fever** (**Heerfordt's syndrome**). It is bilateral and characterized by simultaneous involvement of uveal tract (causing granulomatous anterior uveitis), parotid gland (painful swelling of parotid resembling mumps, causing fever and malaise and cranial nerves (causing facial palsy and ocular motor nerves palsy leading to diplopia). It affects young individuals between 10 and 30 years of age.

Investigations

- *Serum angiotensin-converting enzyme (ACE)* is raised.
- Estimation of *serum lysozyme.*
- *X-ray chest* may show bilateral involvement of hilar lymph nodes in lungs.

- *Skin test:* **Kveim test** (injection of sarcoid tissue suspension into skin of sarcoidosis patient) is positive. *Mantoux test is negative in most patients.* Patient's sarcoidosis often fails to react to intradermal injection of tuberculin.

A strongly positive reaction to tuberculin makes the diagnosis of sarcoidosis highly unlikely.

- Biopsy of lungs, conjunctival nodules, lacrimal glands, lymph nodes or skin lesions.

Treatment

Treatment includes administration of steroids, which may be topical, periocular and systemic. Immunosuppressives (methotrexate or cyclosporin) are rarely required.

■ Viral Uveitis

Herpetic Uveitis

Herpes viruses are:

1. **Herpes simplex virus (HSV),** which has 2 subtypes:
   - HSV-1
   - HSV-2

HSV-1 affects the area supplied by trigeminal or sacral ganglia. *HSV-2* mostly affects genitals. HSV causes *Herpes simplex* which affects human being early in life.

2. **Varicella zoster virus (VZV):** It causes herpes zoster and commonly involves the ophthalmic (1st) division of trigeminal nerve (*Herpes zoster ophthalmicus [HZO]*).

Ocular Manifestations

Herpes viruses cause granulomatous chronic anterior uveitis, acute retinal necrosis (**ARN**) and progressive outer retinal necrosis (**PORN**).

Granulomatous Chronic Anterior Uveitis

Due to HSV—It may occur with or without corneal disease, and iris atrophy is present. Treatment includes:

- Topical steroids: Steroids should never be used in presence of active epithelial keratitis.

- Cycloplegics.
- Systemic acyclovir: 400 mg 5 times a day.

Due to VZV: Anterior uveitis affects patients with HZO, particularly when vesicular eruption (rash) is present on the tip of nose (**Hutchinson sign**). The rash on the tip of nose is due to the involvement of the branch of nasociliary nerve. Anterior uveitis in HZO *usually manifests 10 to 25 days after the onset of rashes.* It is usually mild and asymptomatic and may be associated with sectorial iris atrophy. Treatment includes administration of topical steroids and cycloplegics.

Complications of anterior uveitis:

- Secondary glaucoma due to associated trabeculitis resulting in trabecular obstruction.
- Complicated cataract.
- Iris atrophy which is sectorial and thought to be due to occlusive vasculitis.
- Damage to sphincter pupillae.

Acute Retinal Necrosis (ARN)

It is a rare necrotizing retinitis caused by HSV in younger patients and VZV in older ones. In this condition, anterior granulomatous uveitis and vitritis are universal. Peripheral periarteritis progresses to involve full thickness of retina, leading to retinal necrosis and rhegmatogenous retinal detachment. Posterior pole is usually spared, so visual acuity remains fairly good.

Treatment: *Includes* IV acyclovir—10 mg/kg every 8 hours for 10 to 14 days, followed by oral acyclovir 800 mg 5 times a day for 6 to 12 weeks. This may arrest the disease and reduce the risk of involvement of the fellow eye but it does not prevent retinal detachment. Prognosis is relatively poor as a result of retinal detachment and ischemic optic neuropathy.

Progressive Outer Retinal Necrosis (PORN)

It is *caused by* VZV. It is a rare necrotizing retinitis seen in patients with immunosuppression due to AIDS or immunosuppressive drugs. The necrotizing retinitis is devastating because of immunosuppression of patient. The infection is limited only to outer retina in early stages and there is rapid progression to full-thickness retinal necrosis. PORN affects posterior pole and outer retinal layer. Involvement of posterior pole in PORN results in early macular involvement, leading to rapidly progressive visual loss and minimal anterior uveitis. Involvement of outer retinal layers results in multifocal, yellow–white retinal infiltrates with minimal vitritis.

Rapid progression of disease due to immuno-suppression causes full-thickness retinal necrosis and vitritis. So, vitreous inflammation is usually late and reflects extensive retinal necrosis.

It is diagnosed by vitreous samples for PCR and diagnostic assay of VZV DNA. Treatment includes IV ganciclovir alone or in combination with foscarnet. Thus, the basic difference between ARN and PORN is as given in **Table 8.9**.

Cytomegalovirus (CMV) Retinitis

CMV is an opportunistic pathogen in patients with impaired immune system due to AIDS or immunosuppressives (for leukemia and lymphoma, following organ transplantation).

Ocular Manifestations

CMV retinitis is the most common infection in AIDS. It is a chronic diffuse exudative infection of retina and characterized by yellow–white exudates in retina, representing the areas of retinal necrosis (necrotizing retinitis). It is associated with:

- Vasculitis with perivascular sheathing.
- Retinal hemorrhages.
- Vitreous exudates.

The infective process spreads slowly along retinal blood vessels to involve entire fundus and leads to total retinal atrophy.

Treatment

- IV ganciclovir in the dosage of 5 mg/kg every 12 hours for 2 to 3 weeks, followed by 5 mg/kg every 24 hours for long term. Its side effect is bone marrow suppression.
- IV foscarnet: 60 mg/kg every 8 hours for 2 to 3 weeks, followed by 90 mg/kg every 24 hours for long term. Its side effects are nephrotoxicity and electrolyte disturbance.
- Implantation of ganciclovir slow-release device into vitreous. The implant is sutured to sclera and suspended in vitreous cavity. Its duration of efficacy is 8 months and it is superior to IV therapy with ganciclovir/foscarnet.

A combination of three or four antiretroviral drugs is known as highly active anterior retroviral therapy (**HAART**) and acts at different stages of the HIV lifecycle. Side effects of HAART are bone marrow suppression and nephrotoxicity.

■ Spirochaetal Uveitis

Syphilis

It is *caused by* a spirochete, *Treponema pallidum*, and may be congenital or acquired. Syphilis affects both anterior and posterior uvea. In **congenital syphilis**, fetus acquires infection from infected mother via placenta. It is usually bilateral. Anterior uveitis and interstitial keratitis are common in congenital syphilis. Fundus shows bilateral pigmentary retinopathy (**salt and pepper fundus**). The fundus picture may mimic retinitis pigmentosa.

In adults, syphilis is usually sexually acquired. The *stages of acquired syphilis* in an untreated patient are primary, secondary, latent and tertiary.

Table 8.9 Difference between acute retinal necrosis and progressive outer retinal necrosis	
Acute retinal necrosis	**Progressive outer retinal necrosis**
• It tends to *start in periphery* so macula is usually spared and cause anterior granulomatous uveitis	Its *affects posterior pole* so there is early macular involvement and so anterior uveitis is minimal
• It involves full thickness of retina so results in vitritis and peripheral periarteritis	It affects outer retinal layers, hence it causes minimal intraocular inflammatory signs of vitritis in early stages
• Vision: As macula is spared, visual acuity remains fairly good	Because of early macular involvement, there is rapidly progressive visual loss

Ocular Manifestations

Eye involvement occurs during secondary and tertiary stages. Occasionally, it may be seen during primary syphilis.

Anterior uveitis occurs in the secondary stage of syphilis. It may be *granulomatous or nongranulomatous*. In some cases, iridocyclitis is first associated with dilated iris capillaries termed roseolae, possibly due to treponemal emboli. These roseolae may develop into localized papules and subsequently into larger yellowish, heavily vascularized nodules near pupillary and ciliary border of iris (*but not in intermediate region*) called Gummas (**Gummatous iridocyclitis**). These are associated with exudation and broad synechiae. Posterior uveitis may occur as:

- *Acute syphilitic chorioretinitis* which is characterized by yellow placoid lesions, especially in the macular area.

  This is almost always associated with severe vitritis.
- *Chronic syphilitic chorioretinitis* which consists of depigmented retinal lesions, with pigment aggregated in corpuscles and attenuated vessels, and atrophy of optic disc resembling retinitis pigmentosa. *Symptoms include* defective central vision, night blindness, and irregular and concentric contraction of field and metamorphopsia. Neuroretinitis and periphlebitis are also common. Syphilitic infection is more severe and has a more aggressive course in HIV infection and responds less and slowly to conventional treatment. *It is recommended that tests for both HIV and syphilis be performed if either is found to be positive.*

Differential Diagnosis

It must be differentiated from uveitis due to TB, sarcoidosis, autoimmune disease and serpiginous choroidopathy.

Diagnosis

Following investigations are required to ascertain the diagnosis of syphilis:

- VDRL and RPR: These are nontreponemal tests and detect antibody to lecithin or cardiolipin which is a cholesterol antigen. These tests have lower specificity.
- FTA-ABS test and treponemal hemagglutination test: These are treponemal antibody tests which detect antibodies against treponemal antigens and are more specific.
- Cerebrospinal fluid (CSF) examination for evidence of neurosyphilis is done in all cases of ocular syphilis.

Treatment

Penicillin is used in all stages of syphilis. One of the following regimens may be used:

- IV aqueous penicillin G: 12 to 24 mega units/day for 14 days
- IM procaine penicillin: 2 to 4 mega units/ day for 14 days.

It is supplemented with oral probenecid 2 g daily. It increases and prolongs plasma level of penicillin.

Patients sensitive to Penicillin are treated with:

	Oral tetracycline	– 500 mg q.i.d. for 30 days
or	Oral doxycycline	
or	Oral erythromycin	– 500 mg q.i.d. for 30 days

■ Fungal Uveitis

Fungal uveitis may be:

- Exogenous following penetrating injury with vegetable matter or after intraocular surgery.
- Endogenous transmitted via blood from focus elsewhere in the body.

It may be due to Histoplasma capsulatum, Candida albicans, Coccidiodes immitis, or Cryptococcus.

Presumed Ocular Histoplasmosis Syndrome (POHS)

It is *caused by* Histoplasma capsulatum. Patients with POHS show an increased prevalence of HLA–B7 and HLA–DR2.

Ocular Manifestations

If there is no macular involvement, the patient is asymptomatic. With macular involvement, metamorphopsia occurs. Intraocular inflammation is absent, that is, vitreous cells are not seen in POHS. Types of fundus lesions seen in POHS are:

- Atrophic "punched-out" chorioretinal scars (called **histospots**) are seen in midretinal periphery and posterior pole. These probably represent the healed benign histoplasma lesions of childhood.
- Peripapillary atrophy.
- Macular lesion as exudative maculopathy–Atrophic macular scar causes a hole in the Bruch's membrane with ingrowth of capillaries. It results in development of subretinal choroidal neovascularization and leakage from choroidal new vessels (**CNV**), causing **serous macular detachment**. Serous macular detachment causes visual symptoms (metamorphopsia and decreased central vision), which may regress if fluid gets absorbed spontaneously. It may be complicated by subretinal bleeding from CNV (**hemorrhagic disciform maculopathy**).

Diagnosis

It is confirmed by the histoplasma skin test.

Treatment

Treatment of CNV is done with argon laser photocoagulation. In extrafoveal CNV, treatment is rewarding, while in subfoveal CNV, prognosis is poor.

Candidiasis

It is caused by *Candida albicans*, a frequent commensal of mucous membranes of mouth, gastrointestinal tract (GIT), and vagina. Candida is an opportunistic nonpathogenic fungus. So, candidiasis occurs when immunity is compromised in patients receiving immunosuppressive therapy, and in patients afflicted with AIDS or diabetes. Hematogenous spread occurs from GIT to involve the eye.

Ocular Manifestations

Chorioretinitis with overlying vitritis–Multiple, round, white, slightly elevated lesions with indistinct borders (**cotton ball-like**) develop in retina. These may be associated with retinal hemorrhages. If antifungal therapy is not instituted, these small retinal lesions enlarge and extend into vitreous, giving rise to floating "cotton ball" colonies which may join together to form a "**string of pearls.**"

Treatment

It includes IV amphotericin B or pars plana vitrectomy + intravitreal amphotericin B.

■ Parasitic Uveitis

- Toxoplasmosis.
- Toxocariasis.
- Onchocerciasis.
- Cysticercosis.

Toxoplasmosis

It is caused by *Toxoplasma gondii*, an obligate intracellular protozoan parasite. It has a particular affinity for neural tissues, so it primarily involves CNS and retina. Cats are the definitive hosts of the parasite which excrete oocytes in their feces. Transmission of trophozoites (active form responsible for tissue destruction and the inflammation) via placenta causes infestation of fetus in a pregnant woman. *If mother is infested before pregnancy, fetus will not be affected.* Ocular involvement can be congenital (congenital toxoplasmosis) or acquired (acquired toxoplasmosis).

Congenital Toxoplasmosis

In congenital toxoplasmosis, ocular lesion is usually associated with encephalitis. Inflammatory reaction is more severe in congenital form.

Ocular Features

Parasite causes granulomatous retinochoroiditis which is typically necrotic (necrotizing retinochoroiditis). The lesions are bilateral and particularly involve the macular area. In necrotizing retinochoroiditis, entire thickness of retina and choroid is destroyed, resulting in bilateral punched out, heavily pigmented scar, especially in the macular area (**Fig. 8.21**) which causes defective vision. The lesions resemble macular coloboma.

Encephalitis leads to convulsions. If the infants survive, they show areas of intracranial calcification in brain and mental retardation.

So, the **characteristic triad** (**three C's**) of congenital toxoplasmosis is:
- Convulsions.
- Chorioretinitis.
- Calcification in brain.

Acquired Toxoplasmosis

In adults, ocular infestation can be the result of reactivation of congenital infestation or it can be acquired postnatally. Reactivation of healed lesion is quite common, often at the edge of previous scar. In acquired toxoplasmosis, ocular involvement is usually unilateral, mild, and without CNS involvement.

Reactivation of healed lesion (recurrence): The necrotic retina has encysted parasites at the edge of previous scar. The periodic rupture of cysts releases trophozoites into normal retinal cells. It causes secondary immunological reaction, resulting in fresh lesions commonly at the margins of old scar.

The *primary lesion* is retinitis associated with posterior uveitis, that is, retinochoroiditis. It is usually associated with severe vitritis due to exudation into vitreous with overlying vitreous haze.

Clinical Presentation

It presents as unilateral, sudden onset of floaters, blurred vision and photophobia. Focal retinitis is present which is characterized by yellow–white lesion with fluffy indistinct margins adjacent to the edge of an old inactive pigmented scar (**"satellite lesion"**). The lesion is most commonly solitary. There is also an overlying vitreous haze.

Investigations

- Sabin–Feldman dye test.
- ELISA test for IgG and IgM.
- Indirect hemagglutination test (IHA).
- Immunofluorescent antibody test.

Treatment

Steroids are given in conjunction with antimicrobials.
- **Corticosteroids:** Oral prednisolone—1 mg/kg/day initially, then tapered according to the clinical response.
- **Antimicrobials:**
  - ◊ Sulphatriad (sulphadiazine + sulphathiazole + sulphamerazine) is given in dosage of 1 g every 6 hours for 4 weeks.

  Alternatively,
  - ◊ Cotrimoxazole is a combination of trimethoprim 160 mg + sulphamethoxazole 800 mg is given b.i.d. for 4 to 6 weeks. Side effects of cotrimoxazole are renal stones and Stevens–Johnson syndrome.
  - ◊ Pyrimethamine: Loading dose is 75 to 150 mg followed by 25 mg daily for

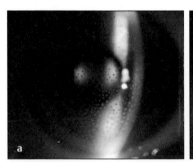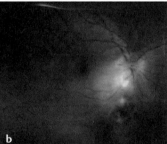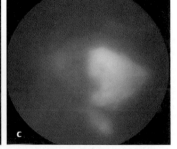

Fig. 8.21 (a–c) Ocular toxoplasmosis. Source: Exam Findings. In: Ehlers J, ed. The Retina Illustrated. 1st Edition. Thieme; 2019.

3 to 4 weeks. It is a *folic acid antagonist,* so it may cause thrombocytopenia and leucopenia. Therefore, weekly complete blood counts and platelet counts must be done. It is given in combination with oral folinic acid 10 mg/day.

Pyrimethamine is avoided in AIDS due to preexisting bone marrow suppression and the antagonistic effect of zidovudine when given with pyrimethamine.

◊ Clindamycin (300 mg q.i.d. for 4 weeks) and sulphadiazine (1 g q.i.d. for 3–4 weeks): These act synergistically. Clindamycin causes clostridial overgrowth and may cause colitis. Sulphadiazine (a sulphonamide) inhibits clostridial overgrowth, so risk of colitis is reduced when clindamycin is used together with a sulphonamide.

Corticosteroids should always be used in conjunction with one or more of the above antimicrobials. If medical measures fail, photocoagulation is done.

Toxocariasis

It is *caused by* Toxocara canis (an intestinal roundworm of dogs) and Toxocara catis (an intestinal roundworm of cats). Children who play with dogs or cats are at particular risk of acquiring the disease.

Ocular Manifestations

Ocular toxocariasis is almost always unilateral and can present as one of the following ocular lesions:

- Chronic Endophthalmitis: It presents as **leucocoria** between the age of 2 to 9 years. So, it mimics retinoblastoma.
- Posterior pole granuloma: Granuloma consists of eosinophils and IgE. It appears as a white lesion and protrudes into the eye from retinal tissue.
- Peripheral granuloma.
- Localized vitreous abscess.

Diagnostic test is ELISA.

Treatment

It includes systemic corticosteroids and pars plana vitrectomy. Indications of pars plana vitrectomy are endophthalmitis and vitreoretinal traction. Antihelminthic drugs are of minimal value and may even result in increased inflammation due to death of toxocara organism.

Onchocerciasis (River Blindness)

It is *caused by Onchocerca volvulus*, a filarial nematode. It is *transmitted by* the bite of black fly simulium (vector). Ocular features include punctate keratitis, sclerosing keratitis, anterior uveitis, floating microfilariae in aqueous, chorioretinitis, usually bilateral, and optic atrophy. Diagnosis is achieved by biopsy of skin nodules. Ivermectin is a very effective drug for its treatment.

Cysticercosis

It is *caused by cysticercus cellulosae,* the larvae form of pork tape worm, Taenia solium.

Ocular Manifestations

It presents as subconjunctival cysts. Larvae may be found in vitreous or subretinal space (**Fig. 8.22**). Live cysticercus (larvae) cause little reaction but dead larva release toxins which produce intense inflammation.

Investigations

As the disease often involves lungs, muscles and brain, so the following investigations are performed:

- X-ray chest and muscle– show calcified cysts.
- ELISA test.
- CT or MRI scan of head for accompanying cysticercus infection in brain. *Presence of cysticercus in the eye is diagnostic.*

Treatment

Medical treatment with **albendazole is not indicated** for ocular disease, since dead larvae may induce intense inflammation, leading to loss of vision. Treatment of choice is surgical removal of cysts. Subretinal cysts may be removed

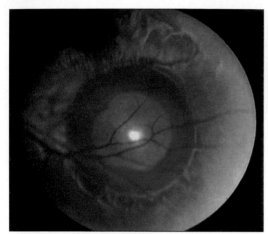

Fig. 8.22 Subretinal cysticercus.

transsclerally and intravitreal cysts are removed by vitrectomy.

■ Immunological Uveitis

Ankylosing Spondylitis

It is a chronic, inflammatory arthritis characterized by calcification and ossification of ligaments, and capsules of joints, leading to progressive stiffening and fusion of axial skeleton. It **involves axial skeleton** (sacro-iliac joint and posterior intervertebral joints). **HLA–B27** antigen is strongly associated with the disease. Males are more affected than females. It affects people between 20 to 40 years of age.

Clinical Features

It presents with pain and morning stiffness in the lower back in early adulthood. Arthritis is also seen mostly affecting sacro-iliac joints and spine. The spine becomes fixed in flexion with reduced mobility of thoracic cage. *Acute anterior uveitis* occurs, which is often unilateral, recurrent and nongranulomatous. Bilateral simultaneous involvement is rare.

Investigations

Following investigations help in reaching a diagnosis:
- ESR is raised.
- Radiology: X-ray sacro-iliac joints reveals sclerosis and ossification. Spinal ligaments are also ossified and called **"bamboo spine."**
- Tissue typing: HLA–B27 is positive in 95% cases.

Treatment

It is treated as usual anterior uveitis, that is, by steroids (topical and systemic) and topical cycloplegics.

Complications

Complicated cataract and glaucoma are the usual complications of ankylosing spondylitis.

Juvenile Chronic Arthritis (JCA)

It is a chronic inflammatory arthritis occurring before the age of 16 years.

Classification

JCA can be classified as pauciarticular onset JCA, polyarticular onset JCA, and systemic onset JCA. *The term* **Still's disease** *is reserved for patients with systemic onset disease.*

Ocular Manifestations

Anterior uveitis in JCA is fairly rare with **polyarticular JCA**. Uveitis itself is not common but is seen as a complication of scleritis. It is extremely rare in **systemic onset JCA** (Still's disease). It develops in **pauciarticular JCA** which is bilateral usually, chronic, of insidious onset and nongranulomatous with minimal signs.

Treatment

Treatment is done by the following:
- Topical steroids.
- Periocular steroids: When there is poor response to topical steroids
- Methotrexate in low dose: When there is steroid resistance.

Complications

Band keratopathy, cataract and secondary glaucoma are the usual complications of juvenile chronic arthritis.

Reiter's Syndrome

It is also known as **reactive arthritis** and characterized by the triad of urethritis (nongonococcal), conjunctivitis, and arthritis. Conjunctivitis follows urethritis and precedes arthritis. It affects mostly young males and is associated with **HLA–B27**.

Ocular Manifestations

- Conjunctivitis: It is bilateral and mucopurulent.
- Acute anterior uveitis: It occurs in 12% cases and is nongranulomatous.
- Keratitis as punctate subepithelial keratitis.

Treatment

Chlamydia have been isolated from urethral discharge in 50% of cases. For urethritis in Reiter syndrome, oral tetracycline 500 mg q.i.d. for 3 to 6 weeks is given. For uveitis, steroids and cycloplegics are given.

Behçet Syndrome

It is an idiopathic multisystem disease characterized by severe uveitis with hypopyon, ulcerative lesion in conjunctival, oral and genital mucosae, neurological manifestations, and articular manifestations. It is strongly associated with **HLA–B51**. It is seen in young adults and rarely presents in childhood or old age. Etiology is unknown. Basic lesion is probably caused by immune complexes.

Ocular Manifestations

These are usually bilateral. The disease involves:

- *Anterior segment* and manifests as acute anterior uveitis, which is bilateral, nongranulomatous and recurrent.

  Uveitis is usually associated with a transient, mobile hypopyon. Hypopyon shifts with gravity as the patient changes head position.
- *Posterior segment* lesions include retinal vasculitis: It may involve both veins and arteries and result in occlusion (**obliterative vasculitis**). Retinal vasculitis leads to vascular leakage, which gives rise to **diffuse retinal edema** involving outer retinal layers, **CME** and **disc edema**.

Treatment

There is no specific treatment. Important points of consideration are:

- Systemic steroids shorten the duration of inflammation.
- Immunosuppressives are suitable for long-term therapy.

Prognosis

It has poor visual prognosis.

Vogt–Koyanagi–Harada (VKH) Syndrome

It is a rare condition which typically affects pigmented races (Asians and Africans).

Etiology

The *cause is* unknown, but it may be an autoimmune response to melanocytes. So, it causes inflammation of melanocyte-containing tissues such as uvea, ears, skin and meninges. The disease is associated with **HLA–DR 1** and **HLA–DR 4** which suggests a immunogenic predisposition. Originally, VKH syndrome was categorized as **Vogt Koyanagi disease,** which is characterized by skin changes (poliosis, vitiligo, and alopecia), chronic anterior uveitis, and **Harada disease,** which is characterized by bilateral posterior uveitis with exudative retinal detachment and neurological features. Now, the two entities are clubbed together as VKH syndrome.

Ocular Manifestations

Ocular features in VKH syndrome include:

- Chronic granulomatous anterior uveitis.
- Posterior uveitis (exudative choroiditis).
- Exudative retinal detachment.
- Depigmentation of fundus lesions ("**sunset glow**" fundus).

Extraocular Features

Inflammation of melanocyte-containing tissues in VKH syndrome affects meninges, skin and ear. *Neurological signs* due to the involvement of meninges include neck stiffness, convulsions, paresis and cranial nerve palsies. *Cutaneous signs* include alopecia (baldness), poliosis (whitening of eyebrows, eye lashes and hair) and vitiligo (patch of skin depigmentation). *Auditory features* include tinnitus, vertigo and deafness.

Neurological and auditory features occur in the prodromal phase of the disease. Uveitis phase occurs within 1–2 days after onset of neurological signs. Skin findings do not precede onset of CNS or ocular disease.

Treatment

Posterior segment involvement is treated with:

- IV steroids: Methyl prednisolone 1 g/day in infusion bottles for 3 days, followed by high-dose oral steroids tapered over months.
- In steroid-resistant cases: Immuno-suppressive drugs (cyclosporin and cyclophosphamide).

■ Miscellaneous Uveitis

Glaucomatocyclitic Crisis (Posner–Schlossman Syndrome)

It is characterized by acute recurrent, mild anterior uveitis associated with raised IOP (secondary glaucoma). The condition is probably due to an accompanying trabeculitis. Inflammation is minimal with no aqueous flare, fine and nonpigmented KPs, no posterior synechiae, and no peripheral synechiae.

Glaucoma is out of proportion to the inflammation and presents with very high IOP (40–60 mm Hg), epithelial edema due to raised IOP, halos in a white eye, and open-angle and unilateral glaucoma. Patients present with diminution of vision and halos around light.

Treatment

Topical steroids are commonly given. Control of IOP is done by timolol maleate and systemic carbonic anhydrase inhibitors.

Fuchs Heterochromic Iridocyclitis

It is a chronic, low-grade anterior uveitis of insidious onset. It presents with the following signs:

- KPs:
  - ◇ Small and white: They never become confluent or pigmented.

  - ◇ Round and scattered throughout the corneal endothelium. Presence of KPs distinguish the condition from congenital heterochromia.
- Aqueous: Cells are often present.
- Iris: Absence of posterior synechiae.
  - ◇ *Diffuse atrophy of iris stroma* lead to:
    - Atrophy of sphincter pupillae resulting in *mydriasis.*
    - Prominent radial iris blood vessels.
    - Loss of iris details resulting in *washed-out appearance* of iris.
  - ◇ Heterochromia iridis: It is an important and common sign.
- Neovascularization of angle of anterior chamber on gonioscopy. So, when paracentesis is done, pressure in anterior chamber is suddenly reduced. These new vessels bleed, and fine filiform hemorrhage occurs from the opposite angle. This is known as **Amsler sign.**

Treatment

- Posterior subtenon injection of triamcinolone.
- Topical steroids.
- *As posterior synechiae do not develop, mydriatics are not required.*

Complications

Cataract and glaucoma are usual complications of Fuchs heterochromic iridocyclitis.

Lens-Induced Uveitis

It is an immune response to **lens proteins** (antigen) following rupture of lens capsule. It is caused by trauma and incomplete cortical aspiration in extracapsular cataract extraction (ECCE). It may present as phacoanaphylactic uveitis and phacogenic uveitis. It presents with blurred vision and pain. Clinical signs seen in a patient include granulomatous anterior uveitis, raised IOP, and lens matter in anterior chamber.

Treatment

Removal of all lens matter followed by topical and systemic steroids.

■ Endophthalmitis

Endophthal (inner eye) itis (inflammation) is an intraocular inflammation involving uveal tissue, retina, vitreous, and anterior chamber. It involves all intraocular structures except sclera. Endophthalmitis is classified into two groups: **infective** (bacterial or fungal) **and noninfective** (sterile). **Infective** endophthalmitis may be **exogenous** (due to exogenous infection elsewhere) or **endogenous** (due to endogenous infection during intraocular surgery). **Noninfective** endophthalmitis may be due to:

- Retained lens matter (induced by lens proteins).
- Toxic material introduced in the body.

■ Bacterial Endophthalmitis

It may be exogenous and endogenous. Exogenous endophthalmitis may be postoperative or posttraumatic. *Source of infection in postoperative endophthalmitis may be* eyelids, conjunctiva and lacrimal sac. Microbes can enter the eye through the filtering bleb after glaucoma surgery. It can develop one to several days after surgery.

In endogenous endophthalmitis, organisms enter the eye through blood stream from the infected focus elsewhere in the body. Risk factors include:

- Diabetes mellitus.
- Patient's receiving steroids or immunosuppressives.
- Meningococcal septicemia.
- AIDS.
- IV drug abusers.
- Urinary tract infection (UTI) (*E. coli*).
- Endocarditis.

Causative Pathogens

Causative pathogens in bacterial endophthalmitis are:

- Staphylococcus (S. aureus and S. epidermidis).
- Streptococcus.
- Pneumococcus.
- Pseudomonas pyocyanea.

- Klebsiella.
- *E. coli*.
- Bacillus cereus especially in IV drug abusers.

The anaerobe propionibacterium acnes produce chronic, low-grade infection and causes delayed onset postoperative endophthalmitis.

Clinical Features

Symptoms of bacterial endophthalmitis include pain, blurred vision, floaters, redness, photophobia, headache, and fever (it is more common with endogenous infection).

Signs of bacterial endophthalmitis include:

Anterior segment:
- Lids: Swollen lids
- Conjunctiva: Circum corneal congestion.
- Cornea: Corneal edema.
- AC: Hypopyon in severe cases and soon becomes full of pus.
- Iris: Anterior fibrinous uveitis.

Posterior segment: Vitreous becomes purulent. Vitreous abscess shows yellow reflex with oblique illumination, and normal red fundus reflex is lost.

In severe cases, destruction of ciliary processes causes decrease in IOP and shrinkage of eyeball.

Investigations

The following investigations help in the diagnosis of bacterial endophthalmitis:

- Complete blood count.
- Blood sugar.
- Urine.
- X-ray chest.
- Aqueous and vitreous tap for:
  - ◊ Smears which are examined by Gram and Giemsa staining.
  - ◊ Cultures on blood and chocolate agar media.
- Blood culture.

Treatment

It includes the use of antibiotics and steroids and then vitrectomy.

Antibiotics

A combination of antibiotics must be used to cover all organisms. Every possible route of administration should be used (intravitreal, topical, subconjunctival, and systemic).

1. **Intravitreal antibiotics** are the treatment of choice. Intravitreal antibiotics are injected after taking a 0.2 to 0.3 mL vitreous aspirate. Vitreous aspirate is used for smears and culture. The regimen to be followed is given below:

   Vancomycin   1 mg in 0.1 mL (for Gram
   +   positive cocci)
   ceftazidime   2.25 mg in 0.1 mL (for
                Gram negative organisms)
                Or
   vancomycin   1 mg in 0.1 mL
   +
   amikacin/   0.4 mg in 0.1 mL (for
   gentamicin   Gram negative organisms)

2. **Topical antibiotics:**

   Eye   fortified cefazolin/
   drops   vancomycin   are used
                               every
            +   1 hour
           gentamicin/amikacin

   They are instilled along with cycloplegics: Atropine 1% or Homatropine 2%

            +

   steroid eye drops–dexamethasone or predacetate

3. **Subconjunctival antibiotics**:

   Vancomycin   25 mg in 0.5 mL

            +

   ceftazidime   100 mg in 0.5 mL

   These are used along with subconjunctival dexamethasone 6 mg in 0.25 mL.

4. **Systemic antibiotics** (for systemic infections):

   Combination of 1 g every
   vancomycin   12 hours   are given
                              intra-
            +   venously
   ceftazidime   1 g every
                  12 hours

Steroids should be withheld where there is strong suspicion of a fungal etiology.

Corticosteroids

There exist two views on the use of steroids: Some recommend use of steroids along with antibiotics from the outset, while others prefer to wait for control of infection by antibiotics therapy and start steroids 24 to 48 hours after the antibiotic therapy. They exert anti-inflammatory effect, so limit the inflammatory damage to intraocular structures.

They can be used either topically (dexamethasone/prednisolone acetate eye drops) or subconjunctivally (dexamethasone injection 0.4 mg in 0.1 mL is optional).

Pars Plana Vitrectomy

- *Indications:*
  ◊ If visual acuity is light perception or worse.
  ◊ If patient does not respond to intravitreal antibiotics within 48 hours.
- *Advantages:*
  ◊ It helps in recovery by removing infected vitreous.
  ◊ Vitrectomy allows better antibiotic penetration following intravitreal injection.
  ◊ It provides vitreous for smear and culture.

■ Fungal Endophthalmitis

It may be exogenous or endogenous. **Exogenous** occurs after intraocular surgery or injury with vegetable matter. It is usually caused by filamentous fungi such as Aspergillus, Fusarium and Penicillium. **Endogenous variety** is metastatic in origin and from a focus within the body. Risk factors are Immunosuppression, IV drug abuse and chronic lung disease such as cystic fibrosis. It is most commonly caused by Candida albicans and mucor.

The progression is much slower and usually manifests within 3 months after surgery.

Clinical Features

Exogenous fungal endophthalmitis usually affects anterior vitreous and anterior uvea with formation of hypopyon.

Endogenous fungal endophthalmitis causes chorioretinal lesions with overlying vitritis and floating "cotton ball" colonies seen after extension into vitreous.

Investigation

Anterior chamber and vitreous taps—Smear and culture samples inoculated onto **Sabouraud medium.**

Treatment

Treatment includes drugs and vitrectomy. **Drug of choice:** Amphotericin B given systemically in IV drip and by intravitreal injection 5 µg in 0.1 mL. Additional oral antifungal agents like fluconazole, ketoconazole, and flucytosine should be given. In fluconazole-resistant candida and fusarium infections, oral voriconazole is given. Systemic steroids are contraindicated in fungal infections. Pars plana vitrectomy with intravitreal Amphotericin B (5 µg in 0.1 mL) is also used.

■ Panophthalmitis

Panophthal (whole eye) itis (inflammation) involves the entire globe. Thus, it is similar to endophthalmitis, except that inflammation also involves outer coat of eye and Tenon's capsule. In severe cases, orbital tissues may also be affected. It usually starts as purulent anterior or posterior uveitis and soon involves the whole eye.

■ Etiology

The following may occur:
- Penetrating ocular injury/postoperative infections (**exogenous** panophthalmitis).
- Infective embolus in retinal or choroidal vessel causing **endogenous** panophthalmitis.

Causative organisms are identical for infective bacterial endophthalmitis:
- Pneumococcus.
- Staphylococcus.
- Streptococcus.
- Pseudomonas pyocyanea.
- *Escherichia coli.*

■ Clinical Features

Symptoms include severe ocular pain, headache and sometimes vomiting, fever, loss of vision, and redness and swelling of eyes.

Clinical signs are as follows:

Lids:
- Intense swelling.

Conjunctiva:
- Chemosis.
- Ciliary as well as conjunctival congestion.

Globe:
- Proptosis may be present.
- Painful and limited ocular movements due to involvement of Tenon's capsule.
- Tender.

Cornea: Cloudy and edematous.

Anterior chamber: Contains massive hypopyon.

IOP: Often raised.

Posterior segment—Purulent retinochoroiditis and vitreous become a bag of pus. Posterior segment cannot be visualized due to hazy media.

In severe cases, perforation of globe takes place usually near limbus and pus oozes out. Thus, pain subsides, IOP falls, and eyeball shrinks.

■ Treatment

- Antibiotics:
  ◇ Systemic.
  ◇ Subconjunctival injections.
- Anti-inflammatory and analgesics.
- Evisceration to avoid risk of intracranial dissemination of infection.

In most cases, a **frill excision** (a collar of sclera is left around optic nerve) can be performed.

■ Complications

If panophthalmitis is not adequately treated in time, infection may spread, leading to orbital cellulitis and consequently cavernous sinus thrombosis. Infection may spread to optic nerve sheath, resulting in meningitis.

■ Pigment Dispersion Syndrome

It is usually a bilateral condition characterized by the liberation of pigment from iris pigment epithelium. The liberated pigment is deposited throughout the anterior segment. Pathogenesis of pigment dispersion syndrome is explained in **Flowchart 8.4**.

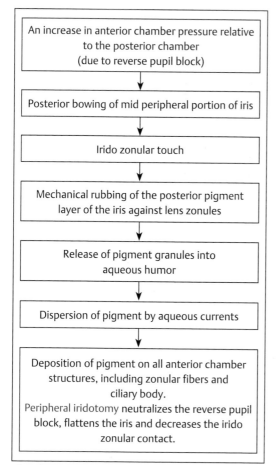

Flowchart 8.4 Pathogenesis of pigment dispersion syndrome.

■ Clinical Features

It affects cornea, iris, and the angle of anterior chamber.

- Cornea: There is pigment deposition on corneal endothelium in vertical spindle-shaped distribution (**Krukenberg spindle**).
- Iris: Pigment epithelial atrophy of iris gives rise to characteristic radial slit-like defects. Partial loss of pupillary frill is common.
- Angle of anterior chamber: There is a wide open angle. Also, there is characteristic midperipheral iris concavity that may increase with accommodation. Trabecular hyperpigmentation is also seen. Pigmentary obstruction of intertrabecular spaces causes rise in IOP.

■ Degenerative Changes in Uveal Tract

Degenerative changes in uveal tract may involve iris or choroid. Degenerative changes in **iris include** essential (progressive) atrophy of iris and iridoschisis. Degenerative changes in choroid could be either primary or secondary. Primary degenerations are localized or general. Localized primary degenerations include:

- Central areolar choroidal atrophy.
- Myopic chorioretinal degeneration.
- Central guttate choroidal atrophy (Tay choroiditis).

General primary degenerations include:

- Gyrate (essential) atrophy of choroid.
- Choroideremia.

■ Degenerative Changes in Iris

■ Essential Atrophy of Iris

It is often unilateral and progressive and affects young females. Etiology is unknown. Because of its progressive nature, a large portion of uveal tissue completely disappears with the development of multiple holes in iris—**pseudopolycoria** (more than one pupil due to secondary holes in iris.

Essential atrophy of iris is a part of iridocorneal endothelial (**ICE**) syndrome. The common feature of ICE syndrome is an abnormal corneal endothelial cell layer which has the capacity to proliferate and migrate across the angle and on to the surface of iris. The down growth of endothelial layer across the angle causes onset of glaucoma and loss of vision. Contraction of membrane produces:

- Peripheral anterior synechiae.
- Ectropion uveae.
- Dyscoria (abnormal shape of pupil).
- Corectopia (displaced pupil or malposition of pupil).

Prognosis is poor, but, fortunately, the disease is unilateral.

Iridocorneal endothelial syndrome (ICE syndrome)

ICE syndrome typically affects one eye of middle-aged women. It consists of three clinical entities:
- Progressive (essential) iris atrophy.
- Cogan–Reese syndrome (iris nevus).
- Chandler syndrome.

Cogan–Reese syndrome (iris nevus) is characterized by dark brown pigmented nodules in the iris stroma.

Chandler syndrome is associated with endothelial disturbances and corneal edema.

Iridoschisis

It is the dehiscence of anterior mesodermal layers of iris. A cleft is formed between anterior and posterior part of iris stroma, with strands of anterior part floating into the anterior chamber. It occurs due to senile degenerative changes or may be a late manifestation of ocular trauma.

■ Degenerative Changes in Choroid

These are more common than degenerative changes in iris and may be:
- Primary choroidal degenerations such as:
  ◇ Central guttate choroidal atrophy (Tay choroiditis).
  ◇ Central areolar choroidal atrophy.
  ◇ Myopic chorioretinal degeneration.
  ◇ Gyrate atrophy of choroid.
  ◇ Choroideremia.
- Secondary choroidal degenerations.

Primary Choroidal Degenerations

Central Guttate Choroidal Atrophy (Tay Choroiditis)

It is characterized by multiple minute, yellowish-white spots in the macular area called colloid bodies (drusen). These are due to the presence of hyaline excrescences on the Bruch's membrane. The condition is bilateral and generally does not cause visual impairment.

Central Areolar Choroidal Atrophy

It is characterized by large circular patch of degeneration in the macular area, owing to retinal pigment epithelial (RPE) atrophy and loss of choriocapillaris at the macula. Choroidal vessels are visible in the degenerative patch. It is genetically determined with autosomal dominant inheritance. Prognosis is poor with severe visual loss.

Myopic Chorioretinal Degeneration

It is commonly seen in pathological myopia. Degenerative changes are more marked around the optic disc and central area of fundus. These include:
- Myopic crescent around temporal border of disc or formation of a complete ring around disc. It is essentially atrophic.
- Chorioretinal atrophy in the central area of fundus (**Fig. 8.23a**).
- Foster–Fuchs spot: This is a circular pigmented lesion developed after macular hemorrhage has been absorbed (**Fig. 8.23b**).
- Lacquer cracks (linear breaks in the Bruch's membrane).

Gyrate Atrophy of Choroid

It is an inborn error of ornithine (amino acid) metabolism. The disease usually begins during the first decade of life. This condition is due to deficiency of enzyme **ornithine keto acid aminotransferase** (the main ornithine degradation enzyme). The deficiency of the enzyme results in an elevated ornithine level in plasma (ornithinemia), urine, CSF and aqueous humor.

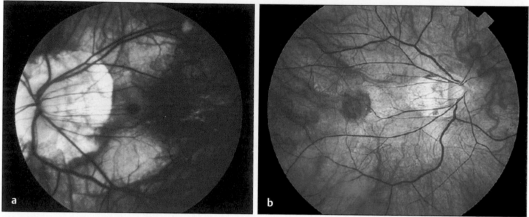

Fig. 8.23 (a) Myopic chorioretinal degeneration. Source: Scott I, Regillo C, Flynn H et al., Vitreoretinal Disease: Diagnosis Management, and Clinical Pearls, 2nd Edition, 2017. **(b)** Fuchs Spot. Source: Myopia. In: Steidl S, Hartnett M, ed. Clinical Pathways In Vitreoretinal Disease. 1st Edition. Thieme; 2003.

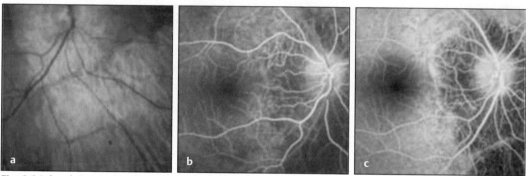

Fig. 8.24 (a–c) Gyrate atrophy of choroid. Source: Choroideremia and gyrate atrophy. In: Heimann H, Kellner U, Forester M, ed. Atlas of fundus angiography. 1st Edition. Thieme; 2006.

It is characterized by progressive atrophy of choroid and RPE with **macular sparing (Fig. 8.24)**. The patches of chorioretinal atrophy are in far and midretinal periphery, resulting in reduction of peripheral vision associated with night blindness. It has autosomal recessive inheritance. In this, electroretinogram (ERG) is subnormal or nonrecordable. Prognosis is generally poor.

Treatment

- Reduction in ornithine levels with an arginine-restricted diet.
- Pyridoxine (Vitamin B_6) may normalize plasma and urinary ornithine levels.

Choroideremia

It has X-linked recessive inheritance with gene located on X-chromosome and affects only males with female carriers. Thus, an affected male cannot transmit the gene to his sons, and all the daughters of the affected father will be carriers.

Clinical Presentation

It is characterized by progressive, diffuse degeneration of choroid, RPE and retinal photoreceptors, and presents in the first decade of life with defective night vision and depigmentation of RPE. Atrophy of choroid and RPE develop in the midperiphery and then spread centrally and toward periphery (**Fig. 8.25**). Because of midperipheral atrophy, the condition presents with defective night vision (as rods are more in periphery and mid periphery) and progressive constriction of visual fields. **Central vision is the last to be affected** as RPE under foveola may remain intact. At the end of the first decade, scotopic ERG is nonrecordable and photopic ERG is severely subnormal. Prognosis is very poor and causes blindness.

So, choroideremia is characterized by:
- Night blindness (nyctalopia).
- Progressive atrophy of choroid and RPE.
- Constriction of visual fields.

Secondary Choroidal Degenerations

These occur following inflammatory lesions (chorioretinitis), resulting in atrophy of choroid and outer retinal layers, with pigmentary changes.

Ophthalmoscopically, jet-black, branched pigment spots resembling bone corpuscles deposits in the perivascular spaces of veins. Thus, the picture resembles retinitis pigmentosa (pigmentary retinal dystrophy).

> In **chorioretinal atrophy** (healed chorioretinitis), pigment resembles bone corpuscles but lie deep to retinal vessels, so retinal vessels can be traced over the pigmentary spots. **In retinitis pigmentosa**, pigment also resembles bone corpuscles but lie anterior to retinal vessels; thereby they hide the course of vessels.

■ Detachment of Choroid

It is the separation of choroid from sclera.

■ Etiology

- It may occur within the first few days following an intraocular surgery as a result of sudden lowering of IOP, for example, trabeculectomy with excessive filtration → sudden lowering of IOP → increased vasodilatation → exudation into outer lamellae of choroid → choroidal detachment.
- Severe choroidal hemorrhage.
- Choroidal tumors.
- Trauma.

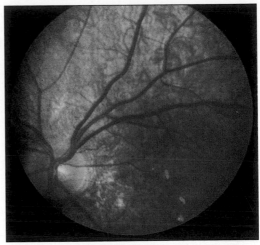

Fig. 8.25 Choroideremia. Source: Scott I, Regillo C, Flynn H et al., Vitreoretinal Disease: Diagnosis Management, and Clinical Pearls, 2nd Edition, 2017.

- Plastic iridocyclitis (in plastic, iridocyclitis exudation from iris and ciliary body is profuse).

> In choroidal detachment, there is no vitreoretinal traction, so photopsia and floaters are absent. Choroidal detachments are limited anteriorly by scleral spur and do not extend to posterior pole because they are limited by firm adhesions between suprachoroidal lamellae, where vortex veins enter their scleral canals.

■ Clinical Signs

- Very low IOP.
- Shallow anterior chamber.
- **Ophthalmoscopically**, dark brown mass is seen through pupil.

If IOP remains low and anterior chamber remains shallow for a long period (e.g., in trabeculectomy with excessive filtration), iris remains long in contact with cornea at the angle of anterior chamber and peripheral anterior synechiae may form. Thus, secondary (obstructive) glaucoma may develop.

■ Treatment

- Postoperative choroidal detachments resolve by itself.

- In trabeculectomy with excessive filtration, ensure that wound or conjunctival flap is not leaking. If it is, it should be repaired.
- If choroidal detachment is not settled, drainage of suprachoroidal fluid through sclera and reestablishment of anterior chamber with balanced salt solution is done.

■ Congenital Anomalies of Uveal Tract

■ Heterochromia of Iris (Hetero = Different; Chromia = Color)

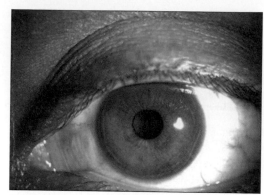

Fig. 8.26 Heterochromia iridis.

Heterochromia is the variation in iris color. Variation in iris color may be in the same iris (when a sector of iris has a different color from the remainder) and the condition is called **heterochromia iridis (Fig. 8.26),** or it may be between two iris (when one iris has different color from the other) and the condition is called **Heterochromia iridium**.

Heterochromia may be congenital or acquired as in Fuch's heterochromic iridocyclitis, siderosis and melanoma of iris.

■ Anomalies of Pupil

Normally, pupil is slightly nasal to the center of cornea. If pupil is abnormally eccentric, it is called corectopia. If more than one pupil is present, the condition is called polycoria.

■ Aniridia (Irideremia)

It is the absence of iris and is usually bilateral. Usually a narrow rim of iris tissue is present at the ciliary border, but it is hidden behind the sclera. Zonules of lens (suspensory ligaments) and ciliary processes are often visible due to aniridia. Anterior chamber angle anomalies in aniridia lead to development of secondary glaucoma.

■ Persistent Pupillary Membrane

It represents the persistence of a part of anterior vascular sheath of the lens; a fetal structure normally disappears before birth. Fine, stellate-shaped spots of pigmented tissue are scattered on the lens surface. These can be distinguished from broken posterior synechiae, as these are stellate in shape and regularly arranged with no signs of iritis.

■ Coloboma of Uveal Tract

A coloboma is the absence of a part of an ocular structure as a result of incomplete closure of the embryonic fissure. In the fully developed eye, **embryonic fissure is inferior and slightly nasal** and extends from the optic nerve to the margin of pupil (anterior part of optic cup). Coloboma may be typical or atypical. Typical coloboma is due to defective closure of embryonic fissure. So, these occur in the **inferonasal** quadrant. It may involve the entire length of fissure (**complete coloboma**), extending from pupil to optic nerve and giving rise to leukocoria, or it may involve only part of fissure, resulting in coloboma of a part (iris, ciliary body, choroid and retina or optic disc). Atypical coloboma is not related with nonclosure of embryonic fissure, so it is found in other positions. Retinal detachment may occur due to break within or outside coloboma.

■ Cysts of Iris

Congenital cysts of iris arise from stroma or pigment epithelium. *Implantation cyst of iris* occurs after performing ocular injury or intraocular surgery. It has a characteristic pearly appearance. *Serous cysts of iris* are due to closure of iris crypts with retention of fluid.

The Pupil

Normal Pupil..213
Afferent Pathway of Pupil..213
Efferent Pathways of Pupil..214
Pupillary Reflexes...215
Examination of the Pupils 217

■ Normal Pupil (PY10.17)

Pupil is the circular aperture in the iris diaphragm. Characteristic features of pupil are given below.

Number: Normally, there is one pupil in each eye. Rarely, there may be more than one pupil in one eye. This congenital anomaly is known as **polycoria**.

Location: Normally, pupil is slightly nasal. Rarely, it may be congenitally eccentric. An eccentric pupil is called **corectopia**.

Size: **Normal size** is 2.5 to 4 mm.

Miotic pupils are <2 mm.

Mydriatic pupils are >7 mm.

During sleep, it is smaller due to parasympathetic dominance. Normally, the two pupils are equal in size. This condition is known as **isocoria**. A difference in pupillary diameter of the two eyes of the same individual by 0.3 mm or more is known as **anisocoria**. The pupillary size is controlled by two muscles of ectodermal origin:

- **Sphincter pupillae**—It constricts the pupil (**miosis**) and is supplied by parasympathetic fibers via the oculomotor (III) nerve originating from the Edinger–Westphal (EW) nucleus. It is arranged in a circular fashion around the pupillary margin.
- **Dilator pupillae**—It dilates the pupil (**mydriasis**) and is supplied by sympathetic fibers. It is arranged radially near the root of the iris.

Shape: Normally, it is circular in shape.

Color: Normally, it is grayish black.

Functions of the pupil
- It regulates the amount of light entering the eye by miosis in light and mydriasis in darkness.
- It improves the visual acuity because it prevents the irregular refraction by the periphery of the cornea and lens, and increases the depth of focus.
- It allows passage of aqueous humour from the posterior chamber to the anterior chamber.

■ Afferent Pathway of Pupil

The afferent pupillary pathway consists of the afferent input from the retina, optic nerve, chiasma optic tract, and midbrain pathways. Afferent pupillary defects in any of the retinal layers, up to midbrain pretectal areas, interfere with the input of light to the pupillomotor system. Thus, defect in afferent pupillary pathway results in decrease in contraction of both pupils to light when given to the damaged eye.

■ First Order Neuron

It *commences at the retinal photoreceptors*. The fibers responsible for pupillomotor excitation pass through optic nerve, partially decussate in the chiasma, and enter the optic tracts. *The pupillary afferents separate from visual fibers in the posterior third of the optic tract* and *terminate in pretectal nucleus*.

The impulses originating in nasal retina will be conducted by the fibers to contralateral pretectal nucleus, and impulses from temporal retina will be conducted by uncrossed fibers to ipsilateral pretectal nucleus.

■ Second Order Neuron

This connects each pretectal nucleus to the EW nucleus on each side. It explains constriction of both pupils on light stimulation of one pupil. The neurons joining pretectal nucleus to EW nucleus are called internuncial neurons. These cross dorsal to the aqueduct. Internuncial neurons are damaged in syphilis and by pinealomas, resulting in light-near dissociation.

■ Efferent Pathways of Pupil

The efferent pupillary pathway is the pupillary motor output from the pretectal nucleus in the midbrain to the ciliary sphincter muscle of the iris. Efferent pupillary defects interfere with contraction or dilatation of the pupil due to damage in the midbrain, and in the peripheral nerve that supplies the iris muscles, causing asymmetrical pupils (anisocoria).

Efferent pathway includes parasympathetic and sympathetic pathways. Efferent pupillary defects may be associated with either damage to the parasympathetic or sympathetic nerves.

■ Parasympathetic Pathway

The fibers start in the EW nucleus in the midbrain and consist of two neurons:
- EW nucleus to ciliary ganglion via oculomotor (III) nerve.
- Ciliary ganglion to sphincter pupillae via short ciliary nerves.

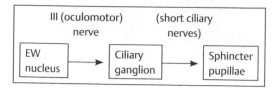

The ciliary ganglion is located within the muscle cone just behind the globe. Although it receives other nerve fiber also, only parasympathetic fibers synapse in the ganglion.

■ Sympathetic Pathway

The sympathetic pathway starts from the posterior hypothalamus (**sympathetic center**). It sends an inhibitory pathway to the EW nucleus and also has connections with the cerebral cortex. It consists of three neurons:
- The **first neuron** (central) starts in the posterior hypothalamus. It descends downward through medulla oblongata to terminate in ciliospinal centre of Budge (C8–T2), which is located in the intermediolateral horn of the spinal cord.
- The **second neuron** (preganglionic) from the ciliospinal center leaves the cord via anterior (ventral) root of C8, T1, T2 to the paravertebral sympathetic chain and terminates in the superior cervical ganglion. During its course, *it is closely related to apical pleura*. These preganglionic fibers may be damaged by bronchogenic carcinoma (pan coast tumour) or during surgery on the neck.
- The **third neuron** (postganglionic) ascends along the internal carotid artery and enters the cavernous sinus. In the cavernous sinus, it joins the ophthalmic division of the trigeminal nerve V1. The sympathetic fibers follow the nasociliary nerve, which they finally leave to enter the long ciliary nerves. The long ciliary nerves run in suprachoroidal space to reach the ciliary

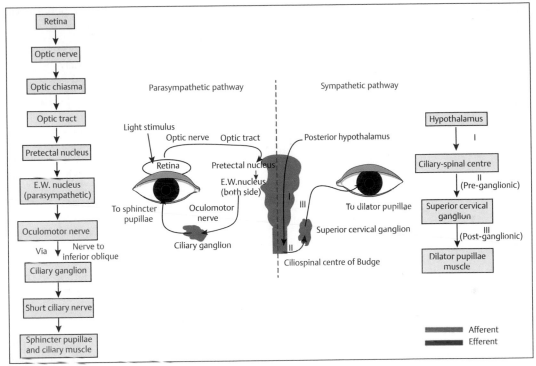

Fig. 9.1 Efferent pathways of pupil.

■ Pupillary Reflexes

Reflexes associated with change in size of pupil are called pupillary reflexes. Three pupillary reflexes are of clinical importance:

- Light reflex.
- Near reflex.
- Psycho sensory reflex.

■ Light Reflex

On flashing the light into the eye, constriction of both pupils takes place (light reflex). There are two types of light reflexes: direct and consensual light reflexes (**Fig. 9.2**).

Direct Light Reflex

When light is thrown into one eye, pupil of that eye constricts. It is known as direct light reflex.

Consensual Light Reflex

When light is thrown into one eye, constriction of pupil occurs in other eye (even though no light falls on that eye). This phenomenon is known as indirect or consensual light reflex. In normal subjects, the direct and consensual reactions are almost, always identical in time, course, and magnitude.

■ Near Reflex

It is synkinesis rather than a true reflex and activated when gaze is changed from distant to a near object. The **near reflex triad** consists of:

- Pupillary constriction to sharpen the image on the retina (miosis).
- Convergence of the optic axis.
- Increased convexity of the lens to increase its refractive power (accommodation).

Stimulus for near reflex: It is the blurring of retinal images when the object is near.

body and the dilator pupillae muscle (**Fig. 9.1**).

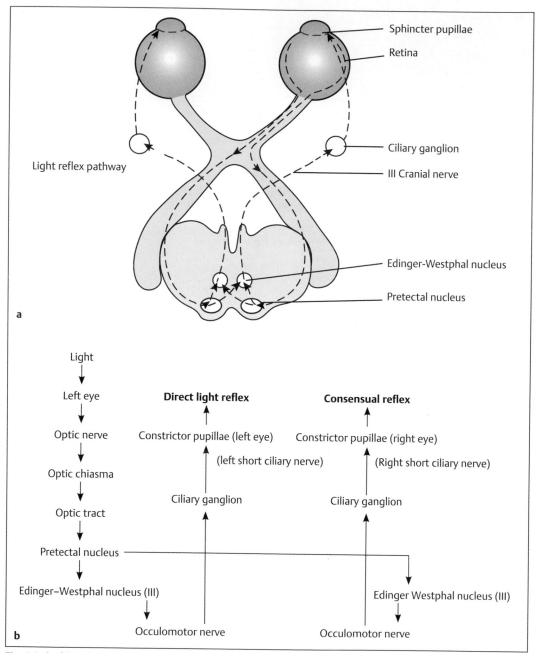

Fig. 9.2 (a, b) Pathway for light reflex.

Afferent Pathway

The accommodation (near) reflex requires the image analysis. Thus, the cerebral cortex must be involved. There are probably two supranuclear influences: the frontal (frontal eye field) and occipital lobes (striate and parastriate areas). Afferent fibers extend retina to parastriate area via visual pathway. Pathway for light reflex dissociates in pretectal area and visual cortex is not required for the light reflex pathway.

Centre for Near Reflex

The centre for near reflex is ill-defined and the fibers do not pass through the pretectal nucleus situated in the midbrain. The midbrain center for the near reflex is probably located more ventrally than the pretectal nucleus.

Efferent Pathway

The final pathways for near and light reflexes are identical.

There is no clinical condition in which the light reflex is present but the near reflex is absent. The compressive lesions such as pinealomas preferentially involve the dorsal internuncial neurons involved in the light reflex, sparing the ventral (near reflex) fibers until late. Therefore, damage to internuncial neurons is responsible for **light-near dissociation** in neurosyphilis and pinealomas.

■ Psycho Sensory Reflex

It refers to dilatation of pupil in response to psychic and sensory stimuli. These are not seen in the newborn but develop fully by the age of 6 months.

Mechanism

It is believed that the mechanism of psychosensory reflexes is a cortical one and pupillary dilatation results from two components:

- Sympathetic discharge to the dilator pupillae.
- Inhibition of parasympathetic discharge to the sphincter pupillae (**Flowchart 9.1**).

Rapid dilatation of pupil is followed by a quick second dilatation due to inhibition of constrictor tone.

■ Examination of the Pupils

Pupils are observed regarding the shape, size, color, and reaction. They react equally to the light.

■ Size of the Pupil

Pupil size is determined by the interaction of the parasympathetic and sympathetic nervous systems which constrict or dilate the pupil. These are controlled by central nervous system inputs that are influenced by light or viewing distance, etc. The pupil constricts in response to light (direct light reflex) and, to a lesser extent, to near accommodation. The other pupil constricts consensually.

When pupillary function is normal, pupils are isocoric (equal-sized). Anisocoria refers to unequal pupils. The variation between size of the pupils of both the eyes should be no more than 1mm. It is necessary to ascertain first which pupil is behaving abnormally.

■ Reaction of Pupil

Three pupillary reflexes should be tested: **light reflex, swinging flashlight test, and near reflex.**

Light Reflex

This assesses the integrity of the pupillary light reflex pathway. Dim the ambient light and ask the patient to fixate a distant target. Illuminate the right eye from the right side and the left from the left side. Note whether there is a direct pupillary response (the pupil constricts when the light is shone on to it) and a consensual response (the other pupil also constricts).

A normal result is a brisk, simultaneous, equal response of both pupils in response to light shone into one or the other eye.

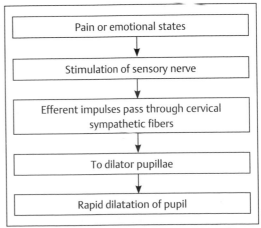

Flowchart 9.1 Mechanism of psychosensory reflex.

Swinging Flashlight Test

It relies on a comparison between the two eyes, and is looking for (and can only detect) an asymmetrical abnormality in the afferent pathway. It compares the difference in the afferent conduction between two eyes, which is called a **relative afferent pupillary defect** (**RAPD**).

Ambient light should be dimmed and check the light reflex in each eye. Move the beam swiftly and rhythmically from eye to eye and note the pupillary constriction of both eyes. When the beam is swung from eye to eye, the bilateral pupil constriction should not change.

If afferent signal from one eye is weaker and light is shone onto this eye, both pupils appear to dilate, that is, direct reaction in weaker eye and consensual reaction in other eye is reduced (RAPD is present). The abnormal response is also known as the **Marcus Gunn pupil**.

RAPD is a useful test in order to determine if visual loss is due to optic nerve defect or a cataract:

- In optic nerve defect, RAPD will be present.
- In cataract, RAPD will not be present.

Near Reflex Test

This assesses the pupillary component of accommodation. In a normally lit room, instruct the patient to look at a distant target. Bring an object (e.g., a finger) to their near point (about an arm's length away) and observe the pupillary reflex when their fixation shifts to the near target. A normal test shows a brisk constriction of pupil.

In near-light dissociation, the patient has a better near reflex than light reflex.

10 The Lens

Anatomy of Lens 219
Physiology of Lens 222
Lens Changes with Age 225
Lens Abnormalities 225
Developmental Cataract 230
Acquired Cataract 235
Management of Cataract 244
Aphakia 249
Intraocular Lenses 252

■ Anatomy of Lens (OP7.1)

The adult human lens is located behind the iris and pupil in the anterior compartment of the eye. The lens is held in place by zonules (suspensory ligaments) which run between the lens and ciliary body. The lens continues to grow throughout life. It is a unique characteristic not shared with any other internal organ.

■ Shape

The lens is biconvex, with the anterior surface being less convex than the posterior surface (**Fig. 10.1**).

■ Radius of Curvature

The radius of curvature of anterior surface is 10 mm, while that of posterior surface is 6 mm.

The poles represent the center points of these two surfaces. The anterior pole is the center of anterior surface and posterior pole is the center of posterior surface of lens. The anteroposterior axis runs from the anterior pole to the posterior pole (polar axis). The anterior and posterior surface meet at the equator which is the circumference of lens. The equatorial axis is at right angle to the anteroposterior axis.

■ Dimensions

Diameter of lens: 8.8 to 9.2 mm.

Thickness (distance from anterior to posterior pole) of lens is 3.5 mm at birth, which reaches up to 5 mm.

■ Refractive Index (RI)

RI of lens = **1.39.**

RI of nucleus (1.41) > RI of cortex (1.386).

RI of anterior capsule > RI of posterior surface.

The change in RI from surface of lens (cortex) to the center (Nucleus) results from changes in the protein content which is highest in the nucleus. Higher the concentration, the greater is the refractive power.

■ Power of Lens

It is approximately **18D**. Refractive power of cornea ($\approx$ 43D) is greater than that of lens ($\approx$ 18D).

■ Transparency

During early stage of embryonic development, lens is opaque, but as development continues and hyaloid vascular supply is lost, lens becomes

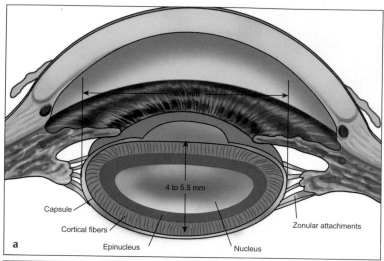

Capsule

Cortical fibers

a Epinucleus

Nucleus

Zonular attachments

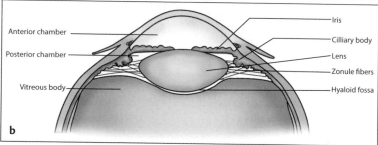

Anterior chamber

Posterior chamber

Vitreous body

b

Iris

Cilliary body

Lens

Zonule fibers

Hyaloid fossa

Fig. 10.1 (a) Surgical anatomy of lens. Source: Divide-and-Conquer Technique and Complications. In: Fishkind W, ed. Phacoemulsification and Intraocular Lens Implantation: Mastering Techniques and Complications in Cataract Surgery. 2nd Edition. Thieme; 2017. doi:10.1055/b-004-140243. **(b)** Shape of the lens and its position in the eye. Source: Basic Knowledge. In: Lang G, ed. Ophthalmology. A Pocket Textbook Atlas. 3rd Edition. Thieme; 2015.

transparent. The lens of the eye has a avascular structure. There are no nerves in the lens.

■ Functions

Lens serves the following functions:

- It transmits and refracts the light. Lens absorbs ultraviolet (UV) light of <350 nm wavelength. Thus, prevents damaging UV radiation from reaching the retina.
- It contributes 35% of refractive power of the eye.
- It helps in accommodation: During accommodation, radius of curvature of anterior capsule decreases while that of posterior capsules remains unaltered. Therefore, the front of lens moves forward during accommodation and depth of anterior chamber decreases.

■ Structure

Histologically, the lens consists of three components: capsule, epithelium, and lens fibers (**Fig. 10.2**).

- **Lens capsule:** Lens capsule is elastic, acellular, and transparent. It is made up of collagen-like material and is digested by collagenase. It is secreted by lens epithelium, so the most superficial part of lens capsule is the oldest. Its *thickest region* is close to the equator on both the anterior and posterior surfaces, while its *thinnest region* is at the posterior pole. The equator and anterior pole are of *intermediate thickness* (**Fig. 10.3**).
- **Lens epithelium:** It is a single layer of *cuboidal cells* beneath the anterior capsule and not present posteriorly, as posterior

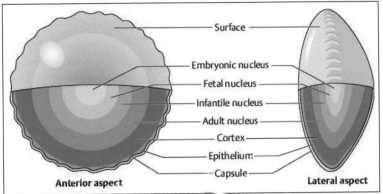

Fig. 10.2 Structure of adult human lens. Source: Lang G, ed. Ophthalmology. A Pocket Textbook Atlas. 3rd Edition. Thieme; 2015.

Surface
Embryonic nucleus
Fetal nucleus
Infantile nucleus
Adult nucleus
Cortex
Epithelium
Capsule
Anterior aspect
Lateral aspect

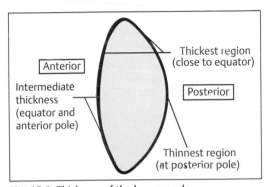

Anterior
Thickest region (close to equator)
Intermediate thickness (equator and anterior pole)
Posterior
Thinnest region (at posterior pole)

Fig. 10.3 Thickness of the lens capsule.

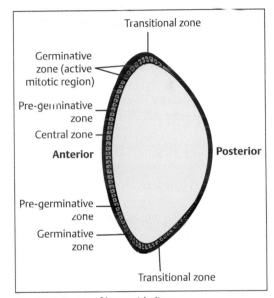

Transitional zone
Germinative zone (active mitotic region)
Pre-germinative zone
Central zone
Anterior
Posterior
Pre-germinative zone
Germinative zone
Transitional zone

Fig. 10.4 Zones of lens epithelium.

epithelial cells elongate to form primary lens fibers. Cells have nuclei and organelles. Lens epithelium is the area of lens with highest metabolic rate and secretes *lens capsule.* Epithelium contains Na^+K^+ ATPase and generates ATP to meet the energy demand of the lens. Lens epithelium regulates transport of metabolites, nutrients, and electrolytes to lens fibers. **Proliferative capacity** of epithelial cells varies according to their location (**Fig. 10.4**):

◊ *Cells in central zone* do not proliferate.
◊ *Cells in pre-germinative zone* rarely divide.
◊ *Cells in germinative zone* (preequatorial area) divide actively and give rise to lens fibers.

• **Lens fibers (lens substance):** Lens fibers are composed of soluble proteins called **crystallins,** which are of the following three types: α-crystallin, β-crystallin and

γ-crystallin. These develop from epithelial cells in the preequatorial germinative zone. These cells divide and get elongated to form lens fibers which lose cell organelles and nuclei (important for transparency of lens). As new fibers are formed, older ones are pushed toward the deeper plane (nucleus of lens), so the youngest lens fibers are most superficial. Thus, *lens substance consists of two parts*: The central part contains the oldest fibers and is called **nucleus,** and the peripheral part consists of the youngest fibers and is called **cortex.** The cortex is composed of all secondary fibers continuously formed after sexual maturation. Nucleus consists of densely compact lens fibers and has a higher RI than cortex. Nucleus can be further divided, according to the period of development, into embryonic, fetal, infantile and adult nucleus. **Embryonic nucleus** contains original primary lens fibers formed in the lens vesicles. Rests are secondary fibers which are added concentrically at different stages of growth by encircling previously formed nucleus. **Fetal nucleus** corresponds to the nucleus at birth, that is, it contains embryonic nucleus and all fibers added to the lens before birth. **Infantile nucleus** contains all fibers added until 4 years of age, that is, embryonic nucleus + fetal nucleus + all fibers added until 4 years of age. The **adult nucleus** is composed of all fibers added before sexual maturation (**Fig. 10.5**).

■ Formation of Sutures

The ends of each lens fiber run toward the poles of both capsular surfaces. Overlapping of the ends of each secondary fibers result in the formation of sutures at both the anterior and posterior poles.

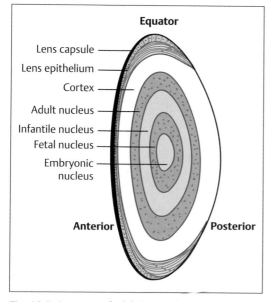

Fig. 10.5 Structure of adult human lens.

No sutures are found between primary fibers in the embryonic nucleus.

Secondary fibers formed *before birth* have anterior suture—"Y-shaped" (erect Y) and posterior suture—"λ-shaped" (inverted Y).

■ Zonules (Suspensory Ligaments of Lens)

Zonules stretch from ciliary body to anterior and posterior lens capsule at the lens equator in a continuous fashion.

The zonules attach to the lens capsule 2 mm anterior and 1 mm posterior to the equator. The anterior fibers arise from anterior ciliary processes and insert posterior to the equator. The middle fibers from ciliary processes insert at the equator, while the posterior fibers arise from pars plana region of ciliary epithelium and insert into lens capsule anterior to the lens equator.

Chemically, they are made of collagen-like glycoprotein and acidic mucopolysaccharide (chondroitin sulfate). Zonules are broken by α–*chymotrypsin*, a proteolytic enzyme. Zonules contain 7% cysteine (amino acid). In **homocystinuria,** *enzyme cystathionine synthetase is absent.* Therefore, amino acid homocysteine is not converted into cysteine, resulting in broken zonules and dislocated lens. Excessive homocysteine is also present in the urine.

■ Physiology of Lens

■ Composition of Lens

The lens is composed of the following:
- Water 66%.
- Proteins 33%: Protein content of the lens is highest amongst body organs/tissues. These comprise:
  ◇ *Soluble proteins* (crystallins): α, β, and γ–crystallins are mostly found in the lens cortex.
  ◇ *Insoluble proteins* (albuminoids) constitute the membranes of lens fibers and are mostly found in the lens nucleus.
- Lipids, carbohydrates, and electrolytes 1%.

■ Transport of Ions

Lens capsule is freely permeable to water, ions, and small molecules.

Lens epithelium is metabolically active and contains Na^+K^+ ATPase and calmodulin regulated Ca^{++}– ATPase for active transport of electrolytes between lens and aqueous.

The Na^+ and K^+ move asymmetrically across the lens. Na^+ and K^+ diffuse through both the anterior and the posterior poles of the lens, down their concentration gradient, and are pumped out/in by Na^+K^+ ATPase in the epithelial layer. The Na^+ removed are exchanged actively for K^+. *There is a net movement of Na^+ ions from posterior to anterior and of K^+ ions from anterior to posterior.*

Ca^{++} level in aqueous and vitreous is higher than that of lens, which plays an important role in the control of membrane permeability to both Na^+ and K^+ ions. Ca^{++} enters the cell down its electrochemical gradient but low-intracellular concentration of Ca^{++} is maintained by calmodulin-regulated Ca^{++}-ATPase which actively pumps Cu^{++} out of the cell.

■ Transport of Amino Acids

Amino acid content of lens is higher than that of surrounding ocular fluids (aqueous and vitreous). Amino acids enter the lens against the concentration gradient through active transport localized to the epithelial layer beneath the anterior capsule and passively "**leak**" out through the posterior capsule.

After involution of hyaloid blood supply to lens, the metabolic needs of lens are met by the aqueous and vitreous humors (**Fig. 10.6**).

■ Lens Metabolism (OP7.1)

Lens, like tissues, require energy to drive various reactions. The fact that aqueous in aphakic eyes contain more glucose than in normal (phakic) eye confirms that glucose is the essential source of energy in the lens. Lens has a respiratory quotient (CO_2/O_2) of 1.0.

Glucose Metabolism

Glucose metabolism occurs through the four mechanisms (**Flowchart 10.1**), namely, glycolysis, pentose phosphate pathway, Kreb's cycle (TCA cycle) and sorbitol pathway. Approximately, 90 to 95% of glucose that enters the normal lens is phosphorylated into glucose-6-phosphate by hexokinase enzyme. Glucose-6-phosphate is used either in the glycolytic pathway (80%) or pentose phosphate pathway (10%).

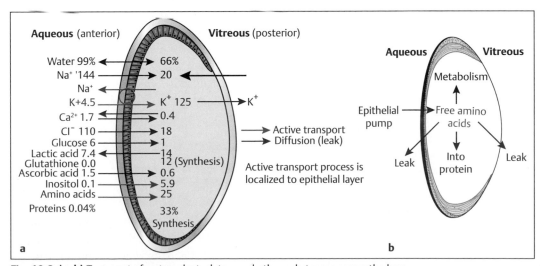

Fig. 10.6 (a, b) Transport of water, electrolytes, and other substances across the lens.

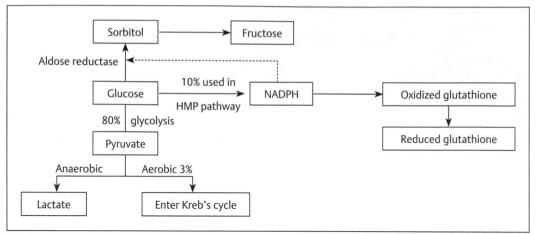

Flowchart 10.1 Pathways of glucose metabolism in lens. Abrreviation: HMP, hexose monophosphate.

Glycolysis: 80% of total glucose is metabolized by anaerobic *glycolysis*, that is, metabolism of lens is anaerobic. Bulk of pyruvate produced by glycolysis is reduced to lactate by lactate dehydrogenase which diffuses into aqueous. So, lactic acid is found in considerable amount in the aqueous of phakic (and not so in aphakic) eyes.

Pentose phosphate pathway or hexose mono phosphate shunt (**HMP shunt**): 10% of total glucose is metabolized in HMP shunt. It does not produce ATP. The primary function of HMP shunt is to produce NADPH (reduced NADP) which maintains lens glutathione in the reduced state and also used in the conversion of glucose to sorbitol. HMP shunt also produces pentose sugars needed for synthesis of nucleic acids. End products of this pathway are converted into glyceraldehydes PO_4 which enters the glycolytic pathway.

Kreb's cycle or tricarboxylic acid cycle (**TCA cycle**): Due to avascularity and low-oxygen content of lens, 70% of lens ATP are produced by anaerobic glycolysis, a relatively insufficient mechanism for the production of ATP. Approximately, 3% of glucose is metabolized aerobically by Kreb's cycle which generates approximately 25% of lens ATP. It occurs more prominently in the lens epithelium.

Sorbitol pathway: Activity of this pathway increases if glucose levels are increased above normal as in diabetes and galactosemia.

Protein Metabolism

Because the lens grows throughout life, protein synthesis also must occur throughout life. It predominantly involves production of crystallins.

Glutathione

It is a polypeptide synthesized in the lens made of three amino acids: glycine, cysteine and glutamic acid. Most of lens glutathione is in the reduced state. Reduced glutathione retains integrity of the lens transport pump (as thiol groups [-SH] are needed for the enzyme *Na⁺ K⁺ ATPase*) and also maintains lens proteins in reduced state. The reduced lens protein prevents formation of high-molecular weight (HMW) crystalline aggregates and, thus, helps to maintain lens transparency.

Antioxidant Mechanisms

Because lens is susceptible to oxidative damage, so lens has a complex antioxidant system which protects against reactive oxygen species (superoxide anion, singlet oxygen, Hydrogen peroxide H_2O_2) produced during photochemical reactions in the lens. Glutathione is synthesized in lens and protects it from oxidative damage. Ascorbic acid (vitamin C) appears to play a major role in the antioxidant system in the lens.

■ Lens Changes with Age

Lens exhibits age-related changes in structure, light transmission, metabolic capacity and enzyme activity. Characteristic changes in lens with age include the following:

- Diameter increases with increasing age.
- Thickness increases with increasing age. Thickness of nucleus decrease with age as a result of compaction, while that of cortex increases as more fibers are added at the periphery. Radius of curvature of anterior surface decreases with increasing age but that of posterior surface remains almost constant.
- Sutures at birth become complex with increasing age.
- Weight of lens increase with increasing age.
- Elasticity of lens decreases with age, leading to decreased accommodation. It results in presbyopia.
- Light transmission decreases with age partly through increased brunescence of the lens.
- Metabolic activity of lens decreases with age.
- Reduction in antioxidant system with age: Lens is more prone to oxidative damage with increasing age.
- Changes in crystallins:
  ◇ Aggregation of lens proteins.
  ◇ Degradation.
  ◇ Increased insolubility.
  ◇ Appearance of lens opacities.

■ Lens Abnormalities

Lens abnormalities may be one of the following:
- Abnormalities in shape and size of the lens:
  ◇ Coloboma of lens.
  ◇ Microspherophakia.
  ◇ Lenticonus and lentiglobus.
- Abnormalities in position of the lens:
  ◇ Subluxation of lens.
  ◇ Dislocation of lens.
- Abnormalities in the lens transparency:
  ◇ Cataract.

■ Abnormal Shape or Size of Lens

These are largely developmental.

Coloboma of Lens

It is characterized by segmental agenesis (notching), usually at the inferior margin, and is due to localized absence of zonules (suspensory ligament of lens). It is usually unilateral and may be associated with coloboma of iris, ciliary body and choroid. It is not a true coloboma as there is no focal absence of a tissue layer due to the failure of closure of the optic fissure.

Microspherophakia

It is a bilateral condition. It is a developmental anomaly with defect in the development of lens zonules (**Flowchart 10.2**). It may occur as an isolated familial defect or may be associated with Marfan's syndrome or Weil–Marchesani syndrome.

Lenticonus and Lentiglobus

These are abnormalities of central lens curvature which are associated with thinning of lens capsule.

Thinning of lens capsule results in protrusion of lens surface. If *protrusion is conical, the* condition is called lenticonus (**Fig. 10.7**) which may be anterior or posterior. If *protrusion is spherical, the* condition is called lentiglobus.

Both lenticonus and lentiglobus may *cause lenticular myopia with irregular astigmatism.*

> *Internal lenticonus*: Surface of capsule has a normal contour but the nucleus within forms a cone. It is very rare.

■ Abnormal Position of Lens

Ectopia lentis refers to the displacement of lens from its normal position. Displacement of lens may be **partial,** termed as subluxation of lens, or

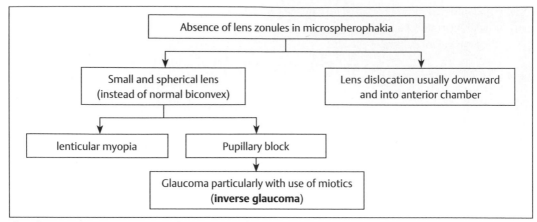

Flowchart 10.2 Etiopathogenesis of microspherophakia.

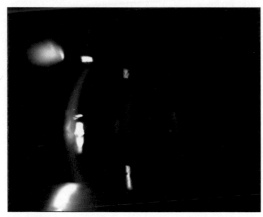

Fig. 10.7 Lenticonus.

complete, termed as dislocation of lens (luxation). When zonules are torn in one segment, the lens is displaced to the opposite segment of torn zonules but still remains in the pupillary area (Subluxation of lens). When all fibers of zonules are torn, the lens is displaced anteriorly or posteriorly (luxation or dislocation of lens). The basic defect involves the breakage or weakening of zonules. The following are the causes of abnormal position of lens:

- **Familial**: It may be associated with iris coloboma, microspherophakia, or aniridia.
- Systemic conditions (due to deficient development of zonules) such as:
  ◇ Marfan's syndrome.
  ◇ Weil–Marchesani syndrome.
  ◇ Homocystinuria.
  ◇ Ehlers–Danlos syndrome.
- Trauma
- Eye diseases (secondary to weakening of zonules) such as:
  ◇ Uveitis.
  ◇ Hypermature cataract.
  ◇ Pseudoexfoliation syndrome.
  ◇ Ciliary body tumors.
    – Displacement of lens may be (**Fig. 10.8**).
- Upward in:
  ◇ Marfan's syndrome.
- Downward in:
  ◇ Weil–Marchesani syndrome.
  ◇ Homocystinuria.
- Anterior in anterior chamber or incarceration in pupil.
- Posterior in vitreous.

Clinical Features

Subluxation of lens presents with poor vision and uniocular diplopia (**Flowchart 10.3**).

Clinical signs depicted in case of subluxation of lens are:
- Irregular depth of anterior chamber.
- Tremulousness of iris (iridodonesis)
- Tremulousness of lens (phacodonesis)

which are accentuated by eye movements.

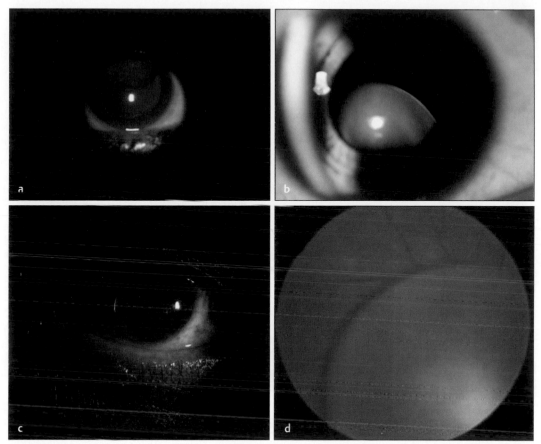

Fig. 10.8 Dislocation of lens. **(a)** In Marfan's syndrome (upward). **(b)** In Weil-Marchesani syndrome (downward). Source: Features. In: Ehlers J, ed. The Retina Illustrated. 1st Edition. Thieme; 2019. **(c)** Anterior dislocation of lens. **(d)** Posterior dislocation (into vitreous).

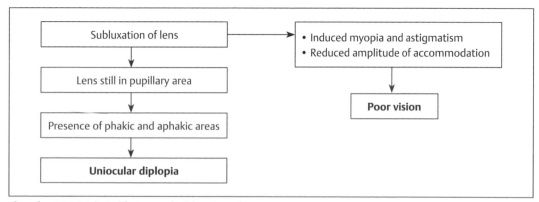

Flowchart 10.3 Clinical features of subluxation of lens.

- Edge of subluxated lens in pupillary area appears as a black crescent on ophthalmoscopy. A clear dislocated lens in the anterior chamber appears like a drop of oil in aqueous.

Complications

Complications include secondary glaucoma (**Flowchart 10.4**) in case of anterior dislocation of lens and lens-induced uveitis due to irritation of ciliary body caused by posterior dislocation of lens.

Treatment

In **subluxated lens**:
- If lens is clear, spectacle correction is done. Aphakic correction gives better visual acuity than phakic.
- If excessive lenticular astigmatism results in poor vision, removal of lens is done.
- If lens is cataractous, removal of lens by pars plana lensectomy or cataract extraction with capsule tension ring (CTR) with IOL implantation is performed.

In **dislocated lens**:
- In anterior dislocation with secondary glaucoma, lens removal after controlling intraocular pressure (IOP) is done.
- In posterior dislocation: If uveitis is present with posterior dislocation, removal of lens via pars plana followed by anterior chamber IOL or scleral fixated IOL is implanted. If there is no uveitis, no treatment is required.

■ Abnormal Lens Transparency: Cataract

The crystalline lens is a transparent structure. Any opacity in the lens that causes it to lose its transparency and/or scatter light is called a **cataract**. A cataract does not necessarily have any demonstrable effect on vision. A cataract may be either developmental cataract or acquired cataract.

Transparency of lens is maintained by multiple factors:
- Avascularity of lens.
- Regular arrangement of lens fibers.
- Dense packing of crystallins.
- Absence of cell organelles and nuclei from lens fibers.
- Reduced glutathione synthesized in lens and vitamin E present in lens membrane, which act as antioxidants and protect lens against oxidative damage.

Many factors that are evident in the process of cataract formation are:
- Alterations in cation permeability: Increase in Na^+ content and decrease in K^+ content of lens correlates with increase in the optical density of lens.

Increase in intralenticular CA^{2+} levels causes increased activity of proteolytic enzymes, which break down the proteins into amino acids. This may cause the lens contents to liquefy.
- Biochemical changes: Alterations in many of the biochemical processes that take place within normal lens can lead into a cataractous lens such as:

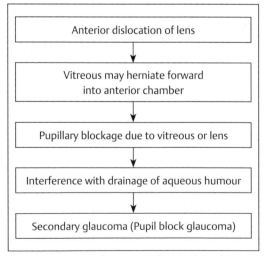

Flowchart 10.4 Pathogenesis of secondary glaucoma as a complication of anterior dislocation of lens.

Changes in protein:
- Soluble protein content decreases.
- Insoluble protein content increases.
- Accumulation of HMW aggregates.

Hydration: It may be due to osmotic changes within lens or changes in semipermeability of capsule, as in diabetes, galactosemia, and trauma. Droplets of fluid gather under capsule. Lacunae between fibers are formed, and entire tissue swells (**intumescence**) and becomes opaque.

Changes in glutathione: Glutathione is found at higher concentration in the lens epithelium. It exists in both oxidized and reduced form. A major percentage (95%) of lens glutathione is found in reduced form. Glutathione is synthesized from L-glutamate, L-cysteine and glycine. Glutathione reductase, an enzyme that uses NADPH, converts oxidized glutathione into reduced glutathione. Glutathione plays following important roles in the lens:
- It maintains protein thiols in the reduced state which maintain lens transparency by preventing the formation of HMW crystallin aggregates.
- It protects against oxidative damage.
- It protects the thiol groups involved in cation transport and permeability (oxidation of thiol group of Na^+K^+ ATPase pump results in increased permeability of these ions).
- It detoxifies hydrogen peroxide which is normally present in the aqueous humor and is a reactive oxygen species. The glutathione peroxidase (found in both epithelial cells and fibers) provide protection against H_2O_2 by detoxifying it.

Reduced activity of glutathione synthetase and depletion of glutathione reductase causes fall in reduced glutathione, which is an antioxidant, and lens is susceptible to oxidative damage.

Antioxidants vitamins such as vitamins C, E, and β-carotene may be important in the prevention of cataract.

- *Fibrous metaplasia of fibers* may occur in complicated cataract.
- *Opacification of lens epithelium in* trauma or chemical injury.

Etiology (OP7.2)

Following are the common etiological factors for the formation of cataract:
- Age-related (senile).
- Trauma:
  ◇ Concussion injury.
  ◇ Penetrating injury.
  ◇ Electric shock.
- Radiation:
  ◇ Ionizing radiations.
  ◇ Nonionizing (infrared) radiations.
  ◇ UV radiations.
- Metabolic disorders:
  ◇ Diabetes mellitus.
  ◇ Galactosemia.
  ◇ Hypoparathyroidism.
  ◇ Lowe's syndrome.
  ◇ Fabry's disease.
  ◇ Wilson's disease.
- Dermatological disorders:
  ◇ Atopic dermatitis.
  ◇ Rothmund syndrome.
  ◇ Ichthyosis.
  ◇ Werner's syndrome.
- Local ocular diseases (complicated cataract):
  ◇ Uveitis.
  ◇ Retinitis pigmentosa.
  ◇ Degenerative myopia.
  ◇ Glaucoma.
  ◇ Retinal detachment.
  ◇ Tumors.
- Toxic causes:
  ◇ Corticosteroids.
  ◇ Miotic drugs.
  ◇ Chloroquine.
  ◇ Phenothiazines.
  ◇ Chemicals.
  ◇ Copper.

◇ Iron.

◇ Gold.

• Systemic disorders:

◇ Dystrophia myotonica.

◇ Down's syndrome.

◇ Alport's syndrome.

• Developmental (congenital).

Classification

Cataract may be classified as follows:

• Developmental: Different types of developmental cataract are as follows:

◇ Nuclear cataract.

◇ Lamellar (zonular) cataract.

◇ Sutural (stellate).

◇ Coralliform cataract.

◇ Floriform cataract.

◇ Coronary cataract.

◇ Blue-dot cataract.

◇ Anterior polar cataract.

◇ Posterior polar cataract.

◇ Membranous cataract.

◇ Central "oil droplet" opacities.

• Acquired—It may be:

◇ Senile.

◇ Metabolic.

• Secondary due to:

◇ Local ocular diseases (complicated cataract).

◇ Trauma.

◇ Radiations.

◇ Systemic diseases.

◇ Skin diseases.

◇ Drugs and chemicals (toxic).

■ Developmental Cataract

The new lens fibers are continuously laid down under the capsule throughout life. The fibers formed earlier lie deeper within the lens substance and the newer ones occupy a more superficial plane. Thus, the central nucleus of lens consists of the oldest fibers and the cortex comprises the youngest ones (**Fig. 10.5**).

The nucleus is subdivided into:

• Embryonic nucleus: It contains the original primary lens fibers formed in the lens vesicle.

• Fetal nucleus.

• Infantile nucleus.

• Adult nucleus.

The fetal, infantile, and adult nucleus are composed of secondary fibers added concentrically at the different stages of growth.

Developmental cataract may be present at birth (congenital, **Fig. 10.9**), and is limited to embryonic or fetal nucleus, or may develop after birth; therefore, it may involve infantile or adult nucleus and deeper cortex. It has a tendency to affect particular fibers, depending upon the time of disturbance in normal development of lens. Thus, the location of developmental cataract may indicate the stage of development at which disturbance occurred. The fibers laid down previously and subsequently are often normally formed and remain clear. *Most development opacities are partial and stationary.*

■ Causes (OP7.2)

• Hereditary:

◇ The most common cause is genetic mutation and is usually autosomal dominant.

◇ Deficient oxygenation due to placental hemorrhage.

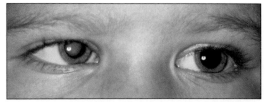

Fig. 10.9 Congenital cataract. Source: Special Considerations in Cataract Surgery in Children. In: Lang G, ed. Ophthalmology. A Pocket Textbook Atlas. 3rd Edition. Thieme; 2015.

- Metabolic disorders of fetus:
  ◇ Galactosemia.
  ◇ Lowe's syndrome.
  ◇ Hypocalcemia.
- Chromosomal abnormalities:
  ◇ Down's syndrome.
- Intrauterine infections such as:
  ◇ Rubella.
  ◇ Cytomegalovirus.
  ◇ Toxoplasmosis.
- Toxic: Maternal drug ingestion during pregnancy, for example, corticosteroids and thalidomide.
- Birth trauma.
- Nutritional deficiency.

■ Morphological Types

Nuclear Cataract

It may exist in nonprogressive and progressive forms:

Nonprogressive form: It is confined to embryonic or fetal nucleus and dominantly inherited. It is a nonprogressive biconvex or spheroid-shaped opacity and consists of fine, white, powdery (pulverulent) dots (**cataracta centralis pulverulenta**).

Progressive form: The progressive form of nuclear cataract is associated with Rubella (German measles) infection in the mother during the second month of pregnancy. Risk to fetus is closely related to the stage of gestation at the time of maternal infection. *After the gestational age of 6 weeks, the virus is incapable of crossing the lens capsule, so that lens is immune.* The lens nucleus is found to be necrotic and a total opacification of lens may occur. *Virus is capable of persisting within the lens for up to 3 years after birth. Unless all the lens matter is removed, aspiration of cataract may be followed by a chronic inflammatory endophthalmitis associated with the presence of residual lens matter.*

Classical manifestations of rubella infection (**Rubella triad**)
- Congenital heart defects: Patent ductus arteriosus.
- Cataract.
- Deafness.

Other malformations in Rubella infection include microcephaly, mental retardation. *Besides cataractous lens*, other ocular features in rubella infections include:
- *Pigmentary retinopathy* represents involvement of cells of RPE (retinal pigment epithelium). Retina has a "**salt and pepper**" appearance.
- Microphthalmos.

Lamellar (Zonular) Cataract

It accounts for nearly 50% of all developmental cataracts.

Etiology (OP7.2)

It is usually dominantly inherited but may have a metabolic or inflammatory cause. Deficiency of vitamin D is apparently a potent factor. Hypoparathyroidism during pregnancy and disturbances of CA++ metabolism may cause a zonular cataract.

Clinical Features

- It is generally, bilateral and symmetrical.
- Occurs usually in the area of fetal nucleus surrounding the clear embryonic nucleus.

Opacity is sharply demarcated and has disc-shaped opacity when viewed from the front (**Fig. 10.10**).

- Lens area within and around the opacity is clear, although linear opacities resembling spokes of a wheel (**called riders**) may run outward toward the equator. Visual impairment is frequently present. With time, opacity is pushed deeper, as normal lens fibers are laid down around it and diameter of opacity decreases with time as nucleus becomes compressed.

Sutural (Stellate) Cataract

It affects one or both fetal sutures, so opacities are Y-shaped. It is almost always bilateral.

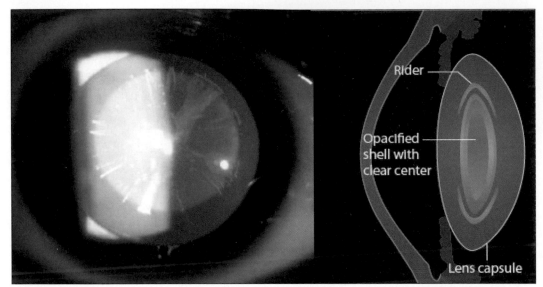

Fig. 10.10 Lamellar cataract. Source: Hereditary Congenital Cataracts. In: Lang G, ed. Ophthalmology. A Pocket Textbook Atlas. 3rd Edition. Thieme; 2015.

It has autosomal dominant inheritance. The opacity consists of bluish dot or a dense chalky band around the sutures and may interfere with vision (**Fig. 10.11**).

Coralliform Cataract

It is also known as fusiform, spindle-shaped or **axial** cataract. It is usually dominantly inherited. It consists of anteroposterior spindle-shaped opacity occurring axially with off shoots and resembling a coral.

Floriform Cataract

It is a bluish-white cataract in the axial region and appears like a flower.

Coronary Cataract

It occurs around puberty and therefore involve deeper layers of cortex and superficial layers of adolescent nucleus. It appears as corona of club-shaped opacities in the periphery of lens, encircling the central axis, and surrounds the nucleus like a crown (**Fig. 10.12**). Axial region and extreme periphery of lens remain clear, so

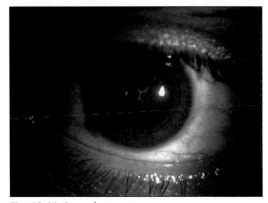

Fig. 10.11 Sutural cataract.

vision is usually unaffected. They are hidden by iris and seen when pupil is dilated. Opacities are nonprogressive.

Blue-dot Cataract (Cataracta Punctata Caerulea)

It consists of punctate opacities appearing as tiny blue dots scattered all over the lens.

It is usually bilateral, nonprogressive and have little effect on vision (**Fig. 10.13**).

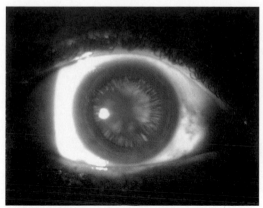

Fig. 10.12 Coronary cataract.

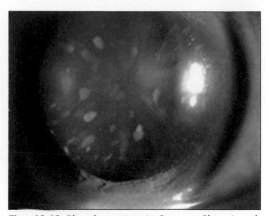

Fig. 10.13 Blue-dot cataract. Source: Glass L, ed. Opthalmology Q&A Board Review. 1st Edition. 2019.

Anterior Polar Cataract (Anterior Capsular Cataract)

The opacities may be caused by imperfect separation of lens from surface ectoderm or incomplete reabsorption of vascular tunic of lens. Most commonly it is acquired and follows the perforation of central corneal ulcer, wherein lens capsule comes in contact with cornea. It *involves the central part of anterior capsule, affecting the vision.*

The opacity may have a conical projection into the anterior chamber like a pyramid (anterior pyramidal cataract).

Sometimes along with the anterior polar cataract, the underlying lens fibers also become opaque, forming anterior cortical cataract. Subsequently, clear lens fibers are laid down by subcapsular epithelium, resulting in separation of capsular and cortical opacities by a transparent zone and both constitute a reduplicated cataract.

Posterior Polar Cataract (Posterior Capsular Cataract)

It is characterized by the presence of opacity at the central part of posterior capsule. Slit lamp examination reveals concentric rings around central opacity (onion peel appearance) and is associated with thin posterior capsule (**Fig. 10.14**). It is nonprogressive. It may be associated with:

- Posterior lenticonus.
- *Mittendorf's dot*: A small, white dot on posterior capsule slightly inferonasally represents attachment of hyaloid vessel to the posterior capsule.

Various forms of cataract are depicted in **Fig. 10.15**.

Membranous Cataract

It is rare and occurs due to partial or complete absorption of lens fibers, leaving behind residual chalky-white lens matter sandwiched between anterior and posterior capsule. It leads to marked visual loss.

■ Management

Management *includes* ocular examination, laboratory investigations, and treatment.

Ocular Examination (OP7.3)

It requires considerations including:

- *Laterality*: Whether cataract is unilateral or bilateral.
- *Density of cataract.*
- *Morphology of cataract*: It can give important clues to possible etiology.

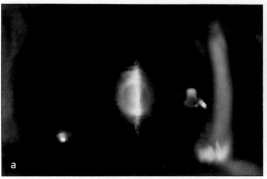
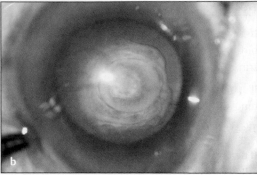

Fig. 10.14 (a, b) Posterior polar Cataract. Source: Fishkind W, ed. Phacoemulsification and Intraocular Lens Implantation: Mastering Techniques and Complications in Cataract Surgery. 2nd Edition. 2017.

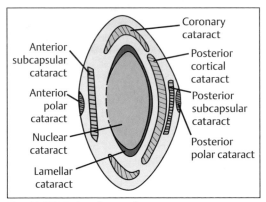

Fig. 10.15 Various forms of cataract.

- *Assessment of visual function*: Visual function can be determined by preferential looking, visually evoked potentials (VEP). Absence of central fixation, nystagmus and strabismus indicate severe visual impairment.
- *Assessment of associated ocular pathology*: Examination under general anesthesia may be required. Recording of IOP and fundus examination under dilation is required to rule out associated diseases. B scan ultrasonography is useful in assessing the posterior segment of eye.

Laboratory Investigations

These are performed to detect underlying etiology in infants with bilateral, nonhereditary cataracts. These include testing of blood and urine samples.

Blood Tests

- Serology (TORCH test) for intrauterine infections such as **T**oxoplasmosis, **R**ubella, **C**ytomegalovirus and **H**erpes simplex (to estimate antibody titer).
- Red blood cell GPUT and galactokinase for galactosemia.
- Serum biochemistry: Blood glucose for hyperglycemia.
- Serum calcium and phosphorous for hypocalcemia.

Urine Tests

- Urine analysis for galactosemia to detect the presence of reducing substances after milk feeding.
- Chromatography for amino acids (if Lowe syndrome is suspected).

Treatment

No treatment is required in a development cataract unless vision is considerably impaired.

Main considerations are density and laterality of cataract. Visual prognosis of unilateral congenital cataract is less favorable than that of bilateral cataract because unilateral visual deprivation often causes irreversible amblyopia.

Treatment for Bilateral Cataracts

If dense: Early surgery within first 6 weeks of birth is performed to prevent development of stimulus deprivation amblyopia.

If partial: Defer surgery and monitor visual function. If vision deteriorates surgery is done.

Treatment for Unilateral Cataracts

If dense: Urgent surgery (within days) is required, followed by aggressive antiamblyopia therapy. Visual prognosis in unilateral cataract is very poor even after timely operation. If cataract is detected after 16 weeks of age, then surgery is inadvisable because amblyopia is refractory.

If partial: It is treated nonsurgically with pupillary dilatation (mydriasis) and part-time occlusion of other eye to prevent amblyopia.

> Development of cataract in galactosemia can be reversed, if discovered in early phase, with elimination of galactose from diet.

Surgical Procedures

In children, cataract can be removed through limbus (by aspiration of lens material through incision) or through pars plana (by lensectomy). Pars plana approach is gradually being abandoned in favor of limbal approach, because the limbal approach allows better preservation of capsular bag for in-the-bag IOL placement.

■ Acquired Cataract (OP7.2)

Acquired cataract may be senile cataract, metabolic cataract and secondary cataract. Secondary cataract may be associated with ocular diseases, trauma, radiations, systemic disorders, skin diseases, drugs and chemicals.

■ Senile (Age-related) Cataract (IM24.15)

Any cataract that occurs after the age of 50 years and has no evident cause is termed senile cataract. It is usually bilateral but often asymmetrical. Both sexes are equally affected. In senile cataract, degeneration of the already formed normal fibers results in opacification. Loss of transparency of lens is due to changes in proteins. It occurs in three forms:

- Cortical cataract.
- Nuclear cataract.
- Sub-capsular cataract.

Cortical Senile Cataract

Biochemical alterations in cortical cataract are:

- Decrease in soluble protein content.
- Increase in insoluble protein content with overall decrease in protein content.
- Coagulation of proteins.
- Increase in content of lens, resulting in hydration of cortex.

Thus, the main processes involved in cataract formation are hydration and replacement of soluble by insoluble proteins. The changes in transparency involve most of the cortex of the lens. Development of cortical senile cataract can be divided into the **following five stages**:

1. Stage of lamellar separation: It is characterized by hydration of cortex. Hydration of cortex increases the refractive index of cortex and hence patient becomes slightly hyperopic. Owing to hydration, there is also collection of fluid between lens fibers, causing lamellar separation (it can only be seen with slit lamp and not by ophthalmoscope).

2. Stage of incipient cataract: Collection of fluid between lens fibers due to hydration of cortex results in formation of ray-like spaces filled with fluid, which are at first transparent and later become opaque. It leads to formation of **wedge-shaped opacities (cuneiform opacities)** with clear areas between them.

These opacities originate *at the periphery* of lens and extend toward the center. The bases of these wedge-shaped opacities are peripheral. They are commonly seen in the *inferonasal quadrant* (**Fig. 10.16**).

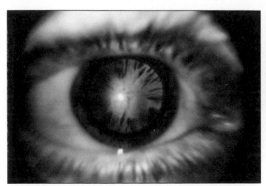

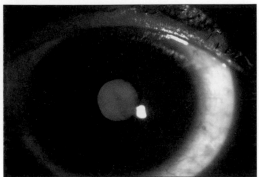

Fig. 10.16 Cuneiform cataract. Source: Biousse V, Newman N, ed. Neuro-Opthalmology Illustrated. 3rd Edition. 2019.

Fig. 10.17 Mature cataract. Source: Cortically Mature Lens: White Cataract. In: Fishkind W, ed. Phacoemulsification and Intraocular Lens Implantation: Mastering Techniques and Complications in Cataract Surgery. 2nd Edition. Thieme; 2017.

They appear *gray on oblique illumination* and black against red glow of fundus when seen with ophthalmoscope. These opacities are present both *in anterior and posterior cortex.*

Since these opacities start at the periphery, initially, it can only be seen with the pupil dilated. Patient feels visual disturbances, especially in evening or night, owing to the dilatation of pupil.

Effect of opacities on vision includes glare due to scattering of light and colored halos. There occur visual disturbances, polyopia (many images of an object) and internal astigmatism also, due to heterogenous lens structure in incipient cortical cataract.

Polyopia is common in conjunction with water clefts that form radial wedge shapes and contain a fluid of lower RI than the surrounding lens.

3. Stage of intumescent cataract: In this stage, progressive hydration of deeper cortical layers takes place and leads to swelling of lens with *more diffuse and irregular lenticular opacities.* This condition of swollen and opacified lens is called "**intumescent cataract.**" Swollen lens pushes the iris forward and the anterior chamber becomes shallow. It may produce *secondary angle-closure glaucoma.* Up to this stage, the lens is partially opaque and clear lens substance

remains between the pupillary margin of iris and lens opacity (**immature cataract).** The iris casts a shadow upon gray opacity, if a beam of light is thrown upon eye obliquely (*iris shadow*). Thus, *iris shadow is seen in immature cataract.*

4. Stage of mature cataract: In this stage, cortex is completely opaque and no clear zone is present between the pupillary margin of iris and opaque lens. Iris does not cast any shadow (*no iris shadow*) and cataract is said to be **mature cataract (Fig. 10.17).**

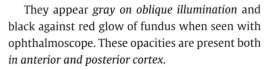

Thus, presence or absence of iris shadow is a useful sign in differentiating immature and mature cataracts.

5. Stage of hypermature cataract: When mature cataractous lens is not extracted from the eye and left in situ, hypermaturity sets in. In some patients, cortex becomes liquefied and appears as a milky fluid. The small, brown nucleus sinks to the bottom of the lens. The nucleus changes its position along with change in position of head. Such a cataract is called **Morgagnian hypermature cataract (Fig. 10.18).**

Sometimes, leakage of water out of lens continues and lens becomes shrunken and wrinkled (**Shrunken cataract** or **sclerotic hypermature cataract.** Due to shrinkage, anterior chamber become deep and iris becomes tremulous (*iridodonesis*).

The anterior capsule becomes thickened due to proliferation of anterior epithelial cells, and a white dense capsular cataract is formed at the anterior pole in pupillary area. The associated degeneration of suspensory ligaments may cause dislocation of the lens.

Nuclear Senile Cataract

In senile nuclear cataract, the normal age-related nuclear sclerosis is intensified, while the cortical fibers remain transparent, so it tends to occur earlier, often soon after 40 years of age. Biochemical alterations in nuclear cataract include increase in insoluble protein content but total protein content remains normal.

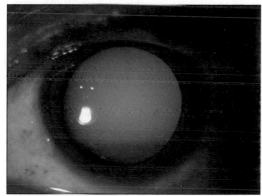

Fig. 10.18 Morgagnian hypermature cataract.

Nuclear sclerosis: In the early stages, it is caused by a yellowish hue due to the *deposition of urochrome* pigment, but when advanced, nucleus may become brown (**brown cataract** or **cataracta brunescens**) or black (**Black cataract** or **cataracta nigra**) owing to the *deposition of melanin* derived from tryptophan amino acid in the lens. In brown or black cataract pupillary reflex appears black (**Fig. 10.19**).

Effect on vision: Nuclear sclerosis increases RI of nucleus and patient becomes myopic, that is, distant vision is blurred more than near vision.

The elder patients, who had emmetropia previously, may be able to read again without spectacles ("second sight of aged"). Initially, the central part of lens becomes completely opaque and opacification spreads gradually toward cortex. The entire lens functions as a nucleus (mature nuclear cataract). However, progress to maturity is usually very slow and hypermaturity generally does not occur in the nuclear cataract. Other differentiating features of nuclear and cortical cataracts are listed in **Table 10.1**.

Subcapsular Senile Cataract

Posterior subcapsular opacity (**cupuliform cataract**) may develop as isolated entity or may be associated with other lens opacities and lie in the posterior cortex just in front of the posterior

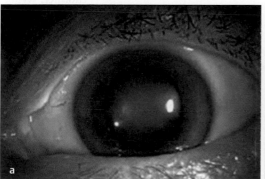
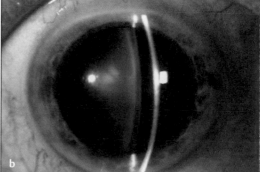

Fig. 10.19 (a) Nuclear sclerosis. Source: Biousse V, Newman N, ed. Neuro-Opthalmology Illustrated. 1st Edition. 2009. **(b)** Brown cataract. Source: Lang G, ed. Opthalmology. A Pocket Textbook Atlas. 3rd Edition. 2015.

Table 10.1 Difference between nuclear cataract and immature cortical cataract

	Nuclear cataract	Immature cortical cataract
• *Site of lens opacity*	Central	Peripheral
• *Shape of lens opacity*	Round or oval	Wedge-shaped
• *Color of lens opacity*	Brown or black	Usually white
• *Vision*	Poor in daytime	Poor in nighttime. In evening or night, due to dilation of pupil, peripheral opacities cause defective vision
• *Improvement of vision*	With minus lenses	With plus lenses
• *Onset*	Often soon after 40 years of age	Usually starts after 50 years of age
• *Progress to maturity*	Usually very slow	Matures relatively
• *Hypermaturity*	Rare	Reaches hypermaturity if mature cataract is left in situ

capsule. These are often axial and progress toward periphery (equator) and not axially toward nucleus.

Appearance: On oblique slit lamp biomicroscopy, posterior subcapsular opacity appear as granular and vacuolated in front of the posterior capsule. On retroillumination with slit lamp, the opacity appears black against red fundus reflex.

Symptoms: Owing to the axial location, posterior subcapsular opacity causes:
- Poor vision in bright light (sunlight and headlights of oncoming vehicles). Constriction of pupil (miosis) takes place in bright light, causing profound effect on vision due to posterior subcapsular opacity.
- Glare.
- On looking at near objects, constriction of pupil occurs (near reflex), and *near vision is frequently impaired more than distance vision.*

An anterior subcapsular cataract lies directly under lens capsule and is associated with fibrous metaplasia of lens epithelium.

■ Metabolic Cataract

Metabolic cataract occurs in endocrine disorders and biochemical abnormalities, of which some are described below.

Diabetes Mellitus

Diabetes mellitus can affect clarity of lens, RI of lens and amplitude of accommodation. Diabetes is associated with two types of cataract:
- *True diabetic cataract*: It is due to osmotic over hydration of lens and appears as white snow flake opacities in the cortex—**"snow flake" cataract**.
- Age-related cataract: It occurs earlier in diabetes and progresses more rapidly than in nondiabetics. Cataract in diabetes depends on its duration. The mechanisms such as glycation, carbamylation of crystallins, and increased oxidative damage may be responsible (**Flowchart 10.5**).

Hypoparathyroidism

It is due to the deficiency of parathormone as a result of inadvertent removal of parathyroid glands during thyroidectomy. Cataractous changes may occur due to hypocalcaemia. The cataract is marked by small discrete opacities in the cortex, which are separated from capsule by a clear zone. These opacities coalesce to form large glistening crystalline flakes.

Galactosemia

It is an inborn, autosomal recessive error of carbohydrate metabolism characterized by

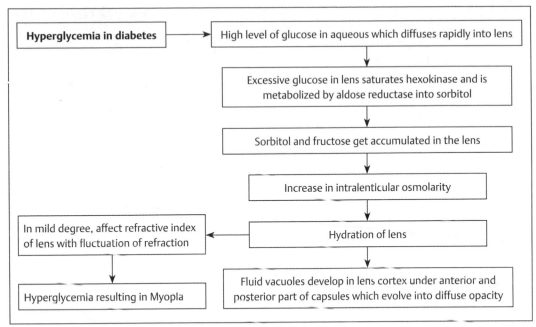

Flowchart 10.5 Etiopathogenesis of cataract in diabetes.

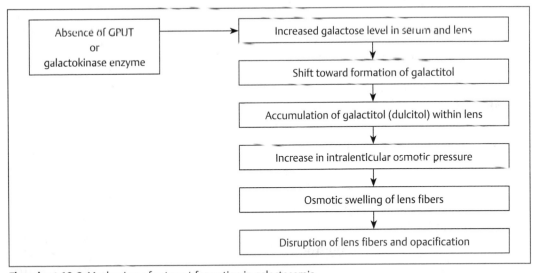

Flowchart 10.6 Mechanism of cataract formation in galactosemia.

inability of infant to metabolize galactose. The cause is the absence of one of the enzymes involved in conversion of galactose into glucose, leading to increase in galactose levels in blood (galactosemia) and accumulation of galactitol. It has autosomal recessive inheritance.

Mechanism of Cataract Formation

Galactose is only indirectly cataractogenic through its reduction to dulcitol (galactitol), the sugar alcohol of galactose (**Flowchart 10.6**).

Deficiency of GPUT is associated with systemic features, while in galactokinase deficiency, galactosemia is associated with cataract but without other systemic manifestations. Galactokinase deficiency is a milder disorder and the affected children are healthy.

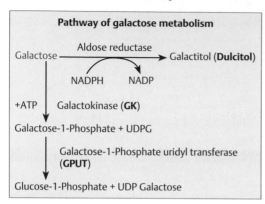

Pathway of galactose metabolism

Galactose —Aldose reductase→ Galactitol (**Dulcitol**)
(NADPH → NADP)

+ATP | Galactokinase (**GK**)

Galactose-1-Phosphate + UDPG

Galactose-1-Phosphate uridyl transferase (**GPUT**)

Glucose-1-Phosphate + UDP Galactose

Clinical Features

Systemic features include failure to thrive, mental retardation and hepatosplenomegaly.

Ocular features include cataract characterized by bilateral "oil droplet" central lens opacities (usually anterior and posterior subcapsular opacity), which later becomes nuclear before it matures. *Exclusion of galactose from diet prevents progression of cataract* and regression may occur if galactose is eliminated from diet in early stage.

Diagnosis

It is done by:
- Red blood cells GPUT level.
- Galactokinase level.
- Presence of reducing substance in urine after drinking milk.

Lowe's Syndrome (Oculo Cerebrorenal Syndrome)

It is an inborn error of amino acid metabolism and predominantly affects boys. It has a X-linked inheritance pattern. It manifests ocular, cerebral, and renal symptoms. *Ocular features* include congenital cataract and congenital glaucoma. It is one of the few conditions in which congenital cataract and congenital glaucoma may coexist. *Cerebral feature* include mental retardation.

Renal features include renal tubular acidosis and renal rickets.

Wilson's Disease (Hepatolenticular Degeneration)

It is an inborn error of copper metabolism. It has an autosomal recessive inheritance pattern. It develops as a result of the *deficiency of alpha-2 globulin*, **ceruloplasmin**. Most of the copper (95%) is tightly bound to ceruloplasmin, while a small fraction (5%) is loosely held to albumin.

Clinical Features

Deficiency of ceruloplasmin results in inadequate copper binding, and free copper in plasma enters the tissues which bind with proteins and gets deposited. Copper deposition *in liver* causes cirrhosis of liver. Copper deposition in lenticular nucleus of brain *leads to* brain necrosis. So, it is also called hepatolenticular degeneration. Copper deposition in kidney causes renal damage. Deposition of metallic copper in eye (**ocular features**) occurs either in cornea or lens capsule. Deposition in cornea manifests as **Kayser–Fleischer ring,** a brown corneal ring at the level of Descemet's membrane which is a characteristic feature (**Fig. 10.20**). Deposition in lens capsule results in typical **"sunflower" cataract.** It is a disc-shaped polychromic opacity in the anterior capsular region, with petal-like spokes that extend toward periphery.

Treatment is with D-penicillamine, a naturally occurring copper chelating agent.

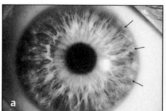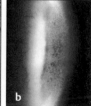

Fig. 10.20 (a) Kayser–Fleischer ring (Deposition of copper). **(b)** Sunflower cataract. Source: Wilson disease (hepatolenticular degeneration). In: Biousse V, Newman N, ed. Neuro-ophthalmology illustrated. 3rd edition. Thieme; 2019.

■ Secondary Cataract

Complicated Cataract (Cataract Associated with Ocular Diseases)

Lens depends for its nutrition on intraocular fluids. A disturbance in nutrition of lens results in the development of complicated cataract. It results due to inflammatory (uveal tissue and retina) or degenerative disease (degenerative myopia, retinitis pigmentosa and gyrate atrophy).

Etiology (OP7.2)

Ocular conditions giving rise to complicated cataract are as follows:

- Inflammatory diseases.
  ◇ Iridocyclitis.
  ◇ Choroiditis.
- Degenerative conditions:
  ◇ Degenerative myopia.
  ◇ Retinitis pigmentosa.
  ◇ Gyrate atrophy.
- Tumors like ciliary body tumors.
- Retinal detachment and surgery due to silicone oil injection and gas tamponade.
- Ischemia as in anterior segment ischemia.
- Glaucoma due to:
  ◇ Use of miotics.
  ◇ Glaucoma drainage surgery.
  ◇ Lens trauma during peripheral iridectomy.

Posterior cortical cataract or posterior subcapsular cataract will be formed in inflammations or degenerations affecting posterior segment, such as in uveitis, retinitis pigmentosa, gyrate atrophy, degenerative myopia, retinal detachment and surgery. In inflammations of anterior segment, opacification appears through the cortex.

Clinical Features

As opacity is situated near the nodal point of eye, vision is markedly impaired. On slit lamp examination, opacity shows the irregular margins extending toward the equator and nucleus. The opacities have an appearance like *bread crumbs*. A characteristic sign of complicated cataract is polychromatic luster (characteristic rainbow display of colors). The *complicated cataract* may remain stationary or progress peripherally and axially to involve the entire lens.

Cataract Associated with Systemic Disorders

Dystrophia Myotonica (Myotonic Dystrophy)

It is caused by delayed muscular relaxation after cessation of the voluntary effort (myotonia). It has an autosomal dominant inheritance pattern.

Clinical Features

Systemic features include the following:
- Difficulty in releasing grip (due to difficulty in relaxation of skeletal muscles).
- Expressionless face due to wasting of facial muscles.
- Slurred speech due to involvement of tongue and pharyngeal muscles.
- Gonadal atrophy.
- Cardiac conduction defects.

Ocular features include the following:
- Early onset cataract develops in 90% of patients.
- Early cataract consists of polychromic dots and flakes in superficial cortex underneath the capsule. As the opacities mature, a *characteristic stellate opacity* appears at the posterior pole, resembling a *"Christmas tree"* (**Christmas tree cataract**) (**Fig. 10.21**).
- Other ocular features include ptosis, mild pigmentary retinopathy, and external ophthalmoplegia.

Down Syndrome (Trisomy 21)

It is the most common autosomal trisomy.

Systemic features include mental retardation, stunted growth, Mongoloid facies and congenital heart defects.

Ocular features include:
- *Cataract* (punctate and subcapsular opacities).
- *Brush field spots* (iris spots)—light colored and spotted irides.
- Narrow and slanted palpebral fissures.

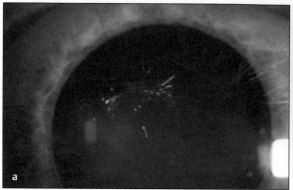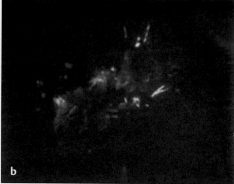

Fig. 10.21 (a, b) Christmas tree cataract. Source: The Diagnosis of Binocular Diplopia. In: Biousse V, Newman N, ed. Neuro-Opthalmology Illustrated. 3rd Edition. 2019.

Other chromosomal abnormalities associated with cataract include Patau syndrome (Trisomy 13) and Edward syndrome (Trisomy 18).

Dermatogenic Cataract (Cataract Associated With Skin Disease)

Both skin and lens share a common embryological origin, the *ectoderm*. Therefore, many skin disorders are associated with cataract formation, while many are inherited. Dermatogenic cataracts are bilateral and occur at a young age. Cataract develops in approximately 10% of patients with atopic dermatitis which is a chronic erythematosus skin disorder associated with increased IgE.

Atopic cataract: It is usually bilateral and develop in the second to fourth decades. "**Shield cataract**" is characteristic. It is a dense, anterior subcapsular plaque which causes wrinkling of anterior capsule because of localized proliferation of lens epithelium. It has radiating cortical riders and may involve the entire lens.

Other skin disorders associated with cataract include Rothmund's syndrome, Werner's syndrome, and ichthyosis.

Traumatic Cataract

It may be due to concussion (contusion or blunt) injury, penetrating injury and electric shock. *In concussion injury, cataract may be formed due to mechanical effect of injury on lens fibers or minute rupture in lens capsule.*

Due to the mechanical effect of injury, lens fibers become edematous and whiten.

The opacities outlining the lens fibers radiate from sutures and a characteristic flower-shaped pattern forms (**rosette-shaped cataract**) (**Fig. 10.22**). It is axial in location and usually involves the posterior cortex, sometimes anterior cortex, or both. *Rupture frequently occurs at the thinnest part of* lens capsule, that is, *at the posterior pole of lens,* leading to hydration of lens fibers and subsequent opacification.

In concussion injury, force of blow drive cornea and iris backward, causing release of pigment from pupillary ruff. Pigment get imprinted on to the anterior surface of lens as a circular ring, called the **Vossius ring**, whose size is nearly identical to the diameter of constricted pupil. A ring-shaped faint anterior subcapsular opacity may underlie the Vossius ring.

> Presence of the Vossius ring is suggestive of blunt trauma.

In *penetrating injury*, lens may be ruptured, resulting in rapid progression to mature cataract. Surgical injury during peripheral iridectomy behaves similarly.

In *electric shock* (due to lightning or live electricity wire), cataract may develop, which usually starts as punctate, subcapsular opacities and matures rapidly. If shock occurs equidistant

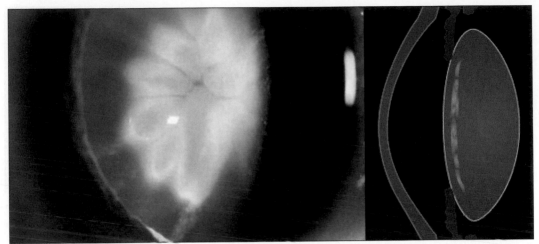

Fig. 10.22 Traumatic cataract. Source: Traumatic Cataract. In: Lang G, ed. Opthalmology. A Pocket Textbook Atlas. 3rd Edition. Thieme; 2015.

between two eyes, bilateral cataracts result. If shock is to one side, cataract develops on that side.

Radiation Cataract

This may be caused by:

- Ionizing radiation such as cosmic rays, gamma-rays and X-rays.
- Nonionizing radiation such as infrared (IR) radiation.
- Heavy charged and uncharged particles such as neutrons.

Ionizing radiations affect the cells with high-mitotic rate such as lens equatorial fibers. An early cataractous change is apparent in the cortex near posterior pole, when the equatorial cells have migrated posteriorly, therefore posterior subcapsular opacities are common.

Nonionizing radiation (as in glass blowers and furnace workers without protective lenses) influences the lens fibers indirectly. Heat is absorbed by the iris pigment epithelium, with increase in its temperature, which influences the lens fibers. A characteristic posterior subcapsular cataract is formed. In addition, true exfoliation of anterior lens capsule may take place, which peels off from periphery and coils up in the anterior chamber. As it is typically seen in glass blowers, so it is also called as **"glass-blower's cataract."**

UV radiation (290 to 320 nm) develops the cortical and posterior subcapsular cataracts.

Toxic Cataract

Many drugs and chemicals may include lens opacities:

- *Corticosteroids:* Prolonged use of cortico-steroids (topical or systemic) may induce posterior subcapsular cataract. Children are more susceptible. Although predni-solone ≤10 mg/day for 1 year is usually regarded as a safe maintenance dose, the role of individual (genetic) susceptibility has been stressed.
- *Anticholinesterase and miotic drugs:* Prolonged use of anticholinesterases for the treatment of chronic open-angle glaucoma may cause anterior subcapsular cataract in the form of vacuoles.
- *Phenothiazines:* Chlorpromazine and thi-oridazine may cause deposition of fine yellow brown granules under the anterior capsule in pupillary zone, finally developing into anterior polar cataract.
- *Antimitotic drugs* (such as busulfan) used in the treatment of chronic myeloid leukemia cause posterior subcapsular cataract.

- *Antimalarial drugs* (chloroquine *but not hydroxychloroquine*) may cause posterior subcapsular cataract.
- *Cigarette smoking:* Cyanide in cigarette smoke causes carbamylation of lens proteins, leading to cataract (nuclear type).
- *Iron:* Retention of foreign body (iron) following penetrating injury may cause flower-shaped cataract.
- *Gold:* It is deposited in the capsule and epithelium as fine, golden anterior capsule deposits.

■ Management of Cataract (OP7.4)

There is no medical treatment for cataract. The only effective treatment of cataract is its surgical removal. The surgery is indicated only when cataract causes difficulty in performing daily essential activities. Visual improvement is the most common indication for cataract surgery. It may be required to improve the clarity of ocular media in fundal pathology, for example, diabetic retinopathy.

■ Preoperative Evaluation (OP7.3)

Any patient undergoing cataract surgery should have general medical and ocular examinations. The following considerations are essential while evaluating the patient preoperatively:
- **General medical examination** must be done to exclude systemic diseases such as:
  ◊ Diabetes.
  ◊ Hypertension.
  ◊ Ischemic heart disease (**IHD**).
  ◊ Chronic obstructive pulmonary disease (**COPD**).
  ◊ Cerebrovascular disease.
  ◊ Source of infection: Urinary tract infection and septic gums.
  ◊ Bleeding disorders.
- **Ocular examination:** A detailed ocular examination is required before cataract surgery.

- **Visual acuity assessment:** The patient with cataract should have, at least, perception of light (**PL**).
- **Refraction** is performed to determine the best corrected visual acuity.
- **Slit lamp examination:** A detailed slit lamp examinations of anterior segment is done to exclude the presence of an active intraocular inflammation, for example, uveitis. Treatment must be directed first to control the uveitis.

The main refracting media are the cornea and lens. Because lens is removed at surgery, a proper corneal examination is important, especially with reference to the *corneal shape* (using **corneal topography**) and endothelial cell count (using **specular microscopy**). Normal endothelial cell count is >2400 cells/mm². Postoperative corneal decompensation is likely in *eyes with low endothelial cell count or due to loss of endothelial cells during cataract surgery.*

So, special precautions should be taken to protect the endothelium during surgery with viscoelastics.
- **Testing of pupil:** Presence of afferent pupillary defect (**APD**) indicates defective retinal and optic nerve function. Visual outcome will be poor after surgery in such cases. Poorly dilated pupil can make cataract surgery difficult.
- **Lens:** The type and grade of lens opacities must be recorded as it is very useful. The cortical opacities tend to be softer, while nuclear opacities tend to be harder. The **grading of nuclear hardness** is useful in planning phacoemulsification (**Table 10.2**).

Table 10.2 Grading of nuclear hardness	
Grade	**Color of nucleus**
1	Grayish (soft)
2	Gray–yellow
3	Brown
4	Black (hardest)

- **Fundus examination**: Patients with senile cataract may also have age-related macular degeneration (**ARMD**) which may affect visual outcome. When fundus cannot be seen in eyes with opaque or very dense cataracts, the following tests (**macular function tests**) give valuable information:
  ◊ *Projection of rays (PR)*: It is tested in a dark room with the opposite eye covered. The patient is asked to look straight and a beam of light is thrown into the cataractous eye from various directions. Patient is asked to point out the direction from which light seems to come.
  ◊ *Two-light discrimination test*: Patient is asked to look at two "point" sources of light 2 inches apart and kept at 2 feet from the eye. If patient appreciates the presence of two lights, macular function is probably good.
  ◊ *Maddox rod test*: Patient is asked to look at a distant light through a Maddox rod. If continuous and unbroken red line is perceived, macular function is probably good.
  ◊ *Entoptic view test*: The eye is closed and a bare lighted bulb of a torch is rubbed on the closed lower eyelid (transillumination). The blood vessels of retina which lie in front of rods and cones cast a shadow on these elements and the vascular tree of retina is visualized. Retinal vessels are seen as black lacework against a red background. The only limitation of this test is that avascular fovea cannot be tested by this method.
  ◊ *Color perception*: Different colored lights are projected from an ophthalmoscope. If the patient identifies different colors, macular function is present.
  ◊ *Laser interferometry*: A beam of **helium–neon laser** is optically split into two and projected through the lens. The laser beams form the interference fringes on the retina. The visual acuity may

be measured by varying the spaces of fringes.
  ◊ *B-scan ultrasonography*: Gross pathology can be detected with B-scan such as vitreous hemorrhage, retinal detachment, intraocular tumors, and posterior staphyloma.
  ◊ *Multifocal ERG*: The technique can be used for almost any disorder which affects retinal function, but this test is not required in routine clinical practice.
  ◊ *Measurement of IOP*: It is mandatory to exclude glaucoma. Raised IOP may be due to preexistent primary glaucoma, phacomorphic glaucoma and phacolytic glaucoma.
  ◊ *Ocular adnexa*: The search for local cause of infection should be made to exclude the possibility of infective complications. Conjunctivitis, blepharitis and dacryocystitis may predispose to endophthalmitis and require preoperative effective treatment.

■ Preoperative Preparation

The following points are noteworthy for preparing the patient for operation:
- **A written informed consent** should be obtained.
- **Conjunctional swab** is sent for culture.
- **Syringing of lacrimal sac**: If regurgitation is found from lacrimal sac, a nasal drainage operation DCR (dacryocystorhinostomy) should be performed first before cataract surgery.
- **Topical antibiotics** such as tobramycin or moxifloxacin or ciprofloxacin eye drops are instilled 3 to 4 times a day × 3 days prior to surgery.
- **Lowering of IOP**: Tab acetazolamide (250 mg) 2 tablets, stat 2 hours before surgery. In glaucomatous patients, hyperosmotic agents like glycerine (orally) or IV mannitol can be given an hour before surgery.

- **Pupillary dilatation** (when required): *For adequate dilatation of pupil,* Tropicamide 1% + Phenylephrine 5–10% eye drops are instilled every 10 minutes 1 hour before surgery. *For sustained pupillary dilatation,* antiprostaglandin eye drops such as flurbiprofen or diclofenac sodium (nonsteroid anti-inflammatory drugs [NSAIDS]) are instilled along with Tropicamide and Phenylephrine. *The flurbiprofen inhibit prostaglandin release from the iris on mechanical stimulation during surgery and prevent intraoperative miosis.* Thus, *with Tropicamide (1%), Phenylephrine (5–10%) and Flurbiprofen (0–0.3%) eye drops adequate and sustained dilatation of pupil is achieved intraoperatively.*
- Preparation of eye to be operated:
  ◊ Trimming of eyelashes before surgery.
  ◊ The eye to be operated should be marked by an adhesive tape.
  ◊ Cleaning of the eye and surrounding skin must be done with povidone–iodine solution.

■ Anesthesia for Cataract Surgery

Cataract surgery can be performed under either local anesthesia (LA) or general anesthesia (GA). Majority of cataract surgery is performed under LA. GA is required for:

- Babies and children.
- Mentally retarded adults.
- Patients with head tremors.
- Anxious and uncooperative patients.

Mechanism of Action of LA

LAs interact with a receptor within voltage sensitive channel and raise the threshold of channel opening. Therefore, entry of ions is decreased in response to an impulse, and depolarization of nerve membrane is prevented. In this way, nerve conduction is blocked, that is, impulses are not conducted along the nerve.

Techniques of LA

LA can be classified into topical (surface) anesthesia and infiltration anesthesia. Infiltration anesthesia may be:

- Retrobulbar block (requires facial block).
- Peribulbar block.
- Parabulbar (subtenon) block.

Drugs used for LA

These are either esters or amides: Ester LAs (proparacaine, cocaine, and tetracaine) have higher risk of hypersensitivity than amide LAs (lignocaine and bupivacaine). So, ester agents are rarely used for infiltration or nerve block but are still used topically.

Proparacaine (0.5%) or Lignocaine (4%) are used for **topical anesthesia**. Cocaine is a good topical anesthetic but is no longer used because of the potential risk of side effects and drug abuse. It should never be injected. Tetracaine (amethocaine) and proparacaine are least toxic to corneal epithelium, while Lignocaine 4% has increased association with corneal toxicity. The most common mixture used for **infiltration anesthesia** is: Bupivacaine 0.75% (5 mL) + Lignocaine 2% (5 mL) + adrenaline 1:200,000 + hyaluronidase 75 units. *Bupivacaine* prolongs action of anesthesia. *Lignocaine* provides early onset of action. *Adrenaline* causes vasoconstriction. Therefore, duration of anesthesia is prolonged, systemic toxicity of LA is reduced and local bleeding is minimized. As it causes vasoconstriction, so it should be avoided in patients with hypertension, ischemic heart disease and generalized atherosclerosis as pressure in ophthalmic artery is decreased. *Hyaluronidase* breaks down C_1–C_4 bonds between glucosamine and glucuronic acid in connective tissue, resulting in more effective diffusion of LA in the tissues. Therefore, the time of onset and the required quantity of LA is reduced. This anesthetic mixture is same for both retrobulbar as well as for peribulbar blocks.

Topical Anesthesia

- *Indications*:
  - ◊ Phacoemulsification in cooperative patients.
  - ◊ Prior to infiltration anesthesia.
- *Relative contraindications*:
  - ◊ Difficult or extended surgery.
  - ◊ Uncooperative patients.
  - ◊ Deafness and language barrier.
- *Aim*: Aim of topical anesthesia is to block the nerve that supplies superficial cornea and conjunctiva, namely, long and short ciliary nerves, nasociliary nerve and lacrimal nerve.
- *Adverse effects*:
  - ◊ Alteration of lacrimation and tear film stability.
  - ◊ Corneal epithelial toxicity.
  - ◊ Allergy (contact dermatitis) is more common.
- *Advantages*:
  - ◊ No risk associated with needle insertion (e.g., piercing the globe/optic nerve).
  - ◊ No risk of periocular hemorrhage.
  - ◊ No postoperative diplopia or ptosis.
- *Disadvantage*:
  - ◊ No akinesia of the eye.
  - ◊ Although analgesia is adequate, there is no true anesthesia, as sensation is still intact.

Recently, intracameral (*in anterior chamber*) preservative-free 1% Lignocaine has been used with topical anesthesia (*usually during hydrodis-section*) to obtain intracameral anesthesia. At present, no side effects have been reported.

Infiltration Anesthesia

Site of Injection

The block is given at the junction of medial 2/3rd and lateral 1/3rd of lower orbital margin (or halfway between lateral canthus and lateral limbus, **Fig. 10.23**). This is a relatively avascular area. The injection is given via skin or inferior fornix by pulling the lower eyelid down. It is same for both retrobulbar as well as peribulbar block. The infiltration of local anesthesia in retrobulbar block is given within the muscle cone, while in peribulbar block, anesthetic agent is injected outside the muscle cone. Therefore, the chance of optic nerve injury is less with peribulbar block and safer. Peribulbar block has now almost replaced retrobulbar block. The needle of 25 gauge is used for the block. The length of the needle should not be more than 31 mm in length for retrobulbar block (to avoid piercing the optic nerve) and 25 mm for peribulbar block (**Table 10.3**). The eye is kept in primary gaze as the optic nerve is directly away from the path of needle.

Technique

With the eye in *primary gaze*, the needle is inserted and advanced first directly *backward*, then slightly *upward* and *medially* toward the apex of orbit (*for retrobulbar block*), and finally advanced parallel to orbital floor for approximately 2.5 cm (*for peribulbar block*). Gentle aspiration of syringe is performed to alleviate possible entry of needle into a blood vessel. After aspiration, the LA is injected slowly. Pressure is applied either by fingers or Honan balloon.

Retrobulbar block anesthetizes the ciliary ganglion and its surrounding structures. Thus, temporary paralysis of extraocular muscles (akinesia) and slight dilation of pupil (because of oculomotor block) occurs. *Some activity may*

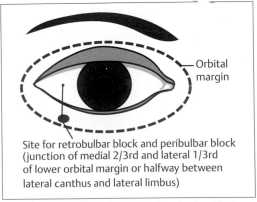

Site for retrobulbar block and peribulbar block (junction of medial 2/3rd and lateral 1/3rd of lower orbital margin or halfway between lateral canthus and lateral limbus)

Fig. 10.23 Site of retrobulbar and peribulbar block.

Table 10.3 Differentiating features of retrobulbar and peribulbar blocks

	Retrobulbar block	Peribulbar block
1. Volume of anesthetic agent injected	2–4 mL	4–6 mL
2. Needle used	Long (31 mm)	Short (25 mm)
3. Anesthesia and akinesia	Excellent	Good
4. Chemosis	Less	More
5. Optic nerve injury	More chances	Less chances
6. Safety	+	+ +
7. Onset of block	Quicker	Takes time
8. Complication rate	More	Less
9. Need of facial block	+	–
10. Infiltration of local anesthetic	Within muscle cone (intraconal block)	Outside muscle cone (extraconal block)

be retained in superior oblique muscle because the 4th cranial nerve (CN) (Trochlear N) is outside the muscle cone.

Complications

Peribulbar block carries low risk of complications. Complications associated with retrobulbar block include:

- Retrobulbar hemorrhage.
- Perforation of globe.
- Injury to optic nerve.
- Respiratory depression or arrest.
- Muscle complications include ptosis from levator aponeurosis dehiscence and diplopia following extraocular muscle injection.
- Oculocardiac reflex is usually produced by pressure on globe. Vasovagal bradycardia is more common.

Sub-tenon Block

To achieve anesthesia, the anesthetic mixture is injected with a blunt cannula into the posterior subtenon space, bathing the nerve and muscles within the cone. It requires low volumes of anesthetic, and vascular or optic nerve injuries are avoided.

Facial Block

It is required with the retrobulbar block but not with peribulbar block.

Principle: It blocks facial nerve, so orbicularis oculi supplied by facial nerve is temporarily paralyzed and the patient cannot squeeze the eyelids.

Techniques: It can be achieved by either O'Briens technique or Van Lint technique. In O'Briens technique, 4 to 6 mL of anesthetic agent is injected near the condyloid process down to the periosteum (position of mandibular condyle is ascertained by asking the patient to open and close his mouth which is located 1 cm anterior to tragus). Massage is applied and facial nerve with its branches is blocked. This technique is associated with unwanted facial paralysis. Van Lint technique blocks terminal branches of facial nerve. So, localized akinesia of orbicularis oculi muscle is produced without facial paralysis. A needle is inserted subcutaneously outside lateral canthus and advanced upward toward brow and downward toward infraorbital foramen. The anesthetic mixture is infiltrated along both paths and branches of facial nerve are blocked.

■ Cataract Surgery

Cataract extraction may be:

Intracapsular cataract extraction (**ICCE**): It is now becoming obsolete.

Extracapsular cataract extraction (ECCE): Different methods of ECCE are:

- Conventional ECCE.
- Small incision cataract surgery (SICS).
- Phacoemulsification.

Nowadays, phacoemulsification is the most popular and preferred method *(surgical details are explained with the chapter 26 [eye surgery])*.

Aphakia

The absence of crystalline lens from its normal pupillary position is called aphakia. It may be surgical, traumatic or due to dislocation of lens as a result of degeneration of zonules. Common terminologies with regard to lens are:

- *Phakic eye*: Eye with normal crystalline lens.
- *Aphakic eye*: Eye without normal crystalline lens.
- *Pseudophakic eye*: Eye with IOL.

Optics of Aphakia

Out of total dioptric power of eye, 75% of power comes from the cornea and 25% from the crystalline lens. So, aphakic eye (eye without crystalline lens) becomes extremely deficient in dioptric power. The eye becomes grossly hypermetropic if the eye was emmetropic or had low-grade of ametropia before removal of lens. In addition to hypermetropia, there is always some astigmatism, owing to the scarring of incision. Astigmatism after cataract extraction is generally "**against the rule**" **(Fig. 10.24)**. There is complete loss of accommodation in the aphakic eye. Refractive power of aphakia eye becomes approximately + 44D from normal + 60D of phakic eye.

If cataract surgery is performed with *superior incision* in its usual location, scarring of superior incision takes place, which results in flattening of *cornea in vertical meridian. It leads to* astigmatism "against the rule" after cataract surgery.

Signs of aphakia (anterior to posterior) are:

1. Limbal scar in case of surgical aphakia.

2. Deep anterior chamber.
3. Surgical iridectomy.
4. Tremulousness of iris (iridodonesis) due to loss of support of lens.
5. Jet black pupil.
6. Absence of third and fourth Purkinje images.

■ Treatment

Aphakic eye becomes extremely deficient in dioptric power due to removal of crystalline lens, which must be corrected to restore vision. Replacement of dioptric power (i.e., optical rehabilitation) can be in the form of:

- Spectacles.
- Contact lenses.
- IOLs (**Table 10.4**).

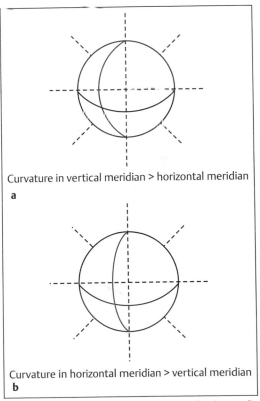

Curvature in vertical meridian > horizontal meridian

a

Curvature in horizontal meridian > vertical meridian

b

Fig. 10.24 (a) Astigmatism "with the rule" (normal). **(b)** Astigmatism "against the rule" (after cataract surgery).

Table 10.4 Treatment modalities for aphakia

Aphakic correction			
	With spectacles	**With contact lenses**	**With IOLs**
1. **Magnification**	About 25%	About 7%	1.5% (with IOL in capsular bag) 2% (with anterior chamber IOL)
2. **Optical aberrations:**			
• Roving ring scotoma	+	–	–
• Jack-in-the-box phenomenon	+	–	–
• Pin cushion distortion	+	–	–
3. **Field of vision**	Restricted	Full peripheral vision	Full peripheral vision
4. **Indications:**	• Aphakia in fellow eye with good vision. • High-axial myopia with IOL power <8D	Young children <2 years	Universal

Abbreviation: IOL, intraocular lens.

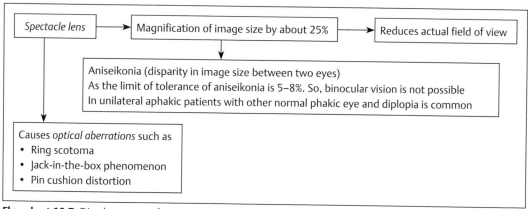

Flowchart 10.7 Disadvantages of spectacle lens in aphakia.

Although each modality can restore the patient's vision, the optical consequences are dramatically different.

Aphakic Correction with Spectacles

Spectacles are placed at a vertex distance of 14 mm from the corneal surface, which causes magnification of image by approximately 25% (**Flowchart 10.7**). There is approximately 2% of magnification for each diopter of power in spectacles. The average aphakic spectacle is therefore 12.5D.

Convex lens can be considered as base-in prism, so light rays at the edge bends toward its

base, and rays in this area are, therefore, not seen. This "blind area" along the edge circumscribes the field of aphakic eye, resulting in **ring scotoma**. It is not a true scotoma but rather an optically produced defect in visual field caused by prismatic effect at the periphery of spectacle lens. Ring scotoma is not stationary. Its movements are initiated by movements of eye, so it is referred to as "roving ring scotoma." If eye rotates temporally (with head fixed), ring scotoma moves nasally or centrally (**Fig. 10.25**).

When an object moves from extreme visual field toward the center of fixation, the object passes through ring scotoma and disappears.

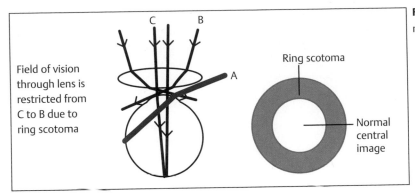

Fig. 10.25 Formation of ring scotoma by spectacle.

Field of vision through lens is restricted from C to B due to ring scotoma

Now, the object moves into central island of vision and is visible again. *This jumping into and out of patient's vision is referred to as* jack-in-the-box phenomenon. So, driving becomes very difficult to perform.

The jack-in-the-box phenomenon may also be appreciated on moving the head toward the object. An object of interest (**A**) appears in the periphery of the patients' visual field. It appears blurred as light does not fall on the fovea. The person moves his head toward the object to see it clearly but the object comes to lie in the area of scotoma (**B**) on turning the head and thus disappears. The person turns his head further, so that the object comes to lie in front of the visible area (**C**) in spectacles. Thus, the object reappears again clear and sharp.

Restriction in field of vision is due to:

- Magnification of image size.
- Ring scotoma.
- Unrefracted field of vision outside spectacle lens because of small size of aphakic lenticular spectacles.

Pin Cushion Distortion

It is a property of all plus lenses with oblique angles of gaze and is proportional to their dioptric power. The corners of a square have a stretched-out appearance and the sides are pushed in. Thus, this distortion makes a square look like a pin cushion. Rectangular objects such as doors and boxes appear like a pin cushion. For an architect, these distortions make the job extremely difficult (**Fig. 10.26**).

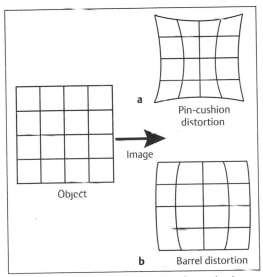

Fig. 10.26 (a) Pincushion distortion from plus lenses to correct hypermetropia. (b) Barrel distortion from minus lenses to correct myopia.

Aphakic Correction with Contact Lenses

Advantages of correction of aphakia with contact lenses are magnification only approximately 7%, no pincushion distortion, no ring scotoma, no Jack-in-the box phenomenon, and full peripheral vision.

Power of Contact Lenses

As the position of optical correction (corneal plane) moves closer to the retina, the required power of contact lens increases.

+ 12.5D at vertex distance of 14 mm in spectacle
≡ + 14.7D in contact lens at corneal plane.

As magnification decreases to 6 to 8% at the corneal plane, which is near the limit of tolerance of aniseikonia (5–8%), so unilateral aphakic patients can have binocular vision with aphakic eye corrected using a contact lens and other normal phakic eye.

Aphakic Correction with Intraocular Lenses (IOLs)

This is the preferred method nowadays. It eliminates most of the disadvantages associated with the use of spectacles or contact lenses. The lens can be implanted in the capsular bag (in case of ECCE) or anterior chamber (in ICCE).

Aphakic Correction with Refractive Surgery

This is a newly emerging treatment for aphakia. Important considerations are listed below:

- *Keratophakia*: A lenticule prepared from the donor cornea is placed within the lamellae of the patient's cornea.
- *Epikeratophakia*: A lenticule prepared from the donor cornea is stitched to the patients' cornea after removing the epithelium.
- *Hyperopic Lasik*.

■ Intraocular Lenses (IOL)

The first IOL was implanted by Sir Harold Ridley. IOLs provide many advantages over spectacles and contact lenses. IOL implantation may be:

Primary: It refers to IOL implantation during cataract surgery.

Secondary: It refers to IOL implantation to correct aphakia in a previously operated eye. Placement sites of an IOL are (**Fig. 10.27**):

- Anterior chamber (AC IOLs).
- Iris-supported IOLs.
- Posterior chamber (PC IOLs).

■ Anterior Chamber Lenses (AC IOLs)

These lie in front of the pupil and iris and are supported by the scleral spur in angle of anterior chamber, for example, Kelman AC IOLs. They are discarded for primary implantation due to complications.

- *Indications*—Following ICCE:
  - ◇ For correcting high myopia.
  - ◇ ECCE with vitreous loss and poor capsular support.
- *Complications*:
  - ◇ Corneal decompensation.
  - ◇ Uveitis-glaucoma-hyphema (UGH) syndrome.
  - ◇ Cystoid macular edema.

■ Iris-supported IOLs

These are held over the surface of iris, for example, worst iris claw lens (**Fig. 10.28**).

■ Posterior Chamber Lenses (PC IOLs)

These may be placed in ciliary sulcus or capsular bag.

Advantages of "in the bag" implantation are:

1. Low incidence of decentration and dislocation.

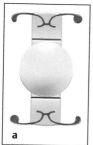
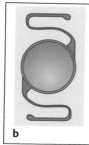
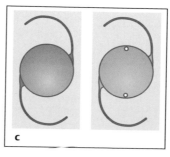

a b c

Fig. 10.27 (a) Crystal lens (accommodating lens). **(b)** Kelman anterior chamber lens. Source: Randleman J, Ahmed I, ed. Intraocular Lens Surgery: Selection, Complications, and Complex Cases. 1st Edition. 2016. **(c)** Posterior chamber IOLs. Abbreviation: IOL, intraocular lens.

2. IOL is positioned in the proper anatomical site.

3. Because of no direct contact with uveal tissue, there is reduced postoperative pigment dispersion from posterior iris pigment epithelium.

4. IOL is positioned at a maximum distance behind the cornea.

5. Posterior capsular opacification (PCO) may be reduced.

Complications:
- Pupillary capture.
- Decentration.

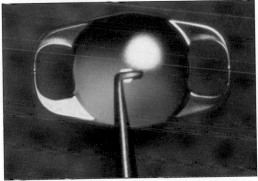

Fig. 10.28 Iris - supported IOLs. Source: History and Design of the Iris Claw Lens. In: Agarwal A, Narang P, ed. Video Atlas of Anterior Segment Repair and Reconstruction: Managing Challenges in Cornea, Glaucoma, and Lens Surgery. 1st Edition. Thieme; 2019.

- Posterior capsular rupture.
- Posterior dislocation.
- PCO.

■ Parts of an IOL

IOL consists of two parts:
- *Optic*: It is the central part overlying the optic axis.
- *Haptics*: These are peripheral arms used for placement and stabilization of IOL.

Optic haptic junction: IOL may be single piece or 3-piece with different haptic angulation relative to the plane of optic. *Usually, PC IOLs have a 10° anterior angulation to keep the optic away from the pupil* (**Fig. 10.29**).

Two other types of IOL are manufactured currently: multifocal and toric, but monofocal IOLs are still most widely used.

■ Magnification by IOL

- Magnification by IOL in capsular bag is 1.5%.
- Magnification by anterior chamber IOL would be approximately 2%.

■ Optic of IOL

Optic in nonfoldable IOLs consists of **PMMA** (polymethyl methacrylate) whose RI is 1.491. Optic in foldable IOLs is made of silicon (with RI 1.41–1.46) and acrylic (with RI 1.55), which may be hydrophilic or hydrophobic (**Fig. 10.30**).

Fig. 10.29 (a, b) IOL parts and design. Abbreviation: IOL, intraocular lens.

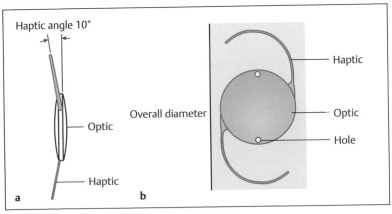

Haptic angle 10°

Optic

Haptic

a

Overall diameter

Haptic

Optic

Hole

b

Holes in optic may be present or absent. Holes assist in positioning of IOL. Size of optic is 5 to 7 mm. Shape of optic may be biconvex, convexoplano, or meniscus. Edge of optic may be square or rounded. *For same refractive power, higher the RI, flatter will be the curvature of lens. So, for the same power, acrylic lens has flattest curvatures and silicone the steepest. So, order of thickness is: acrylic < PMMA < silicone provided all else is equal.* Important differentiating features of hydrophobic and hydrophilic lenses are listed in **Table 10.5**.

Advantages of Biconvex Over Convexo Plano Lens

1. Minimizes effects of tilt, decentration, and spherical aberration.
2. Posterior convex surface reduces migration of lens epithelial cells; hence, the reduced incidence of PCO.

Front surface of biconvex lens is much steeper than back surface, so posterior surface would not be in contact with posterior capsule. Hence, pitting of lens is avoided with YAG laser capsulotomy. Biconvex lenses are used predominantly because of superior optical and mechanical clinical performance.

■ Haptics of IOL

Materials used for haptics are polypropylene, PMMA and acrylic. The haptic is angulated relative to the plane of the optic in different ways. Usually posterior chamber IOL have a 10° anterior angulation to keep the optic away from the pupil, while the anterior chamber lenses have posteriorly angulated haptics to keep the IOL away from the pupil.

■ Optical Transmission

Cornea filters out any wavelength <320 nm.

Crystalline lens filters out any wavelength <400 nm.

So, when crystalline lens is removed, wavelengths of 320 to 400 nm reach the retina. As PMMA lens (Without UV absorbing filter) filters only light below 320 nm, so blue cones

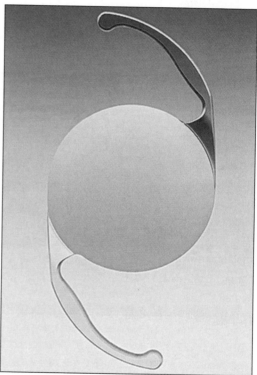

Fig. 10.30 Foldable hydrophobic acrylic IOL with one-piece design. Source: Acrylic: Foldable Hydrophobic. In: Randleman J, Ahmed I, ed. Intraocular Lens Surgery: Selection, Complications, and Complex Cases. 1st Edition. Thieme; 2016. Abbreviation: IOL, intraocular lens.

Table 10.5 Difference between hydrophobic and hydrophilic lenses

Criteria	Hydrophobic lens	Hydrophilic lens
Water content	<1%	18–35%
PCO	Inhibit PCO	Higher incidence of PCO
RI	Higher, so are thinner	Lower than hydrophobic lens

Abbreviations: PCO, postoperative capsular opacification; RI, refractive index.

are bleached out by excessive UV rays, leading to erythropsia (vision appears to be through a red transparency). So, PMMA lenses were modified to filter out wavelengths below 400 nm (*UV light*) just as the crystalline lens does to protect the retina.

■ Power of IOL

12.5D in spectacle ≡ 18D for AC IOL and 21D for in-the-bag IOL.

Calculation of IOL power: It can be calculated by various formulae. The most commonly used formula is Sanders–Retzlaff–Kraff (**SRK**) formula which is:

$$P = A - 2.5L - 0.9\,K$$

Where, P = IOL power to produce emmetropia (D).

A = a constant which is specific for each lens type.

L = Axial length (mm) measured by A-scan ultrasonographic biometry.

K = Average of keratometry readings (measured by keratometer).

It is based upon the correlation between calculated and observed refractive error after IOL implantation.

Closer the lens implant is to the retina, the greater is the A constant. Therefore, the A constant is greatest with PC IOLs.

Other IOL power calculation formulae are:
- Holladay 1: Holladay 2
- SRK 2: SRK-T
- Hoffer Q: Binkhorst 1

■ Choice of Aphakic Correction in Children

Spectacles are prescribed in cases of bilateral aphakia wherein anisometropia does not represent a problem. Most of these patients develop good visual acuity with spectacles.

Contact lenses provide a better optical correction than spectacles. However, management of cataract by contact lenses in children can be very difficult.

IOL: Implanting an IOL in a growing eye is not an ideal solution, but it is currently the most practical one. Residual refractive error is corrected with spectacles.

■ Selection of IOL

The rapid growth of eye during the first 2 years of life makes an effective choice difficult. PMMA lenses are used for children. *Overall diameter should not exceed 12 mm* because average adult ciliary sulcus diameter rarely exceeds 11.5 mm. Oversized IOLs act like loaded springs and can dislocate (**Flowchart 10.8**).

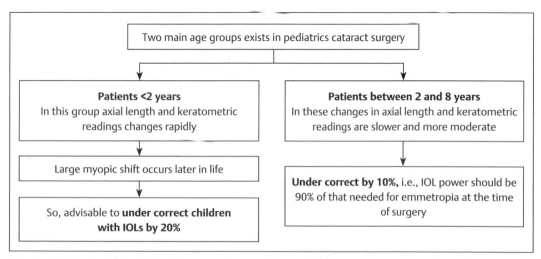

Flowchart 10.8 Algorithm for the selection of IOL in children. Abbreviation: IOL, intraocular lens.

Postoperative Care

Residual refractive error is corrected by spectacles. A patch over sound eye is advised in infants with unilateral pseudophakia and worn for half their waking hours until 4 to 5 years of age. Thereafter, patch time can be reduced gradually until 10 to 12 years of age. At the age of 3 years, bifocal lens with addition of + 3D is prescribed in the pseudophakic eye. Visual outcome depends largely on type of cataract, timing of cataract, quality of surgery and amblyopia management. Binocularity is usually poor in these cases; however, some gross stereosis can be expected.

11 The Glaucoma

Aqueous Humor Dynamics 257

Aqueous Humor 261

Intraocular Pressure 262

Classification of Glaucoma 265

Clinical Examination of Glaucoma 265

Antiglaucoma Drugs 280

Primary Open-Angle Glaucoma 288

Normal-Tension Glaucoma 292

Ocular Hypertension 292

Primary Angle-Closure Glaucoma 293

Secondary Glaucoma 298

Childhood Glaucoma 311

■ Aqueous Humor Dynamics (PY10.17)

Aqueous humor is a clear fluid occupying both anterior and posterior chambers of the eye. It is continuously secreted and drained out of the eye. IOP (intraocular pressure) is determined by the rate of aqueous secretion and rate of its outflow. The study of glaucoma deals primarily with the consequences of elevated IOP. Therefore, aqueous humor dynamics is necessary to understand the pathophysiological mechanism of glaucoma (**Fig. 11.1**). Two main structures related to aqueous humor dynamics are ciliary body, which is the site of aqueous secretion, and limbal region, which is the site of aqueous outflow.

■ Applied Anatomy (AN41.2)

Ciliary Body

The *ciliary processes* are the actual site of aqueous production. Each ciliary process is lined by *outer pigmented epithelial layer* and *inner nonpigmented*

epithelial layer which contain mitochondria, Na$^+$-K$^+$ ATPase, and carbonic anhydrase. Ciliary processes are supplied by branches from major arterial circle which end in capillary network. Capillaries of ciliary processes are fenestrated. The fenestrated capillaries allow easy passage of fluid and macromolecules but tight junctions between adjacent nonpigmented epithelial cells together with nonfenestrated iris vessels constitute the *blood–aqueous barrier* (**Fig. 11.2a**).

To reach posterior chamber, constituents of aqueous must traverse capillary wall, stroma of ciliary processes, and both epithelia.

Limbal Region

Limbus is the transition zone between cornea and sclera with an indentation on its inner surface called *scleral sulcus*. Scleral sulcus has a sharp posterior margin called *scleral spur* and a sloping anterior wall that extends to peripheral cornea. Scleral sulcus is bridged by a sieve-like structure called *trabecular meshwork* which converts the sulcus into a tube called *Schlemm canal*. Where

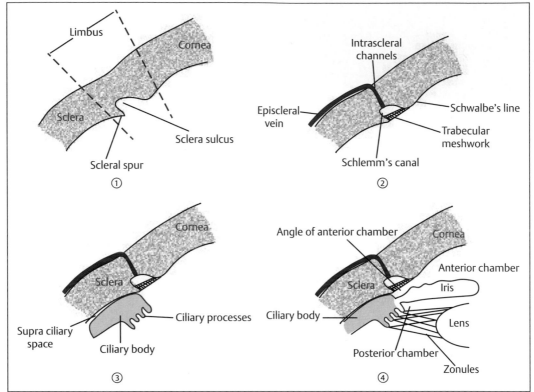

Fig. 11.1 Stepwise construction of structures involved in aqueous humor dynamics. (1) Limbus is the transition zone between cornea and sclera on the inner side of which is an indentation called scleral sulcus. Scleral sulcus has a sharp posterior margin called scleral spur. (2) Trabecular meshwork bridges the scleral sulcus and converts it into Schlemm canal which is connected by intrascleral channels to episcleral veins. A ridge is created at the insertion of meshwork into the peripheral cornea known as Schwalbe line. Thus, the main route of aqueous outflow is formed comprising trabecular meshwork, Schlemm canal, intrascleral channels, and episcleral veins. (3) The ciliary body attaches to scleral spur creating a potential space between itself and sclera called supraciliary space/suprachoroidal space. The ciliary processes are the site of aqueous production at the inner and anterior portion of ciliary body. (4) The iris is inserted into the ciliary body which is visible between the scleral spur and the root of iris. The lens is suspended by the suspensory ligaments from the ciliary body. The angle formed by the iris and cornea is called the angle of anterior chamber.

the trabecular meshwork inserts into peripheral cornea, a ridge is formed called *Schwalbe line.* Schlemm canal is connected by *intrascleral channels* to the *episcleral veins* (**Fig. 11.2b**).

Iris inserts into anterior side of ciliary body leaving a part of ciliary body between root of iris and the scleral spur.

Iris separates aqueous compartment into posterior chamber and anterior chamber.

Angle of anterior chamber is a peripheral recess formed by:
- Root of iris and part of ciliary body—posteriorly.
- Scleral spur and trabecular meshwork—anteriorly.

Longitudinal fibers of ciliary muscle attach at scleral spur which insert into suprachoroidal lamina (fibers connecting choroid and sclera) as far back as equator.

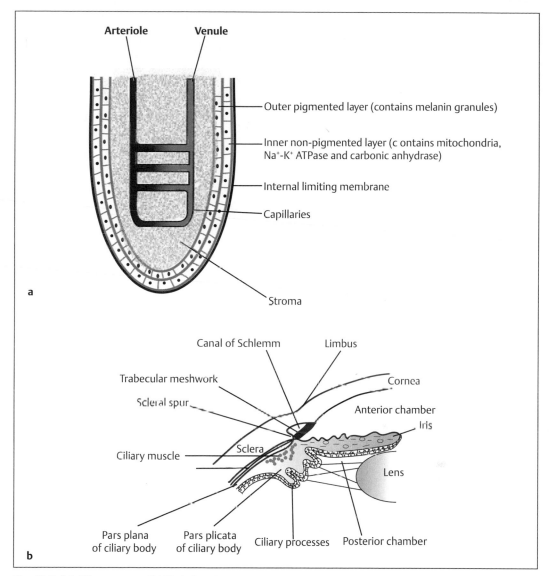

Fig. 11.2 (a) Ciliary process. **(b)** Limbal region.

■ Applied Physiology (PY10.17)

It involves aqueous formation and aqueous outflow.

Aqueous Formation

Aqueous is formed in ciliary processes by two processes, namely, *passive secretion* (by ultrafiltration and diffusion) and *active secretion* (by nonpigmented epithelium) (**Flowchart 11.1**).

Passive Secretion

It constitutes ultrafiltration and diffusion. Ultrafiltration from capillaries of ciliary processes depends on capillary hydrostatic pressure, plasma oncotic pressure, and level of IOP.

Lipid-soluble substances that easily penetrate cell membranes readily move by diffusion.

Active Secretion

Certain substances are actively transported (secreted) across blood–aqueous barrier formed by inner nonpigmented epithelium which contains mitochondria, Na$^+$-K$^+$ ATPase and carbonic anhydrase. Substances that are actively transported include Na$^+$, K$^+$, Cl$^-$, HCO^{3-}, ascorbic acid, and amino acids.

Control of Aqueous Formation

Aqueous formation is subject to endogenous influences. Humoral or neurohumoral mechanisms influence the rate of aqueous formation. Ciliary epithelium is not innervated but ciliary body vessels have a dense adrenergic innervation. Catecholamines released from sympathetic nerve endings diffuse to adrenergic receptors on ciliary epithelium and aqueous humor secretion is regulated. The fluctuation in the rate of aqueous formation accounts for diurnal variations in IOP.

Aqueous Outflow

Aqueous formed by ciliary body is secreted into posterior chamber which circulates into anterior chamber via pupil and is drained out by two routes:

- Trabecular (conventional) route.
- Uveoscleral (unconventional) route.

Trabecular Outflow

It accounts for 75 to 90% of aqueous outflow.

Route

Aqueous escapes through drainage channels at the angle of anterior chamber (**Flowchart 11.2**).

It is a pressure sensitive route so that increasing the pressure head will increase outflow.

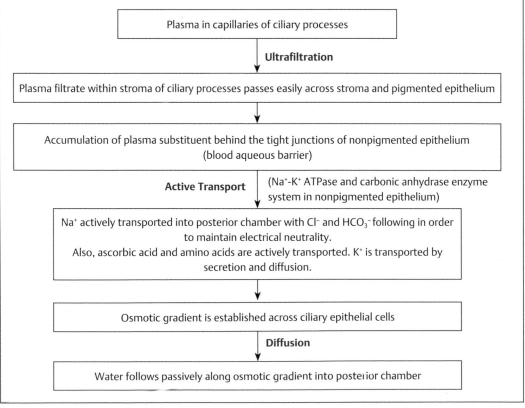

Flowchart 11.1 Algorithm depicting aqueous formation.

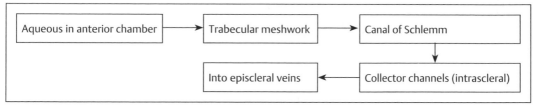

Flowchart 11.2 Main route of aqueous outflow.

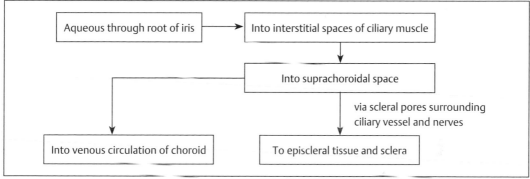

Flowchart 11.3 Uveoscleral route of aqueous outflow.

The spaces in trabecular meshwork sheets progressively decrease in size moving outwards. The extracellular spaces contain mucopolysaccharide, collagen, and elastic components which offer the greatest resistance to the aqueous outflow. Schlemm canal lies circumferentially in scleral sulcus, i.e., it is a 360-degree channel lined by endothelium. Endothelium of its inner wall contains giant vacuoles while the outer wall of the canal contains openings of large collector channels (intrascleral channels). There are two systems (direct and indirect systems) of intrascleral channels connecting Schlemm canal to *episcleral veins*:

Direct system: Intrascleral vessels (aqueous veins) drain directly into episcleral veins.

Indirect system: Intrascleral vessels form an intrascleral plexus before draining into episcleral veins.

Mechanism of Aqueous Outflow

The mechanism of outflow across **inner wall endothelium of Schlemm canal** is partially understood. The most accepted theory is **vacuolation theory**. Initially, the vacuole is formed by the infolding of basal surface of endothelial cell. A progressive enlargement of this infolding leads to the formation of macrovacuolar structure which eventually opens on the luminal aspect of endothelium. Thus, temporary vacuolar transcellular channel are formed which drains the bulk of aqueous humor down the pressure gradient. Finally, the basal infolding is occluded and the cell returns to nonvacuolated stage.

Uveoscleral Outflow

It is an unconventional outflow accounting for remaining 10 to 25% of aqueous outflow. It is a pressure-independent route. **Flowchart 11.3** describes the route of aqueous outflow through uveoscleral route.

Effect of Cholinergic Pathway on Aqueous Outflow

Parasympathetic fibers originate from Edinger–Westphal nucleus to innervate ciliary muscle (**Flowchart 11.4**).

▆ Aqueous Humor

The aqueous humor is a transparent fluid similar to plasma but the blood–aqueous

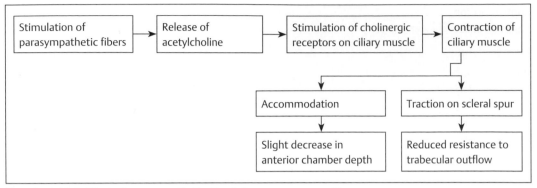

Flowchart 11.4 Effect of parasympathetic stimulation on aqueous outflow.

Table 11.1 Physiological properties of aqueous humor	
Features	**Properties**

• Refractive index
• Functions
 	
• Viscosity
• Density
• Volume
• Osmolarity
• pH
• Composition
	• 1.336, slightly lower than that of cornea.
	• It nourishes avascular structures of the eye (cornea and lens), maintains proper IOP and also provides transparent medium as a part of optical system of eye.
	• 1.025–1.040 relative to water.
	• It is slightly greater than that of water. Specific gravity of aqueous is 1.002–1.004.
	• It is 0.25 mL in anterior chamber and 0.06 mL in posterior chamber.
	• Aqueous is slightly hyperosmotic to plasma.
	• It is 7.2 (*alkaline*) but acidic relative to plasma.
	• **Water** constitutes 99.9% of normal aqueous.
	• Two most striking characteristics of aqueous compared to plasma are:
	  ◇ Marked excess of **ascorbate**: 15 times greater than that of arterial plasma.
	  ◇ Marked deficit of **protein**: 0.02% in aqueous and 7% in plasma. Blood–aqueous barrier normally limits the total protein content of aqueous. A/G ratio is several times higher in aqueous as compared to that of plasma due to exclusion of heavy globulins from aqueous by blood–aqueous barrier.
	• Cornea and lens take up **glucose** from aqueous, so there is slight deficit of glucose in aqueous relative to plasma.
	• **Lactic acid** is released by cornea and lens into aqueous, so there is slight excess of lactic acid in aqueous relative to plasma.
	• **Other constituents** are amino acids, norepinephrine, HCO_3^-, Cl^-, Na^+, K^+, oxygen in dissolved state, urea, nitric oxide, sodium hyaluronate, and tissue plasminogen activator.

barrier is responsible for differences in chemical composition between the plasma and the aqueous humor. Properties of aqueous humor are listed in **Table 11.1**.

■ Intraocular Pressure

Intraocular pressure (IOP, the pressure inside eyeball) is determined by the rate of aqueous formation and the rate of its outflow. Normally, there is a balance between formation and drainage of aqueous. Normal range of IOP is 11 to 21 mm Hg with a mean of 16 mm Hg, and 21 mm Hg is considered the upper limit of normal IOP.

■ Factors Affecting IOP

IOP is dependent on ocular, genetic, systemic and certain other factors.

Ocular Factors

IOP is a function of aqueous formation and its drainage. The changes in IOP are caused either by alterations in aqueous formation or alterations in aqueous outflow.

Alterations in Aqueous Formation

Aqueous formation may increase or decrease. *Normal rate of aqueous formation* is 2.4 ± 0.6 µL/min approx. No condition of excess aqueous formation has been observed.

Increased Aqueous Formation

It depends upon the following factors:

- Capillary hydrostatic pressure: Rise in capillary hydrostatic pressure causes rise in IOP and vice versa.
- Osmotic pressure of blood: Hypotonicity induces rise in IOP as in water drinking test and hypertonicity induces a fall in IOP.
- Permeability of capillaries: **Flowchart 11.5** explains the mechanism of rise in IOP due to increased aqueous formation.

Decreased Aqueous Formation

It results due to the following factors:

- Drugs: For example, β-blockers, carbonic anhydrase inhibitors (CAIs), and sympathomimetics. Sympathomimetics cause vasoconstriction leading to reduced ultrafiltration and decreased aqueous formation.
- Detachment of ciliary body.
- Retinal detachment.

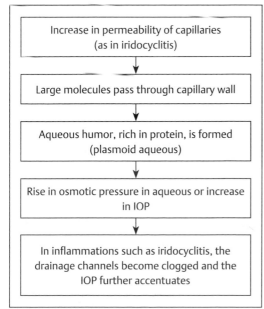

Flowchart 11.5 Effect of iridocyclitis on intraocular pressure (IOP).

- Cyclocryotherapy: It is a cyclodestructive procedure.

Alterations in Aqueous Outflow

Aqueous outflow may increase or decrease.

Increased outflow: Parasympathomimetics (e.g., pilocarpine) cause ciliary muscle contraction which results in traction on scleral spur because of its attachment. IOP decreases due to increased outflow.

Decreased outflow (increased resistance): Aqueous flows from posterior chamber via pupil into anterior chamber and mostly drained through trabecular route. Obstruction to aqueous flow may occur either at pupil or angle of anterior chamber where it may be pre-trabecular, trabecular, or post-trabecular (**Fig. 11.3**).

Genetic Factors

IOP is under hereditary influence so that first-degree relatives of patients with primary open-angle glaucoma (POAG) have higher IOP.

Systemic Factors

Diabetes mellitus and systemic hypertension are the two most common systemic diseases that have been implicated as risk factors for POAG.

Myotonic dystrophy results in reduced aqueous production and increased outflow by uveoscleral route from atrophy of ciliary muscle. So, IOP is markedly low in myotonic dystrophy.

Other Factors

Age—IOP generally increases with age. Thus, increasing age is a major risk factor for glaucoma.

General anesthesia is usually associated with reduction in IOP but ketamine elevate IOP.

Succinyl choline causes extraocular muscle contraction and intraocular vasodilatation resulting in transient increase in IOP.

Corticosteroids may cause IOP elevation.

Exertional influences: Valsalva maneuver elevates episcleral venous pressure (EVP) and IOP. Prolonged exercise lowers the IOP.

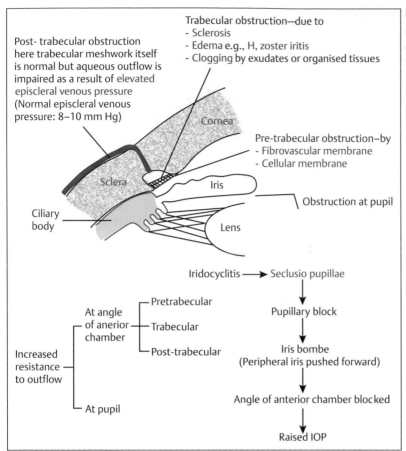

Post- trabecular obstruction here trabecular meshwork itself is normal but aqueous outflow is impaired as a result of elevated episcleral venous pressure (Normal episcleral venous pressure: 8–10 mm Hg)

Trabecular obstruction—due to
- Sclerosis
- Edema e.g., H, zoster iritis
- Clogging by exudates or organised tissues

Cornea

Pre-trabecular obstruction–by
- Fibrovascular membrane
- Cellular membrane

Sclera

Iris

Obstruction at pupil

Ciliary body

Lens

Fig. 11.3 Sites of increased resistance to aqueous outflow. Abbreviation: IOP, intraocular pressure.

Iridocyclitis ⟶ Seclusio pupillae

Increased resistance to outflow ┬ At angle of anerior chamber ┬ Pretrabecular
                               │   ├ Trabecular
                               │   └ Post-trabecular
                               └ At pupil

Pupillary block
↓
Iris bombe
(Peripheral iris pushed forward)
↓
Angle of anterior chamber blocked
↓
Raised IOP

■ Diurnal Variation of IOP

IOP is subjected to cyclic fluctuations throughout the day. Normally, diurnal variation up to 5 mm Hg occurs. Fluctuations in IOP of >8 mm Hg are considered to be pathologic even though the reading may fall within normal limits (21 mm Hg).

IOP is maximum in morning hours between 8 a.m. and 12 p.m. and lower in afternoon and evening. So, a single normal reading, particularly if taken during late afternoon, is of no value and may be misleading (**Fig. 11.4**).

Mechanism of diurnal IOP variation has been related to the diurnal variation of plasma cortisol.

■ Postural Variation of IOP

IOP increases when changing from sitting to supine position.

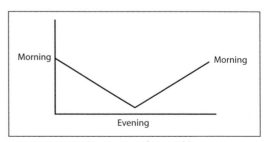

Morning   Morning

Evening

Fig. 11.4 Diurnal variation of IOP. Abbreviation: IOP, intraocular pressure.

Total body inversion (whole body head down tilt) leads to a further increase in IOP (greater in glaucomatous eyes) and appears to be related to the elevated EVP. Thus, obtaining clinical history on the type of exercise (yoga and inversion in particular) may be relevant for the patients with glaucoma.

■ Classification of Glaucoma (OP6.6, 6.7)

Glaucoma is a group of condition associated with characteristic optic neuropathy and visual field defects. Glaucoma is frequently but not invariably associated with raised IOP. Normal range of IOP is 11 to 21 mm Hg. If IOP is more than 21 mm Hg (up to 30 mm Hg) but without any detectable glaucomatous damage, the condition is termed as "ocular hypertension." If IOP is less than 21 mm Hg and characteristic optic disc changes and visual field defects of glaucoma occur with normal or low IOP, the condition is termed as **normal tension glaucoma (NTG)**, also referred to as "low-tension glaucoma." Thus, raised IOP is the most important risk factor for development of glaucoma, but not always. Glaucoma may be developmental or acquired.

Based upon etiology, glaucoma may be primary or secondary glaucoma.

Primary glaucoma: In primary glaucoma, elevation of IOP is not associated with other ocular or systemic disorder. It is typically bilateral and probably has a genetic basis.

Secondary glaucoma: It is secondary to ocular or systemic disorder. It may be unilateral or bilateral. It may be developmental and may have a genetic basis or may be acquired.

Based upon mechanism, glaucoma may be open-angle glaucoma or angle-closure glaucoma.

With an emphasis upon etiology and mechanism, glaucoma can be classified as follows:

- **Primary glaucoma**: It may be:
  ◊ Open-angle glaucoma: *With raised IOP*, it is known as primary open-angle glaucoma (**POAG**).
  ◊ *With normal IOP*, it is known as normal-tension glaucoma (**NTG**).
  ◊ Angle-closure glaucoma: Primary angle-closure glaucoma (**PACG**).
- **Secondary glaucoma**: It may be:
  ◊ Secondary open-angle glaucoma.
  ◊ Secondary angle-closure glaucoma.
- **Developmental glaucoma.**

■ Clinical Examination of Glaucoma (OP6.6, 6.7)

The clinical examination of glaucoma is vital to make the diagnosis, which includes:
- Tonometry to record accurate IOP.
- Gonioscopy to identify angle pathology.
- Optic nerve head (ONH) examination.
- Visual field examination by perimetry.
- Retinal nerve fiber layer (RNFL) analysis by OCT.

■ Measurement of IOP: Tonometry and Tonography

Tonometry is essential for the diagnosis of glaucoma and also for monitoring of antiglaucoma medications.

Assessment of IOP can be done digitally or by an instrument called "Tonometer."

Digital assessment of IOP (digital tonometry) is a qualitative method. The patient is asked to look down and the two fingers (tips of index finger) are placed a short distance from one another just above the superior tarsal plate. IOP is assessed in the same manner by testing the fluctuations.

If fluctuations are feeble or absent, IOP is high and if the globe gives a feeling of water bag, IOP is low.

Assessment of IOP by tonometer works behind the principle that the force necessary to deform a globe is directly related to the pressure within that globe.

According to the shape of deformation, tonometers are of two basic types:
- Indentation tonometer.
- Applanation tonometer.

Indentation Tonometry

It is done by Schiotz tonometer. The shape of deformation with this type of tonometer is a truncated cone. It is based on the principle that a plunger will indent a soft eye more than a hard eye.

Schiotz Tonometer

It consists of the following structures:
- *Foot plate* which rests on the cornea.
- *Weighted plunger,* which moves freely within a shaft, that ends in foot plate. A 5.5 g weight is permanently fixed to plunger, which can be increased 7.5 and 10 g by adding additional weights. Plunger indents the cornea.
- A *bent lever* with *short arm* which rests on upper end of plunger *and* a *long arm* acting as a pointer needle move on a scale (**Fig. 11.5**). The amount of indentation of cornea by plunger is indicated by the movement of pointer needle on the scale and the reading is converted into mm Hg by using a special conversion table. Generally, using the standardized plunger weight of 5.5 g, the normal eyes give scale readings

of **5 to 8 units** and high-pressure eyes read <4 units.

Method of Schiotz Tonometry

Following are the steps of Schiotz tonometry:
- Sterilize foot plate and lower end of plunger with acetone, ether.
- Ask the patient to lie down in supine position (**Fig. 11.6**).
- Cornea is anesthetized with 4% xylocaine or 0.5% proparacaine.
- Patient is asked to look at ceiling and lids are gently retracted.
- Foot plate of tonometer is placed over corneal surface.
- Scale reading is noted and converted into mm Hg with conversion table.

Advantages of Schiotz tonometer are that it is cheap, easy to use, convenient to carry, does not require a slit lamp, and may be used in operation room.

There are potential sources of error with indentation tonometry due to ocular (scleral) rigidity, accommodation, and contraction of extraocular muscles.

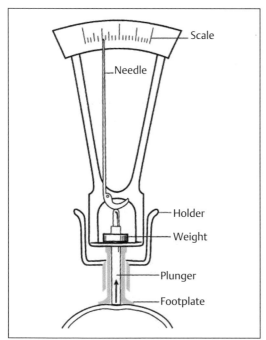

Fig. 11.5 Parts of Schiotz tonometer. Source: Intraocular Pressure and Tonometry. In: Morrison J, Pollack I, ed. Glaucoma: Science and Practice. 1st Edition. Thieme; 2002.

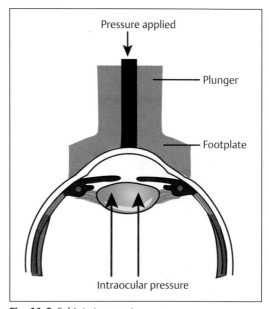

Fig. 11.6 Schiotz tonometry.

Ocular infection or discharge, corneal abrasion, marked nystagmus, corneal scarring, and blepharospasm serve as the probable contraindications of indentation tonometry.

Potential Sources of Error with Indentation Tonometry

- Errors due to ocular rigidity: The indentation is dependent on IOP and the distensibility of the ocular walls (ocular rigidity). Conversion table is based on an "average" coefficient of ocular rigidity. Difference in ocular rigidity among different eyes gives false IOP measurements.

  In *low-ocular (scleral) rigidity*, small force of indentation is required giving the falsely low IOP reading while in high ocular (scleral) rigidity large force of indentation is required and the falsely high IOP is measured. Thus, IOP measured by Schiotz tonometer is inaccurate because of variations in ocular rigidity.
- Errors due to accommodation: Practically, as soon as tonometer is put on cornea there is a tendency of patient to look at the tonometer and accommodation comes into play. The use of miotics also causes accommodation. Accommodation causes contraction of ciliary muscle and pull on trabecular meshwork. It increases the facility of aqueous outflow and results in falsely low IOP reading.
- Errors due to contraction of extraocular muscles (EOM): Contraction of EOM causes false impression of high IOP. So, because of many potential sources of error, Schiotz tonometry largely has been replaced by applanation tonometry.

Applanation Tonometry

It is more accurate than indentation tonometry. It assesses the force required to flatten (or applanate) the standard area of cornea, disturbing relatively little aqueous. **Goldmann applanation tonometer (AT)** is most popular and used with slit lamp. When it flattens (applanates)

the area having a diameter of 3.06 mm, the factor of ocular rigidity is eliminated and a little amount of aqueous is displaced. Thus, AT does not influence the IOP measurement and records IOP more accurately than Schiotz tonometer. It is based on Imbert–Fick principle (**Fig. 11.7**), which states that

Pressure inside the sphere (P) =

$$\frac{Force\ required\ to\ flatten\ the\ surface\ of\ sphere\ (F)}{Area\ of\ flattening\ (A)}$$

$$IOP\ (mm\ Hg) = F(gm) \times 10$$

Grams of force applied to flattened 3.06 mm diameter of cornea multiplied by 10 is directly converted to mm Hg.

The shape of deformation with AT is simple flattening.

Applanation Tonometer

Goldman AT is a very accurate variable force tonometer. It is mounted on a slit lamp. It consists of a plastic biprism attached by a rod to a housing which contains a coil spring and series of levers that are used to adjust the force of biprism against the cornea. Biprism on contact with cornea creates two half circles, one above and one below the horizontal midline. These semicircles are easy to view with a cobalt blue light after fluorescein application in conjunctival sac (**Fig. 11.8**).

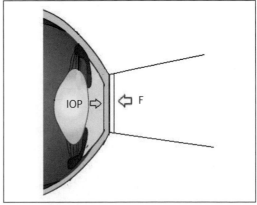

Fig. 11.7 Imbert–Fick principle. F, force required to flatten the surface of sphere; IOP, intraocular pressure.

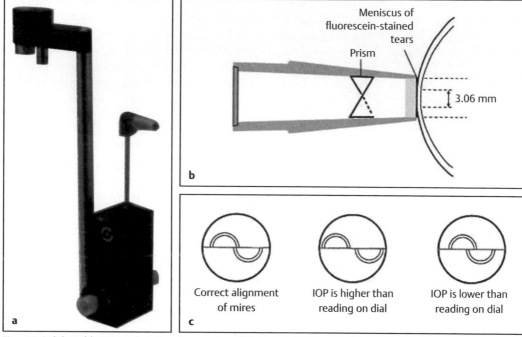

Fig. 11.8 (a) Goldman applanation tonometer. **(b)** The Goldmann applanation tonometer produces a tear film meniscus when the tip contacts the cornea. **(c)** The biprism splits the view of the circular meniscus into semicircles, which are aligned at their inner edges once the tip flattens a corneal area with diameter of 3.06 mm as shown in (b). Source (b, c) (a, b): Intraocular Pressure and Tonometry. In: Morrison J, Pollack I, ed. Glaucoma: Science and Practice. 1st Edition. Thieme; 2002. Abbreviation: IOP, intraocular pressure.

Technique of Using Goldman Applanation Tonometer

- Patient is positioned at slit lamp after anesthetizing cornea with topical preparation.
- Fluorescein strip is applied in conjunctival sac to stain tear film.
- Cobalt blue light from slit lamp is projected obliquely at prism.
- Biprism is advanced until it touches the apex of cornea.
- When biprism touches the cornea, two fluorescent semicircles will be seen. These semicircles represent the fluorescent-stained tear film touching the upper and lower outer halves of prism.

- Force against cornea is adjusted by rotating adjustment knob (dial) until inner margins of semicircles overlap. Inner margins of semicircle overlap when 3.06 mm of cornea is applanated.
- IOP is determined by reading on dial × 10.

Types of Applanation Tonometer

There are two types of AT, namely constant force AT and variable force AT. In constant force AT, a constant force (weight) is applied to the cornea and IOP is estimated by measuring the diameter of flattened area of the cornea, e.g., Maklakov AT. Variable force AT measures the force that is required to flatten a standard area (3.06 mm) of corneal surface. For example, Goldmann AT (slit-lamp mounted) and Perkin AT (handheld tonometer).

Sources of Error in Applanation Tonometry

- *Amount of fluorescein*: Appropriate amount of fluorescein is important because width of semicircles influences the reading. Excessive fluorescein causes thick (wide) semicircles with small radius and falsely high IOP estimation while insufficient fluorescein causes thin semicircles with large radius and falsely low IOP estimation.

  Improper vertical alignment (one semicircle larger than the other) will also lead to a falsely high IOP estimation (**Fig. 11.9**).

- *Central corneal thickness* (**CCT**): Calculations of IOP in Goldmann applanation tonometry assume that average CCT is 530 to 545 μm. Deviations from this value are a source of errors.

  Thick corneas due to corneal edema are associated with *falsely low IOP readings*.

  Thick corneas secondary to other processes (i.e., from increased collagen fibrils) give a *falsely high IOP reading*.

  Thin corneas usually give *falsely low IOP readings*. In refractive surgery (LASIK), cornea becomes thinner and the measured IOP is low.

Other Tonometers

Perkins tonometer: It is a handheld applanation tonometer and uses Goldmann prism. It does not require slit lamp, so can be used in anesthetized patients or reclining patients (**Fig. 11.10**).

Tono-Pen: It is a digital, handheld, portable contact tonometer. It can measure IOP through a soft contact lens as well as in the eyes with scarred or irregular cornea.

Pneumotonometer: It is an electronic tonometer. The cornea is indented by flow of gas against a flexible diaphragm covering the sensing nozzle. Sensor measures air pressure and converts to a record of IOP on a paper strip.

Noncontact tonometer (NCT): It is based on the principle of applanation but, instead of using a prism, puff of air is used to flatten the cornea. The time required to flatten the cornea relates directly to the level of IOP. It may be portable (handheld pulsair NCT) or nonportable. Advantages of using NCT are:

- It does not require topical anesthesia.
- It is useful for screening by nonophthalmologists.

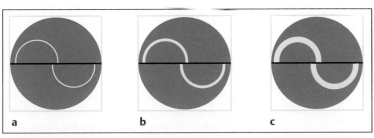

Fig. 11.9 Amount of fluorescein and semicircles during applanation tonometry. **(a)** Too thin semicircles. **(b)** Normal semicircles. **(c)** Too thick semicircles.

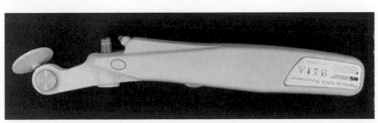

Fig. 11.10 Perkins tonometer.

- There is no risk of infection spread or of corneal abrasion.

Dynamic contour tonometer (DCT): It is a nonapplanating, slit-lamp mounted, contact tonometer and offers IOP measurements independent of corneal biomechanics such as CCT (central corneal thickness). Biomechanical changes induced by LASIK do not affect IOP measurements using DCT. It is based on contour matching. DCT has a contoured tonometer tip surface which contains an electronic pressure sensor. Pressure sensor generates an electric signal, the voltage of which is digitized by an analogue-to-digital converter and pressure in mm is displayed on the digital panel. It aims to match the contour of cornea and, therefore, corneal pathology does not interfere in recording of IOP.

Disease Transmission During Tonometry with Contact Tonometers

There is risk of transmission of infections such as:

- Adenovirus keratoconjunctivitis.
- Herpes simplex virus type I.
- Hepatitis B virus.
- Human immune deficiency virus (HIV)—AIDS.
- Bacterial conjunctivitis.

To reduce the risk of cross-infection, avoid tonometry in individuals with overt infection.

Disinfection of Tonometers

Sterilization of tonometers is essential. Wipe the tonometer tip with 3% hydrogen peroxide or 70% isopropyl alcohol and allow it to dry. It destroys HIV, adenovirus, and hepatitis virus. Other chemical disinfectants are:

- 1:1,000 merthiolate.
- 1:10 sodium hypochlorite.
- Ethylene oxide.

Tonography

It is a form of tonometry in which IOP is measured continuously over the course of 4 minutes with electric Schiotz tonometer placed on cornea. The measurement is recorded graphically as a continuous tracing on a paper strip.

Aim of tonography is to estimate the ease with which aqueous leaves the eye. This estimate is called facility of aqueous outflow (C). C value may be influenced by certain factors like IOP, increase in EVP, and variable ocular rigidity.

The weight of tonometer acts as a force and aqueous is expressed from the eye resulting in lowering of IOP.

■ Gonioscopy

Gonioscopy is the technique to visualize the angle of anterior chamber. The angle of anterior chamber cannot be visualized directly with slit lamp because of total internal reflection (**TIR**). For TIR, the angle must be greater than the critical angle which is 46.5 degree for cornea and the essential condition for TIR is that the light ray must pass from denser to rarer medium (**Fig. 11.11**). Problem of TIR at cornea–air interface is solved with a goniolens (a denser medium) placed in front of cornea. Now the light ray passes from rarer to denser medium.

Thus, goniolens eliminates TIR and angle of anterior chamber can be visualized. The contact lenses used for gonioscopy are called goniolenses. There are two types of goniolenses: direct and indirect types. Direct goniolenses provide direct view of angle, for example, Koeppe lens and Barkan lens. In indirect goniolenses, mirrors are used, so light rays are reflected by mirror in goniolens and provide an image of the opposite angle, e.g., Goldmann single mirror, Goldmann 3-mirror lens, and Zeiss 4-mirror lens (**Fig. 11.12**).

Goldmann 3-mirror lens contains two mirrors for the examination of fundus and one for the examination of angle. Goldmann lenses require

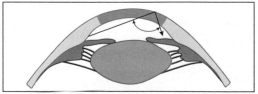

Fig. 11.11 Total internal reflection (TIR) from corneal surface.

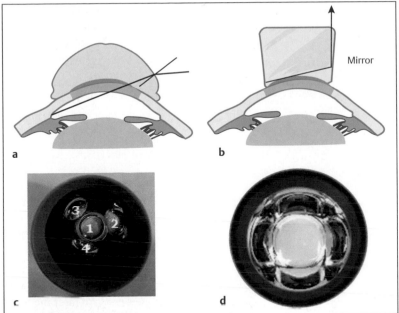

Fig. 11.12 Types of gonio-lenses. **(a)** Koeppe lens (a 50D concave lens). **(b)** Goldmann single-mirror lens. **(c)** Goldmann three-mirror lens. **(d)** Zeiss lens.

Mirror

a

b

c

d

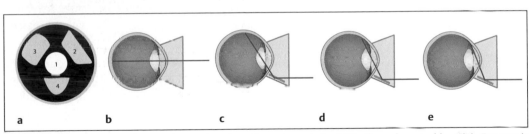

a   b   c   d   e

Fig. 11.13 (a) Parts of Goldmann three-mirror lens. Posterior pole is visible through central lens (1). Equator is visible through 73-degree largest mirror (2). Ora serrata is visible through 67-degree mirror (3). Angle of anterior chamber is visible through 59-degree smallest mirror (4). **(b)** Central lens. **(c)** 73-degree mirror. **(d)** 67-degree mirror. **(e)** 59-degree mirror.

the use of viscous solution to couple this lens to cornea (**Fig. 11.13**).

In *Zeiss 4-mirror lens*, each quadrant of angle is visualized with the opposite mirror. A coupling fluid is not required in Zeiss 4-mirror lens.

> **Goldmann 3-mirror lens** has a contact surface diameter of 12 mm. This large posterior diameter stabilizes the globe and is therefore suitable for laser trabeculoplasty but prevents the luxury of indentation gonioscopy. Contact surface of **Zeiss lens** has a diameter of 9 mm which does not stabilize the globe and *cannot be used* for laser trabeculoplasty but is useful for indentation gonioscopy.

Indentation Gonioscopy (Pressure Gonioscopy)

It is carried out if the angle appears narrowed. In indentation gonioscopy, lens is pressed against cornea and aqueous is displaced into the angle of anterior chamber. The peripheral iris is forced posteriorly, tending to open the angle more widely (**Flowchart 11.6**).

Thus, indentation gonioscopy allows easy distinction between appositional angle closure and synechial closure of angle.

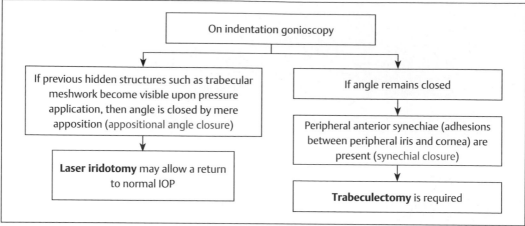

Flowchart 11.6 Significance of indentation gonioscopy.

Purposes of Gonioscopy

Diagnostic gonioscopy: It facilitates the identification of abnormal angle structures and estimation of the width of angle.

Surgical gonioscopy: It is done to visualize the angle during procedures such as laser trabeculoplasty and goniotomy.

Cleaning of Goniolenses

Goniolenses are a potential source of infection. These are disinfected in the same way as tonometer heads.

Gonioscopic Identification of Angle Structures

Starting posteriorly at the root of iris and moving anteriorly toward cornea, following structures can be identified gonioscopically in a normal angle (**Fig. 11.14**):

- Ciliary body band (anteromedial surface of ciliary body): It stands out as a gray or dark brown band.
- Scleral spur: It is usually seen as a prominent white band between ciliary body and trabecular meshwork and represents posterior lip of scleral sulcus. It is a very important landmark because in laser trabeculoplasty application of burns posterior to scleral spur will result in

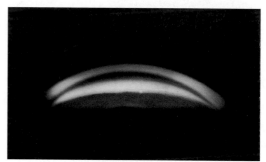

Fig. 11.14 Structures identified on gonioscopy. Source: History. In: Singh K, Smiddy W, Lee A, ed. Ophthalmology Review: A Case- Study Approach. 2nd Edition. Thieme; 2018.

uveitis with early rise in IOP and formation of peripheral anterior synechiae (PAS).
- Trabecular meshwork: It is faintly pigmented.
- Schwalbe line: It is seen as a glistening white line.

Grading of Angle Width

Gonioscopically, angle is graded according to the visibility of various angle structures. Following systems have been suggested to grade the angle width:

- Shaffer system.
- Scheie system.
- Spaeth system.

Shaffer grading system is the most commonly used system. It describes:

- Angle width in degree (angle between iris and trabecular meshwork).
- Anatomical structures visible.
- Type of angle.
- Clinical interpretation.

The system assigns a numerical grade (4–0) to each angle (**Table 11.2** and **Fig. 11.15**).

■ Optic Nerve Head (ONH) Analysis

ONH or intraocular part of optic nerve extends from the retinal surface to the posterior scleral surface. *The term ONH is generally preferred over optic disc because latter suggests a flat structure without depth.* However, the terms "disc" and "papilla" are frequently used for the portion of ONH that is clinically visible by ophthalmoscope.

Divisions of ONH

Optic cup is a central, depressed, pallor area of disc or ONH which represents the volume with partial or complete absence of axons. Its bottom is formed by lamina cribrosa. **Neuroretinal rim (NRR)** is the tissue between outer edge of cup and the disc margin. It represents the location of the bulk of axons. It has an orange-red color because of associated capillaries (**Fig. 11.16**).

Order of the width of NRR: inferior rim > superior rim > nasal rim > temporal rim (remembered by the acronym 'ISN T').

Grade	Angle width	Structures visible	Type of angle	Clinical interpretation
IV	35–45 degree	Ciliary body Scleral spur Trabecular meshwork Schwalbe's line	Wide open angle	Closure is impossible.
III	20–35 degree	Scleral spur Trabecular meshwork Schwalbe's line	Open angle	Closure is impossible.
II	10–20 degree	Trabecular meshwork Schwalbe's line	Moderately narrow angle	Angle closure is possible but unlikely.
I	0–10 degree	Schwalbe's line	Very narrow angle	High risk of angle closure.
0	0	None of the structure is visible (Iridocorneal contact)	Closed angle	Indentation gonioscopy with Zeiss goniolens is necessary to differentiate "appusitional" from "synechial" closure.

Table 11.2 Shaffer grading system of angle width

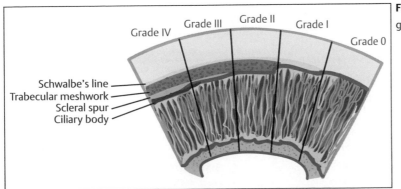

Fig. 11.15 Diagrammatic grading of angle width.

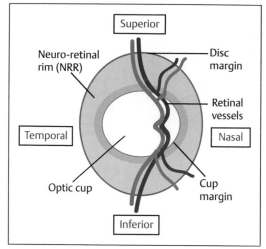

Fig. 11.16 Right normal optic nerve head (ONH).

As inferior NRR is broadest followed by superior, nasal, and temporal rims, so cup is *horizontally oval* in most of normal eyes. *Thus, a vertical cup should be considered suspicious.*

Border between optic cup and NRR is determined by contour and not by pallor. *Pallor* is the area of optic disc lacking small blood vessels or the maximum area of color contrast. *Cupping,* the border of optic cup, is determined by kinking (bending) of blood vessels as they cross the optic disc.

Diameter of optic cup is commonly expressed as a fraction of disc diameter both in vertical and horizontal meridian and is known as **cup-disc ratio (CDR)**.

$$CDR = \frac{\text{diameter of cup}}{\text{diameter of disc}}$$

Normal vertical CDR = **0.3**. CDR is genetically determined. A difference in CDR between two eyes of >0.2 should be regarded with suspicion until glaucoma has been excluded.

> Normally, *optic cup* is horizontal oval, so **in normal eyes**, horizontal CDR **>** vertical CDR. In glaucoma, vertical CDR increases faster than horizontal (because of large fenestrations in superior and inferior portions), so, **in glaucoma**, horizontal CDR **<** vertical CDR. *This is important for diagnosis of glaucoma.*

An enlarged cup may represent a normal physiological variant. An estimation of cup size alone is therefore of limited value in diagnosis of early glaucoma unless it is found to be increasing.

Blood vessels enter the disc centrally and then course nasally and follow the edge of cup. Central retinal artery is usually nasal to the vein.

ONH may be divided into four portions:
- Surface nerve fiber layer (NFL).
- Prelaminar region.
- Lamina cribrosa region: Lamina cribrosa consists of fenestrated sheets of scleral connective tissue through which the nerve fibers pass. Fenestrations in superior and inferior portions are large with thin connective tissue and glial cell support is not well. Therefore, initial damage occurs superiorly and inferiorly at ONH to produce characteristic arcuate defects.
- Retrolaminar region.

Changes in Neuroretinal Rim (NRR)

The disc changes in glaucoma range from focal loss of neural rim tissue with notching of NRR to diffuse rim damage with concentric enlargement of cup. Disc changes are typically progressive and asymmetric. *Order of involvement* in localized tissue loss—Localized loss of neural rim tissue begins usually in inferotemporal region of ONH and to a lesser extent in superotemporal region in early stages. As the glaucomatous process continues, temporal neural rim is typically involved after the vertical poles, with the nasal rim being the last to be affected.

Change in Optic Cup

Following changes are seen in optic cup due to glaucomatous changes:
- There occurs vertical enlargement of cup (vertical oval shape of cup) due to notching of NRR at lower and upper poles. So **vertical CDR > horizontal CDR** (in normal eyes, horizontal CDR > vertical CDR).
- Increase in CDR (normal CDR ≤ 0.3).
- Asymmetry of CDR of > 0.2 between the two eyes.

- Deepening of cup (excavation). There is increase in depth of cup leading to exposure of underlying lamina. The fenestrae of lamina cribrosa become visible due to loss of nerve fibers, referred to as *lamellar dot sign* (as fenestrae of lamina cribrosa have a dotlike appearance on ophthalmoscopy).
- Pallor-cup discrepancy: Initial enlargement may lead to a diffuse, shallow cupping with sloping margins and extending up to disc margins with retention of central pale cup, referred to as saucerization of cup. Thus, area of pallor appears smaller than area of cupping and may be an early sign of glaucoma (**Fig. 11.17**).

Vascular Changes

Following vascular changes are seen due to glaucomatous changes:

- Bayonetting of vessels: If progressive changes of glaucoma are not arrested, advanced glaucomatous cupping with loss of all neural rim tissue occurs. The vessels dive sharply backwards and then ascend up along the steep wall under the overhanging edge of the cup and bend again sharply to emerge at the disc margin (that resemble bayonet of a rifle), i.e., double angulation of blood vessels occur and is referred to as **Bayonetting of vessels**. This total cupping has also been called "bean pot cupping" because cross-sectional view reveals extreme posterior displacement of lamina cribrosa and undermining of disc margin.
- Baring of circumlinear blood vessels: In many normal ONH, one or two vessels may curve to outline a portion of physiologic cup and run along superior and inferior margins of cup (circumlinear vessels). With enlargement of cup, these circumlinear vessels may be "bared" from the margins of cup and come to lie on the floor of the optic cup. Baring of circumlinear vessels is an early sign of rim thinning and thus diagnostic of glaucoma.
- Disc hemorrhages (splinter hemorrhages): These are flame-shaped, usually near the margin of ONH. They typically cross the disc margin and extend on to the NFL. Their most common location is inferotemporal region.

They are *more common in* NTG than in patients with POAG and in glaucoma patients with diabetes, hypertension, and use of aspirin. They precede RNFL defects and visual field defects in glaucoma and are a sign of progressive disease.

■ Visual Field Analysis in Glaucoma

Glaucoma causes damage to ganglion cell axons at ONH which results in loss of retinal nerve fiber bundles. Therefore, *glaucoma causes mostly nerve fiber bundle defects* which may be diffuse, localized, or both. Retina is divided into temporal and nasal halves by a vertical line at fovea. Retina is also divided into superior and inferior halves by a horizontal meridian (raphe) that passes from fovea to temporal periphery. Fibers do not cross the horizontal meridian (**Fig. 11.18**). Important points for consideration in analysing visual field are:

- Fibers from macula pass straight to ONH forming **papillomacular bundle**.
- Fibers arising temporal to macular follow an arcuate path around papillomacular bundle to reach ONH.
- Fibers from nasal retina also pass straight to ONH (**Fig. 11.19**).

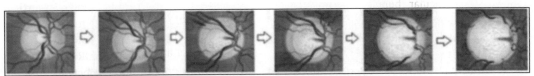

Fig. 11.17 Pictorial representation of the progression of glaucomatous cupping.

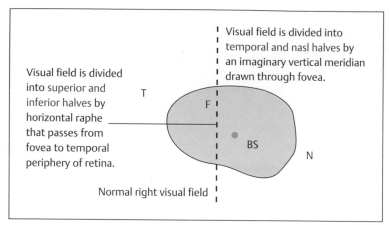

Visual field is divided into superior and inferior halves by horizontal raphe that passes from fovea to temporal periphery of retina.

Visual field is divided into temporal and nasl halves by an imaginary vertical meridian drawn through fovea.

Normal right visual field

Fig. 11.18 Divisions of right visual field. Abbreviations: BS, blind spot; F, foveola of retina.

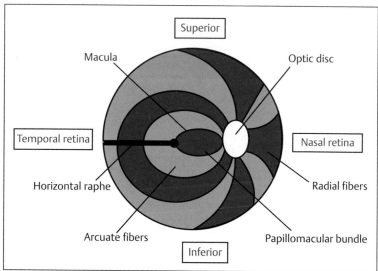

Fig. 11.19 Normal anatomy of retinal nerve fiber layer (RNFL).

Nerve Fiber Bundle (NFB) Field Defects in Glaucoma

The nature of nerve fiber bundle defects relates to the anatomy of RNFL and depends on the location of damaged nerve fibers. Therefore, nerve fiber bundle defects are of three main types: papillomacular bundle defects, arcuate NFB defects and nasal NFB defects. Characteristic features of nerve fiber bundle field defects are:

- NFB visual field defects respect the horizontal meridian especially in nasal portion of visual field corresponding to temporal retina.
- NFB defects have a tendency to be found in Bjerrum area, which is between 10 and 20 degrees from fixation.
- Typically, there is an abrupt change in sensitivity across the horizontal midline.

Papillomacular Defects

Papillomacular fibers are resistant to glaucomatous damage. Therefore, a central island of visual field is retained even in advanced glaucoma. A defect in this bundle of nerve fibers results in one of the following (**Fig. 11.20**):

- Central scotoma: A defect involving central fixation.
- Centrocecal scotoma: A central scotoma connected to the blind spot.
- Paracentral scotoma: These are the small isolated visual field defects between 2 and 10 degrees. Initially, these scotomas are relative but eventually become denser and larger forming an absolute defect in the center surrounded by a relative scotoma.

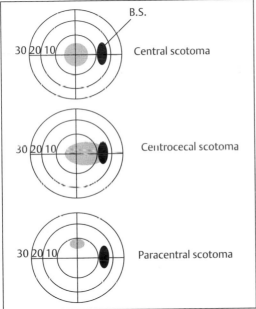

Fig. 11.20 Papillomacular defects, Abbreviation: B.S., blind spot.

Arcuate NFB Defects

Arcuate fibers are most sensitive to glaucomatous damage. Usually lower fibers are affected earlier than upper fibers in glaucoma. Because superior and inferior parts of lamina cribrosa contain larger pores and thinner connective tissue, superotemporal and inferotemporal parts of ONH are most vulnerable. Therefore, arcuate fibers are susceptible to damage and arcuate defects tend to occur first. These fibers do not cross horizontal raphe. Defect of these bundles may cause one of the following (**Fig. 11.21**):

- **Arcuate scotoma:** Arcuate scotoma starts from blind spot to reach the horizontal raphe, arching around fixation. These never cross horizontal raphe and may be superior or inferior arcuate scotoma.
- **Double arcuate** (Ring) **scotoma:** When arcuate scotomas both above and below the horizontal meridian are present, they join to form a double arcuate or ring scotoma.
- **Seidel scotoma:** Occasionally, the paracentral scotoma (early arcuate defect) may connect with blind spot to form a sickle-shaped scotoma, known as seidel scotoma, with concavity toward fixation point.
- **Roenne nasal step:** It is caused by an asymmetry in the rate of nerve fiber loss above and below the horizontal meridian in the nasal field which results in unequal contraction of peripheral isopters. A steplike defect is created where the nerve fibers meet along horizontal meridian.

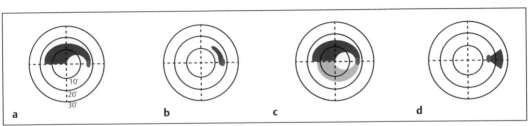

Fig. 11.21 Arcuate nerve fiber bundle (NFB) defects. **(a)** Arcuate (Bjerrum) scotoma. **(b)** Seidel scotoma. **(c)** Double arcuate (ring) scotoma with nasal step. **(d)** Temporal sector defect.

> **Differential diagnosis of arcuate scotomas**
>
> Although arcuate scotoma is usually associated with glaucoma, it is not pathognomonic because it can be found in other conditions too (especially when field and disc do not seem to correlate) such as **chorioretinal lesions (e.g.,** juxtapapillary retinochoroiditis, retinal artery occlusions); **ONH lesions** (e.g., Drusen of ONH, papillitis, colobomas) and **anterior optic nerve lesions** (e.g., pituitary adenoma, optico chiasmatic arachnoiditis).

Nasal NFB Defects

Fibers from nasal retina course in a straight fashion to ONH. A defect in this bundle results in a wedge-shaped temporal scotoma arising from blind spot and does not necessarily respect the temporal horizontal meridian which extends from foveola to temporal retinal periphery.

Other Visual Field Defects in Glaucoma

There are many other causes of these types of VF defects. These are:

- Generalized loss of retinal sensitivity and generalized constriction of visual field.
  ◊ Enlargement of blind spot.
  ◊ Baring of blind spot.

Generalized Constriction of Visual Field

The diffuse reduction in peripheral visual fields along with double arcuate scotoma results in **tubular vision** (only central vision remains). Causes of tubular vision are glaucoma, retinitis pigmentosa, and central retinal artery occlusion with sparing of cilioretinal artery.

Enlargement of Blind Spot

Enlargement of blind spot, due to depression of peripapillary retinal sensitivity, is also considered to be an early glaucomatous field change. However, it may be seen with other optic nerve or retinal disorder. So, it is not pathognomonic sign of glaucoma.

Baring of Blind Spot

Because the reduced sensitivity of peripapillary retina is greater in upper and lower poles, kinetic perimetry with very small test object may show a vertical elongation of blind spot and localized constriction of central visual field to exclude the blind spot (baring of blind spot). It is not specific for early detection of glaucoma as it may also be found in lens opacities, miosis, or aging process (**Fig. 11.22**).

Advanced Glaucomatous Field Defects

Visual field defects in uncontrolled glaucoma gradually progresses both centrally and peripherally except temporally. Therefore, a central island and a temporal island of vision are left in advanced glaucoma. *Temporal island of vision is more resistant* and may persist long after the central vision is lost. Temporal island of vision, too, will eventually be destroyed, if glaucoma is not controlled, resulting in no perception of light.

Diagnosis of a Glaucomatous Field Defect

Visual field loss in glaucoma is considered significant if one of the following is present on Humphrey perimetry:

- Glaucoma hemifield test (GHT) is abnormal. In GHT, sensitivity of five groups of test points above and below the horizontal midline is compared. These groups of points resemble the nerve fiber bundle pattern. The sensitivity is usually asymmetrical about the horizontal meridian in glaucoma.
  ◊ If asymmetry is more than 1% probability in one or more of the five groups, the visual field is abnormal.

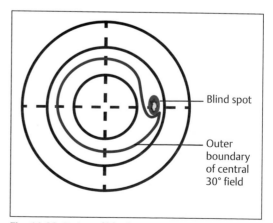

Fig. 11.22 Baring of blind spot.

◊ If asymmetry is within 1% probability in all the five regions but more than 3% in one or more regions, the visual field is regarded as borderline. GHT should be abnormal on at least two consecutive occasions.

- Pattern deviation plot shows three contiguous nonedge points having sensitivity with a probability of <5%, one of which should have a probability of <1%. Pattern standard deviation (PSD) is a measure of focal loss or variability within the field. The probability values indicate the significance of defects and are shown as <5%, <2%, <1%, and <0.5%. The lower the probability value the greater is its clinical significance.

Visual field defects in glaucoma can be graded based on the value of mean deviation (MD). MD is a measurement of overall field loss (**Table 11.3**).

■ Retinal Nerve Fiber Layer (RNFL) Analysis

Evaluation of RNFL is important in early diagnosis of glaucoma because RNFL defects can occur before disc changes and visual field defects. *Thus, RNFL defects due to axonal loss are useful in early detection of glaucomatous damage and in follow up for progression of glaucoma.*

Appearance of NFL

Normal human optic nerve is made up of 1 to 1.2 million axons of retinal ganglion cells which converge at optic disc. These axons make up the RNFL. Because NFL is the innermost retinal layer after internal limiting membrane (ILM), a short wavelength light that focuses more anteriorly

helps bring the RNFL into focus. NFL is best seen with 78D or 90D lens at slit lamp in a red-free light because this light does not penetrate beyond RNFL and is reflected back. In areas of RNFL loss, light gets absorbed by RPE and choroid and a contrast is created between normal and degenerated area. Normal RNFL reflects light and appears as bright striations while the area of RNFL loss provide a dark background due to absorption of light by RPE.

Diffuse loss of RNFL results in decreased visibility of RNFL which may be difficult to detect. There is increased visibility of retinal blood vessels which are normally embedded in NFL and partially obscured.

Thus, another indication of the loss of nerve fibers is increased visibility of retinal blood vessels.

Techniques for ONH and RNFL Analysis

Following techniques are helpful for the analysis of ONH and RNFL:

- *Fundus examination*: *Red-free* (green) *light* used either in direct ophthalmoscope or slit lamp with 78D or 90D lens makes the NFL easier to visualize.
- *Confocal scanning laser ophthalmoscopy* (CSLO): CSLO offers 3D imaging of ONH and NFL by using a focused laser beam. The **H**eidelberg **R**etinal **T**omograph (HRT) is the only commercially available confocal scanning laser ophthalmoscope.
- *Confocal scanning laser polarimetry.*
- *Optical coherence tomography* (OCT): OCT is a noninvasive, noncontact imaging system which provides cross-sectional images of retina and optic nerve. It is analogous to B-Scan ultrasonography but uses light instead of sound waves. OCT involves *low coherence infrared* (≈840 nm) diode light source and is *based on the principle of Michelson interferometry.* OCT images can be displayed as false-color. The different colors correspond to the different degree of reflectivity, *highly reflected light is brighter.*

Table 11.3 Grading of visual field defects in glaucoma on the basis of mean deviation	
Grading of visual field defects in glaucoma	**Value of mean deviation**
• Mild defect	<6 dB
• Moderate defect	<12 dB
• Severe defect	>12 dB

The *principal application of OCT* in glaucoma is:
- Measurement of RNFL thickness.
- Analysis of ONH.
- To monitor progression of glaucoma and response to treatment.

OCT is also used for diagnosis of macular pathology.

Antiglaucoma Drugs

Autonomic nervous system (ANS) has two divisions: sympathetic division (adrenergic neurons) and parasympathetic division (cholinergic neurons). The released neurotransmitters combine with specific receptors on postjunctional membrane and depending on its nature induce an excitatory or inhibitory response (**Flowchart 11.7** and **Table 11.4**).

Fig. 11.23 depicts that β_2-blockers, α_1 agonists, α_2 agonists, and CAIs all reduce secretion of aqueous by ciliary body and their site of action is ciliary process.

Classification of Antiglaucoma Drugs (PH1.58)

Antiglaucoma drugs could be classified as follows:
- **Cholinergic drugs** (direct parasympathomimetics): e.g., pilocarpine.

- **Adrenergic drugs**: These could be subdivided into adrenergic agonists and adrenergic antagonists.
- Adrenergic agonists:
  ◊ Nonselective (and β-agonists), e.g., epinephrine (adrenaline) and dipivefrine.
  ◊ Selective (-selective), e.g., clonidine, apraclonidine, and brimonidine.
- Adrenergic antagonists:
  ◊ Nonselective (blocks β_1 and β_2 receptors), e.g., timolol maleate, levobunolol, carteolol, and metipranolol.
  ◊ Selective, e.g., betaxolol (α β_1-cardioselective blocker).
- **Prostaglandin and prostamide analogues**: e.g., latanoprost, travoprost, bimatoprost, and unoprostone.
- **Carbonic anhydrase inhibitors**: These could be topical (e.g., dorzolamide and brinzolamide) or systemic (e.g., acetazolamide, dichlorphenamide, and methazolamide).
- **Hyperosmotic agents**: e.g., mannitol, glycerol, and isosorbide.

Basic Mechanism of Action of Antiglaucoma Drugs

Glaucoma therapy modulates IOP by decreasing aqueous humor inflow or by enhancing trabecular

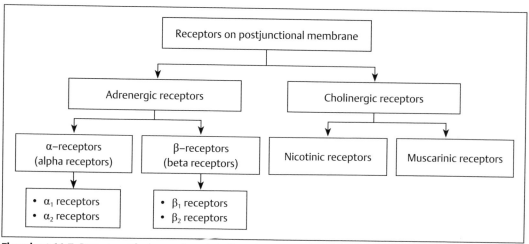

Flowchart 11.7 Receptors of adrenergic and cholinergic neurons on postjunctional membrane.

Table 11.4 Location of various receptors and effect of their stimulation

Receptors	Location	Effect of receptors stimulation
• α_1 **receptors stimulation**	• Radial muscle of iris • Ciliary blood vessels	• Mydriasis • Constriction of ciliary vessels resulting in decreased aqueous formation
• α_2 **receptors stimulation** • β_1 **receptors stimulation before heart muscle** • β_2 **receptors stimulation**	• Muller muscle • Ciliary epithelium • Heart muscle	• Lid retraction • Reduced aqueous secretion • Increased heart rate and cardiac output
• **Nicotinic receptors stimulation**	• Bronchial musculature • Ciliary epithelium • Striated muscle such as levator, orbicularis oculi and extraocular muscles	• Bronchodilatation • Increased aqueous secretion • Nicotinic agonists play no part in treatment of glaucoma
• **Muscarinic receptors stimulation**	• Sphincter pupillae • Ciliary muscle	• Miosis • Stimulation of these receptors causes contraction of ciliary muscle and increased outflow facility resulting in reduction of IOP

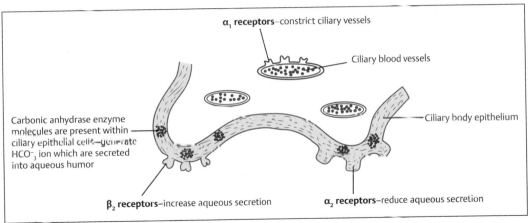

Fig. 11.23 Location of α_1, α_2, and β_2 adrenergic receptors and carbonic anhydrase enzyme molecules.

or uveoscleral outflow (**Flowchart 11.8** and **Fig. 11.24**).

Drugs That Decrease Aqueous Production

β-Blockers (Adrenergic Antagonists)

Mechanism of action: These antagonize the effects of catecholamines at β-receptors (**Flowchart 11.9**).

Efficacy

Initial lowering of IOP with β-blockers is very good but in some patients this pressure response decreases with time (tachyphylaxis). During sleep, there is significant dip in blood pressure with reduced perfusion pressure (Perfusion pressure = BP – IOP) and aqueous flow is normally less than half the daytime flow. Therefore, β-blockers have little effect during sleep.

As a general rule, if patient is already on a systemic β-blocker (oral β-blockers used for hypertension and angina), these also lower IOP and no additional effect is obtained if a topical β-blocker is used in patients on systemic β-blockers.

Side Effects

Ocular side effects include dry eye due to reduced aqueous tear secretion, corneal hypoesthesia, superficial punctuate keratopathy, and stinging.

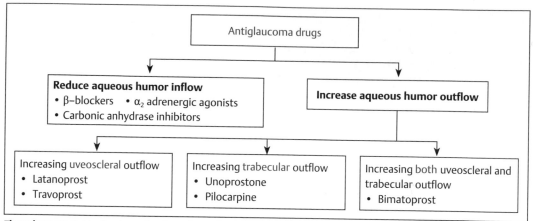

Flowchart 11.8 Mechanism of action of antiglaucoma drugs.

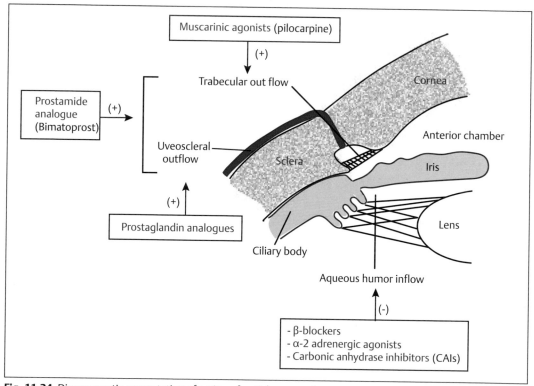

Fig. 11.24 Diagrammatic presentation of action of antiglaucoma drugs.

Systemic side effects occur due to absorption through nasolacrimal duct (NLD). So, these can be reduced by performing punctual occlusion for about 3 min after instillation of drops. Systemic side effects include:

Bronchopulmonary: Bronchospasm due to β_2 blocking action, so *contraindicated in* bronchial asthma and COPD (chronic obstructive pulmonary disease). Betaxolol offers advantage of having less bronchopulmonary side effects.

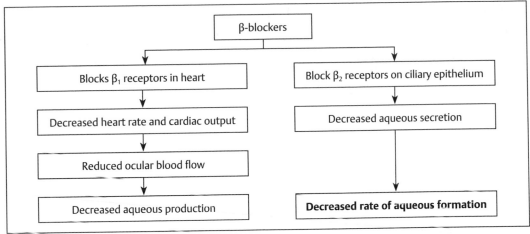

Flowchart 11.9 Mechanism of action of β-blockers.

Cardiac: Bradycardia and hypotension result from β₁ blockade, so contraindicated in congestive heart failure (CHF), bradycardia, and 2- and 3-degree heart block.

Dose

All topical β-blockers are administered twice a day. Long-acting preparations of timolol are also available and administered once daily.

Preparations

Following preparations of β-blockers could be used:

- Timolol maleate 0.25% and 0.5% drops.
- Levobunolol 0.5% drops.
- Carteolol 1% and 2% drops.
- Metipranolol 0.3% drops.
- Betaxolol 0.5% drops.

Adrenergic Agonists

These fall into two categories: nonselective and selective.

Nonselective Adrenergic Agonists

These include epinephrine and dipivefrin.

Epinephrine 1% is an ∝- and β-agonist (nonselective adrenergic agonist). It lowers IOP by increasing the rate of aqueous outflow. It is administered twice daily. It is contraindicated in patients with narrow anterior chamber angles.

Dipivefrin 0.1% (dipivalyl epinephrine) is a prodrug that is converted into epinephrine inside the eye after absorption. Most of the hydrolysis occurs in the cornea. It is more lipid soluble, so penetration of cornea is 17 times than epinephrine. Therefore, it has greater hypotensive effect than epinephrine and decreased incidence of local and systemic side effects.

∝₂-Selective Adrenergic Agonists

∝₂ agonists decrease IOP by decreasing aqueous secretion and increasing aqueous outflow. These include apraclonidine and brimonidine.

Apraclonidine: It is derived from clonidine and less permeable to blood–brain barrier; therefore, it has fewer CNS effects and also produces fewer adverse systemic reactions such as fall in systemic blood pressure. But, when applied topically (0.5–1%), it lowers IOP. It is not suitable for long-term use because of tachyphylaxis; its use is restricted to control of short-term IOP elevation after anterior segment laser surgery, e.g., laser iridotomy, laser trabeculoplasty, and laser capsulotomy.

Side effects: Most significant ocular side effect is follicular conjunctivitis. Systemic side effects include dryness of mouth, drowsiness, and fatigue.

Brimonidine: It is a highly selective ∝₂-agonist. It is indicated both for short-term IOP spikes as well as long-term use in glaucoma. It decreases aqueous secretion and increases uveoscleral outflow, thereby helping in lowering IOP. It also has a neuroprotective effect and may prevent optic nerve damage. Brimonidine does not appear to have an effect on conventional (trabecular) outflow. It is administered twice daily as 0.2% drops. Side effects of its use could be ocular or systemic. Ocular side effects include allergic reaction and conjunctival congestion. Systemic side effects include xerostomia (dry mouth), drowsiness, fatigue (similar to apraclonidine because both act at same receptors). Because of the risks of pronounced CNS depression, brimonidine should not be used in children <5 years of age.

Carbonic Anhydrase Inhibitors (CAIs)

CAIs belong to sulfonamide class of drugs. It is the only class of drugs used systemically (**Table 11.5**) as well as topically in glaucoma therapy.

Topical Carbonic Anhydrase Inhibitors

- Dorzolamide 2% eye drops and administered twice or thrice daily.
- Brinzolamide 1% eye drops are also administered twice or thrice daily.

Systemic Carbonic Anhydrase Inhibitors

Acetazolamide is the only one that can be administrated orally as well as intravenously.

The drug is taken up by serum protein but free amount of the drug determines the pharmacologic effect. So, understanding of protein binding of the drug is important. *Protein binding of acetazolamide is more than methazolamide.* This explains why large doses are required for acetazolamide to achieve its therapeutic effects compared with methazolamide.

Mechanism of Action

All CAIs (topical as well as systemic) share the same basic mechanism of lowering IOP. Carbonic anhydrase is an enzyme that catalyzes the reaction of H_2O and CO_2 in equilibrium with HCO_3^- and H^+.

Carbonic anhydrase:

$$H_2O + CO_2 \rightarrow H_2CO_3 \rightarrow HCO_3^- + H^+$$

Carbonic anhydrase is located in ciliary epithelium and related to the process of aqueous humor production by generating HCO_3^- ions (bicarbonate ions) which are actively transported across the ciliary epithelium with passive water secretion. CAIs decrease the formation of aqueous humor and reduce IOP by inhibiting carbonic anhydrase (CA) enzyme. An important property of carbonic anhydrase is that more than 90% (nearly 100%) inhibition of enzyme is required to produce effects.

Side Effects

Ocular side effects of topical CAIs include burning, stinging, discomfort and superficial punctuate keratitis (SPK). Side effects of systemic CAIs could be ocular or systemic.

Ocular side effects: Transient myopia may be induced with oral CAIs which is a sulfonamide-related reaction (CAIs are chemically related to sulfonamides).

Systemic side effects: Systemic side effects include the following symptoms:
- Renal symptoms: Decreased urinary excretion of citrate or Mg^{++} ions leads to the formation of renal calculi.
- Gastrointestinal symptoms include metallic taste in mouth, gastric irritation and nausea, and diarrhea and abdominal cramps.

Table 11.5 Dosage and preparation of systemic carbonic anhydrase inhibitors		
Drug	**Preparation**	**Dose**
• Acetazolamide		
For oral use:	Available in 250 mg tablets	250 mg 6 hourly
For intravenous use:	Available as powder in vials (500 mg/vial)	5–10 mg/kg body weight
• Dichlorphenamide	Available as 50 mg tablets	50 mg 12 hourly
• Methazolamide	Available as 25 mg, 50 mg tablets	25–50 mg b.i.d.

- Sulfonamide-related reactions cause Stevens–Johnson syndrome and blood dyscrasias.
- CAIs alter the serum electrolyte imbalance causing either HCO_3^- depletion or K^+ depletion. HCO_3^- depletion causes metabolic acidosis leading to malaise-like symptoms, for example, fatigue, anorexia, and depression. K^+ depletion occurs due to increased urinary excretion. This leads to paresthesia (tingling of fingers, toes, hands, and feet).

> To reduce GI symptoms, take CAIs with meals. Due to metabolic acidosis CAIs should be avoided in patients with severe hepatic or renal disease. Methazolamide does not induce systemic acidosis.

Drugs That Increase Aqueous Outflow

These include parasympathomimetic (cholinergic) drugs and prostaglandin analogues (PGAs).

Parasympathomimetic Drugs

Pilocarpine is the only ocular cholinergic agent used worldwide these days. It is obtained from plant *Pilocarpus microphyllus*. It lowers IOP by 20 to 30%. *In general, there is an additive effect of using pilocarpine (Miotic) with other classes of drugs having a different mechanism of action* (brimonidine, timolol, or CAIs) (**Flowchart 11.10**).

Pilocarpine produces parasympathomimetic effect by direct muscarinic receptor stimulation (muscarinic agonists).

Table 11.6 lists the various preparations of pilocarpine along with their duration of action.

The interaction between pilocarpine and PGAs is interesting. Pilocarpine increases trabecular outflow but reduces uveoscleral outflow whereas PGAs increase uveoscleral outflow. Although pilocarpine reduces and PGAs increase uveoscleral outflow, the combination of pilocarpine and PGAs (e.g., latanoprost) demonstrates an additive effect.

Miotic agents (e.g., pilocarpine) can disrupt blood–aqueous barrier with resultant increased permeability to plasma proteins. It may increase inflammation. So, *it should not be used in the patients with uveitis or in presence of anterior segment neovascularization.*

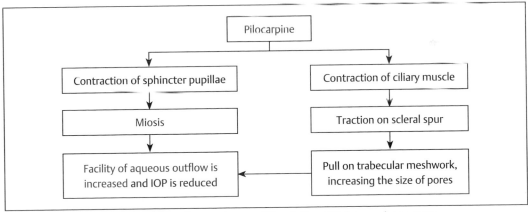

Flowchart 11.10 Pilocarpine and its effect on the eye. Abbreviation: IOP, intraocular pressure.

Table 11.6 Preparations of pilocarpine with duration of action	
Preparation	**Duration of action**
2–4% drops	6–8 h; so, instilled 6–8 hourly but twice a day when used with β-blocker (timolol)
4% gel	18–24 h; so, applied at bed time
Sustained release (in the form of ocuserts)	Release pilocarpine for 7 d at a steady concentration

Side Effects

Ocular side effects of pilocarpine are explained in **Flowchart 11.11**.

In angle recession glaucoma, tear between longitudinal and circular fibers of ciliary muscle takes place. It causes reduction in conventional (trabecular) outflow combined with a tear in ciliary body and shifts the eye to a predominantly uveoscleral outflow, which is known to be impaired by miotics. So, *in angle recession glaucoma miotics are not only ineffective but may also cause paradoxical rise of IOP.*

Prostaglandin and Prostamide Analogues

Prostaglandins (PGs) bind to prostaglandin receptors which are distributed widely in ocular tissues. PGs account for the inflammation in the eye and reduction of IOP.

PGAs include latanoprost, travoprost, bimato-prost, and unoprostone.

Latanoprost and Travoprost

These are ester prodrugs that are hydrolyzed by corneal esterases to become biologically active.

Both these drugs reduce IOP by increasing uveoscleral outflow (**Flowchart 11.12**).

PGAs are a better choice over other drugs because PGAs are as effective at night as during the day, providing uniform round-the-clock IOP reduction whereas timolol (β-blocker) has little effect at night. β-*blockers* decrease aqueous production whereas PGAs increase uveoscleral outflow.

Dosage: Latanoprost 0.005% and travoprost 0.004% are administered once daily. Evening administration is more effective than morning administration.

> Latanoprost exhibits thermal and ultraviolet instability. So, unopened bottles of latanoprost be stored under refrigeration between 2 and 8°C and thus need a cold chain unlike other hypotensive lipids. Once opened, latanoprost may be stored at room temperature for up to 6 weeks.

Drug interactions: PGs have additive effect when combined with timolol, CAIs, or pilocarpine.

> When IOP elevation persists after peripheral iridectomy in patients with PACG, latanoprost is effective in lowering the IOP as it increases uveoscleral outflow.

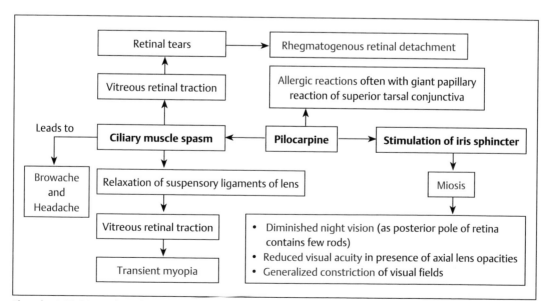

Flowchart 11.11 Ocular side effects of pilocarpine.

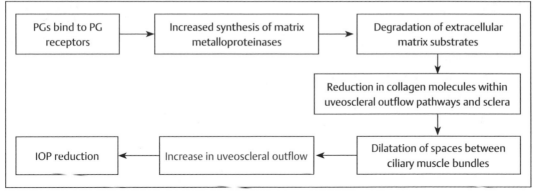

Flowchart 11.12 Mechanism of action of prostaglandin analogues.

Side effects: Following are the side effects of PGAs:

- Conjunctival hyperemia.
- Periorbital skin hyperpigmentation.
- Hypertrichosis (eyelashes may become longer, thicker, and increased in number).
- Allergic contact dermatitis.
- Anterior uveitis. Therefore, PGs should be used with caution in uveitic glaucoma.

Bimatoprost

Bimatoprost is a prostamide. Its structure differs from PGAs and do not bind to prostaglandin FP receptor.

Bimatoprost increases both trabecular and uveoscleral outflow. It decreases IOP by 27 to 33%. It is available in 0.03% strength and administered once daily (OD) at night.

Side effects: Conjunctival hyperemia is more common with bimatoprost than with latanoprost. Other side effects are *eyelash growth* and *increased iris pigmentation.*

Unoprostone Isopropyl

Unoprostone isopropyl (0.15%) mainly increases trabecular (conventional) outflow and lowers IOP by 13 to 18%. It is used twice a day topically.

Hyperosmotic Agents

Osmotic agents remain intravascular and increase blood osmolality. To be effective in the eye, an osmotic agent must be unable to cross

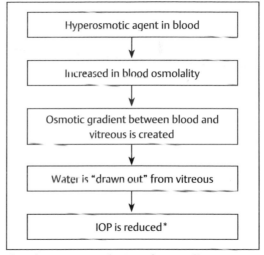

Flowchart 11.13 Mechanism of action of hyperosmotic agents. Note: * The higher the osmotic gradient, the greater is the reduction of IOP.

blood–aqueous barrier. **Flowchart 11.13** explains the mechanism of action of hyperosmotic agents.

If hyperosmotic agent crosses the barrier, osmotic equilibrium is set up and there is no further effect. There may be reversal of osmotic gradient as the compound is cleared from systemic circulation with time resulting in transient rise in IOP. *Therefore, an ideal hyperosmotic agent must have a high molecular weight so that it does not enter the eye.*

In inflammatory glaucomas, permeability of blood–aqueous barrier increases. *Therefore, hyperosmotic agents are of limited value in treatment of inflammatory glaucomas.* These are of great value in acute angle closure glaucoma, lens-induced glaucoma, malignant glaucoma, and traumatic glaucoma. Commonly used hyperosmotic agents are glycerol, mannitol, and isosorbide.

Glycerol: It is given orally as a 50% solution in the dose of 1 to 1.5 g/kg body weight (or 2–3 mL/kg body weight) twice or thrice daily. Glycerol is metabolized to glucose. So, it should be avoided in diabetics. Because of its unpleasant sweet taste, lemon juice is added to it to avoid nausea. It is safer than mannitol based on side effects.

Mannitol: It is an intravenous osmotic agent used as 20% solution in water (as i.v. infusion). Dose: 1 to 2 g/kg of body weight (or 5 mL/kg of body weight) given over a period of 30 to 40 min. It has poor ocular penetration and is distributed in extracellular fluids. Too rapid infusion of mannitol leads to shift of intracellular water into extracellular space. It causes cellular dehydration with risk of hyponatremia, CHF, and pulmonary edema.

So, it should be avoided in patients with cardiac disease and renal diseases. Mannitol may be associated with diuresis, headache, backache, anaphylactic reaction, confusion, and disorientation.

Isosorbide: It is given orally. It is metabolically inert, so it can be given to diabetics. Dose is same as for glycerol, i.e., 1 to 1.5 g/kg body weight.

Primary Open-Angle Glaucoma (POAG) (OP6.6, 6.7)

It is also referred to as:
- Chronic open-angle glaucoma.
- Idiopathic open-angle glaucoma.
- Chronic simple glaucoma.

Features of POAG

POAG is the most common type of glaucoma characterized by features explained in **Table 11.7**.

Although abnormally elevated IOP had long been considered a part of POAG, it is now considered a risk factor for POAG as glaucomatous optic nerve damage can occur despite normal pressure (<21 mm Hg), called NTG (low-tension glaucoma) and IOP may be >21 mm Hg without optic nerve damage or visual field loss is called ocular hypertension.

Risk Factors

Risk factors for POAG include:
- IOP: Raised IOP is the most important risk factor.
- Age: Prevalence of POAG increases with age and is more prevalent between 40 and 75 years of age.
- Race: Blacks > white.
- Family history: POAG is *usually inherited.* First-degree relatives of patient with POAG are at risk of developing POAG.
- Reduction of perfusion pressure (PP): PP = blood pressure – IOP.

An ocular diastolic perfusion pressure of <35 mm Hg is associated with a significant increase in prevalence of glaucoma. There is a significant dip in nocturnal blood pressure which leads to reduction of perfusion pressure to optic nerve, resulting in loss of optic nerve fibers.
- Systemic association: Chances of occurrence increase when associated with diabetes mellitus, hypertension, cardiovascular diseases, and thyroid disorders.

Table 11.7 Features of primary open-angle glaucoma (POAG)

Criteria	Characteristic features
Laterality	• Bilateral but often asymmetrical
Onset	• Adult onset and affects the population over the age of 40 years
IOP	• Elevated IOP >21 mm Hg
Angle	• Open angle
Course	• Chronic, progressive disease
Optic nerve	• Loss of optic nerve fibers with characteristic pattern of optic nerve damage
Visual field	• Typical pattern of visual field loss
Abbreviation: IOP, intraocular pressure.	

- Ocular associations: Myopia and CRVO (central retinal vein occlusion) pose a greater risk for the development of POAG.
- Corticosteroid responsiveness: Patients with POAG are more likely to respond to a 6-week course of **topical** steroid therapy with a significant rise in IOP. **Systemic steroids** most likely induce cataract rather than elevation of IOP.

Pathogenesis

Elevation of IOP in POAG is caused by increased resistance to aqueous outflow in trabecular meshwork. Juxtacanalicular part of trabeculum is thought to be the major site of resistance to aqueous outflow which is the outermost part of trabeculum. Normal trabecular meshwork undergoes several changes with age as follows:

- *The thickening and sclerosis of trabeculae* resulting in narrowing of intertrabecular spaces.
- Loss of trabecular endothelial cells.
- Decrease in the number of giant vacuoles and cells in Schlemm canal.
- Increase in extracellular matrix.

Mechanism of Optic Nerve Damage in Glaucoma

Two theories to account for nerve loss resulting from ganglion cell death include ischemic theory and mechanical theory (**Flowchart 11.14**).

Mechanical theory fails to explain:

- Progression of glaucoma despite normal IOP.
- Etiopathogenesis of normal pressure glaucoma (NTG).

An **immunogenic mechanism** in POAG is supported by the detection of increased X-globulin and plasma cells in trabecular meshwork. In some cases, positive antinuclear antibody reaction has been reported.

Clinical Features

POAG is *usually asymptomatic* until the later stages. Early symptoms may include:

- Progressive and painless decreased vision.
- Mild headache.
- Frequent change of presbyopic glasses— Patient fails increased difficulty in near work due to accommodative failure owing to the pressure upon the ciliary muscle.
- Part of a page missing.
- Constricted visual fields in late stages of disease.

Following are the signs of POAG:

Intraocular pressure (IOP): IOP shows large fluctuations in POAG (normal range 11–21 mm Hg). Diurnal variation in IOP of >8 mm Hg or asymmetry of IOP (>5 mm Hg) between the two eyes should arouse suspicion.

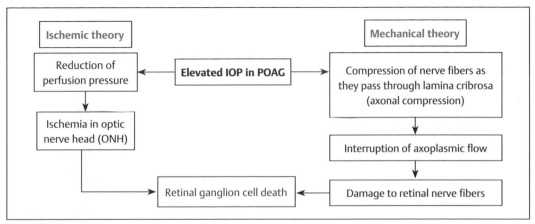

Flowchart 11.14 Theories of optic nerve damage in glaucoma.

Gonioscopy: It shows normal open angle and no PAS.

Signs in optic nerve in POAG are listed in **Table 11.8**.

Peripapillary atrophy is also common in POAG.

Visual fields: The characteristic VF defects include paracentral scotoma, arcuate scotoma, nasal step, altitudinal defect, generalized depression, and temporal wedge.

> Visual field defects that respect **horizontal midline** are nerve fiber bundle defects and are typical of glaucoma.

> Visual field defects that respect **vertical midline** are typical of intracranial lesions at or posterior to chiasm.

■ Differential Diagnosis

POAG must be differentiated from:
- *Ocular hypertension:* Optic nerve and visual fields are normal in ocular hypertension.
- *Physiologic optic nerve cupping:* IOP and visual fields are normal. CDR is enlarged but static.
- *Secondary open-angle glaucoma:* Identifiable cause for open-angle glaucoma (secondary) must be excluded.
- *Normal (low) tension glaucoma (NTG):* Features are same as in POAG except normal IOP.

- *Optic neuropathy:* It is characterized by disproportionately more optic nerve pallor than cupping.
  ◇ IOP is usually normal.
  ◇ Color vision and central vision are usually decreased.

■ Management

Workup or Evaluation

Following workup helps in early diagnosis of POAG:
- History regarding presence of risk factors, chronic steroid use, refractive surgery (it causes change in CCT), ocular trauma and family history of glaucoma is taken.
- Ocular examination includes:
  1. **IOP:** Applanation tonometer is preferred over Schiotz tonometer to measure IOP.
  2. **Measurement of CCT:** Corneal pachymetry should be carried out to measure CCT as CCT affects IOP measurements.
  3. **Diurnal variation in IOP:** Diurnal IOP variation of up to 5 mm Hg occurs in normal eyes. In POAG this fluctuation in IOP is exaggerated (>8–10 mm Hg). Asymmetry of ≥5 mm Hg in IOP between two eyes should arouse suspicion.

Table 11.8 Optic nerve changes in primary open-angle glaucoma (POAG)

Structure	Changes seen in POAG
NRR	• Progressive thinning of neuroretinal rim (NRR) due to progressive enlargement of cup • *Notching of the rim* is *pathognomonic*
Cup	• Enlarged cup with vertical elongation because loss of NRR occurs early at upper and lower poles of disc • Cup-disc ratio (CDR) ≥0.5 (Normal ≤0.3) • Asymmetry of CDR of >0.2 between the two eyes • Deep cup with saucerization
Vessels	• Bayonetting (double angulation of blood vessels) • Nasal displacement of blood vessels • Baring of circumlinear vessels • Splinter or nerve fiber layer (NFL) hemorrhage that crosses the disc margin
Lamina cribrosa	• Lamellar dot sign due to exposure of lamina cribrosa

4. **Gonioscopy:** Angle of anterior chamber is visualized by gonioscopy. It is done to differentiate between primary and secondary glaucoma as well as between open-angle and angle-closure glaucoma.

5. **Evaluation of ONH:** It is done by:
   ◊ Detailed fundus examination.
   ◊ OCT.
   ◊ Heidelberg retinal tomography (HRT).

6. **Analysis of RNFL:** It is performed with the help of OCT.

7. **Assessment of visual fields:** Visual fields are assessed preferably with Humphrey visual field analyzer.

8. **Provocative test (water-drinking test):** The initial IOP of the patient with empty stomach is taken and then asked to drink 1 L of water within 5 minutes. The IOP is measured at 15-minute interval for 1 hour. A rise of IOP >8 mm Hg is pathological and suggestive of POAG.

Treatment

Goal of treatment is to reduce IOP to a level at which it does not cause further damage to the optic nerve fibers. Treatment options for glaucoma include medical therapy, laser trabeculoplasty, and guarded filtration surgery.

Typically, medical therapy is the first-line therapy.

Medical Therapy

Initial treatment is usually with one drug, a β-blocker (e.g., timolol 0.5%) bid OR a PGA (latanoprost, bimatoprost, or travoprost) at night.

β-Blocker should be avoided in patients with asthma, COPD.

PGA should be used with caution in patients with active uveitis, cystoid macular edema and contraindicated in pregnancy.

Additional medications are added or substituted as needed to control IOP adequately. Other medications include:

- Selective α_2-receptor agonists, for example, brimonidine b.i.d.
- Topical CAIs e.g., dorzolamide and brinzolamide.
- Miotics, e.g., pilocarpine.

Patient should be instructed to occlude lacrimal sac punctum by applying pressure for 10 seconds at medial canthus after instillation of a drop. It reduces systemic absorption. Potential adverse effects of drugs should be explained to the patient. IOP should be rechecked in 3 to 4 weeks to evaluate efficacy. Visual fields and OCT are rechecked as needed, often about every 6 to 12 months.

Laser Trabeculoplasty

This includes Argon laser trabeculoplasty (ALT) and selective laser trabeculoplasty (SLT).

Discrete argon or diode laser burns are applied to the trabeculum which produces shrinkage of treated area. Intratrabecular spaces are opened due to stretching of trabecular meshwork and IOP is reduced as a result of increased trabecular outflow. SLT utilizes lower energy and causes less tissue damage. Laser trabeculoplasty causes a transient rise in IOP. So, brimonidine b.i.d is recommended to control post-laser IOP rise.

Indications of laser trabeculoplasty are:
- Poor compliance of patient with medical therapy. Since IOP reduction with laser is approximately 8 mm Hg, an IOP >28 mm Hg is not adequately controlled by laser alone.
- As a substitute for another drug.
- Pigmentary glaucoma.

Filtration Surgery

Filtering surgeries create a fistula between angle of anterior chamber and subtenon space for aqueous to escape from the eye into a 'drainage bleb'. **Trabeculectomy** is most preferred surgical procedure for POAG.

Indications of filtration surgery are:
- Failed medical therapy and/or laser trabeculoplasty.
- Poor compliance to medical therapy.
- Difficult follow-up of the patient.

Adjunctive use of antimetabolites (antifibrotic agents), for example, mitomycin-C, 5-fluorouracil (5-FU) may aid in effectiveness of surgery but increase the risk of bleb leak and hypotony. These are indicated in neovascular glaucoma (NVG) and failed filtering surgery.

■ Prognosis

It depends upon the extent of optic nerve damage and rate of disease progression.

■ Normal-Tension Glaucoma (NTG) (OP6.6, 6.7)

NTG is a variant of POAG in which IOP remains in normal range, that is, POAG without IOP elevation. It is also referred to as low-tension glaucoma.

■ Etiology

The exact cause of NTG is unknown but poor optic nerve perfusion plays an important role as in nocturnal hypotension, vasospasm (as in migraine, Raynaud phenomenon) and prior hemodynamic crisis (as in myocardial infarction, carotid stenosis, acute blood loss). All these conditions decrease ONH perfusion pressure causing ischemic injury to the optic nerve despite normal IOP.

■ Clinical Features

NTG is *asymptomatic*: Patients only notice decreased vision or constricted visual fields in late stages of disease. Clinical signs of NTG are the same as for POAG except that IOP is within normal range. Signs noticed are:

- Normal IOP that is, 21 mm Hg.
- Gonioscopy shows open angle.
- Visual field defects are denser, more localized, closer to fixation than in POAG.
- Optic disc shows progressive optic nerve cupping; optic disc "splinter" hemorrhages and peripapillary atrophy may be found.

■ Differential Diagnosis

- POAG: NTG must be differentiated from POAG presenting with normal IOP because of large diurnal fluctuations or thin cornea.

- Nonglaucomatous optic neuropathy: Optic disc does not show glaucomatous cupping but rather a flat optic atrophy in which area of atrophy exceeds the extent of visual field defect (disc-field disparity).
- Shock optic neuropathy from previous episode of systemic hypotension due to acute blood loss, myocardial infarction, and arrhythmia. Visual field loss should be nonprogressive in these cases.
- Neurological lesions: Compressive lesions of optic nerve or chiasma may produce visual field defects and must be distinguished from glaucomatous field defects. Such lesions also produce optic atrophy without glaucomatous cupping.
- Previous anterior ischemic optic neuropathy, especially the arteritic form.
- Coloboma of ONH.

■ Treatment

NTG is treated on the line of POAG but target IOP is kept low. Lowering of IOP further plays an important role in preventing the progression of NTG.

■ Prognosis

NTG has a worse prognosis than POAG because it is more difficult to treat.

> If a significant nocturnal fall in BP is detected, avoid antihypertensive medications (to lower BP) prior to bed time, and any patient who uses such medication must be checked for such falls in BP.

■ Ocular Hypertension

When a person has a consistently elevated IOP (>21 mm Hg) without optic nerve or visual field damage, the condition is referred to as **ocular hypertension**. The patient with IOP between 20 and 25 mm Hg does not need any treatment unless associated with risk factors.

The term "**Glaucoma suspect**" is used when a person exhibits ONH changes suggestive of glaucoma without raised IOP or visual field changes.

Measurement of CCT is very important as:

- In eyes with *thin cornea* measured IOP < true IOP, and
- In eyes with *thick cornea* measured IOP > true IOP and may be misdiagnosed as having ocular hypertension.

Identification of the **risk factors for developing glaucoma is important.** The most relevant risk factors are:

- Older age.
- High IOP: IOP consistently >30 mm Hg.
- Thin CCT.
- Optic CDR.
- Unilateral POAG in fellow eye.
- Family history of POAG in first-degree relative.
- Additional ocular factors are high myopia, steroid responder, low ONH perfusion pressure.
- Additional systemic risk factors are diabetes mellitus, hypertension, hypothyroidism, and cardiovascular diseases.

■ Treatment

Patients with IOP ≥30 mm Hg need antiglaucoma treatment.

■ Primary Angle-Closure Glaucoma (OP6.6, 6.7)

Angle closure is characterized by apposition of peripheral iris against trabecular meshwork resulting in obstruction of aqueous outflow. Classically, angle closure may be:

Primary angle closure: It results from anatomical predisposition leading to angle closure.

Secondary angle closure: It results from pathological processes in any part of the eye.

Primary angle-closure glaucoma (PACG) *is also known as narrow angle glaucoma.* In PACG the mechanism of angle closure is not thought to be associated with ocular or systemic abnormalities other than anatomical features.

■ Risk Factors for PACG

- *Age*: Prevalence for PACG increases after the age of 40 years.
- *Sex*: Females are affected more than males in the ratio of 4:1.
- *Refractive error*: PACG is higher in persons with hypermetropia.
- *Family history*: As predisposing anatomical factors are often inherited, it is more common in first-degree relatives.

■ Predisposing Factors

The anatomical features predisposing to PACG are:

- *Shallow anterior chamber:* Anterior chamber depth in normal eyes is 2.8 mm while in eyes with PACG it is 1.8 mm.
- *Shorter axial length* having a relative anterior positioning of iris-lens diaphragm.
- *Smaller corneal diameter.*
- *Iris-induced angle closure* may occur if iris base inserts anteriorly on anterior surface of ciliary body. Ciliary processes are displaced anteriorly in the posterior chamber and push the iris base forward into angle recess.

Evaluation of Peripheral Anterior Chamber Depth

Central anterior chamber depth only weakly correlates with angle width and the parameter of greater diagnostic value in context of angle-closure glaucoma is the peripheral anterior chamber depth. The techniques to quantify the anterior chamber depth are:

- *Slit-lamp examination:* Van Herick developed a technique for making this estimation with slit lamp by comparing the peripheral anterior chamber (AC) depth to the thickness of adjacent cornea (**Van Herick grading system**).

  Grade 4   → Peripheral AC depth ≥ corneal thickness.

  Grade 3   → Peripheral AC depth = 1/2 corneal thickness.

Grade 2 → Peripheral AC depth = 1/4 corneal thickness.

Grade 1 → Peripheral AC depth < 1/4 corneal thickness.

Closed angle → Absent peripheral anterior chamber.

- *Gonioscopy:* A ≥180-degree closure of angle (i.e., trabecular meshwork is not visible) constitutes an occludable angle. Compression gonioscopy is important with closed angle to determine whether the closure is appositional or synechial.
- *Ultrasound biomicroscopy.*
- *Optical coherence tomography* (OCT).

■ Mechanism of Angle Closure

Angle closure in PACG may be caused by relative pupillary block or crowding of angle.

Relative Pupillary Block

Pupillary block may be absolute or relative. In *absolute pupillary block* there is no aqueous flow through the pupil as in seclusio or occlusio pupillae. A *relative pupillary block* impedes forward aqueous flow through the pupil which is associated with mid-dilatation of pupil. Mid-dilated pupil of 3.5 to 6 mm is the critical degree of dilatation that seems to bring on the acute attack. Thus, pupillary block and angle closure may be precipitated by the factors that produce mydriasis such as:

- Mydriatic agents.
- Close work in dim illumination conditions.
- Emotional stress (increasing sympathetic tone) (**Flowchart 11.15**).

Crowding of Angle

Angle-closure glaucoma may result from an abnormal anatomic configuration of peripheral iris without pupillary block, also referred to as angle crowding. Angle crowding may occur if iris base inserts anteriorly on anterior surface of ciliary body or ciliary processes are positioned anteriorly in the posterior chamber. Anteriorly positioned/

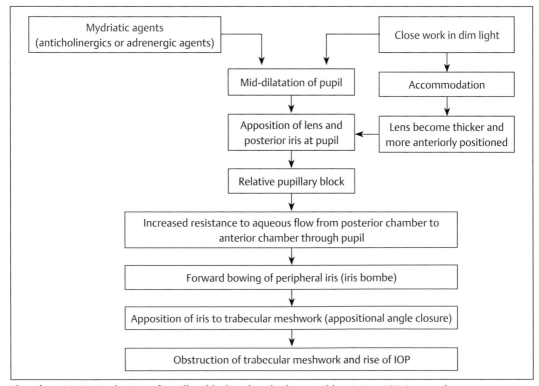

Flowchart 11.15 Mechanism of pupillary block and angle closure. Abbreviation: IOP, intraocular pressure.

rotated ciliary processes cause peripheral iris to be displaced anteriorly into angle recess.

The iris is characterized by a flat plane, so-called **plateau iris** which results in narrow angle recess with a sharp backward iris angulation over anteriorly oriented ciliary processes. On indentation gonioscopy, a characteristic "**double hump**" sign is seen (central hump is due to underlying lens and the peripheral hump results from underlying ciliary processes). *Angle closure is present despite a patent iridectomy or Nd:YAG iridotomy because anterior position of ciliary processes prevents the peripheral iris from falling posteriorly* (**Fig. 11.25**).

Thus, when angle-closure occurs and IOP rises after dilatation, despite a patient peripheral iridectomy and in absence of pupillary block, the **plateau iris syndrome** is suspected which may be diagnosed by ultrasound biomicroscopy. So, plateau iris syndrome is not relieved by iridectomy/iridotomy. Plateau iris syndrome is treated by:

- Miotics–pilocarpine 1% drops.
- Peripheral iridoplasty: Argon laser burns are applied to peripheral iris resulting in contraction of iris tissue and flattening of iris "hump."

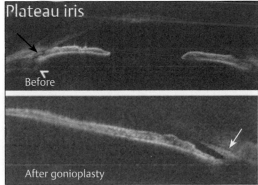

Fig. 11.25 Optical coherence tomography (OCT) of plateau iris, before and after gonioplasty. Source: OCT of the Anterior Segment. In: Agarwal A, Kumar D, ed. Essentials of OCT in Ocular Disease. 1st Edition. Thieme; 2015.

■ Types of Angle Closure

Clinical features depend on the type of angle closure which may be divided into:

- Occludable angle (angle-closure suspect).
- Subacute (intermittent) angle closure.
- Acute angle closure.
- Chronic angle closure.

The angle closure may not progress from one stage to the next in an orderly sequence.

Occludable Angle (Angle-Closure Suspect)

After an acute or chronic angle-closure attack in one eye, the angle in the fellow eye is considered occludable and is prone to develop PACG. Thus, the term implies to an anatomically predisposed eye.

Clinical Features

The symptoms are absent. The slit-lamp biomicroscopy reveals shallow anterior chamber and convex iris lens diaphragm.

Gonioscopy

On gonioscopy without indentation, pigmented trabecular meshwork is not visible in at least three quadrants.

Management

Provocative tests may be used to provoke pupillary block glaucoma to identify the patients for whom treatment should be recommended.

> **Provocative Tests**
>
> **Dark room prone test:** The baseline IOP and gonioscopic findings are recorded. Patient is asked to stay in a dark room in a prone position for 1 hour without sleeping (as sleep can cause miosis). Thereafter, IOP and gonioscopic findings are re-recorded. Dark room causes mydriasis and prone position results in slight anterior shift of lens. Angle closure may develop due to pupillary block. A rise in IOP of ≥8 mm Hg in the presence of closed angle is considered to be a positive test and eyes are predisposed to PACG.
>
> **Mydriatic test:** The baseline IOP is recorded. Pupil is dilated with short-acting parasympatholytic agent or phenylephrine eye drops. IOP is measured at every 30 min for 2 hours. A rise of IOP of ≥8 mm Hg suggests possibility of angle-closure glaucoma. This test is not physiological, so seldom used. Negative provocative test does not rule out angle occlusion.

Careful gonioscopic examination has largely replaced the use of provocative tests to make management decisions about development of angle-closure glaucoma.

Treatment

The condition is managed with prophylactic peripheral laser iridotomy. Clinical course without treatment:

- IOP may remain normal.
- Acute or subacute angle closure may develop.
- Chronic angle closure may develop without passing through subacute or acute stages.

Intermittent (Subacute) Angle Closure

The intermittent pupillary block in a predisposed eye with an occludable angle results in intermittent angle closure with sudden increase in IOP. The pupillary block is then spontaneously relieved and IOP returns to normal.

The attack may be precipitated by:

- Dim illumination: Watching TV in a dark room causes mydriasis and angle closure.
- Emotional stress: Increased sympathetic activity due to emotional stress leads to mydriasis and angle closure.
- Prone or semiprone position during reading or sewing causes physiological shallowing of anterior chamber and angle closure.

- Drugs: Anticholinergic and adrenergic drugs cause mydriasis and angle closure.

Attacks usually subside spontaneously by physiological miosis. Exposure to bright sunlight or sleep results in physiological miosis and spontaneous resolution of pupillary block.

Clinical Features

There is transient blurring of vision. Colored halos around lights due to corneal epithelial edema are transient. Frontal headache is also transient. The slit-lamp biomicroscopy reveals shallow anterior chamber. There is sudden increase in IOP.

Treatment

Prophylactic peripheral laser iridotomy to check future attacks of angle-closure glaucoma.

Acute Angle Closure

Sudden, angle closure with acute rise in IOP causes acute angle-closure glaucoma.

Clinical Features

Symptoms are sudden and severe with pain, blurred vision, colored halos around lights due to corneal edema, frontal headache, nausea and vomiting, red eye, and photophobia. Pain is due to stretching of sensory nerve (5th CN) and radiates over its distribution.

Clinical signs of acute-angle glaucoma are listed in **Table 11.9**.

Table 11.9 Signs of acute-angle glaucoma

Structure	Signs seen in acute-angle glaucoma
• Conjunctiva	Ciliary injection
• Cornea	Corneal epithelial edema
• Anterior chamber (AC)	Shallow

• Pupil
   Size
   Shape
   Reaction
	
	Mid-dilated owing to the pressure on sphincter pupillae
	Vertically oval
	Nonreacting

• IOP	Markedly raised
• Eyeball	Tender

The effects on different ocular structures following **raised IOP in acute PACG** are:

- Ischemic necrosis of sphincter and dilator pupillae causing permanently dilated and fixed (nonreacting) pupil.
- Focal necrosis of lens epithelial cells causing anterior subcapsular lens opacities in pupillary zone (Glaukomflecken).
- Ischemia of iris resulting in patchy iris atrophy and release of pigment. So, fine pigment granules are found on corneal endothelium.

Gonioscopy

Gonioscopy after resolution of corneal edema reveals closed angle in the affected eye and occludable angle in the fellow eye. Indentation gonioscopy is important because it can differentiate between an appositional and synechial (due to PAS) angle closure.

Differential Diagnosis

Acute primary acute congestive glaucoma (PACG) must be differentiated from other causes of acute red eye such as acute conjunctivitis and acute anterior uveitis.

Treatment

Acute angle-closure glaucoma is an ophthalmic emergency and requires immediate treatment. Treatment should be approached in two stages:

- Reduction of IOP.
- Relief of angle closure.

Reduction of IOP: It can be achieved with:

- Systemic CAIs: e.g., acetazolamide.
- Hyperosmotic agents: e.g., orally as glycerol or IV Mannitol.
- Topical IOP reducing drugs.

Relief of angle closure: It is achieved with a miotic (pilocarpine 2%) to break the pupillary block and open the angle of anterior chamber and should be started after IOP lowering because *miotic therapy is usually ineffective when IOP is high (>40–50 mm Hg) due to pressure-induced ischemia of iris which leads to paralysis of sphincter muscle.*

After the control of IOP, peripheral iridotomy with Nd:YAG laser (laser iridotomy) is the procedure of choice or incisional iridectomy is done, if necessary. Prophylactic laser iridotomy in the fellow eye is also performed at the same sitting or within a few days to prevent a future acute angle-closure attack. If iridotomy does not restore a normal IOP in long term, eye is then treated with medication or guarded filtering surgery, if required.

Topical steroids are given to reduce accompanying inflammation.

Chronic Angle Closure

In chronic PACG, IOP is chronically raised and is caused by:

- Gradual and progressive synechial angle closure in which slow PAS formation develops circumferentially (creeping angle closure) which is usually asymptomatic.
- Recurrent attacks of intermittent or acute PACG. Patients may give a history of intermittent eye pain, headache and blurred vision.

Diagnosis

Optic disc:

- Ophthalmoscopy shows optic disc changes similar to those in POAG.
- Disc cupping (glaucomatous).
- *Visual field*: Visual field defects typical of glaucoma become evident.
- *IOP*: Moderate rise in IOP.
- *Gonioscopy*: It reveals narrow angles with PAS. *Gonioscopic evaluation differentiates between chronic angle-closure glaucoma and POAG.*

Treatment

Laser iridotomy to eradicate element of pupillary block. Medical treatment for residual elevation of IOP. Trabeculectomy, if medical treatment fails.

Absolute Glaucoma

If PACG is untreated, it gradually passes into the stage of absolute glaucoma. It is the end stage of glaucoma. The eye is painful and blind with no PL (perception of light). Clinical signs of absolute glaucoma are listed in **Table 11.10**.

Treatment

Cyclocryotherapy to reduce the aqueous secretion and thereby lowering the IOP. Retrobulbar (70%) alcohol injection to destroy the ciliary ganglion and to relieve the pain. Enucleation of eyeball is also done, if the pain is not relieved.

■ Secondary Glaucoma (OP6.6, 6.7)

Secondary glaucoma means glaucoma secondary to some ocular or systemic disease and can be classified on the basis of etiology and mechanism as follows:

- Secondary glaucoma based upon etiology: Glaucoma may be associated with:
  ◇ Disorder of corneal endothelium:
    - Iridocorneal endothelial (ICE) syndrome.
    - Fuchs endothelial corneal dystrophy.
  ◇ Disorder of iris and ciliary body:
    - Pigmentary glaucoma.
  ◇ Disorder of lens (lens-induced glaucoma):
    - Phacolytic glaucoma effusion.
    - Phacomorphic glaucoma.
    - Phacoanaphylactic glaucoma.
    - Glaucoma associated with dislocated lens.
  ◇ Disorder of retina, choroid, and vitreous:
    - NVG.

◇ Intraocular inflammation (inflammatory glaucoma):
  - Associated with uveitis.
  - Associated with keratitis, scleritis, or choroiditis (due to associated secondary uveitis).
◇ Intraocular tumors:
  - Malignant melanoma.
  - Retinoblastoma.
  - Metastatic carcinoma.
◇ Steroids administration (steroid-induced glaucoma).
◇ Elevated EVP.
◇ Ocular trauma (traumatic glaucoma).
◇ Intraocular hemorrhage.
◇ Intraocular surgery (postoperative glaucoma).
◇ Pseudoexfoliation syndrome.

- Secondary glaucoma based upon mechanism:
  ◇ Secondary open-angle glaucoma: Obstruction to aqueous outflow may be pre-trabecular, trabecular, or post-trabecular.
  ◇ Secondary angle-closure glaucoma: It may occur with or without pupillary block.

Secondary angle-closure glaucoma **with pupillary block** causes obstruction to aqueous from passing through pupil into anterior chamber. It results in forward pushing of peripheral iris leading to secondary angle-closure glaucoma. Pupillary block may be caused by phacomorphic glaucoma, total posterior synechiae (seclusio pupillae), due

Table 11.10 Signs of absolute glaucoma	
Structure	**Signs seen in absolute glaucoma**
• Conjunctiva	Perilimbal reddish-blue zone due to dilated anterior ciliary veins
• Cornea	Hazy and insensitive; it may develop bullous keratopathy or filamentary keratopathy
• Anterior chamber	Very shallow
• Iris	Atrophic patches are present
• Pupil	Fixed and dilated
• Optic disc	Glaucomatous optic atrophy
• IOP	Extremely high; eyeball is stony hard

to vitreous (in aphakia), NVG, PAS due to uveitis. All the conditions pull iris diaphragm anteriorly over trabeculum.

Secondary angle-closure glaucoma **without pupillary block** may be caused by choroidal effusion, suprachoroidal hemorrhage and tumors. All of the causes push lens-iris diaphragm forward. ICE may also cause secondary angle-closure glaucoma. Glaucoma is due to synechial angle closure secondary to contraction of abnormal corneal endothelial cell layer proliferating and migrating to the surface of the iris through the angle.

▪ Glaucoma Associated with Disorders of Corneal Endothelium

Iridocorneal Endothelial (ICE) Syndrome

It is a group of disorders characterized by abnormal corneal endothelium, which has the capacity to proliferate and migrate across the angle and onto the surface of iris that is responsible for iris atrophy, secondary angle-closure glaucoma, and corneal edema.

Treatment

Medical treatment is ineffective. Late failures are frequent with filtration surgery (trabeculectomy)

due to fistular (bleb) endothelialization, and glaucoma drainage devices are eventually required which has been used as a primary procedure.

▪ Glaucoma Associated with Disorders of Iris and Ciliary Body

Pigmentary Glaucoma

It is a form of open-angle glaucoma characterized by disruption of iris pigment epithelium with deposition of pigment throughout the anterior segment. It is a bilateral condition and affect mostly young myopic males.

Clinical Features

- Secondary open-angle glaucoma in young myopic males.
- Deposition of pigment granules on the corneal endothelium in a vertical spindle pattern called **Krukenberg spindle.**
- Deposition of pigment granules in trabecular meshwork called **Sampaolesi line.**
- Iris transillumination shows characteristic radial spoke-like defects in midperiphery.

Pathogenesis

A "reverse pupillary block" mechanism has been postulated for pigmentary glaucoma (**Flowchart 11.16**).

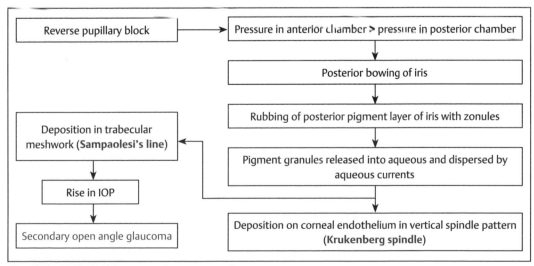

Flowchart 11.16 Pathogenesis of pigmentary glaucoma.

Treatment

- Medical treatment: *Pilocarpine* causes miosis resulting in decreased contact between iris and lens zonules. It relieves mechanism of pigment dispersion and prevents progressive development of pigmentary glaucoma. *Pilocarpine* also causes increased aqueous outflow and lowering of the IOP.

> **Disadvantage of pilocarpine:**
> Pilocarpine causes accommodation leading to induced myopia. So, pilocarpine is usually not tolerated by young patients with myopia. Alternative medications (PGAs, topical CAIs, and brimonidine) are nonmiotic drugs. So, IOP is reduced but mechanism of continued pigment dispersion is not eliminated.

- Peripheral iridotomy with laser: It neutralizes reverse pupillary block and flattens the iris. Thus, contact between iris and zonules decreases.
- Filtration surgery (trabeculectomy).

■ Glaucoma Associated with Disorders of Lens (Phacogenic Glaucoma)

Lens-induced glaucoma is also known as phacogenic glaucoma. It could be associated with subluxated or dislocated lens, where the condition is known as phacotopic glaucoma. It could also be associated with cataract formation leading to three different forms of glaucoma, namely, phacolytic, phacoanaphylactic and phacomorphic glaucomas.

Phacotopic Glaucoma

A dislocated or subluxated lens may induce glaucoma by causing herniation of vitreous into pupil or anterior dislocation of lens into pupil or anterior chamber. In both cases, pupillary block occurs, which, in turn, leads to the development of acute congestive glaucoma.

Pupillary block is particularly common with microspherophakia (small and spherical lens) as in Weill–Marchesani syndrome *because of loose zonules of lens.*

Treatment

- In dislocation of lens into anterior chamber, early surgery is warranted. Constrict the pupil to prevent the back-fall of lens into vitreous followed by surgical removal.
- In pupillary block by a microspherical lens (as in Weill–Marchesani syndrome) *miotics are contraindicated* and should be avoided as miotics cause accommodation due to ciliary muscle contraction leading to relaxation of zonules and hence there is worsening of the pupillary block.

Pupillary block is relieved with mydriatics as mydriatics cause zonules to become taut causing lens to be pulled posteriorly and hence pupillary block is relieved.

Definitive treatment in microspherophakia is laser iridotomy or surgical iridectomy. Fellow eye should undergo prophylactic laser iridotomy.

Phacolytic Glaucoma

It is usually associated with hypermature cataract or damage of lens and causes open-angle glaucoma (**Fig. 11.26**). Pathogenesis of phacolytic glaucoma is explained in **Flowchart 11.17**.

Clinical Features

It presents with acute onset of unilateral pain, redness, and gradual reduction in visual activity. Clinical signs are described as follows:

- Conjunctiva: Hyperemia (ciliary congestion).
- Cornea: Corneal edema.
- Anterior chamber:
  ◊ Flare in anterior chamber is present.
  ◊ Contain iridescent particles (macrophages laden with lens protein in anterior chamber appear as iridescent particles) and are helpful diagnostic sign in phacolytic glaucoma.
- IOP: Elevated.
- Lens: Shows hypermature cataract (Morgagnian).

Treatment

It consists of control of IOP (with hyperosmotic agents, CAIs, topical β-blockers); topical steroids to reduce inflammation and extraction of lens with thorough irrigation of anterior chamber to remove all proteinaceous material.

Phacoanaphylactic Glaucoma

It is due to the hypersensitivity to patient's own lens protein, especially the nucleus. Pathogenesis of phacoanaphylactic glaucoma is explained in **Flowchart 11.18**.

Treatment

It includes steroid therapy to control uveitis, antiglaucoma treatment to control IOP, and removal of retained lens matter.

Phacomorphic Glaucoma

It is caused by intumescent or swollen lens (**Fig. 11.27**).

Pathogenesis

Swollen (intumescent) lens causes pupillary block and iris to be pushed forward. The pupillary block leads to iris bombe, which in association with forward pushing of iris results in obliteration of angle of anterior chamber. It leads to secondary angle–closure glaucoma (**Fig. 11.28** and **Fig. 11.29**).

Clinical Features

It presents with pain, redness, and diminution of vision. Clinical signs are as follows:
- IOP: Raised IOP.
- Lens: Unilateral intumescent cataract.
- Anterior chamber: Anterior chamber is shallow in the center than that of fellow eye.

Treatment

It includes Control of IOP with hyperosmotic agents like I.V. mannitol; oral CAIs, e.g., acetazolamide and topical β-blockers. Once the IOP is controlled, cataract extraction is done.

■ Glaucoma Associated with Disorder of Retina, Vitreous, and Choroid

The most common glaucoma associated with diseases of retina is NVG, although it may be associated with other ocular or extraocular conditions.

Neovascular Glaucoma

NVG is a form of glaucoma which occurs as a result of new vessels proliferation (**neovascularization**) on the surface of iris (rubeosis iridis) and anterior chamber angle. Neovascularization follows extensive retinal ischemia (**Fig. 11.30**).

Etiology

It includes the conditions predisposing to the development of rubeosis iridis such as ischemic central retinal vein occlusion (CRVO), central retinal artery occlusion (CRAO), diabetic retinopathy, intraocular tumors, Sickle cell retinopathy etc.

Pathogenesis

NVG occurs in three stages:
- Preglaucomatous stage (stage of rubeosis iridis).
- Open-angle glaucoma stage (due to neovascularization of angle).
- Angle-closure glaucoma stage (due to contracture of fibrovascular membrane at angle).

Conditions causing retinal hypoxia/ischemia stimulate production of angiogenic factor, vascular endothelial growth factor (VEGF), by hypoxic retina in an attempt to revascularize hypoxic areas. The new vessels proliferate in retina and iris. Vessels grow over the surface of iris towards the angle and neovascularization of anterior chamber angle takes place. It results in raised IOP (secondary open-angle glaucoma).

The peripheral iris is pulled over trabecular meshwork due to contraction of fibrovascular

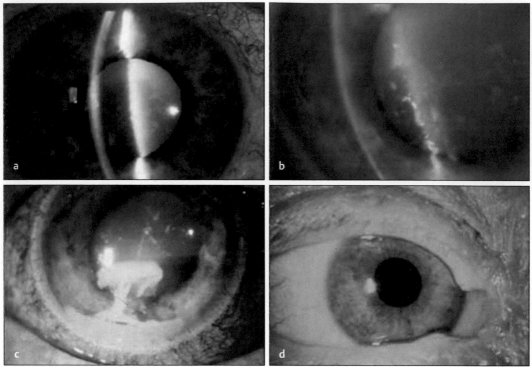

Fig. 11.26 Phacolytic glaucoma. **(a)** Ciliary congestion. **(b)** Corneal edema. **(c)** Hypermature cataract (Morgagnian). **(d)** Extraction of lens. Source: Lens-Induced Glaucoma. In: Morrison J, Pollack I, ed. Glaucoma: Science and Practice. 1st Edition. Thieme; 2002.

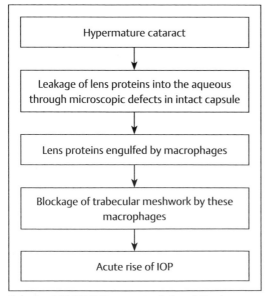

Flowchart 11.17 Pathogenesis of phacolytic glaucoma. Abbreviation: IOP, intraocular pressure.

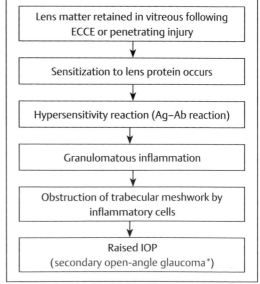

Flowchart 11.18 Pathogenesis of phacoanaphylactic glaucoma. Note: * presence of keratic precipitates distinguishes it from phacolytic glaucoma. Abbreviation: ECCE, extracapsular cataract extraction.

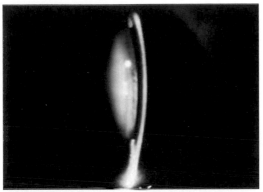

Fig. 11.27 Phacomorphic glaucoma. Source: Lens-Induced Glaucoma. In: Morrison J, Pollack I, ed. Glaucoma: Science and Practice. 1st Edition. Thieme; 2002.

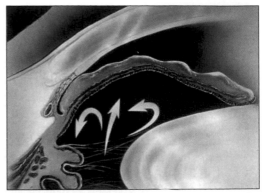

Fig. 11.28 Pupillary-block glaucoma with iris bombé and angle closure. Source: Angle-Closure Glaucoma. In: Morrison J, Pollack I, ed. Glaucoma: Science and Practice. 1st Edition. Thieme; 2002.

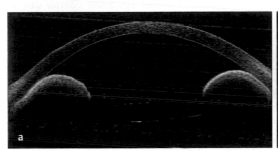
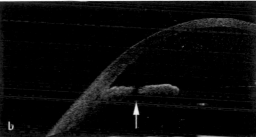

Fig. 11.29 Iritis and pupillary block due to posterior synechiae. **(a)** Anterior segment OCT before laser iridotomy shows iris bombé. **(b)** Anterior segment OCT after laser iridotomy (*arrow*) with opening of the anterior chamber angle. Source: Singh K, Smiddy W, Lee A, ed. Ophthalmology Review: A Case-Study Approach. 2nd Edition. 2018.

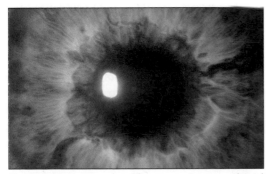

Fig. 11.30 Neovascular Glaucoma. Source: Clinical Features and Diagnosis. In: Scott I, Regillo C, Flynn H et al., ed. Vitreoretinal Disease: Diagnosis, Management, and Clinical Pearls. 2nd Edition. Thieme; 2017.

membrane and causes the formation of PAS. The synechial closure of angle leads to secondary angle-closure glaucoma. The radial traction along the surface of iris due to contraction of fibrovascular membrane results in ectropion pupillae.

Clinical Features

Initially, rubeosis iridis is present with normal IOP but 8 to 15 weeks after the vascular occlusive event IOP rises. It has been called **90-day glaucoma** because the average time interval was thought to be 3 months. Aqueous reveals flare and cells. Gonioscopy shows open angle with

- *Periocular injection* of a long-acting steroid is the most dangerous route. Use of repository steroids is particularly dangerous because of prolonged duration of action.
- *Intravitreal steroid* use (triamcinolone injection to treat intraocular neovascular or inflammatory disease) can also cause a rise in IOP.

Pathogenesis

Steroids administration causes reduction in aqueous outflow and IOP elevation. The precise mechanism responsible for obstruction to the outflow is not known but following theories have been postulated:

- *Influence on extracellular matrix* (Francois theory): Glycosaminoglycans (GAG) are a component of extracellular matrix in trabecular meshwork. GAG in polymerized form become hydrated. Hydrolase in lysosomes depolymerizes GAG. Steroids inhibit the release of hydrolases by stabilizing the lysosomal membrane and GAG in polymerized form gets accumulated. Thus, water in the extracellular space is retained. It leads to narrowing of trabecular openings and resistance to aqueous outflow.
- *Influence on phagocytosis* (phagocytic theory): Endothelial cells lining the trabecular meshwork have phagocytic properties and phagocytose the debris from aqueous. Corticosteroids suppress phagocytic activity so debris in aqueous accumulates in trabecular meshwork leading to its blockage, thereby resulting in decreased aqueous outflow.
- *Prostaglandin (PGs) theory:* PGs, PGE and PGF increase aqueous outflow and lower the IOP. Corticosteroids inhibit synthesis of both PGs E and F.

Clinical Features

Clinical picture resembles that of POAG and patients are usually asymptomatic. It includes white and painless eye, open angle, elevated IOP, ONH changes and visual field defects.

Much less often, patient may have acute presentation with very high IOP with corneal epithelial edema resulting in blurred vision and colored halos, ciliary congestion and pain.

Treatment

Steroids should be stopped immediately. Once steroids have been ceased, IOP almost always returns to baseline within 4 weeks. Medical treatment of glaucoma is essentially the same as for POAG.

- Potent steroids (betamethasone, dexamethasone, and prednisolone) have a significant tendency to produce steroid-induced glaucoma. Weak steroids (fluorometholone and loteprednol) have low potency for inducing IOP rise.
- To reduce chance of provoking such an increase in IOP, steroid use should be minimized with respect to type of steroid prescribed, frequency of instillation, and duration of use. NSAIDs do not cause an elevation of IOP and can be used in high responders. *When more potent steroids are invariably required for the management of significant uveitis, monitoring of IOP in all patients receiving steroids is necessary.*

■ Glaucoma Associated with Elevated Episcleral Venous Pressure

Normal EVP is 8 to 10 mm Hg. It is one of the important factors that influences IOP. Elevated EVP obstructs the aqueous outflow. Elevated EVP results from raised pressure in venous drainage system due to:

- **Venous obstruction:** As seen in superior vena cava syndrome, thyroid ophthalmopathy, retrobulbar tumors, and cavernous sinus thrombosis.
- **Arteriovenous fistulas:** As seen in carotid cavernous sinus fistula, Sturge–Weber syndrome and orbital varices.

Clinical Features

Tortuous and dilated episcleral vessels are the most consistent feature. Rise in IOP is approximately equal to the rise in episcleral venous pressure (EVP). Gonioscopy shows open angle and blood in Schlemm canal. Other features are inconsistent and depend on the underlying cause of elevated EVP and include chemosis, proptosis, and orbital bruit and pulsations.

Treatment

It should be directed toward eliminating the cause of elevated EVP.

■ Glaucoma Associated with Ocular Trauma (Traumatic Glaucoma)

Ocular trauma may be blunt trauma (contusion injuries) and penetrating injuries.

Blunt Injury

Blunt injury to the eye can cause tearing of tissues near the anterior chamber angle. Blunt injury may cause:

- *Tear in the root of iris* near the angle (iridodialysis).
- *Tear in the face of ciliary body* (the portion that lies between iris root and sclera spur), i.e., tear between the longitudinal and circular fibers of ciliary muscle. It results in retro displacement of iris root and recession of the angle of anterior chamber (angle recession). The resistance to outflow is the result of concomitant trabecular meshwork damage (**late-onset glaucoma**).
- *Separation of ciliary body from scleral spur* (cyclodialysis).
- *Tear in the trabecular meshwork.*
- *Tearing of zonules* resulting in subluxation and dislocation of lens. It leads to *pupillary block* and raised IOP.
- Blunt injury may cause hyphema (blood in anterior chamber). IOP rises due to trabecular block by RBCs (**early onset glaucoma**). The usual source of bleeding is a tear in the face of ciliary body resulting in disruption of branches of major arterial circle.

Therefore, early onset glaucoma in blunt injury is due to hyphema but late-onset glaucoma is due to trabecular meshwork damage.

Diagnosis

It is diagnosed by gonioscopy and ultrasound biomicroscopy. Gonioscopy shows irregular widening of ciliary body band and scarring and pigment within angle recess.

Treatment

Hyphema is treated by drugs reducing aqueous production, topical steroids which manage inflammation, and mydriatics and cycloplegics which increase uveoscleral outflow.

> *Miotics should be avoided* as they may increase pupillary block and IOP.

After blunt trauma, conventional outflow is reduced due to trabecular damage and uveoscleral mechanism of aqueous outflow becomes predominant, which is known to be impaired by miotics resulting in paradoxic IOP rise.

Treatment of angle recession glaucoma: Medical treatment is frequently unsatisfactory and laser trabeculoplasty is ineffective. Trabeculectomy with antimetabolite therapy is the most effective procedure.

Penetrating Injury

Mechanism of formation of glaucoma due to penetrating injury is explained in **Flowchart 11.20**.

Treatment

Treatment includes wound repair, antibiotics to prevent infection, steroids to prevent inflammation, mydriatics and antiglaucoma medication. If medical therapy fails, filtering surgery is done. Laser trabeculoplasty is usually not possible because of PAS.

■ Glaucoma Associated with Intraocular Hemorrhage

Intraocular hemorrhage includes hyphema and vitreous hemorrhage. Common causes of intraocular hemorrhage are trauma, surgery, and spontaneous in association with several ocular disorders.

Intraocular hemorrhage may be associated with different types of glaucoma, for example, red cell glaucoma, hemolytic glaucoma, ghost cell glaucoma, and hemosiderotic glaucoma.

Red Cell Glaucoma

It is associated with fresh hemorrhage in anterior chamber. If IOP is not relieved, blood staining of cornea may develop within a few days.

Hemolytic Glaucoma

Intraocular hemorrhage (hyphema) causes RBCs to lyse due to hemolysis. Lysed RBCs are engulfed by macrophages which obstruct the trabecular meshwork and cause raised IOP.

Ghost Cell Glaucoma

It occurs in aphakic or pseudophakic eyes with vitreous hemorrhage. It is secondary open-angle glaucoma. Its pathogenesis is explained in **Flowchart 11.21**.

Hemosiderotic Glaucoma

Iron in hemoglobin causes siderosis which causes secondary glaucoma due to tissue alterations in trabecular meshwork. It results in obstruction to aqueous outflow.

Treatment

It includes:
- Treatment of hyphema.
- Treatment of elevated IOP.
- Anterior chamber irrigation, if required.

Use of aspirin can increase frequency of rebleeding.

■ Glaucoma Associated with Intraocular Surgery (Postoperative Glaucoma)

It may occur after cataract surgery, vitreoretinal surgery, or incisional surgery for angle-closure glaucoma.

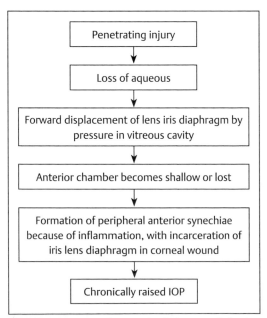

Flowchart 11.20 Pathogenesis of glaucoma following penetrating injury.

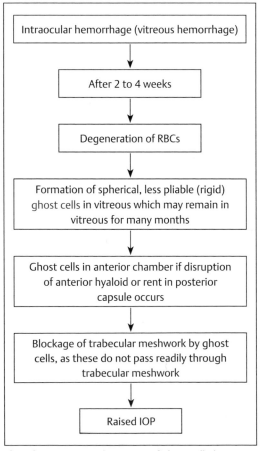

Flowchart 11.21 Pathogenesis of ghost cell glaucoma.

Glaucoma in Aphakia or Pseudophakia

After cataract surgery, glaucoma may develop due to:

- Use of viscoelastics causing temporary obstruction of trabecular meshwork.
- Pupillary block by herniation of anterior vitreous face in aphakia and anterior chamber or iris-supported IOLs.
- Postoperative hemorrhage.
- Postoperative inflammation resulting in pupillary block due to posterior synechiae and obstruction of trabecular meshwork by inflammatory cells.
- Wound leak resulting in flat anterior chamber and angle-closure glaucoma.
- Nd:YAG laser capsulotomy (for posterior capsular opacification) causing obstruction of trabecular meshwork by capsular debris and inflammatory cells.
- Wound dehiscence or delayed wound closure facilitates the epithelial down-growth in anterior chamber which invades trabecular meshwork leading to obstruction of aqueous outflow.

Management

It is managed by the following measures:

- Control of IOP (by CAIs, hyperosmotic agents).
- Steroids (in presence of inflammation).
- Mydriatics (to break early posterior synechiae).
- Multiple laser iridotomies (for pupillary block).
- Reformation of anterior chamber without any delay.

Glaucoma Associated with Retinal Surgery

Vitreoretinal surgery involves:

- **Scleral buckling with encircling bands** which causes *occlusion of vortex veins* by the encircling band. It will cause elevation of EVP and raised IOP.

- **Injection of air or long-acting expansile gases** (such as sulfur hexafluoride SF_6, perfluorocarbons) into vitreous cavity to temponade retina which causes angle closure and raised IOP.
- **Silicone oil** is occasionally used as a retinal temponade in unusually difficult vitreoretinal procedures. Use of silicone oil causes *pupillary block and* raised IOP. Silicone oil in anterior chamber causes *obstruction of trabecular meshwork leading to raised IOP.*

Management

- Glaucoma after scleral buckling procedures is managed by release of band and use of atropine relieving ciliary muscle spasm and pushing iris lens diaphragm back.
- Removal of expansile gas or silicone oil.
- When silicone oil is used, an iridectomy may relieve pupillary block mechanism (**Fig. 11.31**). *Because silicone oil rises to the top of eye, the iridectomy should be placed inferiorly and this should be standard part of all vitreoretinal procedures that include use of silicone oil.*

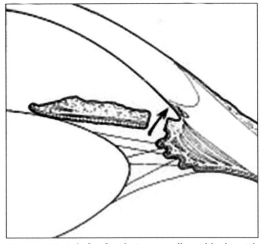

Fig. 11.31 Relief of relative pupillary block with iridectomy. Source: Definition. In: Zimmerman T, Kooner K, ed. Clinical Pathways in Glaucoma. 1st Edition. Thieme; intraocular pressure. 2000.

Patient with gas-filled eye and air travel: Patients with a gas-filled eye should be cautioned regarding air travel. During ascent, expansion of gas and accelerated aqueous outflow results in no significant IOP rise. On descent, eye may become hypotonic and drugs that reduce aqueous production should be avoided because they may prolong the hypotony leading to uveal effusion.

Malignant Glaucoma

It is also called **ciliary block glaucoma** or **aqueous misdirection syndrome**. It typically follows incisional surgery for angle-closure glaucoma such as iridectomy or filtering surgery. In phakic eyes, it can also occur after cataract extraction, anterior segment laser surgery (capsulotomy or iridotomy).

Clinical Features

It presents with symptoms like redness, severe pain and blurring of vision. These are commonly seen after surgery for acute angle-closure glaucoma.

Clinical signs of malignant glaucoma are:
- Shallow or flat anterior chamber (both centrally and peripherally) despite patent iridectomy.
- No iris bombe.
- Marked raised IOP.

There is poor response to conventional therapy, hence called malignant. It is worsened by miotics and relieved by cycloplegics and mydriatics.

Pathogenesis

It is due to posterior pooling of aqueous in the vitreous which pushes the iris lens diaphragm forward. It results in shallow/flat anterior chamber with raised IOP (**Flowchart 11.22**).

Differential Diagnosis

Diagnosis of malignant glaucoma requires exclusion of pupillary block glaucoma, choroidal detachment and suprachoroidal hemorrhage.

In *pupillary block glaucoma,* anterior chamber is deep in the center and shallow/flat peripherally, whereas in malignant glaucoma, anterior chamber is shallow/flat both centrally and peripherally. In *choroidal detachment*, IOP is low and suprachoroidal fluid is present on B-scan ultrasonography while in malignant glaucoma IOP is elevated. In *suprachoroidal hemorrhage*, bullous, dark reddish-brown choroidal elevation is seen on ophthalmoscopy.

Treatment

There is poor response to conventional therapy, hence called malignant. It is worsened by miotics and relieved by cycloplegics and mydriatics.

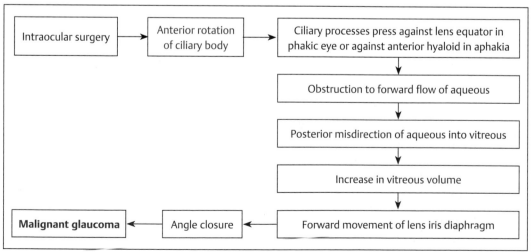

Flowchart 11.22 Pathogenesis of malignant glaucoma.

- First line of therapy involves use of mydriatic–cycloplegic agents such as atropine 1% and phenylephrine 10%. These deepen the anterior chamber. Aqueous production is decreased by topical β-blockers, CAIs, and α_2 agonists. To shrink (dehydrate) vitreous hyperosmotic agents (IV mannitol 20%) are used. Miotics are contraindicated.
- Second line of treatment is laser therapy (**Nd:YAG laser**) to create peripheral iridotomy and to disrupt anterior vitreous face in aphakia and pseudophakia to release trapped aqueous from vitreous.
- If conservative measures fail pars plana, vitrectomy with or without lensectomy is done to reduce volume of vitreous.

■ Pseudoexfoliation Glaucoma

Pseudoexfoliation is a basement membrane disorder, identified in skin and visceral organ as well as in the eye. So, pseudoexfoliation syndrome (PEX syndrome) is a systemic disorder.

Pseudoexfoliation material is a gray-white, dandruff-like fibrillogranular material produced by abnormal basement membrane of equatorial lens capsule, iris, ciliary body and trabeculum, and then deposited on anterior lens capsule except central region, zonules, iris, ciliary body, trabeculum, and anterior vitreous face (**Fig. 11.32**).

When an eye with pseudoexfoliation develops secondary open-angle glaucoma, the condition is referred to as **pseudoexfoliation glaucoma**. Glaucoma associated with pseudoexfoliation is also known as **glaucoma capsulare**.

Pathogenesis

Deposition of pseudoexfoliation material and pigment released from iris on trabeculum causes blockage of trabecular spaces leading to elevation of IOP (secondary open-angle glaucoma).

Clinical Features

- Deposition of dandruff-like material on pupillary border of iris and anterior lens capsule in the region where anterior capsule is rubbed upon by iris. So, *axial region of capsule is free.*
- IOP elevation.
- Gonioscopy shows commonly open angle with increased trabecular meshwork pigmentation.

Differential Diagnosis

It must be differentiated from other forms of lens exfoliation (true exfoliation) and other causes of pigment dispersion (pigmentary dispersion syndrome and pigmentary glaucoma).

- True exfoliation (**capsule delamination**): It occurs due to trauma and exposure to intense heat (glass blowers). It involves lamellar splitting of lens capsule. It is not associated with secondary glaucoma.
- Pigment dispersion and pigmentary glaucoma: There is absence of exfoliated material.

Treatment

Medical treatment is same as for POAG. Laser trabeculoplasty and trabeculectomy are also advised if medical treatment fails.

■ Childhood Glaucoma (OP6.6, 6.7)

Childhood glaucoma is caused by developmental abnormalities of anterior chamber angle.

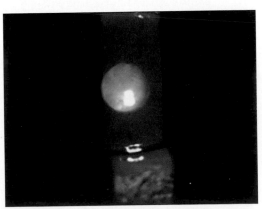

Fig. 11.32 Pseudoexfoliation of lens capsule.

■ Classification

Developmental abnormalities of anterior chamber angle may be (**Flowchart 11.23**):

- Unassociated with any other ocular or systemic developmental anomalies, i.e., congenital anomalies are limited to trabecular meshwork (isolated trabeculodysgenesis) termed as **primary developmental glaucoma**.
- Associated with a variety of ocular and/or systemic developmental anomalies, i.e., **developmental glaucoma associated with congenital anomalies**.

■ Primary Congenital Glaucoma (PCG)

Depending upon the severity of trabeculodysgenesis, the resultant raised IOP may occur at birth or anytime thereafter. According to the age of onset, PCG may be:

- Early onset PCG: It is also called congenital or infantile glaucoma.
- Late-onset PCG: It is also called juvenile glaucoma.

Congenital Glaucoma

It is an early onset glaucoma that arises between birth and the age of 3 years. It is bilateral in up to 75% cases, although involvement is frequently asymmetrical. It is more common in boys than in girls (**Fig. 11.33**).

Etiology

It is characterized by incomplete differentiation of trabecular meshwork during embryogenesis (**trabeculodysgenesis/Barkan membrane**) not associated with other ocular or systemic developmental anomaly.

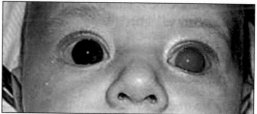

Fig. 11.33 Congenital glaucoma. Source: Examination. In: Gallin P, ed. Pediatric Ophthalmology: A Clinical Guide. 1st Edition. Thieme; 2000.

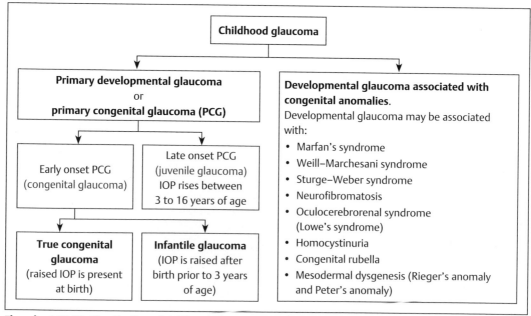

Flowchart 11.23 Classification of childhood glaucoma. Abbreviation: IOP, intraocular pressure.

Pathogenesis

Angle remains closed by persistent embryonic tissue due to abnormal development of trabecular meshwork. Obstruction to drainage of aqueous humor leads to rise in IOP.

Genetics

Most of the cases are sporadic, in 10% cases hereditary pattern is evident and inheritance is *autosomal recessive* with incomplete penetration. The abnormal genes causing congenital glaucoma have been identified on chromosomes 2p21 and 1p36.

Clinical Features

Infants and young children with glaucoma usually present when parents notice enlarged globe and corneal haze. Raised IOP causes corneal edema resulting in lacrimation, photophobia, and blepharospasm (classical triad of symptoms).

Clinical signs: Immature and growing collagen that constitutes cornea and sclera responds to raised IOP by stretching. The eye is distensible up to the age of 3 years. *All parts of the globe may stretch in response to raised IOP until 3 years of age* so that gradual enlargement of globe occurs. This stretching and enlargement may mask the raised IOP on clinical examination (**Table 11.11**).

The globe enlargement in congenital glaucoma can be differentiated from congenital megalocornea by features listed in **Table 11.12**.

Diagnosis

Evaluation of glaucoma in infants requires examination under anesthesia. It includes:

- IOP measurement by handheld applanation tonometer.
- Gonioscopy by Koeppe lens for assessment of anterior chamber angle.

Table 11.11 Signs of congenital glaucoma

Globe	• The hallmark of congenital glaucoma is *enlargement of globe* (**Buphthalmos** = Bull's eye). The eye appears bluish owing to the stretching of sclera and visualization of underlying uvea.
Cornea	• Horizontal *corneal diameter* in normal neonate is 10–10.5 mm and increases about 0.5–1 mm in first year of life; a diameter >12 mm in first year of life is a highly suspicious finding. • *Corneal edema.* • *Haab striae*: These represent healed breaks in Descemet membrane and appear as lines with a double contour. They are characteristically oriented horizontally concentric to limbus (**Fig. 11.34**).
IOP	• It is *elevated* and measured during general anesthesia. IOP >21 mm Hg is suspicious for glaucoma. Range of normal intraocular pressure (IOP) in infants with normal eyes is 11–14 mm Hg.
Refractive error	• *Axial myopia* results due to increase in axial length.
Anterior chamber	• Anterior chamber is *characteristically deep.* Lens does not participate in general enlargement but is flattened and displaced backwards. Iris may become tremulous due to the removal of support (*iridodonesis*). Myopia is compensated due to flattening and backward displacement of lens to some extent.
Optic disc	• *Cupping of optic nerve head* occurs more rapidly in infants than in adults due to stretching of scleral canal and posterior bowing of lamina cribrosa. Cupping is reversible in childhood if IOP is lowered early enough. *Reversibility of cupping is one of the hallmark of successful management of glaucoma.*

Table 11.12 Differential diagnosis of corneal enlargement in congenital glaucoma

Features	Congenital glaucoma	Congenital megalocornea
Vision	Markedly impaired	Not impaired
Corneal transparency	Corneal haze	Not affected
Intraocular pressure (IOP)	Raised	Normal
Cup disc ratio (CDR)	Cupping present	No cupping
Inheritance	Autosomal recessive	X-linked recessive

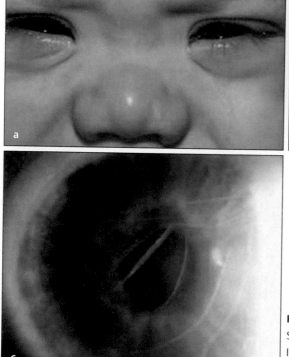
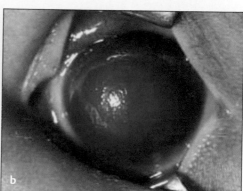

Fig. 11.34 (a–c) Splits in Descemet membrane. Source: Childhood Glaucoma. (In: Morrison J, Pollack I, ed. Glaucoma: Science and Practice. 1st Edition. Thieme; 2002).

- Measurement of horizontal corneal diameter with calipers.
- Pachymetry for measurement of CCT.
- Ultrasonography to measure axial length.
- Retinoscopy to assess refractive error.
- Ophthalmoscopy to examine ONH for cupping.
- Fundus photography.

Optic disc should be examined first followed by measurement of IOP, corneal diameters, and finally gonioscopy.

Intravenous ketamine should be used for general anesthesia since other agents may lower IOP; ketamine may falsely increase IOP.

Treatment

Definitive treatment of congenital glaucoma is surgical. Antiglaucoma medication has limited value in its management and used as a temporary measure before surgery to reduce corneal edema and help clear the cornea to facilitate angle surgery. "**Angle surgery**" may be achieved with:

Goniotomy (an incisional surgery by an *internal approach*) **or trabeculotomy** (an incisional surgery by an *external approach*). In goniotomy, a goniotomy knife is passed through limbus and swept round the angle of anterior chamber under gonioscopic visualization. It is easiest to perform goniotomy over nasal 120-degree of angle using a temporal approach. *Results are poor if corneal diameter is ≥14 mm because in such eyes Schlemm canal is obliterated.* Trabeculotomy is performed *if cornea is not clear* because corneal clouding prevents visualization of angle in goniotomy *or when repeated goniotomy has failed.* In trabeculotomy, a partial thickness flap of sclera is made at upper limbus, exposing the Schlemm canal. Thus, Schlemm canal is opened from a scleral (external) approach.

Table 11.13 Differential diagnosis of congenital glaucoma w.r.t. ocular symptoms

	Lacrimation (epiphora)	Photophobia	Blepharospasm	Red eye	Discharge
Primary congenital glaucoma	+	+	+	−	−
Nasolacrimal duct (NLD) obstruction	+	−	−	−	+
Conjunctivitis	+	+	−	+	+
Uveitis/keratitis	+	+	+	+	−
Corneal abrasion	+	+	+	+	−

Note: (+) denotes presence and (−) denotes absence

In *primary congenital glaucoma, either goniotomy or trabeculotomy is the procedure of choice (success rate is about 90%).* Goniotomy requires a clear cornea for adequate visualization of anterior chamber angle. Trabeculotomy may be performed if cornea is hazy or opaque. If angle incision operations fail, trabeculectomy or drainage implant surgery may be performed.

Prognosis

The age of onset appears to have prognostic implications. If glaucoma is present at birth, prognosis is worse. If glaucoma develops few months after birth (2 months–1year of age), prognosis is good if managed promptly.

Differential Diagnosis of Ocular Symptoms in Congenital Glaucoma

Congenital glaucoma must be differentiated from (**Table 11.13**):

- NLD obstruction.
- Conjunctivitis.
- Uveitis, keratitis.
- Corneal abrasion.

Juvenile Glaucoma

Glaucoma that manifests between 3 and 16 years of age is called late-onset primary congenital glaucoma or juvenile glaucoma. In these cases, trabecular anomalies are not as severe. The structures are poorly differentiated; hence, decreased aqueous outflow occurs. It is least common form of PCG.

Clinical Features

The child is often asymptomatic. Corneal enlargement usually is not the predominant sign but child often presents with decreased vision usually from induced myopia and insidious visual field loss. ONH may reveal enlarged optic cup.

> Although elevated IOP produces corneal enlargement limited to first 3 years of life, sclera stretching persists for approximately 10 years producing progressive myopia and often astigmatism.

Treatment

Treatment is surgical (trabeculotomy or trabeculectomy).

CHAPTER 12

Vitreous Humor

Anatomy of Vitreous 316
Vitreous Detachment...317
Vitreous Opacities..318
Vitreous Bands and Membranes 319
Persistent Hyper Plastic Primary Vitreous...320
Vitreous Hemorrhage 320
Vitreoretinal Degenerations 321

■ Anatomy of Vitreous

Vitreous is a transparent gel, a jelly-like structure filling the space bounded by lens, ciliary body, and retina. It is an avascular structure and has a volume of approximately 4 mL. It consists of water (99%), network of collagen fibrils, hyaluronic acid, peripheral cells (hyalocytes) which synthesize hyaluronic acid, and mucopolysaccharides. Its refractive index is 1.336. Importance of vitreous lies in the following functions:

- It serves optical functions.
- It provides structural integrity to the eye.
- It is a pathway for nutrients to be utilized by the lens and retina.

The interaction between hyaluronic acid and collagen fibrils is responsible for the gel form of vitreous. It possesses all the properties of a hydrophilic gel.

Inorganic ion content of vitreous contains sodium (146.7 mmol/L), potassium (5.73 mmol/L), chloride (121.6 mmol/L), calcium (1.13 mmol/L), and magnesium (0.9 mmol/L).

Unlike aqueous humor, which is continuously replenished, the gel in the vitreous chamber is stagnant. Therefore, if blood, cells, or other byproducts of inflammation get into the vitreous, they will remain there unless removed surgically. These are known as **floaters**.

After death, the vitreous resists putrefaction longer than other body fluids. The vitreous potassium concentration rises so predictably within the hours, days and weeks after death that vitreous potassium levels are frequently used to estimate the time-of-death (postmortem interval) of a corpse.

■ Parts

Vitreous has three parts: Peripheral cortical vitreous, definitive vitreous, and vitreous base.

Peripheral Cortical Vitreous

The density of collagen fibrils is greater in the peripheral part. The condensation of these fibrils on the surface gives rise to the appearance of a boundary membrane called **hyaloid membrane**.

Internal limiting membrane (ILM) separates retina from vitreous and there exists a potential space between the two called **subhyaloid space**.

Main Mass of Vitreous (Definitive Vitreous)

It consists of collagen fibrils which are less dense. Sodium hyaluronate molecules fill the space between fibrils. Developmentally, primary (primitive) vitreous is a vascular structure having a hyaloid system of vessels. Secondary (definitive) vitreous is an avascular structure. When secondary vitreous fills the cavity, primary vitreous is concentrated into the center and forms the **canal of Cloquet**. Primary vitreous with hyaloid vessels ultimately disappears.

Vitreous Base

It is the part of vitreous 4 to 6 mm wide across the ora serrata. It is firmly attached to posterior 2 mm of the pars plana and the anterior 2 to 4 mm of retina. An incision through the midpart of pars plana will usually be located anterior to vitreous base. The cortical vitreous is strongly attached at the vitreous base.

■ Vitreous Attachments

The peripheral cortical vitreous is loosely attached to the ILM. The firm attachment occurs at following sites:

- *Vitreous base*—Attachment is very strong at the vitreous base around ora serrata.
- *Margin of optic disc*—Attachment is fairly strong, forming a ring around optic disc.
- *Around fovea*—Attachment is fairly weak, forming a ring.
- *Along peripheral blood vessels*—Attachments are usually weak.

Anteriorly, it is attached to the posterior surface of the lens by hyaloidocapsular ligament of Wieger in childhood and adolescents, but later a concave space, Berger's space, separates the lens and the vitreous.

■ Changes in Vitreous with Age

Vitreous gel shows the following changes with age:

- Liquefaction of gel (**synchysis**).
- Contraction and shrinkage (**syneresis**).

- Separation of cortical vitreous from ILM of sensory retina (**vitreous detachment**).

■ Vitreous Detachment

Detachment of vitreous occurs as shown in **Flowchart 12.1**.

Vitreous detachment may be:
- Posterior vitreous detachment (**PVD**).
- Basal vitreous detachment.
- Anterior vitreous detachment.

■ Posterior Vitreous Detachment (PVD)

It is the separation of cortical vitreous from ILM of sensory retina posterior to vitreous base (**Fig. 12.1**).

Aetiopathogenesis

1. Degenerations:
   - Senile vitreous degeneration.
   - Myopic degeneration.
2. Ocular trauma
3. Inflammations:
   - Intermediate uveitis.
   - Chorioretinitis.

The above causes may result in liquefaction of vitreous gel (synchysis). Some eyes with synchysis develop a hole in the posterior hyaloid membrane, and the liquefied vitreous gains access to newly formed retrohyaloid space through this defect. Posterior vitreous surface detaches from ILM of sensory retina up to posterior margin of vitreous base.

It is more common among diabetics and elderly patients. People with myopia > 6D are at higher risk of PVD. PVD may also occur in cases of cataract surgery.

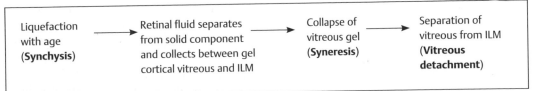

Flowchart 12.1 Mechanism of vitreous detachment

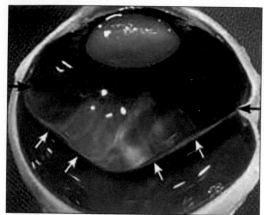

Fig. 12.1 Posterior vitreous detachment. Source: Vitreous detachment. In: Lang G, ed. Ophthalmology. A pocket textbook atlas. 2nd edition. Thieme; 2006..

Types

PVD is of two types:
- Acute PVD (sudden onset).
- Chronic PVD (develops gradually).

Clinical Features

When PVD occurs, there is a characteristic pattern of symptoms:
- Flashes of light (**photopsia**)—It is common in the temporal visual field and occurs due to vitreoretinal adhesions and provoked by ocular movements.
- **Floaters**—If PVD occurs over optic nerve head (optic disc), patient complains of a ring-like opacity (**Weiss ring**).

Complications

In PVD, sensory retina is no longer protected by stable vitreous cortex. Detached vitreous may cause dynamic traction on retina during ocular movements, resulting in retinal tear. The risk of retinal tear associated with vitreous detachment is higher in patients with myopic retinal degeneration and lattice degeneration. Retinal tear may cause:
- Retinal detachment (RD):
  a. Rhegmatogenous RD—is associated with *acute* rhegmatogenous PVD (acute PVD).
  b. Tractional RD—is typically associated with *chronic*, incomplete, nonrhegmatogenous PVD.
  c. Exudative RD—is usually unassociated with PVD.
- Vitreous hemorrhages if retinal tear involves the retinal vessels. If a retinal vessel is torn, the leakage of blood into the vitreous cavity is often preserved as a "shower of floaters."

Therefore, patients with a history of floaters or photopsia must be carefully examined.

Treatment

- If PVD is not associated with retinal tear (i.e., uncomplicated PVD), patient must be reassured and treatment is not required.
- If there is evidence of retinal tear, prophylactic barrage laser photocoagulation or cryopexy of retina is performed.

■ Detachment of Vitreous Base and Anterior Vitreous

These usually occur secondary to trauma. These are often associated with vitreous hemorrhage.

■ Vitreous Opacities

The fibrils of vitreous gel become condensed within liquefied vitreous, so that they are less transparent than the rest of the vitreous. These appears as black spots floating before eyes and mistaken for small flying insects. These are called **muscae volitantes** or **floaters**.

■ Causes

- Developmental: Developmental opacities are located in Cloquet's Canal and represent remnants of hyaloid system.
- Degenerations such as old age or myopia. Some of the other degenerative conditions are asteroid hyalosis, synchysis scintillans, and amyloid degeneration (amyloidosis).
- Inflammation such as pars planitis and chorioretinitis.

- Vitreous hemorrhage.
- Neoplasms—Neoplastic cells in retinoblastoma and reticulum cell sarcoma form the vitreous opacities.

Asteroid Hyalosis

It is often *unilateral* and found in *elderly* individuals. It is characterized by multiple, white round bodies in vitreous gel. The condition is *asymptomatic* but may cause difficulty in fundus examination. These are composed of **calcium-containing phospholipids** attached to collagen fibrils in vitreous. These are suspended throughout the vitreous and unaffected by gravity. If it causes impairment of vision, vitrectomy may be considered, otherwise treatment is rarely required.

Synchysis Scintillans

This degenerative condition is characterized by multiple, yellowish white, crystalline bodies floating in the vitreous. These are composed of **cholesterol crystals**. It occurs in eyes which have suffered from trauma, vitreous hemorrhage, or inflammatory disease in the past, so it may occur at any age. Vitreous in such cases is liquefied, so the bodies float in vitreous and settle down in vitreous cavity due to gravity but can be thrown up by ocular movements and appear as shower of golden crystals. No treatment is indicated. Differentiating features between asteroid hyalosis and synchysis scintillans are listed in **Table 12.1**.

Amyloid Degeneration (Amyloidosis)

It is a *heredofamilial* disease.

Inheritance

It is transmitted as an autosomal dominant trait. It is a systemic disease with amyloid deposition in the collagen fibers of heart, thyroid, pancreas, peripheral nerves, and muscles, and produces symptoms related to affected organs.

Ocular Features

Both eyes are involved and the ocular features include the following:
- External ophthalmoplegia.
- Proptosis.
- Diplopia.
- Diminution of vision.
- Perivasculitis.
- Retinal hemorrhages and exudates.
- Vitreous opacities which are classically linear with footplate attachments to retina and posterior surface of lens, which is a diagnostic feature. These cause severe visual impairment.

Treatment

Pars plana vitrectomy with guarded prognosis.

■ Vitreous Bands and Membranes

Vitreous bands and membranes often develop after PVD or massive vitreous hemorrhage.

Table 12.1 Difference between asteroid hyalosis and synchysis scintillans		
Features	Asteroid hyalosis	Synchysis scintillans
1. Age	In elderly	At any age
2. Laterality	Unilateral	Bilateral
3. Color of bodies	White	Yellowish-white
4. Composition	Calcium-containing phospholipids (hence, white)	Cholesterol Crystals
5. Condition of vitreous	Gel	Liquefied
6. Effect of gravity	Because of gel vitreous, asteroid bodies are suspended in vitreous and unaffected by gravity	As fluid bodies float and settle due to gravity

They originate from hyalocytes or endothelial cells of capillaries.

If a **band** is adherent to retina, traction on retina is likely, producing photopsia and retinal edema/hemorrhage, and may produce retinal break or detachment.

Preretinal or epiretinal membrane (ERM) lines the inner surface of retina. It may be thin and look like a sheet of cellophane or resemble a sheet of tissue when it is thick. Contraction of ERM results in macular pucker.

Treatment includes vitrectromy. ERM may cause impairment of central vision and meta-morphopsia and may be removed by vitrectomy, that is, pars plana vitrectomy + epiretinal membrane stripping which is effective especially in treating macular pucker.

■ Persistent Hyper Plastic Primary Vitreous

It is a developmental disorder of vitreous. In PHPV, structures within primary vitreous fail to regress, that is, there is *persistence of fetal vasculature*.

■ Presentation

- It is unilateral and usually associated with microphthalmos.
- It typically presents with white pupillary reflex (**leucocoria**), seen shortly after birth in full-term infant.

■ Types

It is seen in two forms:
- Anterior PHPV.
- Posterior PHPV– less common.

Anterior PHPV

It is characterized by presence of retrolental mass with long and extended ciliary processes. Later, contraction of retrolental tissue pulls the ciliary processes inward.

It may later be associated with the following:
- Cataract.

- Glaucoma.
- Vitreous hemorrhage.

Diagnosis

It is diagnosed by ultrasonography and CT scan.

Treatment

If diagnosed early, treatment consists of aspiration of lens (pars plana lensectomy)

+

Pars plana anterior vitrectomy

+

Excision of retrolental membrane

Visual Prognosis

It is poor.

Differential Diagnosis

It must be differentiated from other causes of leucocoria, especially:
- Retinoblastoma.
- Congenital cataract.
- Retinopathy of prematurity (ROP).

Posterior PHPV

It is characterized by **persistent hyaloid artery** with a large stalk extending to the peripheral retina from the optic disc. It does not reach the lens, thus usually not causing cataract. It may be associated with tractional retinal detachment.

■ Vitreous Hemorrhage

Vitreous hemorrhage may be located in preretinal or subhyaloid space, vitreous cavity, or both.

Common causes of vitreous hemorrhage are depicted in **Fig. 12.2**.

■ Clinical Features

Symptoms
- Sudden onset of floaters.
- Sudden and painless diminution or loss of vision.

Signs
- **Subhyaloid (preretinal) hemorrhage:** Blood never clots in subhyaloid hemorrhage

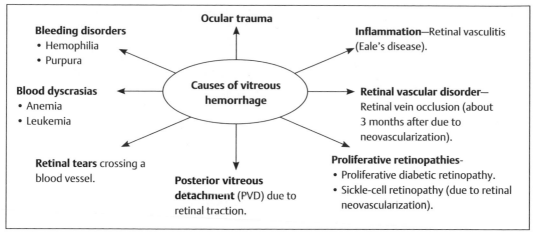

Fig. 12.2 Common causes of vitreous hemorrhage.

and moves with gravity. Blood cells settle down and appear as boat-shaped.

- **Blood in vitreous gel:** It clots and moves with the gel. Blood of long-standing duration in vitreous loses color and becomes a white opaque mass. When vitreous hemorrhage is massive, there is no red reflex.

All cases of vitreous hemorrhage must be carefully examined with indirect ophthalmoscope and slit-lamp biomicroscope to look for a cause.

■ Diagnosis

B-scan ultrasonography is particularly helpful in confirming the diagnosis.

■ Complications

Recurrent vitreous hemorrhage may lead to the following:

- Vitreous degeneration.
- Hemolytic or ghost cell glaucoma.
- Hemosiderosis bulbi.
- Tractional retinal detachment.

■ Treatment

Conservative

- *Bed rest* with elevation of patient's head, which minimizes dispersion of blood within gel and allows the blood to settle down under the influence of gravity. It may be possible to discover the cause and treat accordingly.
- If vitreous fails to clear, a 2-month follow-up is advised.

Surgery

Pars plana vitrectomy is performed. Surgical intervention is required if:

- Blood does not clear within 6 months
- Vitreous hemorrhage is due to trauma.
- Vitreous hemorrhage is associated with retinal detachment.

■ Vitreoretinal Degenerations

Hereditary vitreoretinal degeneration is characterized by early onset cataract, vitreous anomalies, coarse fibrils, and retinal detachment. Additional ocular and systemic features may be present depending on the underlying cause. These include:

- Wagner disease.
- Stickler syndrome.
- Favre–Goldmann syndrome.

■ Wagner Disease

It is a bilateral condition.

Inheritance—It is transmitted as autosomal dominant trait.

Signs

Vitreous—It is liquefied and shrinks (syneresis). Vitreous cavity is optically empty, leaving a thin layer of formed cortex on the surface of retina.

Retina—Retina shows:

- Peripheral retinal degeneration.
- Narrow and sheathed retinal vessels.
- Chorioretinal atrophy.

Complication—Cortical cataract is a late complication.

■ Stickler Syndrome

It is also known as *hereditary arthroophthalmopathy*. It is a connective tissue disorder, resulting in the involvement of eyes, joints, ears, and orofacial abnormalities. It is a relatively common disorder and is, in fact, the most common inherited cause of retinal detachment in children.

Inheritance—It is transmitted as an autosomal dominant trait.

Signs—It is a variant of Wagner disease. Other important features include:

- Arthropathy—It is characterized by stiff, painful, prominent and hyperextensible large joints.
- Ear—Deafness (sensorineural).
- Orofacial abnormalities—These include midfacial flattering, cleft palate, and bifid uvula.
- Ocular findings are same as in Wagner disease which are associated with retinal detachment, that is:

◇ Liquefaction and syneresis of vitreous.
◇ Peripheral retinal degeneration.
◇ Sheathed and narrow retinal vessels.
◇ Myopia.
◇ Cataract.

- Retinal detachment

■ Favre–Goldmann Syndrome

It is a bilateral and familial disorder manifesting features of retinoschisis and pigmentary retinopathy resembling retinitis pigmentosa.

Inheritance—It is transmitted as an autosomal recessive trait.

Signs

- Vitreous—It shows syneresis but cavity is not optically empty.
- Retinoschisis—It is both central, affecting macula, as well as peripheral.
- Pigmentary dystrophy—Pigmentary degeneration resembling retinitis pigmentosa is marked.
- White dendritiform peripheral retinal vessels are also frequent.
- Cataract.

Presentation—The condition presents with progressive loss of vision in childhood due to retinoschisis, pigmentary dystrophy, and cataract.

Electroretinogram (ERG)—It is markedly abnormal. When pigmentary changes are marked, ERG is extinguished.

Prognosis—It is poor with no satisfactory treatment.

CHAPTER

13

The Retina

Anatomy of Retina...323
Symptoms and Signs in Retinal Diseases..327
Evaluation of Retinal Diseases...331
Retinal Photocoagulation..337
Congenital and Developmental Anomalies..338
Vascular Disorders of Retina..339
Vascular Retinopathies...345
Inflammation of Retina..359
Retinochoroidopathies..362
Important Macular Disorders..365
Degenerations of Retina...371
Dystrophies of Retina...378
Phakomatoses...384
Retinal Detachment..386

■ Anatomy of Retina

Retina is the innermost layer of eyeball. It extends from the margin of optic disc to ora serrata, which is 7 mm from the limbus.

■ Microscopic Structure

Retina consists of 10 layers (**Fig. 13.1**). It comprises three layers of cells: photoreceptor cells, bipolar cells and ganglion cells. Layers of retina from *out inwards* are:

1. **Retinal pigment epithelium (RPE):** It is the single layer of hexagonal cells *containing melanin granules* which lies between the Bruch's membrane of choroid and outer segment of photoreceptor cells (rods and cones).

2. **Layer of rods and cones (photoreceptors):** Rods and cones are the end organs of vision, which are nourished by choriocapillaris (**Table 13.1**). Rods and cones contain:

   - *Outer segment:* It consists of membranous discs containing visual pigment.
   - *Inner segment:* It is rich in mitochondria.
   - *Nuclear region:* It forms outer nuclear layer.
   - *Synaptic terminal:* It forms outer plexiform layer.

3. **External limiting membrane (ELM):** It is formed by glial tissue and perforated by rods and cones.

4. **Outer nuclear layer (ONL):** It is formed by nuclei of rods and cones.

5. **Outer plexiform layer (OPL):** It is formed by synapse between: rods and cones, bipolar cells and horizontal cells.

6. **Inner nuclear layer (INL):** It consists of cell bodies of bipolar cells, horizontal cells and amacrine cells. *Bipolar cells*

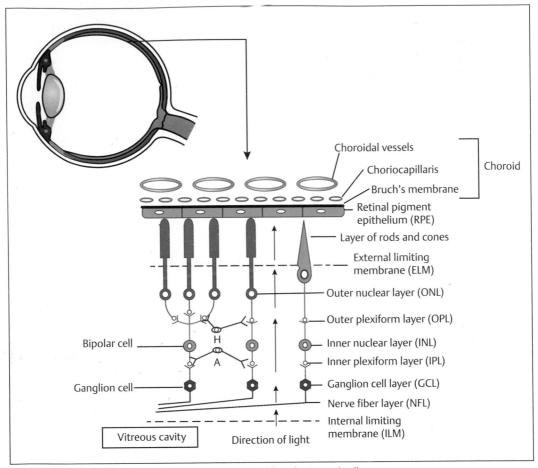

Fig. 13.1 Layers of retina. Abbreviations: A, amacrine cell; H, horizontal cell.

Table 13.1 Characteristic features of rods and cones		
Features	**Rods**	**Cones**
Number	120 million	6 million
Distribution	Mainly in peripheral retina	Occupy central retina
Function	• Responsible for vision in dim light (scotopic vision). • Cannot detect color. • In periphery (extra foveal region) rods synapse with a bipolar cell. Hence, receptive field is more with less resolution.	• Responsible for vision in bright light (photopic vision). • Responsible for color vision. • At fovea there is 1:1 correspondence between cones and bipolar cells. Hence, resolution is more and visual acuity is better.
Loss of function	Leads to night blindness.	Leads to color blindness.
Neurotransmitter	Glutamate	Glutamate

constitute *1st order neurons. Horizontal cells* connect one receptor cell to another. *Amacrine cells* synapse with bipolar cells and ganglion cells.

7. **Inner Plexiform Layer (IPL):** It is formed by synapses between axons of *bipolar cells,* dendrites of *ganglion cells and* processes of *amacrine cells.*

8. **Ganglion cell layer (GCL):** It contains cell bodies of ganglion cells. Ganglion cells are the 2nd order neurons of visual pathway.

9. **Nerve fiber layer (NFL):** It is formed by axons of ganglion cells which are nonmyelinated.

10. **Internal limiting membrane (ILM):** It separates retina from vitreous. It is the innermost layer of retina which is formed by glial tissue.

The various layers of retina are bound together by neuroglia and *vertical fibers of Müller,* which have supportive as well as nutritive functions. To excite rods and cones, incident light has to traverse the tissues of retina. Information flows vertically from photoreceptors (rods and cones) to bipolar cells and then to ganglion cells, as well as laterally via horizontal cells in OPL and amacrine cells in IPL.

The retina comprises of RPE and neurosensory retina. The Bruch's membrane separates RPE from choriocapillaris. RPE contain villous processes which reach out toward the outer segments of photoreceptors. The adhesion between RPE and neurosensory retina is weaker than that between RPE and the Bruch's membrane. So, RPE can separate from neurosensory retina by fluid. This separation is called retinal detachment and the fluid in between the two layers is referred to as subretinal fluid (SRF).

■ Division of Retina

Retina is divided into two parts by retinal equator which is considered to lie in the line with exit of four vortex veins. Retina posterior to retinal equator is called **posterior pole** which can be examined by direct ophthalmoscope and slit lamp

with + 90D lens. Retina anterior to this equator is called **peripheral retina** which can be examined by indirect ophthalmoscope and slit lamp with three-mirror contact lens (**Fig. 13.2**).

Posterior pole of retina includes two distinct areas: optic disc and macula lutea.

Optic Disc

At optic disc, fibers of NFL pass through lamina cribrosa and run in the optic nerve. So, optic disc is also known as optic nerve head (ONH). All other layers of retina terminate at the optic disc, therefore the optic disc has no photoreceptors. The object is not seen if the image falls on optic disc, hence optic disc is a **blind spot** in the visual field. Its diameter is 1.5 mm = 1DD (1 disc diameter). A depression in the disc is called physiological cup. Retinal vessels emerge through this cup (**Fig. 13.3a**).

Macula Lutea (Yellow Spot)

It is a circular area which appears darker than the surrounding retina and contains xanthophyll pigment. It is 5.5 mm in diameter. The center of macula is situated approximately 3 mm (2DD) away from the temporal margin of optic disc and approximately 1 mm below the horizontal meridian. *Clinical landmarks within macula are as follows:* fovea, foveola, and foveal avascular zone (FAZ) (**Fig. 13.3b**).

Fovea (fovea centralis) is a depression in inner retinal surface at the center of macula having a diameter of 1.5 mm (1 DD). **Ophthalmoscopically,**

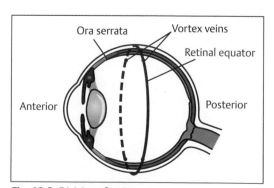

Fig. 13.2 Division of retina.

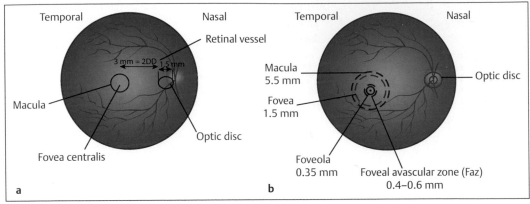

Fig. 13.3 **(a)** Posterior pole of retina. **(b)** Macula lutea.

it is recognized by an *oval light reflex.* Parafoveal region (region around fovea) is the thickest part of retina containing several layers of ganglion cells.

Foveola is a small depression at the center of fovea and is the thinnest part of retina. It is 0.35 mm in diameter and is devoid of ganglion cells. It *contains only cones.* Other layers of retina are almost absent. *This enables the most acute vision at foveola.* Each cone relays to a single ganglion cell.

FAZ is an avascular area, that is, it does not contain any retinal blood vessel. It is 0.4 to 0.5 mm in diameter. Thus, it is located within fovea (1.5 mm) but extends beyond foveola (0.35 mm). Its exact limit can only be determined by fluorescein angiography (FA).

The eye is designed to focus the visual image on retina with minimal optical distortion. RPE cells contain melanin which absorbs any light not captured by the retina. It prevents light from being reflected off to the retina again.

In order to optimize light transmission to the foveolar cones, all retinal elements have to be displaced laterally out of the light path. Hence, light has a direct pathway to photoreceptors, and visual image received at foveola is the least distorted. **Due to lateral displacement of retinal layers in the center of fovea,** nerve fibers in outer plexiform (Henle's) layer run almost parallel with the retinal surface before synapsing with the cells

in INL (**Fig. 13.4**). *Therefore, exudates within OPL (Henle's layer) assume a star-shaped configuration (macular star), owing to this radial arrangement of fibers.*

■ Blood Supply of Retina

Arterial Supply

Outer layers of retina up to ONL, that is, RPE, photoreceptors, ELM and ONL get their nutrition by diffusion from choriocapillaris.

Inner layers of retina are supplied by central retinal artery (CRA) and its branches. CRA is a branch of the ophthalmic artery.

Central retinal artery divides at or near the surface of the disc into two branches:
- *Superior trunk:* It divides into superior temporal (ST) and superior nasal (SN) branches.
- *Inferior trunk:* It divides into inferior temporal (IT) and inferior nasal (IN) branches (**Fig. 13.5**).

Each of these branches divide dichotomously, spreading over retina and reaching the ora serrata. These are the *end arteries,* as they do not anastomose with each other. The only place where retinal system anastomoses with ciliary system is in the region of lamina cribrosa.

Choroidal vessels anastomose freely, whereas retinal vessels do not anastomose at all.

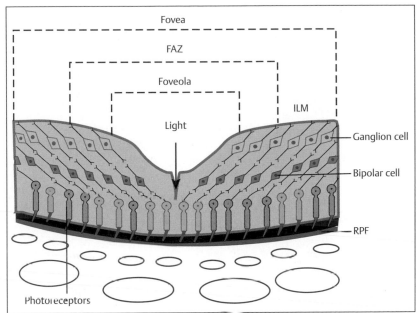

Fig. 13.4 Cross-section of fovea. Abbreviations: FAZ, foveal avascular zone; ILM, internal limiting membrane; RPE, retinal pigment epithelium.

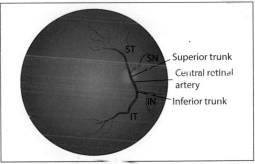

Fig. 13.5 Arterial supply of retina. Abbreviations. IN, inferonasal; IT, inferotemporal; SN, superonasal; ST, superotemporal.

Macular region is supplied by branches from ST and IT arteries. Occasionally, cilioretinal artery from ciliary system enters the eye near the edge of disc and runs temporally toward macula.

Venous Drainage

The outer retinal layers are drained by vortex veins, while the inner layers of retina are drained through retinal veins.

The retinal veins do not accurately follow the course of arteries. At the disc, they join to form the central retinal vein (CRV) which follows the course of CRA. The CRA communicates with choroidal circulation in the prelaminar region.

Arteries are brighter red and narrower, while veins have purplish tint and are more tortuous.

In normal conditions, no pulsations can be seen in retinal arteries. In 80 to 90% of people, *pulsations seen at the disc are venous* due to the effect of intraocular pressure (IOP).

■ Symptoms and Signs in Retinal Diseases

Retinal affections may be congenital or developmental. Diseases of retina rarely occur in isolation. It is frequently affected with systemic diseases or involvement of adjacent structures (choroid, optic nerve, vitreous). *The retina is richly supplied by blood vessels, therefore it is frequently involved in systemic vascular disorders. Retinal manifestation of a systemic vascular disorder is termed as* **retinopathy**.

Retinal disorders may be classified into vascular, inflammatory, degenerative, neoplastic and detachment. Retinal affections, in general, give rise to the following symptoms and signs.

■ Symptoms of Retinal Disorders

1. Diminution of vision.
2. Scotomas corresponding with the areas affected.
3. Metamorphopsia, that is, distortion of perceived images. It is a common symptom of macular disease and not present in optic neuropathy.
4. Micropsia, that is, decrease in image size. It is caused by the spreading apart of foveal cones.
5. Macropsia, that is, increase in image size. It is due to the crowding together of foveal cones.
6. Flashes of light in front of the eyes due to traction on retina.
7. Floaters (black spots in front of eyes).
8. Nyctalopia (night blindness). It is attributed to the interference with function of retinal rods. It may be congenital or found in retinitis pigmentosa and other tapetoretinal degenerations.
9. Hemeralopia (day blindness). It may be due to congenital deficiency of cones (rare).
10. Pain is invariably **absent**.

■ Signs of Retinal Disorders

The retinal changes originate from retinal vascular changes affecting retinal arteries and arterioles, capillaries, veins and venules. In retinal capillaries, endothelium lacks fenestrations and forms inner blood–retinal barrier. Outside endothelium is a thick basement membrane. Within this membrane are the intramural pericytes (**Fig. 13.6**).

Capillaries are distributed within inner layers of retina including INL. Outer layers have no blood vessels which are nourished by choriocapillaris.

Various signs in retinal diseases are (**Flowchart 13.1**):
- Microaneurysms.
- Retinal hemorrhages.
- Exudates.
- Cotton-wool spots.
- Arteriovenous (A–V) shunts.
- Neovascularization.
- Changes in retinal vessels.

Microaneurysms

These appear as small, round, red dots and **located in the INL** of retina. Location of microaneurysms indicates areas of capillary nonperfusion. These may become thrombosed or may leak, resulting in formation of hard exudates, frequently arranged in rings. So, the *center of ring of hard exudates usually contain microaneurysms.*

Retinal Hemorrhages

These may be preretinal hemorrhages (subhyaloid hemorrhage) or intraretinal hemorrhages (hemorrhage within retinal tissue). Intraretinal hemorrhages could be further divided into superficial and deep hemorrhages.

Preretinal hemorrhage lies in the potential space between retina and vitreous. *It never coagulates.* Initially, preretinal hemorrhage is round and becomes hemispherical with straight upper border (**boat-shaped hemorrhage**), as red blood cells (RBCs) settle down inferiorly. The lower cellular portion of hemorrhage is darker than the serum-containing upper portion.

Superficial hemorrhages are **located in the NFL**, so they have a feathery or **flame-shaped** appearance, corresponding to NFL. These arise from large, superficial precapillary arterioles.

Deep hemorrhages are **located in the compact deeper layer of retina**. So, they have a **"dot and blot"** appearance. These arise from the venous end of capillaries in deeper layers (**Fig. 13.7**).

Retinal Edema

Retinal capillaries are located in the INL and inner layers of retina, therefore edema is located between the OPL and INL of retina initially, and later it may also involve IPL and NFL. Retinal edema may be diffuse or localized. A localized edema in the macular region assumes a

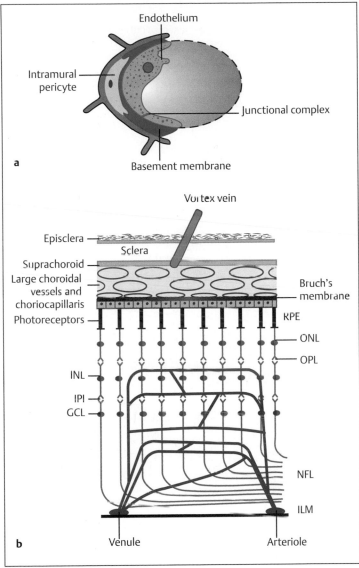

Fig. 13.6 (a) Capillary wall in retina; **(b)** Retinal capillaries and choriocapillaris. Abbreviations: GCL, ganglion cell layer; ILM, internal limiting membrane; INL, inner nuclear layer; IPI, inner plexiform layer; NFL, nerve fiber layer; ONL, outer nuclear layer; OPL, outer plexiform layer; RPE, retinal pigment epithelium.

star-shaped configuration, owing to the formation of radiating folds. This configuration corresponds to the radial arrangement of fibers in OPL (Henle's layer).

Hard Exudates

These are waxy, yellow lesions with relatively distinct margins. These are **located mainly within the OPL** (Henle's layer). They develop at the junction of normal and edematous retina.

These are composed of lipoprotein and lipid-filled macrophages. Lipoproteins are thought to leak from microaneurysms. *Exudates within Henle's fiber layer (OPL) in the macular region typically assume a star-shaped configuration, corresponding to the radial arrangement of fibers* (macular star) (**Fig. 13.8**). When leakage ceases, phagocytosis of their lipid content results in spontaneous absorption of exudates but exudates enlarge if the leakage is chronic.

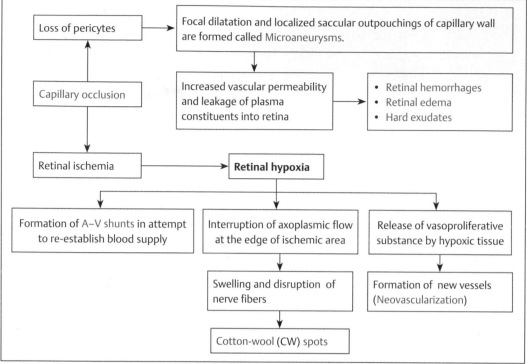

Flowchart 13.1 Pathogenesis of retinal affections.

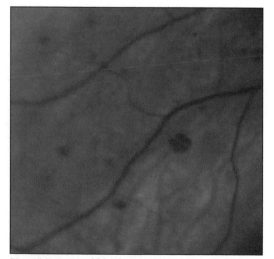

Fig. 13.7 Dot and blot hemorrhages. Source: Diabetic retinopathy. In: Tabandeh H, Goldberg M, eds. The Retina in Systemic Disease: A Color Manual of Ophthalmoscopy. 1st ed. Thieme; 2009.

Cotton-Wool Spots

These are composed of accumulations of neuronal debris **within the** NFL as a result of retinal ischemia. So, cotton-wool spots are fluffy, gray–white, and superficial (in NFL) with ill-defined margins (**Fig. 13.9**). Being superficial, they obscure underlying blood vessels. They disappear rapidly, as debris is removed by autolysis and phagocytosis. Retinal hypoxia leads to formation of A–V shunts and neovascularization in an attempt to re-establish blood supply.

Arteriolar–Venular Shunts/Intraretinal Microvascular Abnormalities (IRMA)

These are the shunt vessels running from the arterioles to venules (bye passing the capillary bed) formed in an attempt to re-establish blood supply. A–V shunts do not leak on FA.

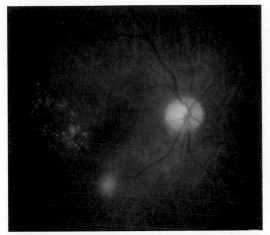

Fig. 13.8 Hard exudates.

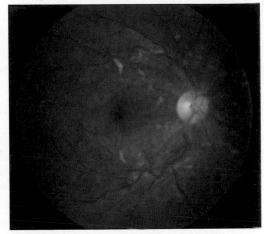

Fig. 13.9 Cotton-wool spots.

Neovascularization (Formation of New Vessels)

Hypoxic retinal tissue elaborates vasoproliferative substance (such as vascular endothelial growth factor [**VEGF**]) in an attempt to re-establish blood supply, which results in the formation of new vessels. The new vessels leak protein and bleeds easily. VEGF can promote neovascularization on:

- Disc: Neovascularization at disc (**NVD**).
- Retina: Neovascularization elsewhere away from disc (**NVE**).
- Iris: Rubeosis iridis (**Fig. 13.10**).

Changes in Retinal Vessels

Ratio of retinal vessels caliber (artery: vein) is 2:3. *Veins are crossed by arteries.* The changes in retinal vessels in various retinal diseases are venous tortuosity, venous dilatation, arteriolar narrowing and changes at A–V crossings. These changes at AV crossings are commonly associated with arteriosclerosis and include:

- Nipping and tapering of veins on both sides of crossings is known as **Gunn's sign.**
- Banking of veins distal to A–V crossings is known as **Bonnet's sign.**
- Right-angled deflection of veins at A–V crossings is known as **Salus' sign.**

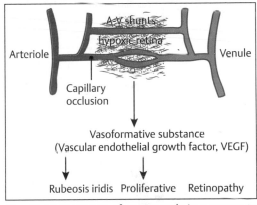

Fig. 13.10 Formation of new vessels in response to hypoxic retina.

▬ Evaluation of Retinal Diseases

- Retinal diseases can be evaluated by the following investigations:
- Electrophysiological tests: These include electroretinography (**ERG**), electro-oculography (**EOG**) and visually evoked potential (**VEP**).
- Fundus angiography: These include **FA** and indocyanine green angiography (**ICGA**).
- Optical coherence tomography (**OCT**).
- Ocular ultrasonography.

◼ Electrophysiological Tests

The objective recordings of visual functions can be achieved by certain tests which are known as electrophysiological tests. These tests include ERG, EOG and VEP.

Electroretinography (ERG)

Normal ERG is biphasic and consists of:
- **α-Wave:** It is a negative wave and arises from photoreceptors.
- **β-Wave:** It is a positive deflection and represents electrical activity in bipolar cells (although generated by Müller cells) (**Fig. 13.11**).

Significance

ERG is useful in detecting functional abnormalities of outer retina up to the bipolar cell layer. ERG gives the indication of activity of rods and cones. ERG is normal in diseases involving ganglion cells and NFL. Focal ERG by using sharply focused light can provide information about macular function. It can assess retinal function in the presence of dense cataract.

Electro-Oculography (EOG)

EOG measures the resting potential between the electrically positive cornea and electrically negative back of eye (retina) with horizontal eye movements. It reflects activity of RPE and photoreceptors, so lesions proximal to photoreceptors will have a normal EOG.

Significance

As EOG is based on the activity of RPE and photoreceptors, it is subnormal or flat in case of retinitis pigmentosa, degenerative myopia, macular dystrophies and vitamin A deficiency.

Visually Evoked Potential (VEP)

It is also called VER (visually evoked response). VEP is the recording of electrical activity of visual cortex, which is generated by stimulation of retina. *VEP is the only objective test to assess functional status of visual system beyond retinal ganglion cells.* So, abnormal VEP with normal ERG and EOG suggests an organic lesion in the pathway between and including GCL and visual cortex.

◼ Fundus Angiography

Fundus angiography may be FA or ICGA. The former is excellent for demonstration of retinal circulation against the dark background of RPE. It is not helpful in delineating the choroidal circulation. To study the choroidal circulation, ICGA is of particular value as it provides better resolution of the choroidal vasculature. ICGA is a useful adjunct to FA.

Fluorescein Angiography

Features of Dye Used in Fluorescein Angiography

Dye used: Fluorescein dye.

Excitation peak of dye—490 nm (blue part of spectrum).

Emission peak of dye: 530 nm (green part of spectrum).

Dose: 5 mL of 10% OR 3 mL of 25% aqueous solution of sodium fluorescein.

Adverse effects: Allergy to Fluorescein results in laryngeal edema, bronchospasm and anaphylactic shock.

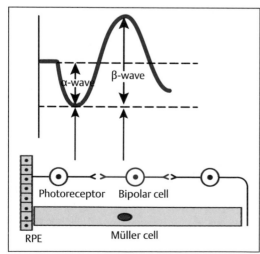

Fig. 13.11 Electroretinography. Abbreviation: RPE, retinal pigment epithelium.

Contraindications:

- Allergy to Fluorescein.
- Diabetic nephropathy.
- Chronic renal failure.
- Opaque media in the eye, preventing proper evaluation.

Dye in Circulation

A significant percentage (70–80%) of **Fluorescein** bind to serum albumin (bound Fluorescein) and the rest remain unbound (free Fluorescein). Major choroidal vessels are impermeable to both bound and free Fluorescein. Choriocapillaris contain fenestrations, so free Fluorescein escape into extravascular space and pass across the Bruch's membrane but tight junctions (zonula occludens) between RPE cells prevent passage of free Fluorescein molecules across RPE and maintain **outer blood–retinal barrier**. Passage of Fluorescein across RPE is, therefore, abnormal. Tight junctions between endothelial cells in retinal capillaries form **inner blood–retinal barrier**.

It prevents leakage of dye, and Fluorescein is confined within the lumen of retinal capillaries. Any leakage from retinal circulation is, therefore, pathological (**Fig. 13.12**).

Thus, **FA** is an excellent method *for studying retinal circulation*. It is not helpful in delineating choroidal circulation, as Fluorescein leaks from choriocapillaris, producing choroidal fluorescence.

Technique of Fluorescein Angiography (FA)

Dilate the pupil and inject fluorescein dye into the antecubital vein of the patient. Arm-to-retina circulation time is about *10 second*, so serial photographs are taken by fundus camera 8 to 10 seconds after commencement of dye injection. Late-phase photographs yield the most useful information in ICGA because the dye remains in neovascular tissue after leaving the retinal and choroidal circulations. Normal angiogram consists of four overlapping phases.

> A cilioretinal artery, if present, fills during the choroidal phase because it is derived from posterior ciliary circulation.

Normal Angiogram

Normal angiogram consists of four overlapping phases.

1. Prearterial/choroidal phase is characterized by filling of choroidal circulation.

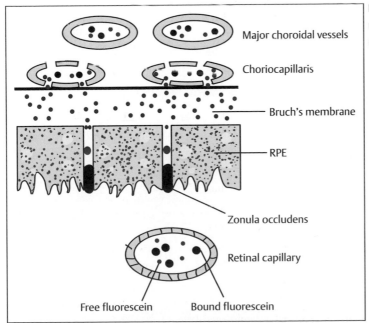

Fig. 13.12 The outer blood–retinal barrier. Abbreviation: RPE, retinal pigment epithelium.

Major choroidal vessels

Choriocapillaris

Bruch's membrane

RPE

Zonula occludens

Retinal capillary

Free fluorescein   Bound fluorescein

2. Arterial phase shows appearance of dye in retinal arterioles.

3. A–V/capillary phase is characterized by complete filling of arterioles, filling of capillaries, and laminar flow in retinal veins.

4. Venous phase shows venous filling with arteriolar emptying (**Flowchart 13.2**).

Dye is absent from angiogram after 5 to 10 minutes. The late phase demonstrates late staining of disc.

Appearance of fovea on FA: *Fovea appears dark on FA* due to:

- Absence of blood vessels in FAZ.
- Increased density of xanthophyll pigment at fovea.
- Heavily pigmented RPE cells with melanin at fovea.

Abnormal Angiogram

It is based on blood–retinal barriers. Outer blood–retinal barrier at the level of choroidal circulation (**RPE barrier**) provides information regarding integrity of RPE. Inner blood–retinal barrier at the level of retinal circulation provides information regarding integrity of retinal vessels. Abnormal fluorescence may be:

- Hyperfluorescence (increased fluorescence).
- Hypofluorescence (decreased or absent fluorescence).

Causes of hyperfluorescence are as follows:

1. **Increased transmission** or **RPE window defect (Fig. 13.13a)**: It is caused by atrophy of RPE as in atrophic age-related macular degeneration (ARMD) which results in unmasking of normal background choroidal fluorescence.

2. **Breakdown of outer blood–retinal barrier** (breakdown of RPE tight junctions): It results in pooling of dye in subretinal space as in central serous retinopathy (**CSR**) (**Fig. 13.13b**).

3. **Breakdown of inner blood–retinal barrier** as in cystoid macular edema (**CME**).

4. **Leakage from abnormal vessels**: Leakage of dye may occur from abnormal choroidal vessels such as

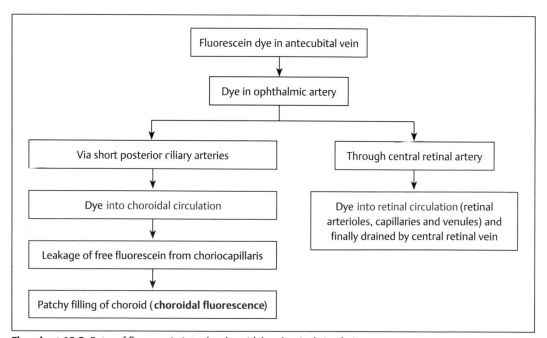

Flowchart 13.2 Entry of fluorescein into the choroidal and retinal circulations.

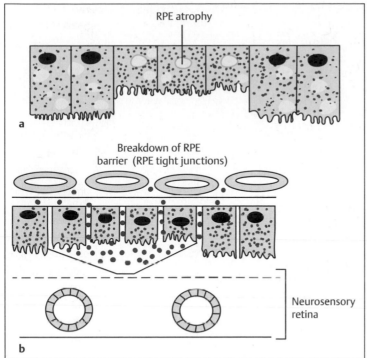

Fig. 13.13 (a) RPE "window" defect as in atrophic ARMD. **(b)** Pooling of dye in subretinal space as in CSR. Abbreviations: ARMD, age-related macular degeneration; CSR, central serous retinopathy; RPE, retinal pigment epithelium.

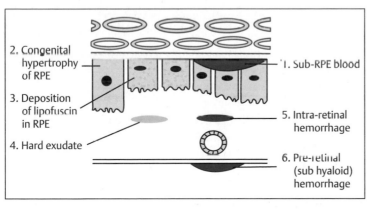

Fig. 13.14 Lesions causing blocked fluorescence.

choroidal neovascularization (**CNV**) or retinal vessels as neovascularization in proliferative diabetic retinopathy (PDR).

5. **Staining of tissues**: Staining due to prolonged retention of dye as in drusen or fibrous tissue.

Hypofluorescence could be due to blockage of normal fluorescence (blocked fluorescence, **Fig. 13.14**) or inadequate perfusion of tissues (filling defects) (**Table 13.2**).

Indocyanine Green Angiography

Features of Dye Used in Indocyanine Green Angiography (ICGA)

Dye used: ICG dye.

Excitation peak of dye: 805 nm (infrared [IR] spectrum).

Emission peak of dye: 835 nm (IR spectrum).

Dose: 25 to 40 mg ICG powder is dissolved in 2 mL of aqueous solvent (40 mg in 2 mL).

Table 13.2 Causes of hypofluorescence

Blocked fluorescence	Filling defects
Blockage of background choroidal fluorescence only: It may be seen in subretinal or sub-RPE lesions such as blood and congenital hypertrophy of RPE.	Vascular occlusion involving choroidal or retinal circulation.
Blockage of retinal as well as choroidal fluorescence: It may be seen in preretinal lesions such as subhyaloid hemorrhage and hard exudates in neurosensory retina.	Loss of vascular tissue as in choroideremia, myopic degeneration.
Abbreviation: RPE, retinal pigment epithelium.	

Adverse effects: These are less common than Fluorescein.

Contraindications: Because dye contains 5% iodine, it should not be given to the patients allergic to any iodine compound and seafood.

Dye in Circulation

A major percentage (98%) of **ICG molecules** bind with serum albumin. So, dye remains within choriocapillaris, as fenestrations of chorio-capillaris are impermeable to albumin. Thus, **ICGA** provides better resolution of choroidal vasculature, and hence it is used *for studying the choroidal lesions*.

Causes of abnormal fluorescence in ICGA (hyper or hypofluorescence) are identical to FA, except in RPE detachment (pigment epithelial detachment). RPE detachment shows hyperfluorescence on FA, but hypofluorescence on ICGA.

■ Optical Coherence Tomography (OCT)

OCT is a noninvasive, noncontact imaging system which provides cross-sectional images of retina, optic nerve head and anterior segment with a high-resolution. OCT is an optical analog of B-scan ultrasound, where instead of sound, IR light is used to image the layers of retina. The coherent light penetrates ocular tissues; reflected images are analyzed by a camera based on reflectivity of tissues, and a color code is assigned for interpretation.

It is based on the principle of Michelson low-coherence interferometry. In the retina, OCT is used to diagnose macular pathology such as:

- Macular hole.
- Macular edema.
- Pigment epithelial detachment (PED).
- Epiretinal membrane (ERM).
- ARMD.

OCT should be avoided in media opacities such as:

- Moderate to dense cataract.
- Vitreous hemorrhage.
- Posterior capsule opacification.

■ Ultrasonography

Diagnostic ultrasound is used in cases of opacification of ocular media. Ultrasonography uses high-frequency sound waves (10 MHz). The sound waves produce echoes on striking the interfaces between acoustically different structures. Different pulse echo techniques are A-scan and B-scan. The sound is coupled to the eye by means of a saline bath or directly through a transducer.

A-Scan

The sound is transmitted from the transducer into eye and echoes are received by the same transducer, which are recorded as spikes. It produces a unidimensional display of vertical spikes along a base line. The height of spikes is proportional to the strength of the echo, and the position of spike indicates the time of receiving the echo. The linear distance between individual spikes is used to measure the anterior chamber depth, lens thickness and axial length. A-scans are used for biometry in intraocular lens (IOL) calculations.

B-Scan

In B-scan, the echoes are plotted as dots instead of spikes. The more sound reflected, the brighter the dot. It provides a two-dimensional (2D) ultra-sonography and delineates intraocular structures in eyes with opaque media, intraocular and orbital mass lesions. The frequency of the transducer determines which part of the globe or orbit is examined. Low-frequency transducers are useful in detecting orbital pathology, while the moderate frequency transducers (7–10 MHz) are used to examine the globe for RD, posterior intraocular tumors and detection of calcification in retinoblastoma and optic disc drusen. The high-frequency transducer (30–50 MHz) images the anterior segment but only to a depth of 5 mm. Dynamic ultrasound scanning is performed by moving the eye but not the probe and allows differentiation of RD and vitreous detachment. The addition of a color Doppler's facility allows the evaluation of blood flow.

■ Retinal Photocoagulation (OP8.2)

Photocoagulation is essentially a destructive form of therapy (**Fig. 13.15**). It depends upon absorption of laser light energy by ocular pigments. Ocular pigments are:

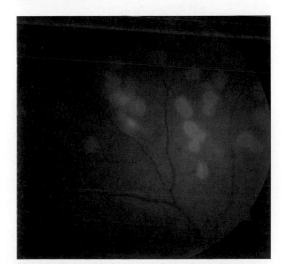

Fig. 13.15 Retinal photocoagulation laser spot.

1. Melanin (present in cells of RPE and choroid).
2. Hemoglobin (present in blood).
3. Xanthophyll (yellow pigment present in inner retinal layers of macula).

The absorbed light is converted into heat energy which is utilized for coagulation of new blood vessels, chorioretinal adhesion and destruction of RPE.

Laser (LASER = **L**ight **A**mplification by **S**timulated **E**mission of **R**adiation) can be delivered to the eye through:

- Slit lamp.
- Indirect ophthalmoscope.
- Fiber optic probe during pars plana vitrectomy (i.e., endophotocoagulation).

■ Laser Used for Photocoagulation

Main photocoagulators are:

1. Argon green laser.
2. Krypton laser.
3. Diode laser—is also used for photodynamic therapy (PDT).
4. Frequency-doubled Nd: YAG laser (Nd: YAG = Neodymium: Yttrium-aluminum-garnet).

■ Principles of Retinal Photocoagulation

The light energy emitted by **argon laser** is *absorbed by all three ocular pigments.*

The light energy emitted by **krypton laser** is *absorbed well by melanin but poorly or not at all by hemoglobin and xanthophyll. So, the main effect of krypton laser is on choroid and RPE containing melanin.*

- *Photocoagulation of lesions inside FAZ*: Xanthophyll in macular area absorbs argon laser light energy and becomes a heat source. So, *when argon laser is applied close to fovea (inside FAZ), it becomes dangerous.* The main advantage of krypton over argon is that it is not absorbed by xanthophyll pigment.

- Because krypton is not absorbed by hemoglobin, it may be possible to treat retina through vitreous hemorrhage with krypton but not with argon.
- *Treatment in presence of nuclear sclerosis*: As krypton is not absorbed by xanthophyll pigment in the lens, so krypton is more effectively transmitted through nuclear sclerosis than argon.
- Smaller the spot size, the greater is the energy. So, when changing to a smaller spot size during photocoagulation, the power level must be turned down and vice versa.

■ Indications of Photocoagulation

- Diabetic retinopathy (DR).
- Other causes of retinal neovascularization.
- Sealing of retinal breaks.
- Macular disorders.

■ Complications of Laser Photocoagulation

Complications of posterior segment include foveal burn, macular pucker, retinal and choroidal hemorrhages. Complications of anterior segment include:
- *Cornea:* Burn, erosion, and superficial punctate keratopathy.
- *Iris:* Absorption of heat by posterior pigment epithelium of iris increases the temperature of aqueous which results in damage to the corneal endothelium.
- *Lens:* Lens opacities (due to energy absorbed by posterior pigment epithelium of iris).

■ Congenital and Developmental Anomalies

■ Coloboma of Retina

A typical coloboma is inferonasal, as embryonic fissure is inferior and slightly nasal (**Fig. 13.16**). The coloboma found in other direction is called atypical. Characteristic features of coloboma of retina are:
- **Fundus examination:** Coloboma appears as an oval, white depressed defect with a

rounded apex toward the disc. Few vessels are seen over the surface.
- **Visual field:** There is scotoma in the field corresponding to coloboma.
- **Complications:** There is high risk of RD.
- **Prophylaxis:** Prophylactic laser delimitation along the edges of coloboma may be done.

■ Myelinated Nerve Fibers (Medullated Nerve Fibers)

Myelination of optic nerve progresses from the brain toward periphery. In normal eyes, myelination of optic nerve stops at lamina cribrosa. It may continue beyond the optic disc to involve NFL and appear as opaque nerve fibers (myelinated nerve fibers of retina, **Fig. 13.17**). Myelination is usually completed shortly after birth. So, strictly speaking medullated nerve fibers (MNFs) are not congenital. Characteristic features of MNF are:
- **Fundus examination:** They appears as white patches with feathery margins

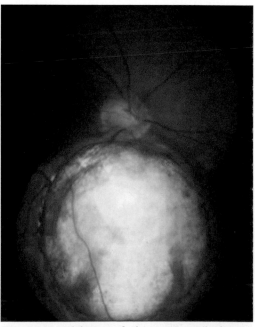

Fig. 13.16 Coloboma of the retina and choroid. Source: Coloboma. In: Lang G, ed. Ophthalmology. A Pocket Textbook Atlas. 3rd ed. Thieme; 2015.

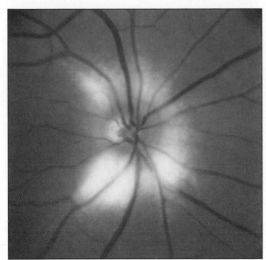

Fig. 13.17 Myelinated nerve fibers. Source: Differential diagnosis of disc edema. In: Biousse V, Newman N, ed. Neuro-Ophthalmology Illustrated. 3rd ed. Thieme; 2019.

covering the retinal vessels. Usually, they are contiguous with disc, and occasionally they are isolated. They are mistaken for cotton-wool spots.

- **Visual field** shows enlargement of blind spot when contiguous with disc or scotoma, corresponding to the position of patch when they are isolated.

Medullary sheath disappears if glaucoma or optic atrophy causes the fibers to degenerate, or in case demyelinating disorder such as multiple sclerosis is present.

■ Vascular Disorders of Retina (OP8.1, OP8.2, OP8.4)

Vascular disorders of retina arise due to:
- Obstruction of arterial circulation: It may be central retinal artery occlusion (CRAO) or branch retinal artery occlusion (BRAO).
- Obstruction of venous circulation: It may be central retinal vein occlusion (CRVO) or branch retinal vein occlusion (BRVO).
- Retinal telangiectasias.

■ Retinal Artery Occlusion (OP8.1, OP8.2, OP8.4)

Obstruction may affect central retinal artery itself (*CRAO*) or a peripheral branch (*BRAO*). Central retinal artery is occluded almost always at lamina cribrosa where vessels normally become slightly narrow. In CRAO, entire retina is involved, but in BRAO, only the area supplied by the branch is affected.

Etiology

Obstruction of a retinal artery is due to atheroma, arteritis, embolus from heart, embolus from carotid arteries and raised IOP.

1. *Obliteration of artery due to atheroma (atherosclerosis):* Thrombosis at the level of lamina cribrosa is the most common cause of CRAO. The risk factors for atherosclerosis include age, hypertension, smoking, diabetes, obesity, and raised low density lipoprotein–cholesterol (LDL–cholesterol) in serum.
2. *Obliteration of artery due to arteritis:* Disorders that may give rise to retinal arteritis include giant cell arteritis, systemic lupus erythematosus (SLE), and polyarteritis nodosa.
3. *Obliteration due to embolus from heart (cardiac embolism):* It results from cardiac valvular diseases comprising calcium (*calcific emboli*) or *septic emboli* from cardiac valves in bacterial endocarditis.
4. *Obliteration due to embolus from carotid arteries (carotid embolism):* Embolus arises from an atheromatous plaque at the bifurcation of common carotid artery. Emboli may be cholesterol emboli (**Hollenhorst plaques**) containing cholesterol, or fibrinoplatelet emboli consisting of platelet and fibrin. Since ophthalmic artery is the first branch of internal carotid artery (ICA), embolus from heart or carotid arteries has a fair chance to occlude retinal artery.

5. *Obliteration due to raised IOP*: It is seen in acute angle closure glaucoma and excessive pressure on globe during RD surgery or neurosurgical procedures.

Clinical Features

Clinical features in arterial occlusion will depend on the size and location of obstructed vessel.

Central Retinal Artery Occlusion (CRAO)

In CRAO, there is sudden, painless loss of vision. Transient loss of vision (amaurosis fugax) due to occlusion by minute emboli may be the premonitory symptom.

> If macula and papillomacular bundle is supplied by a cilioretinal artery, arising from posterior ciliary circulation, central vision may be preserved. The remainder of the field of vision is lost.

Clinical signs of CRAO are:
- Pupil: There is no direct pupillary light reaction, that is, relative afferent pupillary defect (**RAPD**) is present.
- Fundus reveals the following findings:
  1. *Retinal arteries* appear thread-like but no change in caliber of retinal veins.
  2. *Retina* becomes milky white and edematous.

3. **Cherry red spot** at fovea, since the vascular choroid is visible underneath in contrast to the surrounding cloudy-white retina (**Fig. 13.18** and **Flowchart 13.3**).
4. If occlusion is incomplete, a gentle pressure upon globe may break up the blood column in retinal veins into red beads (segmentation of blood

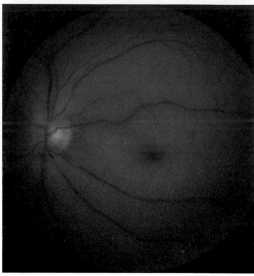

Fig. 13.18 Cherry red spot in CRAO. Abbreviation: CRAO, central retinal artery occlusion.

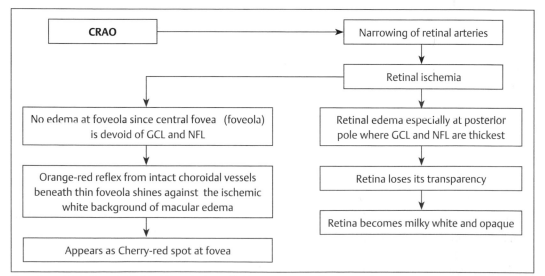

Flowchart 13.3 Signs in CRAO. Abbreviations: CRAO, central retinal artery occlusion; GCL, ganglion cell layer; NFL, nerve fiber layer.

column), moving in a jerky way. The beads of blood column in the veins move sometimes in normal direction of blood flow and sometimes in opposite direction–"**cattle-truck**" **appearance**.

Cherry red spot is seen in: **C**RAO
- **T**rauma (Berlin's edema).
- **N**iemann-Pick disease.
- **G**aucher's disease.
- **T**ay-Sach's disease.
- **S**andoff's disease.

Mnemonic–**C**herry **T**ree **N**ever **G**row **T**all in **S**and

---

After several weeks, retinal cloudiness and cherry red spot gradually disappear as retinal edema subsides. Retina regains its transparency but its inner layers are completely atrophic. However, retina appears nearly normal owing to the viability of its outer layers which receive their nourishment from the choroid. Optic disc becomes atrophic because of the atrophy of NFL, so there is no direct pupillary reaction to light.

Branch Retinal Artery Occlusion (BRAO)

BRAO causes ischemia with edema in the area supplied by the obstructed artery. The ischemic retina appears white, with narrowing of arterioles. The atrophy of inner layers of involved retina causes permanent sectorial visual field defect.

Investigations

The following investigations are helpful to determine arterial occlusion:
- Carotid artery imaging by color Doppler ultrasonography.
- Serum lipid profile.
- Echocardiogram: To evaluate cardiac valves.
- Full blood count and erythrocyte sedimentation rate (ESR).

Treatment

Treatment is very unsatisfactory but attempts should be made to restore retinal circulation by dislodging emboli. Calcific emboli are much more dangerous than cholesterol and fibrin–platelet emboli. Retinal tissue cannot survive ischemia for

than a few hours. So, the following treatment may be tried if patient reports early:
- Massaging the globe intermittently for at least 15 minutes.
- Anterior chamber paracentesis.
- IV acetazolamide (500 mg) to lower IOP.
- Inhalation of amyl nitrite produces vasodilatation.
- Systemic steroids in high dosage if giant cell arteritis is the underlying cause.

To confirm giant cell arteritis, ESR is measured, and biopsy of temporal artery is performed.

Complications

Some eyes with CRAO develop rubeosis iridis and neovascular glaucoma (NVG).

■ Retinal Vein Occlusion (OP8.1, OP8.2, OP8.4)

Both arterial and venous diseases contribute to retinal vein occlusion.

Predisposing Factors

Predisposing factors for retinal vein occlusion are arteriosclerosis, hypertension, hyperviscosity of blood (as a result of hypercellularity in polycythemia vera or leukemia or as a result of changes in plasma proteins in macroglobulinemia or myeloma), hyperlipidemia as in hypothyroidism, occlusive periphlebitis retinae as in sarcoidosis and Behcet's disease, raised IOP as in primary open-angle glaucoma, and diabetes mellitus. There are some miscellaneous causes too, for example, oral contraceptives, secondary hypertension (e.g., Cushing syndrome) and smoking.

An artery (or arteriole) and a vein share a common adventitial sheath at A–V crossings in retina and just behind lamina cribrosa. Thickening of an artery (or arteriole) compresses the vein, resulting in retinal vein occlusion. Therefore, arteriosclerosis is an important causative factor for retinal vein occlusion.

At A–V crossing posterior to lamina cribrosa, central retinal vein is compressed, resulting in

CRVO. At A–V crossings in retina, arteriosclerosis of retinal arteriole compresses the venule and results in **BRVO**.

Thus, retinal vein occlusion may be CRVO or BRVO.

Central Retinal Vein Occlusion (CRVO)

According to clinical features and prognosis, CRVO may be divided into nonischemic and ischemic forms. In nonischemic CRVO (venous stasis retinopathy) or partial CRVO, there is venous stasis with delayed venous drainage, so there is no retinal ischemia. Complete CRVO is accompanied with retinal ischemia, hence the name ischemic CRVO (**Table 13.3**).

Nonischemic CRVO

It is the most common type and occurs in young persons. The cause is unknown. It probably results from phlebitis affecting central retinal vein within ONH. Patient complains of unilateral, mild-to-moderate fogginess of vision.

Fundus Examination

During early stages, venous stasis causes nonischemic CRVO, disc edema, engorged, tortuous and dilated veins and retinal hemorrhages (superficial and deep) more in peripheral retina than at posterior pole (**Fig. 13.19**).

In late stages when venous stasis is chronic (6–12 months), fundus reveals cotton-wool spots and chronic CME. Vitreous hemorrhage is never present.

Fluorescein Angiography (FA)

FA shows venous stasis with delayed A–V transit time (i.e., delayed venous drainage) and good retinal capillary perfusion.

Treatment

Systemic corticosteroids are withheld unless there is macular edema. Intravitreal triamcinolone is given for chronic macular edema.

Prognosis

It is reasonably good. Visual acuity returns to normal or near normal. Main cause for poor vision is chronic CME.

Ischemic CRVO

It usually occurs in elderly people with cardiovascular disorders. It is characterized by sudden complete occlusion of central retinal vein just behind lamina cribrosa due to thrombus formation. Patient complains of sudden and severe, painless visual impairment (it is not as sudden as found in CRAO). There is relative afferent pupillary conduction defect in affected eye which is marked.

Fundus Examination

In early stage, fundus reveals the following:
- Markedly engorged and tortuous retinal veins.
- Disc edema and hyperemia.

Table 13.3 Differentiating features between nonischemic and ischemic CRVO

	Nonischemic CRVO	Ischemic CRVO
1. Visual impairment	++	++++
2. Afferent pupillary conduction defect	±	++
3. Vitreous hemorrhage	Never	Frequent
4. Prognosis	Reasonably good	Extremely poor

Abbreviation: CRVO, central retinal vein occlusion.

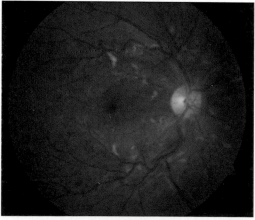

Fig. 13.19 Nonischemic CRVO. Abbreviation: CRVO, central retinal vein occlusion.

- Retinal hemorrhages. These are so extensive that entire retina is covered with them (**splashed tomato appearance**).
- Cotton-wool spots.
- Retinal and macular edema (**Fig. 13.20**).
- In late stage: Marked NVE and NVD are seen (**Flowchart 13.4**).
- Sheathing around veins and collateral around disc are found.

Fluorescein Angiography (FA)

No useful information can be obtained because of marked retinal hemorrhages. In less severe cases, there are extensive areas of capillary nonperfusion.

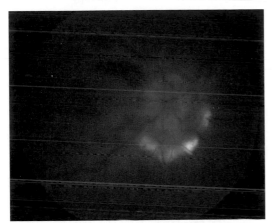

Fig. 13.20 Ischemic CRVO. Abbreviation: CRVO, central retinal vein occlusion.

Clinical Course of Disease

Acute signs resolve after 6 to 12 months. Retina undergoes atrophy and pigmentary changes. Macular degeneration (cystoid degeneration) occurs. Neovascularization may be seen at disc (NVD) or elsewhere in retina (NVE). Cilioretinal collaterals at disc can be seen.

Treatment

No treatment is effective. Laser pan retinal photo-coagulation (laser PRP) should be performed to prevent development of NVG. If media is hazy, anterior retinal cryopexy may prevent NVG.

Prognosis

It is extremely poor.

Complications

Complicated CRVO results in optic atrophy, recurrent vitreous hemorrhage and NVG. Vitreous hemorrhage occurs due to neovascularization of retina. NVG occurs following rubeosis iridis and neovascularization at the angle of anterior chamber. It appears in 50% cases within 3 months of occlusion, so it is also known as 90-day glaucoma.

Branch Retinal Vein Occlusion (BRVO)

BRVO is common in *superotemporal branch* due to numerous crossings by artery.

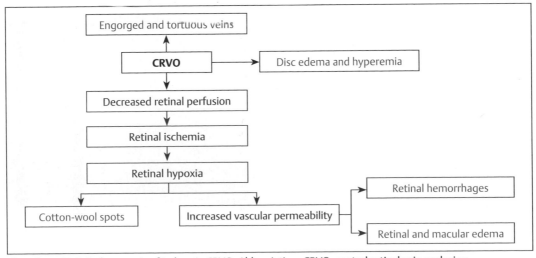

Flowchart 13.4 Pathogenesis of ischemic CRVO. Abbreviation: CRVO, central retinal vein occlusion.

■ Diabetic Retinopathy (DR) (OP8.1, OP8.2, OP8.4)

Diabetes mellitus occurs in two forms:

- Type 1 or insulin-dependent diabetes mellitus (**IDDM**).
- Type 2 or noninsulin-dependent diabetes mellitus (**NIDDM**).

Diabetes mellitus (DM) results in:

- *Macrovascular complications* affecting heart, brain and limbs.
- *Microvascular complications* (due to microangiopathy) affecting kidneys, eyes and peripheral nerves.

Ocular signs in diabetes mellitus are listed in **Table 13.4**.

Risk Factors

Risk factors for the development of DR include:

1. Type of diabetes: **DR** is commoner in type 1 than in type 2.
2. Duration of diabetes: DR develops in approximately 15 years and rarely develops within 5 years of the onset of diabetes.

3. Poor glycemic control: Poor glycemic control (raised HbA1c) is relevant to the development and progression of retinopathy.
4. Conditions like hypertension, poor renal status (nephropathy) and smoking also pose as a risk factor for the development of diabetic retinopathy.

Pathogenesis

DR is essentially a microangiopathy involving retinal precapillary arterioles, capillaries and post-capillary venules. DR includes both, microvascular occlusion and leakage. Retinal capillaries have two types of cells: endothelial cells and pericytes.

Vascular changes in diabetes mellitus are (**Flowchart 13.5**).

- Capillaropathy: It includes loss of pericytes, thickening of capillary basement membrane, proliferation of endothelial cells and progressive closure of retinal capillaries.
- Hematological changes: This includes changes in RBC (deformation and rouleaux formation) and also changes in platelets (increased stickiness and aggregation of platelets).

Table 13.4 Ocular signs in diabetes mellitus	
1. *Transient change in refraction*	**Hyperglycemia** → Increased sorbitol in lens cortex ↓ Imbibition of water with increased thickness of lens ↓ Refractive index of lens increases ↓ **Myopic shift** of refraction **Hypoglycemia** → refractive index of lens decreases ↓ **Hypermetropic shift** of refraction
2. *Ocular movements*	Third nerve palsy with pupillary sparing.
3. *Lids*	Stye or internal hordeolum.
4. *Cornea*	• Infective keratitis with delayed healing. • Decreased corneal sensation due to trigeminal neuropathy.
5. *Lens*	Snowflake cataract, posterior subcapsular cataract.
6. *Vitreous*	Vitreous hemorrhage.
7. *Retina*	Diabetic retinopathy, CRVO.
8. *IOP*	Increased incidence of POAG and NVG.
Abbreviations: CRVO, central retinal vein occlusion; IOP, intraocular pressure; NVG, neovascular glaucoma; POAG, primary open-angle glaucoma.	

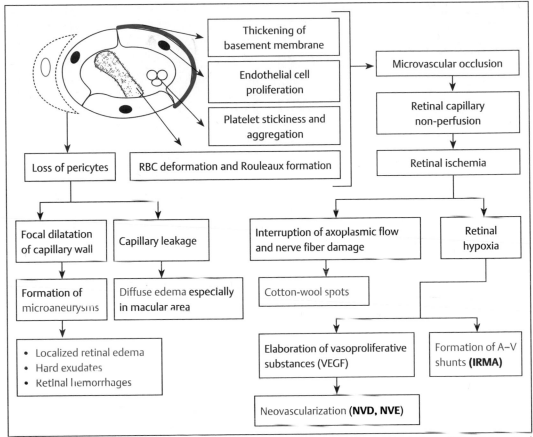

Flowchart 13.5 Pathogenesis of vascular changes in diabetic retinopathy. Abbreviations: IRMA, intraretinal microvascular abnormalities; NVD, neovascularization at disc in retina; NVE, neovascularization elsewhere in retina; RBC, red blood cells; VEGF, vascular endothelial growth factor.

Classification

Previously, DR has been classified as:
- Background DR.
- Preproliferative DR.
- PDR.
- Diabetic maculopathy.
- Advanced diabetic eye disease.

But, presently following classification of DR is adopted:
- Nonproliferative diabetic retinopathy (**NPDR**):
  ◇ Mild NPDR.
  ◇ Moderate NPDR.
  ◇ Severe NPDR.
  ◇ Very severe NPDR.
- Proliferative diabetic retinopathy (**PDR**):
  ◇ Early PDR.
  ◇ High-risk PDR (advanced PDR).
- Diabetic **maculopathy.**
- Advanced diabetic eye disease (**ADED**).

Nonproliferative Diabetic Retinopathy (NPDR)

In NPDR, there are only intraretinal microvascular changes. *Microaneurysms* are the earliest sign (1st detectable lesion) of DR. Leakage from micro-aneurysms leads to retinal hemorrhages both superficial (flame shaped) and deep (dot and blot), retinal edema, and hard exudates (**Fig. 13.23**). As capillary closure become extensive, there is increased formation of microaneurysms and many intraretinal hemorrhages. Also, increased

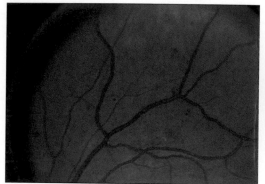

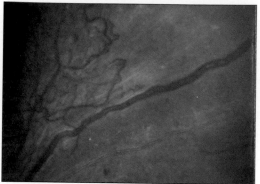

Fig. 13.23 Nonproliferative diabetic retinopathy. Source: Medical Management. In: Singh K, Smiddy W, Lee A, ed. Ophthalmology Review: A Case-Study Approach. 2nd Edition. Thieme; 2018.

Fig. 13.24 Proliferative diabetic retinopathy. Source: Vitreous detachment. In: Lang G, ed. Ophthalmology. A pocket textbook atlas. 2nd edition. Thieme; 2006.

nonperfusion due to capillary closure causes increased retinal ischemia and retinal hypoxia. It results in cotton-wool spots, venous beading (dilated segments of retinal veins) and IRMA (A–V shunts). As A–V shunts clinically resemble focal areas of retinal neovascularization or dilated preexisting capillaries, so clinically they have been referred to as IRMA.

Thus, *NPDR is characterized by* microaneurysms, retinal edema, hard exudates, retinal hemorrhages, venous changes, cotton-wool spots, and IRMA.

The severity of IRMA, intraretinal hemorrhages and venous beading is directly associated with increasing nonperfusion and resulting ischemia. **Severity of NPDR** is expressed by the 4:2:1 rule.

4:2:1 Rule

- Intraretinal hemorrhages and microaneurysms in all four quadrants.
- Venous beading in two quadrants.
- IRMA in one quadrant.

On the basis of severity, NPDR has been classified as:
- *Mild NPDR:* At least one microaneurysm/intraretinal hemorrhage.
- *Moderate NPDR:*
  ◇ Moderate microaneurysms/intraretinal hemorrhages.

◇ Early mild IRMA.
◇ Hard exudates.
◇ Cotton-wool spots (soft exudates).
- *Severe NPDR:* Presence of any one feature of the 4:2:1 rule represents severe NPDR.
- *Very severe NPDR:* Presence of any two features of the 4:2:1 rule indicates very severe NPDR.

Proliferative DR (PDR)

Incidence of PDR in type 1 diabetes is 60% after 30 years. The **hallmark** of PDR is neovascularization (**Fig. 13.24**).

Pathogenesis

Hypoxic retina elaborates angiogenic growth factor such as **VEGF** in an attempt to revascularize. It results in NVD and NVE away from disc and new vessels on iris (rubeosis iridis).

Natural Course of PDR

Over 1/4th of retina (one quadrant) has to be nonperfused before NVD will appear. Predilection for NVD may partially be due to the absence of ILM over optic disc.

NVE will eventually break through retinal ILM, resulting in new vessels in potential space between ILM and posterior hyaloid face. *Proliferation of new vessels is accompanied by fibrous proliferation as the mesenchyme from* which new vessels are derived is also the source of *fibroblasts*. This fibrovascular tissue may lie flat on the retina, attach to vitreous face, or proliferate in vitreous gel:

- If fibrovascular tissue lies flat on retina, tangential traction due to contraction of fibrovascular tissue causes dragging of macula.
- If fibrovascular tissue attaches to vitreous face, vitreous traction due to posterior vitreous detachment (PVD) can cause tearing of new vessels, resulting in preretinal hemorrhage.
- If fibrovascular tissue proliferates in vitreous gel, its contraction into vitreous gel results in tractional RD and vitreous hemorrhage.

If extension of neovascularization process takes place in the anterior segment, neovascularization of iris (rubeosis iridis) and angle of anterior chamber results in **NVG**.

Severity of PDR

It is determined by the area covered with new vessels in comparison with the area of disc (**Table 13.5**).

Diabetic retinopathy study (DRS) group described the **high-risk characteristics** which signify high-risk of severe visual loss, if untreated. These are as follows:

- Mild NVD with hemorrhage (vitreous or preretinal hemorrhage).
- Severe NVD without hemorrhage.
- Severe NVD with hemorrhage.
- Severe NVE with hemorrhage.

On the basis of high-risk characteristics PDR can be:

- Early PDR (PDR without high-risk characteristics).

- Advanced PDR/high-risk PDR (PDR with high-risk characteristics).

Advanced Diabetic Eye Disease

It occurs in patients who have not had laser therapy or in whom photocoagulation has been unsuccessful. One or more of the following complications may occur such as:

- Persistent vitreous hemorrhage.
- Tractional RD.
- Tractional retinoschisis.
- Rubeosis iridis, if severe, it may lead to neovascular glaucoma.

Diabetic Maculopathy

Diabetic maculopathy is the involvement of fovea by edema, hard exudates, or ischemia. It is the commonest cause of diminution of vision in DR and more frequent with type 2 diabetes.

Increased permeability of retinal capillaries leads to leakage of fluid and plasma into macular area, which results in macular edema and hard exudates.

Macular edema is defined as clinically significant macular edema (**CSME**) if any of the following features is present:

- Thickening of retina (retinal edema) within 500 microns of the center of fovea.

or

- Hard exudates within 500 microns of the center of fovea, which are associated with thickening of adjacent retina

or

- Retinal edema one disc area or larger, any part of which is within 1 disc diameter (1 DD) of the center of fovea.

CSME is best recognized by slit lamp biomicroscopy using a +78D or +90D lens.

Table 13.5 Severity of PDR

Severity of PDR	NVD	NVE
Mild PDR	If NVD is <⅓ disc area in extent	If extent of NVE is <½ disc area
Severe PDR	If NVD is >⅓ disc area in extent	If extent of NVE is >½ disc area
Abbreviations: PDR, proliferative diabetic retinopathy; NVD, neovascularization at disc; NVE, neovascularization elsewhere.		

Types

Maculopathy may be focal, diffuse or ischemic.

Focal maculopathy: When leakage from microaneurysms and dilated capillaries is focal, it results in focal maculopathy. It is characterized by mild macular edema and surrounding hard exudates. FA reveals focal leakage with good macular perfusion (**Fig. 13.25a**).

Diffuse maculopathy: When leakage is diffuse from dilated capillaries, it results in diffuse retinal thickening. It may be associated with microcystic spaces (CME). FA shows diffuse hyper fluorescence due to leakage, which may assume a *"flower petal"* pattern of leakage, if CME is present (**Fig. 13.25b**).

Ischemic maculopathy: It occurs due to closure of perifoveal capillary network. The signs are variable. In ischemic maculopathy, photocoagulation is not helpful and should not be attempted.

Management

The aim of treatment is to prevent visual loss from DR. A periodic eye and physical examination is very important for timely management in order to prevent visual loss from DR. The management of DR depends upon its stage/type.

Management of Mild NPDR

It requires no treatment but should be reviewed annually. The management consists of the following:

- Good metabolic control of diabetes.
- Proper management of hypertension.
- Take photographs of entire fundus for documentation and future comparison on follow-up.

Management of Moderate and Severe NPDR

- Watch closely because of the risk of PDR.
- Because some IRMAs are difficult to differentiate from retinal neovascularization, FA is recommended.
- *Reliable patients,* who can be expected to keep follow-ups, observe severe NPDR every 4 to 6 months.
- In an *unreliable patient,* treat at least one eye having severe NPDR with pan retinal photocoagulation (PRP).

Management of PDR

Laser photocoagulation is beneficial at this stage. A good response to PRP is the regression of neovascularization leaving only *"ghost"* vessels or fibrous tissue.

Aim of PRP: Laser therapy is aimed at inducing involution of new vessels. Laser photocoagulation converts hypoxic retina into anoxic one resulting in decreased metabolic demand. Release of VEGF is reduced leading to regression of new vessels.

Technique of PRP: PRP is done in PDR with high-risk characteristics. This is done using a *retinal laser lens.* A circular area of a radius of

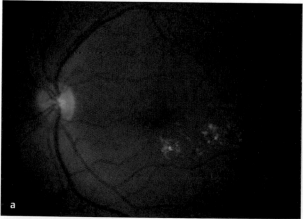
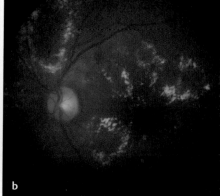

Fig. 13.25 (a) Focal maculopathy. **(b)** Diffuse maculopathy.

2.5 disc diameter (DD) with fovea at its center is left untouched.

Photocoagulation burns: These are applied with argon laser, frequency-doubled Nd: YAG 532 or diode laser. Size of spot burn is 200 to 500 μm. Duration of burn is 0.1 to 0.2 seconds. The total number of burns is 2000 to 3000 applied over 3 to 4 sessions, because PRP completed in a single session carries a slightly higher risk of complications (**Fig. 13.26**).

Management of Advanced Diabetic Eye Disease

Pars plana vitrectomy is indicated for treating:
- Persistent vitreous hemorrhage.
- Tractional RD which is treated by:
    ◇ Excising fibrovascular tissue from retinal surface.
    ◇ Sealing any retinal break.
    ◇ Internal tamponade.

Management of Diabetic Maculopathy

Intravitreal anti-VEGF agents: These are used to control the neovascularization. Several anti-VEGF agents are bevacizumab (Avastin) and ranibizumab (Lucentis).

Intravitreal steroids: Intravitreal injection of triamcinolone acetonide (4 mg in 0.1 mL) is given for diffuse macular edema that fails to respond to conventional laser photocoagulation. Complications of intravitreal steroids are endophthalmitis, intraocular hemorrhage, RD, and raised IOP.

Laser photocoagulation: It is done using krypton and diode lasers. It is indicated in CSME and contraindicated in ischemic maculopathy which carries a poor prognosis.

Main advantage of krypton over argon is that it is not absorbed by xanthophyll pigment of macula. So, lesions inside FAZ can be treated with lesser risk.

Technique of macular laser photocoagulation includes two methods:

1. Focal laser photocoagulation: All leaking microaneurysms (in the center of ring of hard exudates) located 500 microns (500 μm) from the center of macula must be treated by focal laser photocoagulation. Its spot size is 100 to 200 μm and exposure time is 0.1 second.
2. Grid pattern of photocoagulation (**grid treatment**): Diffuse capillary leak, as in cystoid maculopathy, is treated by the grid pattern of photocoagulation. Spots of low/moderate intensity are applied to macula-avoiding FAZ. Burns are applied to areas >500 μm from the center of macula. Its spot size is 100 to 200 μm (**Fig. 13.27**).

■ Hypertensive Retinopathy (OP8.1, OP8.2, OP8.4)

Two aspects of systemic hypertension are considered: Severity of hypertension and duration of hypertension.

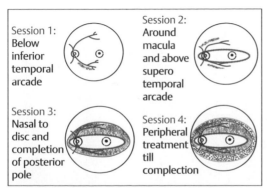

Fig. 13.26 Sessions of laser photocoagulation.

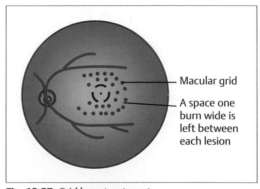

Fig. 13.27 Grid laser treatment.

Severity of hypertension is reflected by hypertensive vascular changes which involve vasoconstriction (narrowing of retinal arterioles) and increased vascular permeability due to disruption in the inner blood–retinal barrier.

Duration of hypertension is reflected by arteriosclerotic vascular changes which manifest as *changes at A–V crossings*. Mild changes at A–V crossings are seen in older patients with *involutional sclerosis* in the absence of hypertension.

Hypertensive narrowing in its pure form can only be seen in young individuals, but in older patients, rigidity of retinal arterioles (because of involutional sclerosis) prevents an identical degree of narrowing seen in young individuals.

Clinical Picture

Fundus picture of hypertensive retinopathy is characterized by:
- Cotton-wool spots.
- Retinal hemorrhages (superficial).
- Retinal edema.
- Hard exudates.
- Changes at A–V crossings (**Flowchart 13.6**).

Hypertensive retinopathy may occur in four circumstances:
- In simple hypertension without sclerosis.
- In hypertension with involutionary (senile) sclerosis.
- In hypertension with compensatory arteriolar sclerosis.
- In malignant hypertension.

Hypertensive Retinopathy in Simple Hypertension Without Sclerosis

It is seen in younger patients. When there is no sclerosis, minimal signs of A–V crossings are encountered. In hypertension, there is constriction of arterioles, so arterioles appear pale and straight with acute-angled branching. Superficial flame-shaped hemorrhage and cotton-wool spots may also occur. **Hard exudates** are **absent.**

Hypertensive Retinopathy in Hypertension with Involutionary (Senile) Sclerosis

It is seen in older patients. Due to sclerosis, the fundus picture is characterized by arteriosclerotic vascular changes, that is, changes at A–V crossings are diagnostic.

Hypertensive Retinopathy in Hypertension with Compensatory Arteriolar Sclerosis

It occurs in younger patients. This condition is seen in patients with systemic hypertension associated with chronic diffuse glomerulonephritis and is known as **renal retinopathy** or **albuminuric retinopathy**. Arterioles show proliferative and fibrous changes in T. media (compensatory arteriolar sclerosis) due to hypertension

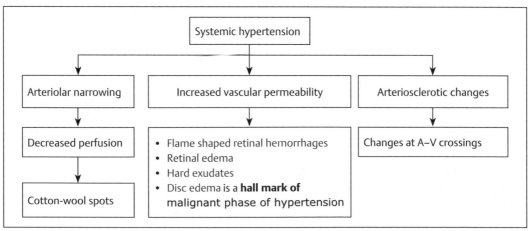

Flowchart 13.6 Signs in hypertensive retinopathy.

associated with chronic glomerulonephritis. *Thus, the fundus picture is characterized by*:

- Constriction of arterioles.
- Nicking at A–V crossings (**Fig. 13.28**).
- Retinal hemorrhages (flame-shaped).
- Retinal edema.
- Hard exudates.
- Cotton-wool spots.

It often causes marked diminution of vision.

Hypertensive Retinopathy in Malignant Hypertension

Malignant hypertension is an expression of rapid progression of hypertension in a patient with arterioles *without sclerosis*. Therefore, the fundus picture is characterized by hypertensive vascular changes, that is:

- Marked *arteriolar narrowing*.
- Increased vascular permeability, leading to generalized *retinal edema* and *hard exudates*. Deposition of hard exudates around the fovea in Henle's layer may lead to radial distribution in the form of macular star. *Disc edema* is a **hallmark** of malignant hypertension. Multiple *cotton-wool patches*

and superficial/flame-shaped *retinal hemorrhages* are also present (**Fig. 13.29**).

Grading

Grading of retinopathy has *prognostic significance*. It also determines the efficacy of treatment. Keith, Wagner and Barker divided the hypertensive retinopathy into four grades as given in **Table 13.6**.

■ Retinopathy in Toxemia of Pregnancy

Toxemia of pregnancy (TOP) occurs late in pregnancy (6–9 months) and is characterized by hypertension, proteinuria and generalized edema. It is always accompanied with hypertension. So, it has features similar to hypertensive retinopathy. The fundus picture shows narrowing of retinal arterioles leading to retinal hypoxia, which results in retinal edema, superficial retinal hemorrhages and cotton-wool spots.

Exudation may be so profuse that a bilateral, exudative RD may develop resulting in profound loss of vision. If pregnancy is allowed to continue,

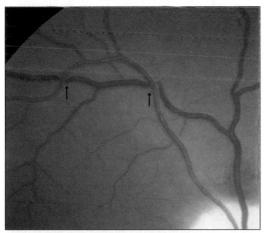

Fig. 13.28 Arteriovenous nicking (*arrows*) being characterized by narrowing of the retinal vein at the site of crossing of an artery. Source: Systemic Hypertension. In: Tabandeh H, Goldberg M, ed. The Retina in Systemic Disease: A Color Manual of Ophthalmoscopy. 1st Edition. Thieme; 2009.

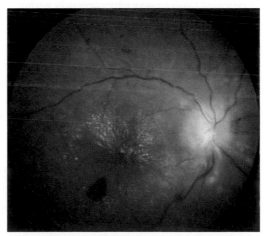

Fig. 13.29 Fundus photo showing marked arteriolar attenuation, multiple hard exudates, retinal hemorrhages, and disc edema in a case of malignant hypertension.

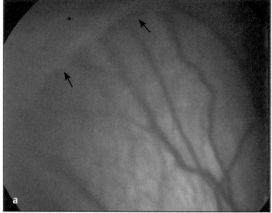

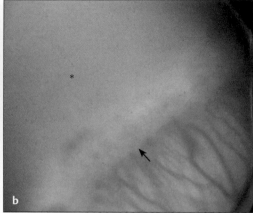

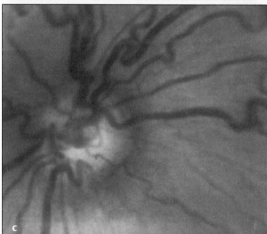

Fig. 13.32 **(a)** Retinopathy of prematurity (stage 2). **(b)** Retinopathy of prematurity (stage 3). **(c)** Retinopathy of prematurity (plus disease). Source: Retinopathy of Prematurity. In: Tabendah H, Goldberg M, ed. The Retina in Systemic Disease: A Color Manual of Ophthalmoscopy. 1st Edition. Thieme; 2009.

Table 13.7 Differential diagnosis of ROP

	PHPV	ROP	Retinoblastoma
1. Age at presentation	Neonatal period	Neonatal period	Average age of presentation is 18 months
2. History of: • Prematurity • Birth weight • Oxygen exposure	– Normal –	+++ Low +++	– Normal –

Abbreviations: PHPV, persistent hyperplastic primary vitreous; ROP, retinopathy of prematurity.
Note: (+) denotes presence and (–) denotes absence.

Screening should be done in a neonatal ICU as low-birth weight baby is highly prone to infections.

Treatment

It is treated by laser photocoagulation or cryotherapy (**Table 13.8**). Laser therapy is preferred over cryotherapy due to the following reasons:

- Laser can be done under topical anesthesia and infants do not need intubation.
- With laser, we can treat posterior ROP.
- Postoperative reaction is minimal with laser when compared with cryo treatment.
- Laser induces less myopia.

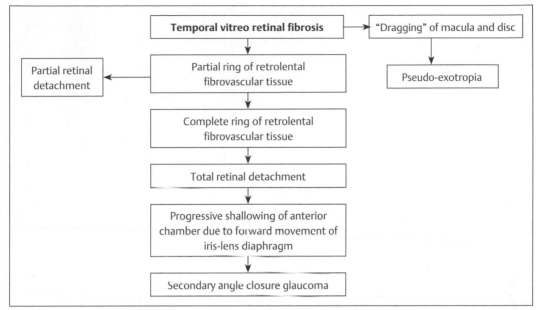

Flowchart 13.8 Sequelae of retinopathy of prematurity.

Table 13.8 Treatment of various stages of ROP

Stage	Treatment
Stage 1 and 2	Only weekly examination is recommended since, spontaneous resolution occurs in 80% of cases.
Stage 3	Laser photocoagulation of avascular immature retina.
Stage 4A	Laser photocoagulation + treatment for tractional retinal detachment.
Stage 4B and 5	Vitreoretinal surgery (lensectomy + vitrectomy).
Abbreviation: ROP, retinopathy of prematurity.	

Prevention of ROP

Reduce the frequency of premature low-birth weight baby through good antenatal and obstetrical care. Monitor proper blood gas chemistry, especially oxygen, and maintain in normal range to prevent the risk of ROP.

PaO_2 level in blood from umbilical artery should be monitored, with levels of 50 to 100 mm Hg being regarded as unlikely to produce constriction of immature retinal vessels.

The key diseases which have been identified as causes of avoidable blindness in children include:
- Corneal problems, for example, vitamin A deficiency, corneal ulcer, keratomalacia, etc.
- Congenital cataract.
- Congenital glaucoma.
- ROP.

■ Sickle-Cell Retinopathy

Normal hemoglobin: Hemoglobin (Hb) contains hem and globin. Globin consists of 4 polypeptide chains—2α and 2β polypeptide chains. Normal adult hemoglobin (**HbA**) is designated as $\alpha 2$ and $\beta 2$. *In β-chain,* glutamic acid *is present at the 6th position in HbA.* Hemoglobin may be abnormal (**Fig. 13.33**).

Abnormal Forms of Hemoglobin

Hemoglobin S (HbS) or sickle-cell Hb: In HbS, valine amino acid is present instead of glutamic acid at the 6th position of chain.

Hemoglobin C (HbC): In HbC, lysine amino acid is present instead of glutamic acid at the 6th position of β-chain.

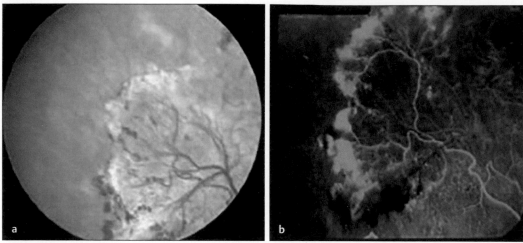

Fig. 13.33 (a, b) Sea fan neovascularization as seen in sickle cell retionopathy. Source: Uveitis. In: Glass L, ed. Ophthalmology Q&A Board Review. 1st Edition. Thieme; 2019.

When hemoglobin S (**HbS)** is reduced (deoxygenated), it becomes insoluble and undergoes a change in its shape. It causes the normal discoid RBC to adopt a characteristic sickle shape. The deformed RBCs tend to obstruct capillaries, particularly in the periphery of retina, resulting in retinal hypoxia.

Sickling disorders are as follows:
- Sickle-cell anemia (SS): It is characterized by severe chronic hemolytic anemia, vaso-occlusive disease (infarctive crises), and mild ocular manifestations.
- Sickle-cell trait (AS): It is the mild form and usually requires severe hypoxia to produce sickling.
- Sickle-cell HbC disease (SC disease): It is characterized by no normal Hb (HbA), hemoglobin consisting of HbS and HbC, and severe retinopathy and hemolytic anemia.

In sickling disorders, these abnormal forms of hemoglobin (HbS and HbC) may occur in combination with normal hemoglobin (HbA) or in association with each other.

Ocular Features

The most characteristic conjunctival sign is isolated commas or corkscrew-shaped dark red vascular segments in sickling disorders. SC disease is the most important haemoglobinopathy because of its manifestations in the eye as sickle-cell retinopathy. Sickle-cell retinopathy can be both proliferative and nonproliferative. Sickle-cell retinopathy begins with occlusion of peripheral arterioles and is divided into five stages (**Table 13.9**).

Treatment

Sector photocoagulation to cause involution of neovascularization. *Pars plana vitrectomy* for tractional RD.

■ Retinopathy in Blood Disorders

Retinopathy in Anemia

Severe anemia causes marked decrease in the Hb level. Fundus examination reveals pale background, dilated retinal veins, and retinal hemorrhages (dot blot and flame-shaped). Roth spots (retinal hemorrhages with white center) are not uncommon.

Retinopathy in Leukemia

Ocular involvement is more common in the acute form than chronic form.

Table 13.9 Staging of sickle-cell retinopathy	
Stage 1	Occlusion of peripheral arterioles resulting in ischemia.
Stage 2	Peripheral arterio venous (A-V) anastomoses.
Stage 3	Sprouting of new vessels from anastomoses which have a "sea-fan" configuration (**"sea-fan" neovascularization**).
Stage 4	Vitreous hemorrhage.
Stage 5	Extensive fibrovascular proliferation and retinal detachment due to vitreous traction.

Fundus picture: Leukemia results in the following:

- Anemia: Therefore, fundus background is pale and orange.
- Thrombocytopenia: It causes intraocular bleeding, and characteristic **Roth spots** are present.
- Hyperviscosity: It causes vascular occlusion and retinal hypoxia, resulting in cotton-wool spots.
- Infections.

Optic nerve infiltration may cause swelling of the optic disc. Other manifestations in leukemia are iritis and pseudo-hypopyon, hyphema, and subconjunctival hemorrhage.

<table>
<tr><td align="center">

Valsalva retinopathy

In Valsalva maneuver, there is forceful exhalation against a closed glottis

↓

Sudden increase in intrathoracic and intra-abdominal pressure

↓

Associated sudden increase in venous pressure

↓

Perifoveal capillaries may rupture

↓

Unilateral or bilateral premacular hemorrhage
(**Fig. 13.34**)

</td></tr>
</table>

■ Inflammation of Retina

Inflammation of retina is called retinitis. Inflammation of retina is often associated with inflammation of choroid and is known as chorioretinitis. When inflammation involves retinal vessels, it is known as retinal vasculitis.

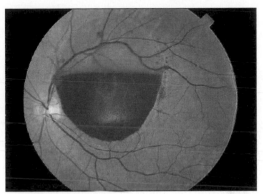

Fig. 13.34 Valsalva retinopathy. A boat-shaped retinal hemorrhage is present. Source: Vitreous Hemorrhage. In: Steidl S, Hartnett M, ed. Clinical Pathways In Vitreoretinal Disease. 1st Edition. Thieme; 2003.

■ Retinitis

Inflammation of retina may be:

- Purulent retinitis: It is caused by pyogenic organisms. It may be acute or subacute (septic retinitis of Roth).
- Specific retinitis.

Acute Purulent Retinitis

It occurs due to organisms lodging in the retina during septicemia (pyemia) and may lead to metastatic endophthalmitis or panophthalmitis.

Subacute Infective Retinitis (Septic Retinitis of Roth)

It occurs due to septic emboli lodging in the retina, typically in patients with subacute bacterial endocarditis (SABE) and sometimes in puerperal septicemia. It is characterized by multiple, superficial retinal hemorrhages at the posterior part of fundus. The characteristic feature is the presence of hemorrhages having a white center. These white-centered hemorrhages are called **Roth's spots**. The general reaction in retina can cause retinal edema or disc edema.

Specific Retinitis

It is usually associated with choroiditis and may be due to:

- Bacterial infections, for example, tuberculosis and leprosy.
- Viral infections, for example, cytomegalovirus (CMV) retinitis, AIDS, Rubella, herpes virus retinitis (causes acute retinal necrosis [ARN] and progressive outer retinal necrosis [PORN]).
- Spirochetal infection, for example, syphilis.
- Parasitic infections, for example, toxoplasmosis and toxocariasis.
- Sarcoidosis.

■ Retinal Vasculitis

It is the inflammation of retinal vessels. It may be classified as:

- Primary: "Eales" disease.
- Secondary:
  ◇ Secondary to systemic/ocular infections: tuberculosis, syphilis, and toxoplasmosis.
  ◇ Secondary to systemic inflammation: Behcet's disease, sarcoidosis, and SLE.
  ◇ Secondary to ocular inflammation: pars planitis and ARN.

Investigations

Investigations carried in case of retinal vasculitis are FA (reveals leakage from sheathed vessels), total leucocyte count (TLC), differential leucocyte count (DLC), erythrocyte sedimentation rate (ESR), X-Ray chest, serum angiotensin-converting enzyme (ACE) levels, serum lysozyme levels, Mantoux test, and venereal disease research laboratory (VDRL) test.

Treatment

For noninfectious causes of retinal vasculitis:

- Systemic steroids: 1 mg/kg of body weight and are tapered 10 mg per week.
- Periocular steroids.
- Immunosuppressives (like cyclophosphamide or azathioprine) in cases not responding to systemic steroids.
- Laser photocoagulation: To manage neovascular complications.

For infectious causes:

- Specific treatment of underlying cause such as tuberculosis, toxoplasmosis, and ARN.

Eales' Disease (Periphlebitis Retinae)

It is an idiopathic inflammation of peripheral retinal veins and occurs typically in young adults, usually males. Its etiology is not known exactly. It is suggested that hypersensitivity reaction to tuberculoproteins may be the cause of vasculitis. It is a bilateral disease and presents with recurrent vitreous hemorrhage in young males.

Clinical Features

Patient complains of sudden, painless loss of vision and floaters (black spots) in front of the eye. Clinical signs of Eales disease include:

- Peripheral vascular sheathing (**Fig. 13.35**).
- Retinal hemorrhages, cotton-wool spots and retinal edema.
- Peripheral neovascularization at the junction of perfused and nonperfused retina.
- Recurrent vitreous hemorrhage (**Flowchart 13.9**).

Investigations

FA reveals shunt vessels, leakage of Fluorescein dye from vessels, and area of capillary nonperfusion (capillary dropout) (**Fig. 13.36**).

Treatment

It consists of systemic steroids in the early stage of vasculitis, laser photocoagulation of peripheral nonperfused area, and vitreoretinal surgery in cases of persistent vitreous hemorrhage or tractional RD.

Prognosis

Visual prognosis is good in majority of cases.

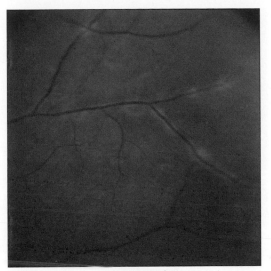

Fig. 13.35 Eales disease (periphlebitis retinae). Source: Multiple Sclerosis. In: Biousse V, Newman N, ed. Neuro-Opthalmology Illustrated. 3rd Edition. Thieme; 2019.

Complications

The clinical manifestations of Eales' disease largely depend upon the extent of retinal vasculitis and obliteration of affected vessels, especially capillaries. However, some eyes may be complicated by tractional RD, rubeosis iridis, NVG and complicated cataract.

■ Macular Inflammations

Macular inflammations comprise photoretinits (retinitis from bright light) and central vision. **Central chorloretinitis** may occur in toxoplasmosis, histoplasmosis, tuberculosis and syphilis.

The symptoms are defective central vision and concentric contraction of the field with central, paracentral, or ring scotomata. Metamorphopsia or distortion of perceived images is a common symptom of macular disease.

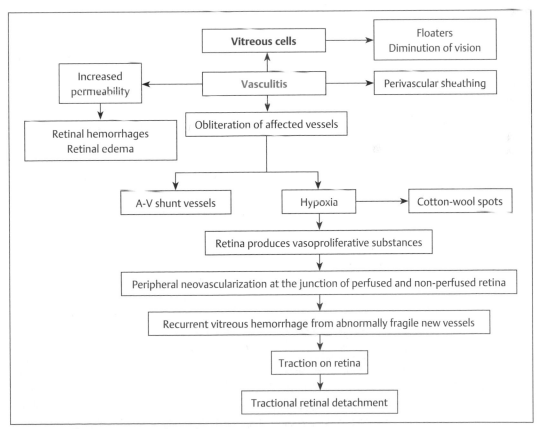

Flowchart 13.9 Clinical course of vasculitis.

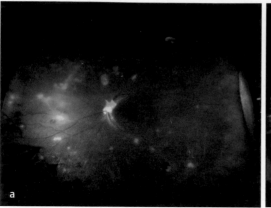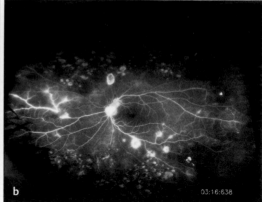

Fig. 13.36 (a) Fundus photo showing peripheral occluded vessels, small fibrovascular proliferation over disc, and few peripheral laser scars. **(b)** FFA showing leakage of dye from nasal inflamed vessels, few neovascularization elsewhere, and temporal capillary nonperfused area. Abbreviation: FFA, fundus fluorescein angiography.

Photoretinitis

Causes of retinal phototoxicity are:

- Gazing at solar eclipse directly or indirectly with inadequately protected eyes, called solar retinopathy/eclipse retinopathy.
- Accidental exposure to welding arc without protective glasses.
- Strong focused light of operating microscope during cataract surgery with posterior chamber lens implantation.

Pathogenesis

All visible rays, ultraviolet (UV) radiations and infrared rays passing to retina are absorbed by RPE. Photochemical retinal injury by UV radiations takes place, which is enhanced by thermal effects of infrared radiations and results in retinal burn. Thus, severity of lesions varies with degree of pigmentation of fundus and duration of exposure.

In young persons with clear crystalline lens, there is higher risk of retinopathy, while in patients with high-refractive error, risk is smaller.

Clinical Features

A persistence of after-image occurs soon after the exposure, progressing later to impairment of central vision, positive central scotoma and metamorphopsia. Initially, a small yellow spot is seen at fovea. Later, thermal effect causes a central burnt out hole in the RPE. The yellow spot gets replaced by a red dot, surrounded by deposits of pigment, or even a lamellar macular hole may develop.

Prognosis

Prognosis is guarded as some defect usually persists.

Treatment

No effective treatment is available.

Prevention

As there is no effective treatment, so emphasis should be on prevention by using protective glasses (which absorb UV and infrared radiations) or viewing of light source should be discouraged.

▪ Retinochoroidopathies

As choroid and outer layers of retina are nourished by choriocapillaris, so inflammatory disorders involving choriocapillaris also involve choroid, RPE and sensory retina.

Retinochoroidopathies are inflammatory disorders of unknown etiology involving choriocapillaris, choroid, RPE and sensory retina. Characteristic lesions of retinochoroidopathies are multiple, small or confluent, cream-colored, yellow or grayish-white, ill-defined, and located at the level of inner choroid or outer retina. Inactive lesions are characterized by RPE changes with areas of depigmentation and clumping.

Clinical entities of retinochoroidopathies include:

- Acute posterior multifocal placoid pigment epitheliopathy (APMPPE).
- Birdshot retinochoroidopathy.
- Serpiginous choroidopathy.

■ Acute Posterior Multifocal Placoid Pigment Epitheliopathy (APMPPE)

These lesions are idiopathic, usually bilateral and affect young adults. Primary lesion appears to be the obstructive vasculitis of choriocapillaris, resulting in ischemia and focal swelling of RPE cells and then the characteristic cream-colored placoid lesions appear (**Fig. 13.37**).

Course and Prognosis

It is a self-limiting condition with good visual recovery.

Clinical Features

The patient has subacute visual impairment. Within a few days, the fellow eye usually becomes affected. The condition is characterized by the following features (remembered by the mnemonic APMPPE):

Acute—*sudden onset.*

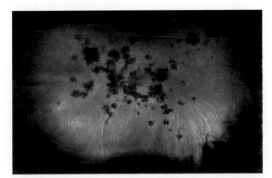

Fig. 13.37 Acute post multifocal placoid pigment epitheliopathy (APMPPE). Source: Uveitis/ Vasculitis. In: Ehlers J, ed. The Retina Illustrated. 1st Edition. Thieme; 2019.

Posterior—involvement of *posterior pole* and posterior equatorial retina.

Multifocal— *multiple* lesions.

Placoid—*placoid*, cream-colored lesions.

Pigment Epitheliopathy—*lesions at the level of RPE.*

Alteration in RPE is permanent. Acute lesions are replaced by RPE changes with multifocal areas of depigmentation and clumping. Visual improvement is not immediate but continues several weeks after the apparent ophthalmoscopic improvement.

Investigations

FA (of active lesions): Initially, obstructive vasculitis of choriocapillaris causes nonperfusion of choriocapillaris and dense hypofluorescence. Choroidal filling is irregular and patchy, outlining the placoid lesions which mask the background fluorescence of choroid.

In later stages, there is hyperfluorescence, due to staining of lesions with Fluorescein and leakage of dye is not significant.

> **ICG** is superior to Fluorescein in demonstrating nonperfusion of choriocapillaris.

Differential Diagnosis

APMPPE should be differentiated from multifocal choroiditis, acute retinal pigment epithelitis and primary RPE detachment.

Treatment

No effective treatment is available.

■ Bird Shot Retinochoroidopathy (Vitiliginous Retinochoroiditis)

These lesions are idiopathic, bilateral, multifocal, and recurrent. It affects middle-aged individuals who are +ve for HLA-A29. It is usually seen in females. Lesions are *postequatorial* and flat *creamy-yellow spots* (due to focal hypopigmentation). Retinal vessels pass over the lesions and larger choroidal vessels can be seen within each lesion (**Fig. 13.38**).

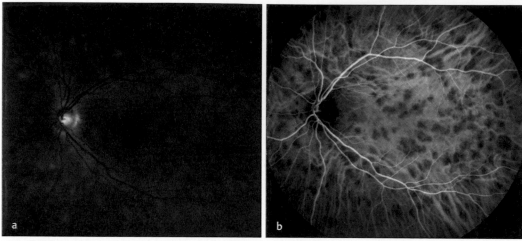

Fig. 13.38 (a, b) Birdshot retinochoroiditis. Source: Indocyanine Green Angiography and Ultra-Widefield Indocyanine Green Angiography. In: Ethers J, ed. The Retina Illustrated. 1st Edition. Thieme; 2009.

Clinical Features

Patient presents with vitreous floaters and blurring of vision. Distribution of lesion in retina resembles the pattern of bird shot scatter from a shotgun.

Treatment

The disease may respond to steroids and immunosuppressives.

■ Serpiginous Choroidopathy (Geographical Choroidopathy)

These lesions are idiopathic, recurrent, and bilateral but have asymmetrical involvement. It affects people between 30 to 70 years of age. It follows a chronic course. It involves choriocapillaris and RPE.

Clinical Presentation

Acute lesions are cream-colored, irregular patches at the level of RPE or inner choroid. They usually start around optic disc (i.e., in peripapillary region) and spread in a snake-like manner in all directions. *As the lesion is peripapillary, patient is asymptomatic unless fovea is involved.* The lesions become inactive, leaving the areas of RPE and choroidal atrophy. Large choroidal vessels are seen at the base of atrophic area.

Recurrence

Fresh acute lesions usually arise as extensions from old inactive scars. It is a progressive disease and involvement of fovea cause a profound and permanent impairment of central vision.

Investigations

- FA: Old inactive lesions show atrophy of choriocapillaris. Decreased choroidal background fluorescence results in early hypofluorescence. Later, due to diffusion of dye from normal choriocapillaris at the margins of atrophic areas, late hyperfluorescence at the margins of atrophic areas is seen.
- ERG is abnormal.

Differential Diagnosis

it should be differentiated from placoid pigment epitheliopathy and pigment epithelitis.

Treatment

There is no effective treatment. The disease may progress despite aggressive therapy with steroids or immunosuppressives.

Prognosis

Prognosis is poor.

■ Important Macular Disorders

Few important macular lesions are:
- Central serous chorioretinopathy.
- CME.
- Macular hole.
- Macular pucker and macular epiretinal membrane.
- Toxic maculopathies (drug-induced maculopathy).

Outer blood–retinal barrier is formed by tight junctions between RPE cells, and inner blood–retinal barrier is formed by tight junctions between retinal capillary endothelial cells (located in inner nuclear layer of retina).

> **Break down of outer blood–retinal barrier** results in **CSR**, while the **breakdown of inner blood–retinal barrier** results in **CME**.

■ Central Serous Chorioretinopathy (CSR)

It is characterized by localized detachment of neurosensory retina at macula secondary to focal RPE defects (i.e., breakdown of outer blood–retinal barrier) (**Fig. 13.39**). It is usually unilateral, typically affects young males, and usually self-limiting. Its etiology is unknown.

Factors reported to induce CSR include:
- Emotional stress.
- Untreated hypertension.
- Elevated blood levels of steroids due to:
  ◇ Administration of systemic steroids.
  ◇ Cushing's disease.
  ◇ Organ transplantation.

Clinical Features

- Blurring of vision: It is sudden in onset, unilateral and painless.

Visual acuity is usually modestly reduced. It is associated with relative positive scotoma, that is, black shadow before the eye. In CSR, elevation of neurosensory retina leads to acquired hypermetropia. So, visual acuity is often correctable by use of convex lenses ("plus lenses").
- Metamorphopsia (distortion of objects).
- Micropsia (**Flowchart 13.10**).

The affected area is raised above the level of retina due to edema. There is a round/oval swelling in the macular area which is demarcated by a characteristic ring-shaped reflex. There is loss of foveal reflex. The SRF may be clear or turbid and few exudative dots can be seen on the posterior surface of detached neurosensory retina.

Investigations

OCT shows elevation of sensory retina, separated from RPE layer by an optically empty zone.

FA shows that CSR is caused by a breakdown of outer blood–retinal barrier which allows the passage of Fluorescein molecules into subretinal space. FA shows one of the following patterns:
- **Smoke-stack appearance:** The dye leaks through RPE and the Fluorescein dye reaches the subretinal space. The small hyperfluorescent spot ascends vertically (like a smoke stack) to the upper limit of detachment. Now, the dye spreads laterally, forming a mushroom or umbrella pattern (**Fig. 13.40a**).
- **Ink-blot appearance:** In this pattern, a small hyperfluorescent spot appears which gradually increases in size until the entire subretinal space is filled (**Fig. 13.40b**).

Course and Prognosis

Spontaneous resolution occurs within 3 to 6 months in most cases and visual acuity returns

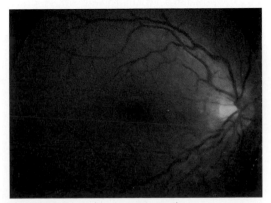

Fig. 13.39 Central serous retinopathy.

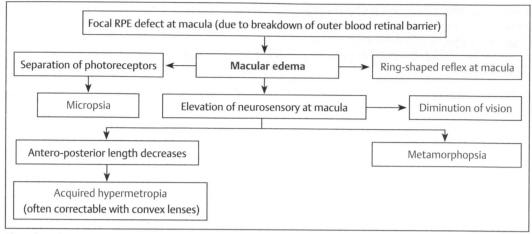

Flowchart 13.10 Symptoms in central serous retinopathy.

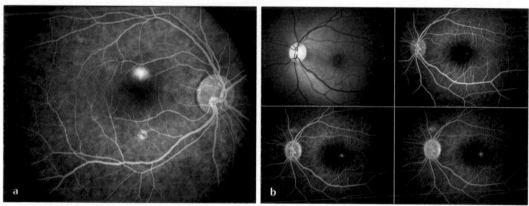

Fig. 13.40 FA showing smoke stack appearance **(a)** and ink blot appearance **(b)**. Abbreviation: FA, fluorescein angiography.

to normal but some subjective symptoms (mild changes in color and contrast sensitivity) may persist.

Prognosis is good in patients with non-involvement of fovea and detachment <1 DD in size. Recurrences are frequent. Recurrences cause extensive degeneration of RPE (RPE decompensation), and permanent impairment of visual acuity results.

Treatment

Most of the cases do not require treatment. Systemic steroids should be avoided. Laser photocoagulation to the site of leakage is indicated in the following circumstances:

1. If edema persists for 4 months or longer.
2. Recurrent episodes of CSR.
3. Permanent visual impairment in other eye due to CSR.

The aim of treatment is to produce a burn just sufficient to blanch the RPE. *Laser photocoagulation is contraindicated if the leak is near or within FAZ.* Photodynamic therapy (PDT) may be beneficial in CSR with subfoveal leaks. *Uncommon side effect* of treated eyes includes development of choroidal neovascularization (CNV).

■ Cystoid Macular Edema (CME/CMO)

It is the accumulation of fluid in the OPL = Henle's layer and INL of macula with the formation of fluid-filled microcysts. It develops following breakdown of inner blood–retinal barrier (**Flowchart 13.11**).

Etiology

CME may be associated with:

- Ocular surgical procedures.
- Diabetic retinopathy.
- Retinal vein occlusion.
- Intermediate uveitis (pars planitis).
- Retinitis pigmentosa.
- Drugs: Topical 2% Adrenaline or Latanoprost in glaucoma.

Ocular surgical procedures such as cataract surgery (**Irvine–Gass syndrome**), glaucoma filtration surgery, and vitrectomy may be associated with CME. It is less frequent following extracapsular cataract extraction (ECCE) than intracapsular cataract extraction (ICCE) with incarceration of vitreous into incision.

Clinical Features

Patient presents with impairment of central vision and a positive central scotoma. On slit lamp biomicroscopy with + 90D lens, the fundus picture reveals macular edema with multiple cystoid spaces which gives a "honeycomb appearance" to macula. There is loss of foveal reflex.

Investigations

FA: Accumulation of dye within microcystic spaces in OPL (Henle's layer) of retina demonstrates "flower-petal" pattern of hyperfluorescence due to radial arrangement of Henle's fibers at fovea (**Fig. 13.41a**).

OCT shows collection of hyporeflective spaces within retina and thickening of macula, with loss of foveal depression (**Fig. 13.41b**).

Advantage of OCT over FA

- Unlike FA, it can also be used *in eyes with opaque media.*
- Serial OCTs may be used *to assess response to treatment.*
- It can be used *to assess lamellar hole formation.*

Treatment

It includes:

- Treatment of causative factor, for example,
  ◇ Anterior vitrectomy (for incarceration of vitreous into incision which is responsible for CME after intraocular surgeries).

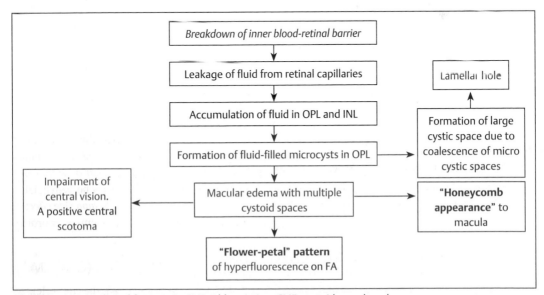

Flowchart 13.11 Clinical features in CME. Abbreviation: CME, cystoid macular edema.

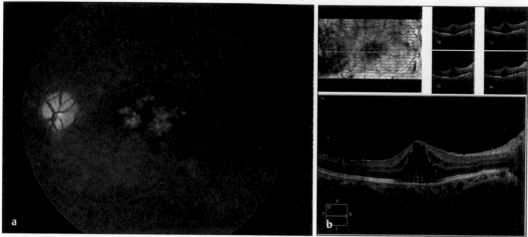

Fig. 13.41 **(a)** Flower-petal pattern of hyper fluorescence seen on FA. **(b)** OCT in CME. Abbreviations: CME, cystoid macular edema; FA, fluorescein angiography; OCT, optical coherence tomography.

◇ Laser photocoagulation (for CME due to diabetes and retinal vein occlusion).

◇ Cessation of medication (If CME is drug-induced).

• Steroids– topical, periocular and systemic.

• Intravitreal triamcinolone may reduce CME in cases unresponsive to subtenon injections.

• Intravitreal Avastin (anti-VEGF agent) injections and grid photocoagulation for chronic CME.

Complications

In long-standing CME, fluid-filled microcystic spaces coalesce and large cystic spaces are formed. It results in formation of lamellar hole at fovea with irreversible damage to central vision.

■ Macular Hole

Foveal region is susceptible to hole formation because of its thinness, avascularity and lack of support.

Etiology

Macular hole results due to ocular trauma, with age (age-related macular hole) or as a sequel to intraocular inflammation. Vitreous gel has a firm attachment to macula. With aging or trauma, vitreous degenerates and separates from retina. Traction on macula may result in partial loss of retinal layers (**lamellar hole**) or loss of entire sensory retina (**full-thickness hole**) (**Fig. 13.42** and **Table 13.10**).

Clinical Features

There is significant reduction in visual acuity due to loss of neurosensory retina in the region of hole. The earliest sign of an impending macular hole is flattening of foveal depression and loss of foveolar reflex. A macular hole is characterized by (**Fig. 13.43**):

• Multiple yellow deposits in the base of hole at the level of RPE.

• Round defect in neurosensory retina surrounded by a rim of RD.

Lamellar holes do not have a surrounding RD.

Differential Diagnosis

• Pseudohole at macula (a hole in the ERM covering the fovea): In patients with pseudohole, vision is better than the macular hole, and yellow deposits at the level of RPE are not found in pseudohole.

• Early yellow lesion of solar retinopathy: A history of sun gazing should be searched to exclude solar retinopathy.

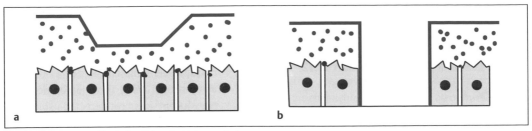

Fig. 13.42 (a) Lamellar hole. **(b)** Full-thickness hole.

Table 13.10 Differentiating features between lamellar and full-thickness variant of macular hole		
Features	**Lamellar hole**	**Full- thickness hole**
Vision	Distorted and blurred.	Severe impairment of central vision.
FA	As RPE is normal, so there is no RPE window defect.	Due to RPE window defect, background choroidal fluorescence is unmasked and FA shows an area of hyperfluorescence.
Abbreviations: FA, fluorescein angiography; RPE, retinal pigment epithelium.		

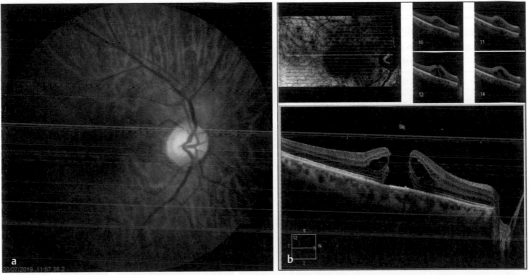

Fig. 13.43 (a) Macular hole (full thickness). **(b)** OCT showing full thickness macular hole. Abbreviation: OCT, optical coherence tomography.

- Foveal detachment due to CSR may be mistaken for an impending macular hole. FA can distinguish these two disorders.

Treatment

- For impending macular hole: Release of vitreomacular traction could stop the progression of disease.

- For full-thickness macular hole: It involves
  ◇ Removal of perimacular cortical vitreous to relieve vitreomacular traction.
  ◇ Peeling of ILM: ILM is invisible, so peeling of invisible ILM is assisted by staining it with ICA.
  ◇ Internal gas tamponade by SF_6 or C_3F_8 followed by strict postoperative face down position.

◼ Age-Related Macular Degeneration (ARMD) (OP8.1, OP8.2, OP8.4, IM24.15)

It is a nonhereditary degeneration also known as senile macular degeneration. It is the most common cause of irreversible central visual loss in persons over 50 years of age.

Risk factors associated with ARMD are age (main risk factor), family history, smoking, obesity, hypertension, cardiovascular disease, and exposure to sun light.

ARMD is caused by sclerosis of arteries nourishing the retina. The earliest clinical finding of ARMD is the appearance of drusen in the macular area.

> Drusen appear as small, discrete, yellowish-white, slightly elevated spots beneath the RPE at posterior pole. They are rarely clinically visible before the age of 45 years.

Histopathologically, drusen are thickening of the Bruch's membrane (localized but diffuse) due to discrete deposition of abnormal material between basal lamina of RPE and inner collagenous layer in the Bruch's membrane.

Pathogenesis: RPE functions as a pump as well as a barrier. With advanced age, arteries nourishing the retina are sclerosed and retinal tissue is deprived of oxygen and nutrients. It results in dysfunction of RPE with failure to clear the debris derived from metabolic products of photoreceptors and RPE. Deposition of abnormal material (lipid-rich) between basal lamina of RPE and inner collagenous layer of the Bruch's membrane (called drusen) takes place and results in localized and diffuse thickening of inner aspects of the Bruch's membrane (**Fig. 13.46**).

Types of drusen: Drusens are mainly of two types (**Fig. 13.47**):

Hard drusen: These are discrete, small, round, yellowish white spots which have *distinct borders*.

Soft drusen: These are larger than hard drusen and have *indistinct margins*. They frequently become confluent.

Calcified drusen represent calcification in hard or soft drusen and have a glistening appearance.

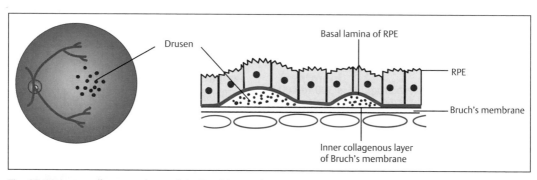

Fig. 13.46 Inner collagenous layer of the Bruch's membrane.

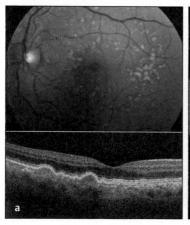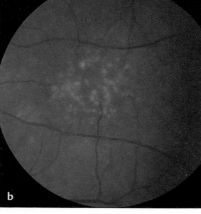

Fig. 13.47 (a) Hard drusen. Source: Vitreoretinal interface disorders. In: Agarwal A, Kumar D, ed. Essentials of OCT in ocular disease. 1st Edition. Thieme; 2015. **(b)** Soft drusen, Source: Scott I, Regillo C, Flynn H et al., ed. Vitreoretinal disease: Diagnosis, management, and clinical pearls, 2nd Edition. Thieme; 2017.

Table 13.11 Differentiating features between dry and wet ARMD

	Dry (atrophic) ARMD	Wet (exudative) ARMD
Prevalence	More common	Less common than dry ARMD
Visual impairment	• Mild to moderate • Gradual over months or years	• More serious visual loss • Sudden, painless within a few days

Abbreviation: ARMD, age-related macular degeneration.

ARMD presents in two forms: Dry (Atrophic) ARMD and wet (exudative or neovascular) ARMD (**Table 13.11**).

Atrophic (Dry) ARMD

It presents with diminution of vision, which is gradual, usually bilateral but often asymmetrical. *Clinical signs in early stage:* Retinal tissue is deprived of oxygen and nutrients due to sclerosis of arteries nourishing retina with advancing age. There is progressive atrophy of RPE cells and depigmentation, pigment clumping with focal hyperpigmentation in macula, and loss of choriocapillaris (**Fig. 13.48a**).

Clinical sign in late stage: During the late stages, the larger choroidal vessels become visible within atrophic areas and preexisting drusen disappear (geographical atrophy, **Fig. 13.48b**).

Investigations

FA is used to diagnose ARMD. In the early phase, *window defect* due to atrophy of RPE overlying drusen leads to unmasking of background choroidal fluorescence, resulting in **hyperfluorescence**. As drusen retain Fluorescein dye for a long period, *staining of drusen* in late phase also results in **hyperfluorescence**.

Treatment

There is no effective treatment. Low-visual aids may be useful.

Prophylaxis

To lower the risk for or decrease the progression of ARMD, the measures taken includes:

- Combination of antioxidant vitamins and zinc. Antioxidant vitamins include vitamin C (500 mg), vitamin E (400 IU) and β carotene 15 mg. Zinc supplement is given

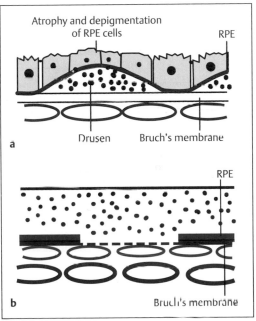

Fig. 13.48 (a) Signs in early stages of dry ARMD. **(b)** Signs in late stages of dry ARMD. Abbreviations: ARMD, age-related macular degeneration; RPE, retinal pigment epithelium.

as zinc oxide- 80 mg and 2 mg of copper as cupric oxide to prevent zinc-induced anemia.
- Patients with ARMD must be encouraged to quit smoking and use sunglasses outdoors.
- There is also some evidence that use of lutein may also be of benefit.

Taking β-carotene is not suitable for a person who smokes due to increase in the risk of lung cancer.

Exudative (Wet or Neovascular) ARMD

It is due to the leakage of fluid from a neovascular growth beneath the retina known as **choroidal**

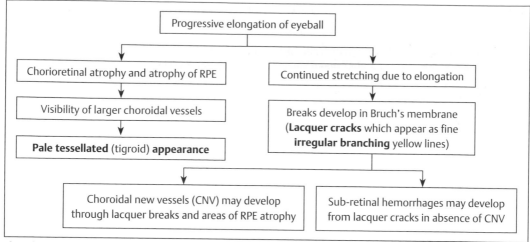

Flowchart 13.14 Clinical features in pathological myopia.

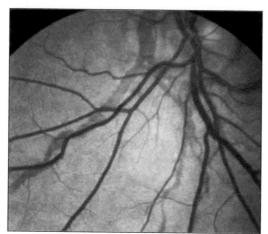

Fig. 13.50 Angioid streaks. Source: Angioid Streaks. In: Tabendah H, Goldberg M, ed. The Retina in Systemic Disease: A Color Manual of Ophthalmoscopy. 1st Edition. Thieme; 2009.

Treatment

Because angioid streaks are generally asymptomatic and visually insignificant, no treatment is warranted. If a CNVM develops, laser photocoagulation should be considered. Laser photocoagulation for extrafoveal or juxtafoveal membranes is beneficial. No role exists for prophylactic photocoagulation of angioid streaks. Repeated treatment may be necessary, as the recurrence rate appears to be high.

■ Peripheral Retinal Degenerations

Peripheral retinal degenerations may be:
- *Benign* peripheral retinal degenerations *do not lead to retinal breaks.*
- Degenerations *associated with retinal breaks.*

Benign Peripheral Retinal Degenerations

- **Paving stone degeneration:** It consists of discrete yellow–white areas caused by focal chorioretinal atrophy. It is present in a high-percentage of normal eyes (**Fig. 13.51**).
- **Microcystoid degeneration:** It consists of tiny vesicles with indistinct boundaries on a grayish-white background. It is present in all adult eyes and increases in severity with age.
- **Honeycomb (reticular) degeneration:** It looks like a honeycomb and is characterized by a fine network of perivascular pigmentation.
- **Equatorial drusen:** These are clusters of small pale lesions frequently having a pigmented border. They are similar to drusen at the posterior pole.
- **White with pressure:** It is a translucent gray appearance of retina *induced by* indenting the sclera. It is frequently seen in normal eyes which do not develop retinal breaks.

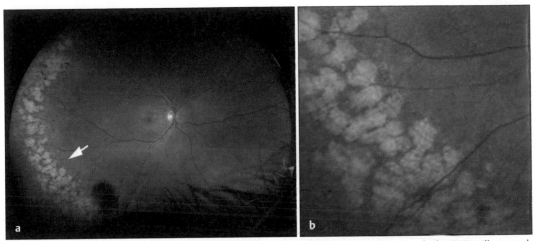

Fig. 13.51 (a, b) Paving stone/cobblestone degeneration. Source: Features. In: Ehlers J, ed. The Retina Illustrated. 1st Edition. Thieme; 2019.

Degenerations Associated with Retinal Breaks

Lattice Degeneration (OP8.1, OP8.2, OP8.4)

It is not an age-related disease. It consists of well-demarcated, spindle-shaped areas of retinal thinning. A characteristic feature is an arborizing network of white lines in the lesion. An associated feature in lattice degeneration is hyperplasia of RPE, hence abnormal pigmentation is often present (**Fig. 13.52**).

Orientation: It is circumferential, that is, its long axes are parallel to ora serrata.

Location: It is located between equator and ora serrata and is more common superiorly than inferiorly.

Prevalence: It is more common in moderate (> –3D) myopes.

Complication: Traction on lattice by vitreous may result in retinal tear and RD.

Prophylaxis: To reduce the risk of development of RD, lattice is treated prophylactically by laser photocoagulation or cryopexy (transconjunctival).

Snail Track Degeneration

It closely resembles lattice degeneration. It consists of sharply demarcated areas of white snowflakes which give the retina a white,

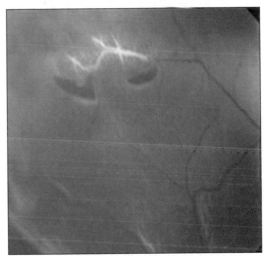

Fig. 13.52 Lattice degeneration with horseshoe-shaped tears. Source: Retinal Detachment. In: Taben deh H, Goldberg M, ed. The Retina in Systemic Disease: A Color Manual of Ophthalmoscopy. 1st Edition. Thieme; 2009.

frost-like appearance. *White lines (characteristic feature of lattice) are absent.*

White Without Pressure

It is a translucent gray appearance of retina even without scleral indentation. It is thought to be due to vitreous traction which could result in the formation of retinal break.

Treatment

There is no effective treatment. Genetic counselling is helpful to reduce incidence of the disease. Counsel the patient for:

- No consanguineous marriages.
- Affected individuals should be advised not to have children unless they are suffering from autosomal dominant disease (having benign course and best prognosis).

■ Atypical Forms of RP

A few atypical forms of RP are listed below:

- *RP sine pigmento:* It is a variant of retinitis pigmentosa characterized by all clinical features of typical RP, except visible pigmentation of retina. It must be differentiated from congenital stationary night blindness which is stationary throughout life. RP sine pigmento is progressive and leads to optic atrophy.
- *Retinitis punctata albescens:* It is characterized by the following features:
  ◇ Small, white dots scattered all over the fundus.
  ◇ Arteriolar attenuation.
  ◇ Night blindness.
  ◇ Constriction of visual fields.
- *Sectorial RP:* It is characterized by involvement of one or two sectors of retina.
- *Pericentric RP* (**inverse RP**): It is similar to typical retinitis pigmentosa, except that pigmentary changes are confined to pericentral retina, sparing the retinal periphery.
- *Unilateral RP:* Only one eye is affected. It may occur occasionally.

■ Systemic Diseases Associated with Retinitis Pigmentosa

RP may be associated with systemic diseases. Important associations are:

- *Laurence–Moon–Bardet–Biedl syndrome:* It is characterized by RP, obesity, hypogonadism, mental retardation, and polydactyly.

- *Usher syndrome:* It is characterized by RP and sensorineural deafness (congenital and nonprogressive).
- *Refsum's syndrome:* It is a hereditary disorder of metabolism due to *deficiency of phytanic acid hydroxylase,* resulting in the accumulation of phytanic acid in blood and body tissues.

It is characterized by RP (usually "salt and pepper" type rather than a classic "bone corpuscle" seen in typical RP), deafness, cerebellar ataxia, and polyneuropathy. It is treated by plasma exchange (plasmaphoresis) and phytanic acid-free diet.

- **Cockayne's syndrome**—It comprises:
  ◇ RP.
  ◇ Dwarfism.
  ◇ Mental retardation.
  ◇ Ataxia.
  ◇ "Bird-like" facies.
- **Kearns–Sayre syndrome**: The **characteristic triad** consists of:
  ◇ RP.
  ◇ Chronic progressive external ophthalmoplegia.
  ◇ Heart block.
- **Friedreich's ataxia**: It comprises of RP, posterior column diseases, cerebellar ataxia and nystagmus.
- **NARP syndrome**: It is characterized by **N**europathy, **A**taxia and **R**etinitis **p**igmentosa.

■ Macular Dystrophies

Juvenile Retinoschisis

It is a bilateral macular dystrophy. In 50% of cases, there is associated peripheral retinoschisis.

Basic defect is in Müller cells. Splitting of retina occurs at the level of NFL (in senile/acquired retinoschisis splitting occurs at OPL). Inheritance is sex-linked recessive. It presents between 5 to 10 years of age with reading difficulties and is *characterized by* cystoid spaces with radial striae (**bicycle-wheel pattern**). ERG is subnormal while **EOG** is normal.

Stargardt Disease and Fundus Flavimaculatus

Stargardt disease (Stargardt macular dystrophy) and fundus flavimaculatus are regarded as variants of same disorder (**Table 13.12**); fundus flavimaculatus is usually seen later than Stargardt disease. It is inherited as an autosomal recessive disorder (**Fig. 13.54**).

Familial Dominant Drusen

It is also called Doyne's honeycomb dystrophy (Tay's choroiditis). It is inherited as autosomal dominant disorder. It appears in 3rd decade of life. Initially patients are asymptomatic. Later CNV or geographic atrophy may develop and visual acuity decreases. It is characterized by round, discrete yellow-dots or flecks arranged in mosaic or honey

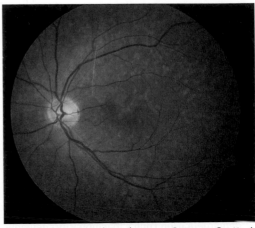

Fig. 13.54 Stargardt's disease. Source: Scott I, Regillo C, Flynn H et al., ed. Vitreoretinal disease: Diagnosis, management, and clinical pearls, 2nd edition. Thieme; 2017.

Table 13.12 Differentiating features between Stargardt disease and fundus flavimaculatus		
Features	**Stargardt disease**	**Fundus flavimaculatus**
Onset	Juvenile onset macular dystrophy.	Appears in adult life (usually third or fourth decade of life).
Symptoms	It presents with bilateral gradual diminution of central vision.	In absence of macular involvement, the condition is asymptomatic. If fovea is involved, central vision is impaired.
Signs	In early stages fovea appears normal. With passage of time, an oval atrophic lesion develops in foveal region giving it a **"beaten-bronze"** appearance. Yellowish-white flecks usually surround this oval zone of atrophy. In final stages, extensive chorioretinal atrophy at posterior pole results with poor vision.	It is characterized by bilateral, yellow-white deep retinal lesions with fuzzy outlines (flecks). These may be round, oval or pisciform (resembling fish tail). They are scattered throughout posterior pole of both eyes and never extend beyond equator.
ERG		
• Photopic • Scotopic	Normal to subnormal Normal (as there are no rods on fovea)	Normal to subnormal Normal
EOG	Subnormal	EOG is based on activity of RPE and photoreceptors. EOG is subnormal, indicating diffuse involvement of RPE.
Fluorescein angiography	It shows a "dark choroid." There is no leakage of dye. With chorioretinal atrophy, there is window defect at macula.	Histological examination reveals an accumulation of lipofuscin like substance in RPE. So, there is absence of normal background in early stages due to lipofuscin deposits in RPE—"dark choroid' effect. In advanced stages of disease, atrophic changes in RPE causes window defect and hyperfluorescence.
Prognosis	Final outcome is atrophic changes in RPE and secondary changes in photoreceptors at macula. Visual acuity tends to decrease rapidly and is seldom worse than 6/60.	Relatively good.
Abbreviations: EOG, electro-oculography; RPE, retinal pigment epithelium.		

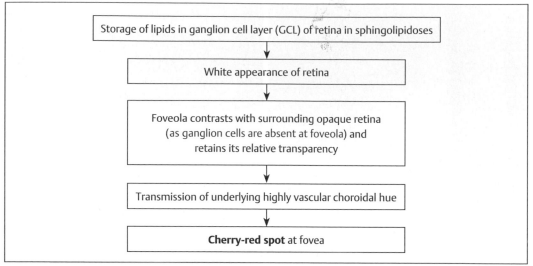

Flowchart 13.15 Development of cherry-red spot in sphingolipidoses.

Phakomatoses

Phakomatoses comprise a group of familial diseases having a tendency for development of neoplasms in the central nervous system (CNS), skin and eye. These are transmitted as autosomal dominant traits. Phakomatoses include:

- Angiomatosis retinae.
- Tuberous sclerosis.
- Neurofibromatosis.
- Sturge–Weber syndrome.

Angiomatosis Retinae

Angiomatosis (formation of angiomas) of retina may occur in isolation. The clinical entity is termed as **angiomatosis retinae** (von Hippel disease).

In 25% of patients, angiomatosis of retina is associated with angiomatosis of CNS (involving cerebellum, medulla or spinal cord), kidneys and adrenals. The clinical entity is termed as **von Hippel–Lindau disease**.

Angiomatosis retinae manifests in the third and fourth decades of life and is more frequent in males than females. It is characterized by the presence of a round orange–red mass (**retinal angioma**) with dilatation and tortuosity of supplying artery and draining vein. Later, extravasation from tumor and vessels leads to massive exudation (resembling exudative retinopathy of coats). Exudative retinal detachment is a sequel of the disease (**Fig. 13.56**).

Treatment is unsatisfactory but laser photo-coagulation or cryotherapy of angioma in early stages may be beneficial.

Tuberous Sclerosis (Bourneville Disease)

It is characterized by development of hamartomas (benign tumor-like nodule) in multiple organ systems: skin, CNS, retina and viscera.

- Nodular lesions of skin, particularly on the face (adenoma sebaceum), consist of fibroangiomatous red papules around nose and cheeks and are universal (**Fig. 13.57a**).
- Cerebral lesions lead to epilepsy and mental retardation.
- Retinal nodular tumors: These are actually astrocytomas, particularly near the ONH (**Fig. 13.57b**). Prognosis is poor.

The classic diagnostic triad of tuberous sclerosis is adenoma sebaceum, epilepsy and mental retardation. Although it is only present in few patients, but it is diagnostic when present.

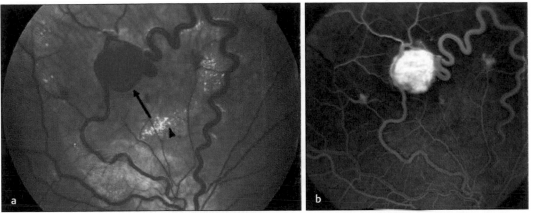

Fig. 13.56 (a, b) Angiomatosis retinae. Source: Hemangiomas. In: Lang G, ed. Ophthalmology. A Pocket Textbook Atlas. 3rd Edition. Thieme; 2015.

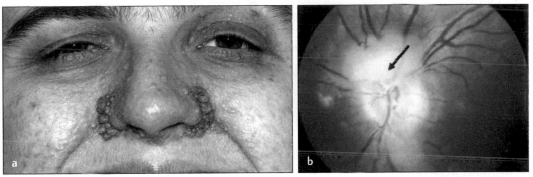

Fig. 13.57 (a) Tuberous sclerosis. Source: Benign Eyelid and Periocular Tumors. In: Leatherbarrow B, ed. Oculoplastic Surgery. 3rd Edition. Thieme; 2019. **(b)** Astrocytoma in tuberous sclerosis (Bourneville's disease). Source: Intraocular Optic Nerve Tumors. In: Lang G, ed. Ophthalmology. A Pocket Textbook Atlas. 3rd Edition. Thieme; 2015.

■ Neurofibromatosis (von Recklinghausen's Disease)

It is characterized by multiple tumors involving CNS, peripheral nerves, skin lesions and bone defects.

It presents with tumors of CNS (meningiomas and gliomas); tumors of peripheral nerves (neurofibromas, as it may also involve internal organs); skin lesions (like café-au-lait spots, which are light brown macules [hyperpigmented patches] commonly found on the trunk); bone defects (the greater wing of sphenoid bone is most commonly involved which is absent) and ocular lesions like optic nerve glioma, neurofibromas of lids, iris, choroid and retina, prominent corneal nerves and pulsating exophthalmos (due to absence of the greater wing of sphenoid bone).

■ Sturge–Weber Syndrome

(Encephalofacial Angiomatosis/ Encephalotrigeminal Angiomatosis)

As the name suggests, it is marked by angiomas of meninges and face, therefore it involves face, leptomeninges (piamater and arachnoid) and eyes.

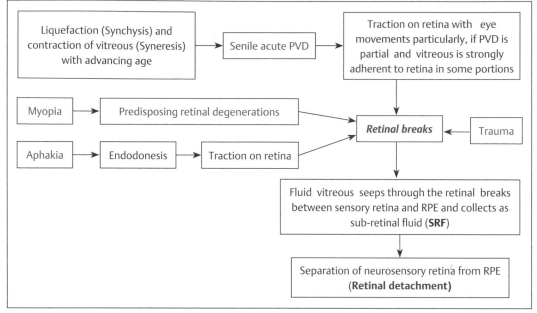

Flowchart 13.16 Predisposing factors of retinal breaks and retinal detachment. Abbreviation: PVD, posterior vitreous detachment.

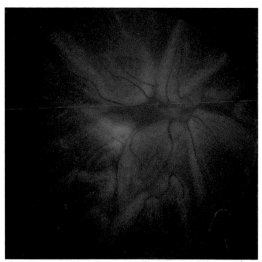

Fig. 13.60 Rhegmatogenous RD with proliferative vitreoretinopathy. Abbreviation: RD, retinal detachment.

Avulsion of a peripheral blood vessel resulting in vitreous hemorrhage in absence of retinal tear formation is rare.

SRF tends to gravitate downward in the upper quadrant retinal break. Retinal detachment in the upper quadrant progresses quickly, resulting in lower field defect, and the patient complains of "curtain" **ascending** in front of eye.

SRF ascends against gravity in the lower quadrant retinal break. So, RD in inferior quadrants takes longer to involve macula, resulting in upper field defect, and patients narrate that a "curtain" has **descended** in front of the eye.

Thus, a lower field defect (retinal break in upper quadrant) is usually appreciated more quickly by the patient than an upper field defect (retinal break in lower quadrant).

Location of primary retinal breaks will be in the opposite quadrant of visual field in which the field defect first appears.

Loss of central vision (sudden and painless) is due to involvement of fovea by SRF or obstruction of visual axis by a large upper bullous RD.

Characteristic signs seen in rhegmatogenous RD are:
- Marcus–Gunn pupil (*Relative Afferent Pupillary Defect*) is present when RD is extensive.
- IOP is usually lower.

If IOP is extremely low, suspect the presence of an associated choroidal detachment. If an eye with an extensive RD has normal IOP, suspect the presence of primary open-angle glaucoma coexisting with RD.

- Tobacco dust: Fine pigmented cells or "tobacco dust" in the anterior vitreous are seen (**Shaffer's sign**). When there is no past history of ocular trauma, inflammation or intraocular surgery, *it is pathognomonic of a retinal break.*

If "tobacco dust" is absent, suspect a simulating lesion such as retinoschisis.

The clinical features in different types of RD are compared in **Table 13.13**.

Examination of Retina in RD

Retina is examined by direct ophthalmoscope or by indirect ophthalmoscope using scleral depressor. Examination after full mydriasis is necessary to discover the retinal break. *Retinal breaks* appear usually red because of color contrast between neurosensory retina and underlying choroid. These are frequently found in the upper temporal quadrant, although these may involve any quadrant. Retinal signs depend on the duration of RD:

- **In fresh RD,** detached retina assumes a white or gray discoloration with corrugated appearance as a result of intraretinal edema. These folds or corrugations oscillate on ocular movements. Detached retina has a convex configuration. Retinal blood vessels coursing over the detached retina appear darker than in the flat retina. In flat retina, all retinal vessels have a bright silvery streak due to reflection of light from convex cylindrical surface, while in detached retina, blood vessels have *no central light streak and appear darker.*

- **Retina in long-standing RD,** retina becomes thin due to atrophy and subretinal demarcation lines (high-water marks) develop due to proliferation of RPE cells

Table 13.13 Comparative study of different types of RD

	Rhegmatogenous RD	Tractional RD	Exudative RD
Symptoms			
• Photopsia	+	Absent	Absent as no traction
• Floaters	+	Absent, as it is not associated with acute PVD	Present if associated vitritis is there
Signs			
Vitreous signs			
• Tobacco dust	+	–	–
• PVD	Universal finding and is acute	PVD is gradual chronic and incomplete	–
Retinal signs			
• Retinal breaks	+	–	–
• Retinal configuration	Convex	Concave	Convex
• Mobility of retina	+	Severely reduced	Marked
• Shifting fluid	–	–	Present and is the hallmark
• Signs of long-standing RD: Retinal thinning and subretinal demarcation lines	+	–	–
• PVR	+	+	–

Abbreviations: PVD, posterior vitreous detachment; PVR, proliferative vitreoretinopathy; RD, retinal detachment.
Note: (+) denotes presence and (–) denotes absence.

- Subretinal demarcation lines are absent.
- PVR is absent.

Treatment

Treatment should be for the causative disease. Some exudative RDs resolve spontaneously, while others require systemic corticosteroids, for example, VKH disease and posterior scleritis. Neoplastic lesions require special attention.

Uveal Effusion Syndrome

It is an idiopathic condition *characterized by* ciliochoroidal detachment followed by exudative RD which may be bilateral.

Pathogenesis

Transudation of fluid from vascular uvea with extravasation from choriocapillaris into suprachoroidal space and within uveal tissues results in bilateral ciliochoroidal detachment with subsequent exudative RD.

Diagnosis

It is made after excluding all other inflammatory and hydrostatic causes of uveal effusion.

Course

The resolution is spontaneous. Following resolution, RPE shows a characteristic residual mottling—"**leopard spot**" changes.

The Optic Nerve

Anatomy and Physiology 393
Optic Nerve Dysfunction...394
Diabetic Papillopathy 409
Hereditary, Nutritional and Toxic Optic Neuropathies 411
Optic Atrophy 415
Congenital Anomalies of Optic Nerve...418

■ Anatomy and Physiology

■ Anatomy (OP8.5)

Optic nerve consists of axons arising from ganglion cells of retina, terminating in the lateral geniculate body. It also contains afferent fibers of pupillary light reflex (pupillomotor fibers). Optic nerve (2nd cranial nerve) carries approximately 1.2 million afferent nerve fibers (axons) which are 2nd order neurons in visual pathway. Although termed as a nerve, optic nerve is actually a tract. It extends from optic disc to optic chiasma. It is approximately 50 mm long.

Parts

It is divided into four parts (**Fig. 14.1**):
- Intraocular (1 mm).
- Intraorbital (25–30 mm).
- Intracanalicular (5–9 mm).
- Intracranial (10–16 mm).
- **Intraocular part (optic nerve head):** It is visible as optic disc on fundus examination and extends to posterior scleral surface. Its vertical diameter is 1.5 mm. It is mostly *transscleral*. The optic nerve fibers pass through a sieve-like structure, lamina cribrosa, which bridges across the scleral

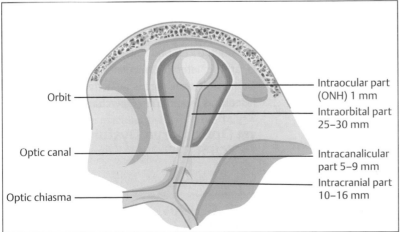

Fig. 14.1 Parts of optic nerve (horizontal section).

Orbit

Optic canal

Optic chiasma

Intraocular part (ONH) 1 mm
Intraorbital part 25–30 mm
Intracanalicular part 5–9 mm
Intracranial part 10–16 mm

Table 14.2 Differentiation of optic nerve disease from macular diseases

	Optic nerve disease	Macular disease
By history		
• Pain	Sometimes with eye movements	Rare
• Metamorphopsia	–	+
By visual function		
• Visual acuity	Variably reduced	Markedly reduced
• Afferent pupillary defect (APD)	+	–
• Brightness sense	Very reduced	Slightly reduced
• Color vision	Very reduced	Slightly reduced
• Visual field	Variable	Central scotoma
By special tests		
• Amsler chart	Central scotoma	Metamorphopsia
• VER	Prolonged latency	Small latency
• Photo stress test	Normal	Abnormal

Abbreviation: VER, visually evoked response.
Note: (+) denotes presence and (–) denotes absence.

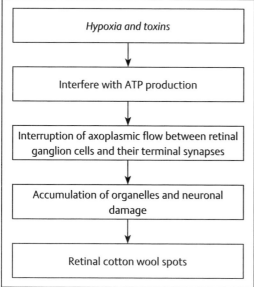

Flowchart 14.1 Physiology of axoplasmic transport.
Abbreviation: ATP, adenosine triphosphate.

referred to as **disc edema**. Disc edema may be unilateral or bilateral. Causes of disc edema include the following:

1. Ocular diseases:
   • Posterior uveitis.
   • Central retinal vein occlusion (CRVO).
   • Ocular hypotony.
2. Inflammatory:
   • Papillitis.
   • Papillophlebitis (or optic disc vasculitis).
   • Neuroretinitis.
3. Infiltrative disorders:
   • Lymphoma.
   • Sarcoid.
4. Vascular:
   • Anterior ischemic optic neuropathy (AION).
5. Orbital causes:
   • Orbital tumors.
   • Orbital cellulitis.
   • Meningioma of optic nerve.
   • Thyroid ophthalmopathy (advanced Grave's disease).
   • Metastatic orbital masses.
6. Increased intracranial pressure (**papilloedema**).

Disc edema due to ocular and orbital lesions is usually unilateral.

- *Ocular lesions include* CRVO, ocular hypotony, papillitis, papillophlebitis, and anterior ischemic neuropathy.
- *Orbital lesions* include orbital tumors, orbital cellulitis, and meningioma of optic nerve.
- *Foster–Kennedy syndrome:* It is the atrophy of optic nerve on the side of the lesion due to direct pressure and papilloedema on the other side due to raised intracranial pressure. It is associated with frontal lobe tumors, particularly meningioma of olfactory groove.

In cases with raised intracranial pressure, disc swelling is bilateral **(Fig. 14.3)**.

- Intracranial lesions include tumors, aneurysms, cavernous sinus thrombosis, and carotid-cavernous fistula.
- Systemic causes include malignant hypertension, diabetic papillopathy, advanced Grave's disease, and anemia.

Papilloedema

Papilloedema is the edema of optic disc *due to* raised intracranial pressure. Causes of papilloedema (or raised intracranial pressure) include:

- Intracranial space occupying lesions (**ICSOLs**): *Tumors of anterior fossa tend to produce papilloedema later than those in the posterior fossa.* Thus, tumors of midbrain, parieto-occipital region, and cerebellum produce papilloedema more rapidly.
- Other intracranial causes include the following:
  ◊ Diffuse cerebral edema from blunt head trauma.
  ◊ Cavernous sinus thrombosis.
  ◊ Pseudotumor cerebri (idiopathic intracranial hypertension).
  ◊ Subarachnoid hemorrhage.
  ◊ Disturbances with CSF circulation.
- Hypersecretion of CSF by choroidal plexus tumor.
- Obstruction to CSF flow in ventricular system or at exit foramina (foramina of Luschka and Magendie) of 4th ventricle, for example, *stenosis of aqueduct of Sylvius.*
- Impairment of CSF absorption via arachnoid villi which may be damaged by *meningitis and subarachnoid hemorrhage.*
- Brain abscess.

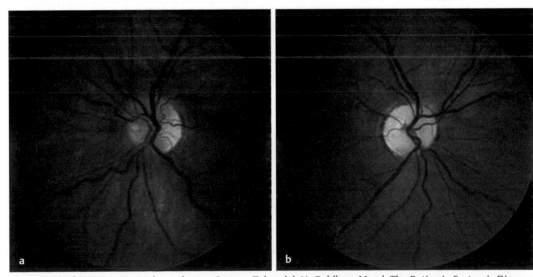

Fig. 14.3 (a, b) Foster–Kennedy syndrome. Source: Tabandeh H, Goldberg M, ed. The Retina in Systemic Disease: A Color Manual of Ophthalmoscopy. 1st Edition. Thieme; 2009.

When measuring the elevation of disc (degree of disc edema) with direct ophthalmoscope, a difference in dioptric power is found between the focus of edematous disc and normal nonedematous retina. Three dioptres of disc elevation denotes 1 mm of elevation.

- Edema of NFL: Edema spreads into surrounding retina, leading to blurring of NFL, and retinal vessels at disc margin become hazy (as retinal vessels course in NFL).
- Paton's lines: As the edema spreads, retinal folds concentric to disc may develop, especially temporally known as Paton's lines. It is one of the surest signs of true disc edema. As the edema increases, Paton's lines are no longer seen (**Flowchart 14.4**).

Any cause of edema can produce Paton's lines, so their presence only signifies edema. These are not seen with drusen of ONH (pseudopapilloedema).

- Hyperemia of ONH and loss of venous pulsations: Hyperemia is due to capillary dilatation in ONH. There is loss of normal previous spontaneous venous pulsations.

However, in 20% of normal individuals, spontaneous venous pulsations are absent. So, loss of venous pulsations is helpful only if they are previously present.

- Venous congestion: Retinal veins become congested and tortuous.
- Peripapillary retinal hemorrhages: Vascular engorgement and stasis leads to hemorrhages within NFL which are flame-shaped and marked around the disc.
- CW spots: These are fluffy patches due to NFL infarcts.
- Hard exudates: Hard exudates appear on disc surface and in the retina itself. These may radiate from the center of fovea in the

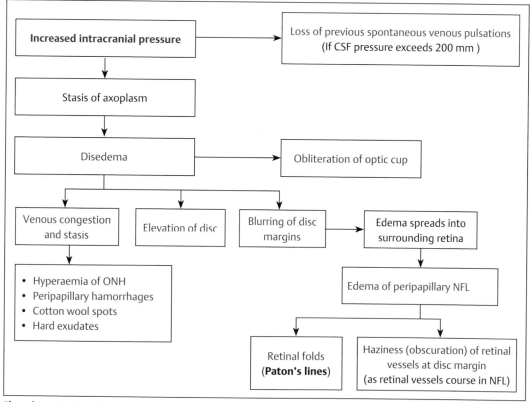

Flowchart 14.4 Pathogenesis of signs of papilloedema. Abbreviation: CSF, cerebrospinal fluid; ONH, optic nerve head; CSF, cerebrospinal fluid; NFL, nerve fiber layer.

form of a "**macular fan**": An incomplete star with temporal part missing.

Stages

Clinically, papilloedema can be described in **four stages**:

1. **Early papilloedema:** This is characterized by the following (**Fig. 14.5a**):
   - Disc hyperemia.
   - Blurring of disc margins and NFL.
   - Mild elevation of disc.
   - Visual symptoms are absent.
   - Loss of venous pulsations, if present.
2. **Established/fully developed papilloedema:** This is characterized by the following (**Fig. 14.5b**):
   - Transient visual obscurations.
   - Disc hyperemia-marked.
   - Gross elevation of ONH.
   - Venous engorgement.
   - Obliteration of physiological optic cup.
   - Peripapillary hemorrhages.
   - Retinal folds (Paton's lines).
   - Hard exudates with CW spots.
   - Enlargement of blind spot (on visual field examination).
3. **Chronic papilloedema:** This is characterized by the following (**Fig. 14.5c**):
   - Optic cup remains obliterated.
   - CW spots and hemorrhages resolve.
   - ONH takes on the appearance of a "champagne cork."
   - Less disc hyperemia is seen.
   - Visual fields begin to constrict.
   - Drusen-like crystalline deposits (corpora amylacea) may be present on disc surface.
4. **Atrophic papilloedema:** This is characterized by the following (**Fig. 14.5d**):
   - Optic disc appears dirty gray and blurred secondary to gliosis (secondary optic atrophy).
   - Retinal arterioles are narrowed with white sheathing.
   - Disc swelling subsides.

Diagnosis

It is done by:
- Fundus examination.
- Neuroimaging: MRI or CT scan.
- Lumbar puncture with manometry.
- Fluorescein angiography (FA): It is useful to distinguish true disc edema from pseudopapilloedema.

However, it does not distinguish among the different causes of disc edema.

Differential Diagnosis

Papilloedema must be distinguished from the following:
- Pseudopapilloedema: It occurs due to drusen of optic disc and hypermetropia
- Disc edema without raised intracranial pressure: It occurs due to the following causes:
  ◊ Papillitis.
  ◊ AION.
  ◊ CRVO.
  ◊ Compressive optic neuropathies in orbital lesions.
  ◊ Papillophlebitis (optic disc vasculitis).
  ◊ Juvenile diabetic papillopathy.
  ◊ *Other causes*: Hypotony and malignant hypertension.
- **Drusen of optic disc:** It may be confused with early papilloedema. Differentiating features of both are provided in **Table 14.3**.
- **Hypermetropia:** In hypermetropia, optic disc is small and nerve fibers from surrounding retina are heaped up on ONH. Therefore, margins appear swollen and blurred. In hypermetropia:
  ◊ Swelling is never >2D.
  ◊ No venous congestion.
  ◊ No edema or exudates.
  ◊ Blind spot not enlarged.
  ◊ No leakage on FA.
- **Papillitis:** It is the inflammation of intraocular part of optic nerve that gives rise to disc edema, which is indistinguishable from that in papilloedema. In papillitis:

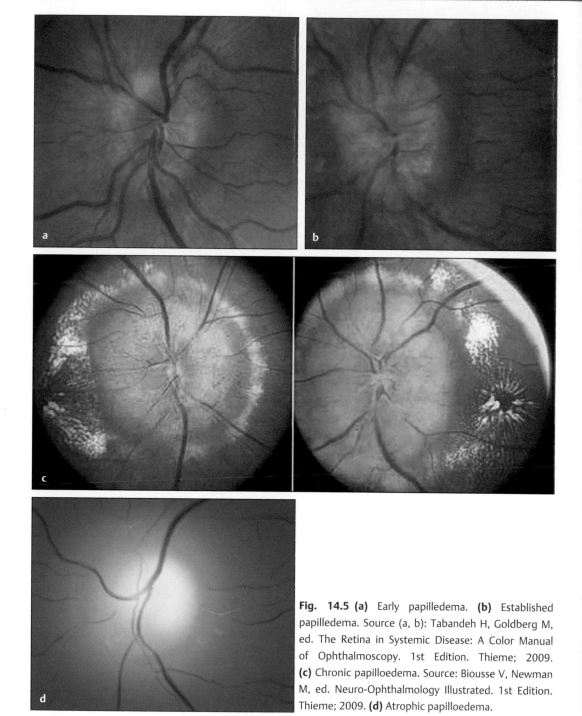

Fig. 14.5 (a) Early papilledema. **(b)** Established papilledema. Source (a, b): Tabandeh H, Goldberg M, ed. The Retina in Systemic Disease: A Color Manual of Ophthalmoscopy. 1st Edition. Thieme; 2009. **(c)** Chronic papilloedema. Source: Biousse V, Newman M, ed. Neuro-Ophthalmology Illustrated. 1st Edition. Thieme; 2009. **(d)** Atrophic papilloedema.

Table 14.3 Differentiating features of papilloedema and pseudopapilloedema

Features	Papilloedema	Drusen of optic disc (Pseudopapilloedema)
1. Color of optic disc	Hyperemic, so bright red	Not hyperemic, so pink or yellow
2. Spontaneous venous pulsations	Absent	Present (in 80% of cases)
3. Peripapillary NFL	Edematous and opacified	Normal
4. Peripapillary hemorrhages	+	–
5. Exudates or CW spots	+	–
6. Retinal veins	Dilated (venous engorgement)	Normal
7. Fluorescein angiography	Early leakage of dye	Show auto fluorescence and stain during late stages
8. Vessels over disc margin	Obscured	Not obscured

Abbreviations: CW, cotton wool spots; NFL, nerve fiber layer.
Note: (+) denotes presence and (–) denotes absence.

◊ Impairment of vision is sudden and marked.
◊ Features of raised intracranial pressure are absent.
◊ Pain on ocular movements is present.
◊ Afferent pupillary defect is present.
◊ Cells in vitreous are present.
◊ Visual field defects usually show central scotoma more for colors.

■ Pseudotumor Cerebri

It is also known as idiopathic intracranial hypertension (IIH) or benign intracranial hypertension.

It is *defined as* the presence of raised intracranial pressure in the absence of ICSOL or enlargement of ventricles due to hydrocephalus with normal CSF composition. It *occurs in* young, obese females of child-bearing age.

Clinical Features

Clinical features are those of raised intracranial pressure. Symptoms include headache, transient blurring of vision, and diplopia. Characteristic signs include papilloedema, 6th nerve palsy (manifested as diplopia), and large blind spot on visual field examination.

Diagnosis

Four criteria to diagnose pseudotumor cerebri are:

1. Increased intracranial pressure.
2. Normal-sized ventricles on neuroimaging (CT or MRI scan).
3. Normal CSF composition: Lumbar puncture shows CSF with no inflammatory cells, normal CSF glucose, and protein.
4. Papilloedema.

Treatment

It is essentially the treatment of cause:

• Diuretics, especially carbonic anhydrase inhibitors (acetazolamide), are the first line treatment for headache and visual field loss.
• Weight reduction in cases of pseudotumor.
• Optic nerve sheath decompression which involves incision of meningeal sheath around the optic nerve. The effect is remarkable if timely performed.
• Lumboperitoneal shunt may be performed.

■ Inflammation of Optic Nerve (OP8.5)

Inflammation of optic nerve is known as **optic neuritis.** Depending upon the part affected by inflammation, optic neuritis can be categorized into:

• **Papillitis:** It is the inflammation of ONH.
• **Neuroretinitis:** It is the inflammation of ONH with adjacent retinal inflammation, that is, *papillitis with retinitis.*
• **Retrobulbar neuritis** is the inflammation of optic nerve behind the eyeball.

Etiology

- Demyelinating disorders are the most common cause and include multiple sclerosis, neuromyelitis optica (*Devic's disease*), and isolated optic neuritis.
- Associated with infections (*infectious optic neuritis*): The infection may be local or systemic.

Local infection may be intraocular (as in endophthalmitis) or contiguous spread from *meninges* (meningitis as in tuberculosis and syphilis), *sinuses* (sinusitis, particularly of sphenoid and ethmoid sinuses), or *orbit* (orbital cellulitis). Systemic (endogenous) infection may be:

Viral:
- Measles, mumps, chickenpox, herpes zoster, and influenza.

Bacterial:
- Tuberculosis, syphilis, and cat-scratch fever.

Fungal:
- Cryptococcosis and histoplasmosis.

Protozoal:
- Toxocariasis and toxoplasmosis.

Parasitic:
- Cysticercosis.
- Noninfectious optic neuritis: It includes systemic autoimmune diseases such as sarcoidosis, systemic lupus erythematosus (SLE), and polyarteritis nodosa.
- Idiopathic.

> White matter of central nervous system (CNS) (brain and spinal cord) consists of myelinated nerve fibers, and gray matter consists of nonmyelinated nerve fibers. In demyelination, myelinated nerve fibers lose their myelin sheath (myelin is phagocytosed by microglia and macrophages, subsequent to which astrocytes lay down fibrous tissue). Therefore, nervous conduction is disrupted within white matter tracts in brain and spinal cord but peripheral nerves are not involved. The involvement of visual pathway results in optic neuritis. Involvement of brain stem result in:
> - Gaze palsies.
> - Ocular motor cranial nerve palsies.
> - V and VII nerve palsies.
> - Nystagmus.
>
> **Neuroretinitis is not seen in demyelinating disease** (multiple sclerosis) as nerve fiber layer is nonmyelinated and is commonly due to an infectious etiology.

Clinical Features

Symptoms

It typically affects patients between 20 and 40 years of age. Symptoms include:

- *Loss of vision:* It is sudden, progressive, and usually maximum approximately 1 week after the onset. It is usually monocular but may be bilateral, particularly in children.
- *Mild pain:* Visual symptoms are accompanied or preceded by periocular pain, usually aggravated by eye movement and *especially in upward and inward direction* due to attachment of some fibers of superior and medial rectus to the nerve sheath. It is increased by pressure on the globe (tenderness is present in the region of superior rectus insertion). It is more marked in retrobulbar neuritis than in papillitis.
- *Decreased light brightness* (reduced perception of light intensity).
- **Fading of colored objects** (*typically red desaturation*), that is, *dyschromatopsia*.

Occasionally, patient may observe impaired depth perception, particularly for moving objects (**Pulfrich phenomenon**) or worsening of impairment of vision with increase in body temperature due to exercise or hot bath (**Uhthoff's phenomenon**).

Signs

- **Visual acuity** is decreased. The severity of visual loss varies from mild to severe.
- **Color vision** is usually severely impaired even in patients with relatively good visual acuity.
- **Contrast sensitivity** is impaired in almost all cases.
- **Pupil:** Pupil of affected eye reacts to light but constriction is not sustained. It slowly dilates even in presence of bright light, that is, ill-sustained pupillary reaction. Such a reaction is known as **relative afferent pupillary defect** (**RAPD**) or *Marcus Gunn pupil.* It is of great diagnostic significance.

- Ophthalmoscopic features as mentioned below:
- *In papillitis*:
  Disc: Hyperemic, swollen with blurred margins.
  Veins: Dilated and tortuous.
  Physiological cup: Obliterated.
  Vitreous: Fine inflammatory cells in vitreous are present.
  Exudates and peripapillary flame-shaped hemorrhages may be present on disc (**Fig. 14.6a**).
- *In retrobulbar neuritis*: Because the site of involvement is behind the globe, optic disc and NFL are normal (**Fig. 14.6b**).

In neuroretinitis: It is the papillitis with involvement of neighboring retina. So, it is characterized by disc edema with retinal exudates in the NFL. So, radial orientation results in formation of macular fan or star (**Fig. 14.6c**).

> Normal fundus in presence of decreased vision is seen in:
> - Retrobulbar neuritis (RBN).
> - Cone degeneration.
> - Toxic optic neuropathy.
> - Amblyopia.
> - Hysteria.

- **Visual field defects**: These may be diffuse or focal. In diffuse visual field defects, there is depression of sensitivity in entire central 30 degrees. Focal field defects include central scotoma, centrocaecal scotoma, and nerve fiber bundle defects.

Most common field defects are central or centrocaecal scotomas. *The field defects are more marked in red color than white.*

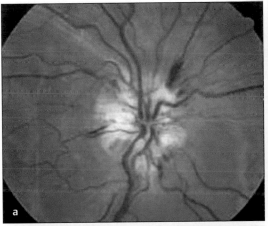

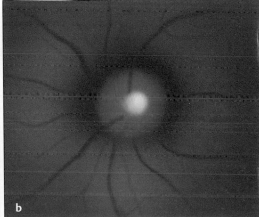

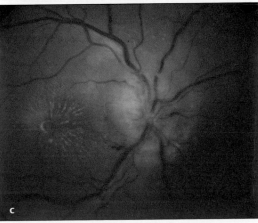

Fig. 14.6 (a) Papillitis. Source: Lang G, ed. Ophthalmology. A Pocket Textbook Atlas. 2nd Edition.Thieme; 2006. **(b)** Retrobulbar neuritis. **(c)** Neuroretinitis. Source: Biousse V, Newman M, ed. Neuro-Ophthalmology Illustrated. 1st Edition. Thieme; 2009.

Transient visual loss is extremely unusual in the nonarteritic form.

Associated symptoms include systemic features of giant cell arteritis. These include headache, and jaw claudication which is *pathognomonic*. It is caused by ischemia of the Masseter muscle and causes pain on speaking and chewing. Scalp tenderness or temporal artery tenderness is noticed when combing hair. Temporal artery is thickened, nodular, palpable, and non-pulsatile. Other symptoms are nonspecific anorexia, weight loss, and fever.

> In giant cell arteritis, severity of involvement is associated with quantity of elastic tissue in media and adventitia. Intracranial arteries possess little elastic tissue, so they are usually spared.

Signs: Pallor is associated with disc edema (**pallid disc edema**) and has been described as a hallmark of AION (**Fig. 14.8**). Over 1 to 2 months, swelling gradually resolves and severe optic atrophy ensues. A relative apparent pupillary defect (**RAPD**) is present. Short postciliary arteries vasculitis results in:

- Anterior ischemia of ONH which, in turn, causes disc edema and disc pallor.
- Choroidal ischemia which then leads to peripapillary pallor and edema deep to retina.

Diagnosis

The following investigations are helpful in ascertaining the diagnoses of AION.

1. ESR is raised to 70 to 120 mm/hour.
2. CRP in serum is raised, which is another acute phase protein and may aid in diagnosis.
3. Temporal artery biopsy (TAB) is confirmatory and shows intimal thickening and giant cell granulomatous vasculitis involving all coats of vessel wall. *Temporal artery biopsy should ideally be performed within 3 days of commencing steroids.*
4. FA shows delayed filling of optic disc with choroid due to impaired perfusion. It is a consistent feature.

Treatment

- High-dose systemic steroids: **IV methylprednisolone** 1 gm/day × 3 days followed by **oral prednisolone** 60 to 100 mg/day. Duration of treatment is 1 to 2 years. If there is no response to treatment, an alternate disease process should be considered.

Prognosis

It is very poor because visual loss is usually permanent.

NAION

NAION has been reported in association with several diseases that could predispose to reduced perfusion pressure or increased resistance to the flow within ONH, for example:

- Hypertension.
- Diabetes mellitus.
- Hypercholesterolemia.
- Collagen vascular disease.
- Migraine.
- Hyper homocystinemia.
- Sudden hypotension.
- Smoking.

Clinical Features

It occurs in a relatively younger age group (mean age 60 years). Sudden, painless, monocular visual loss is frequently reported upon awakening, suggesting that nocturnal systemic hypotension may be the contributing factor. Visual loss is

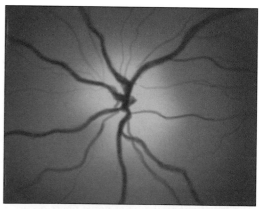

Fig. 14.8 Pallid disc edema.

unassociated with premonitory transient visual symptoms. Bilateral simultaneous involvement is rare. Usually, there are no associated systemic symptoms.

Signs are evident in optic disc. Disc shows **hyperemic disc edema,** which is associated with flame-shaped hemorrhages (**Fig. 14.9**). Pale edema occurs less frequently than it does in AAION.

Optic disc in the fellow eye is small with a small or absent physiological cup. It leads to crowding of axons associated with mild disc elevation and blurred disc margin without overt edema. Disc swelling gradually resolves and pallor ensues.

Investigations

FA: It demonstrates delayed disc filling, suggesting impaired optic disc perfusion.

Treatment

There is no effective treatment for NAION. Oral steroids are not beneficial. It is extremely important to exclude the possibility of occult giant cell arteritis.

Optic nerve sheath decompression, hyperbaric oxygen, systemic aspirin, and oral levodopa were attempted but has not been shown to be of benefit.

Prognosis

Fellow eye is affected in <30% cases. When the fellow eye becomes involved, optic atrophy in one

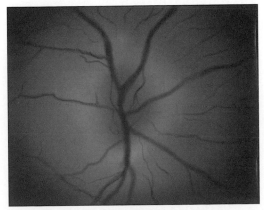

Fig. 14.9 Hyperemic disc edema.

eye and disc edema in other, it gives rise to the "pseudo Foster–Kennedy syndrome."

Differential diagnosis of AION
- Idiopathic optic neuritis.
- Infiltrative optic neuropathy.
- Compressive optic neuropathy (anterior orbital lesions producing optic nerve compression).
- Diabetic papillopathy.
- Optic disc vasculitis (papillophlebitis).

Differentiating features of AAION and NAION are listed in **Table 14.6**.

Posterior Ischemic Optic Neuropathy

PION is much less common than AION.

Etiology: It is caused by ischemia of the retrolaminar portion of the optic nerve which is supplied by surrounding small pial vessels.

Features: It is sudden in onset and shares the features of AION; bilateral involvement is common.

Diagnosis: Diagnosis of PION is made after other causes of retrobulbar optic neuropathy (compression or inflammation) has been excluded.

■ Diabetic Papillopathy

It is an uncommon condition seen in patients suffering from juvenile insulin-dependent (Type-I) diabetes. The patient presents with unilateral or bilateral blurring of vision. Disc swelling, hyperemia, and also telangiectatic vessels over disc surface are usually seen. *The presence of telangiectatic vessels overlying swollen disc is characteristic of the disease* (**Fig. 14.10**). Visual field defects like central scotoma or acute scotoma are seen.

■ Criteria for Diagnosis

- Presence of diabetes mellitus.
- Optic disc edema.
- Only mild optic nerve dysfunction.
- Absence of ocular inflammation.
- Absence of elevated intracranial pressure.

Table 14.6 Comparison of arteritic and non-arteritic AION

Feature	Arteritic AION	Non arteritic AION
Age (mean)	70 years	60 years
Sex ratio	Female > male	Female = male
Symptoms		
Visual loss	Sudden, usually severe	Sudden, usually moderate
Premonitory transient visual obscuration	Occasional	Rare
Associated symptoms	Headache, scalp tenderness, jaw claudication, polymyalgia	Occasional Periorbital pain
Signs		
Optic disc	Pale > Hyperaemic oedema	Hyperaemic > pale oedema
Optic cup	Normal	small
Investigations		
ESR (mm/hour)	70–120	20–40
Temporal artery biopsy	Giant cell granulomatous vasculitis	Not indicated if features do not suggest arteritis
Fluorescein angiography	Disc and choroidal filling delayed	Disc filling delayed
Natural history	Improvement is rare fellow eye involvement (95%)	Improvement in up to 43% fellow eye involvement (<30%)
Treatment	Corticosteroids	No effective treatment

Abbreviation: AION, anterior ischemic optic neuropathy; ESR, erythrocyte sedimentation rate.

Table 14.7 Differentiating features of diabetic papillopathy and AION

	Diabetic papillopathy	AION
Optic nerve dysfunction (evidenced by afferent pupil defect and visual field loss)	Mild	Significant
Disc	Hyperaemic edema	Pale disc oedema
Laterality	Simultaneously bilateral	Initially unilateral but may become bilateral.

Abbreviation: AION, anterior ischemic optic neuropathy.

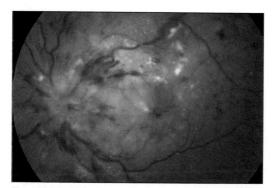

Fig. 14.10 Diabetic papillopathy. Source: Tabandeh H, Goldberg M, ed. The Retina in Systemic Disease: A Color Manual of Ophthalmoscopy. 1st Edition. Thieme; 2009.

■ Differential Diagnosis

It includes:

1. Papilloedema: It is differentiated by absence of symptoms of increased intracranial pressure in diabetic papillopathy.
2. Hypertensive papillopathy: Telangiectasia is absent and blood pressure is raised.
3. AION: Its differentiating features are listed in **Table 14.7**.

Pale disc edema is highly suggestive of AION and not of diabetic papillopathy

4. Pseudotumor cerebri: If diabetic papillopathy is bilateral, neuroimaging is mandatory to rule out ICSOL.

■ Course

If untreated, disc edema resolves in 2 to 10 months with spontaneous improvement. In some cases, there is mild to moderate visual loss.

■ Treatment

No treatment is recommended.

■ Hereditary, Nutritional, and Toxic Optic Neuropathies (OP8.5)

Optic neuropathies are described in **Flowchart 14.5**.

■ Pathogenesis

The clinical picture found in different nutritional deficiencies, toxic, and hereditary optic neuro-pathies, is very similar.

These act by way of a common pathway, *interference with mitochondrial oxidative phosphorylation*. Oxidative phosphorylation in mitochondria leads to ATP synthesis (**Flowchart 14.6**).

■ Ocular Manifestations

The following ocular manifestations are quite similar for LHON, and nutritional and toxic optic neuropathies:

- *Visual loss*: In LHON, it typically begins with *sudden, painless, and monocular loss of central vision*. Later, the fellow eye becomes affected in similar fashion within weeks or months.

In toxic or nutritional optic neuropathy, there is *simultaneous involvement of both eyes* and loss of central vision is *slowly progressive*.

- *Dyschromatopsia* (disturbed color perception).
- *Visual field defects*: These consist of *centrocecal scotoma* which is the hallmark of these disorders. It begins at nasal to blind spot and extends to involve fixation. Centrocecal scotoma is *larger with red light* than white light.

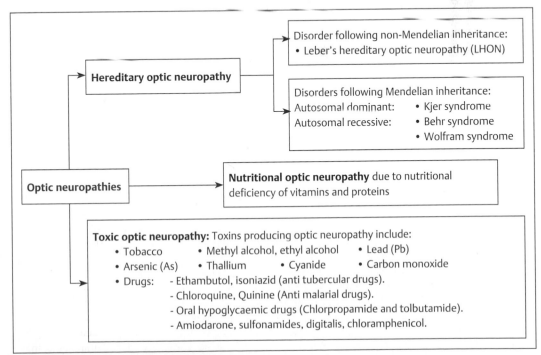

Flowchart 14.5 Types of optic neuropathies.

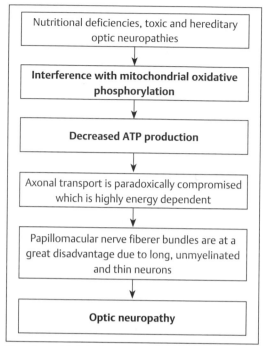

Flowchart 14.6 Pathogenesis of different hereditary, nutritional, and toxic optic neuropathies. Abbreviation: ATP, adenosine triphosphate.

Later, a temporal pallor of disc (due to degeneration of papillomacular bundle fibers) becomes evident.

■ Hereditary Optic Neuropathy

All disorders in this group ultimately lead to optic atrophy.

LHON

Age: It manifests at approximately 20 years of age.

Sex: It typically affects males; nearly 10% daughters are also affected.

Etiology: It is the result of point mutation in mitochondrial DNA.

Inheritance: It is maternally inherited. Transmission of LHON is generally *through unaffected females to males. Affected males do not transmit the trait or carrier state to any of their offspring,* thus transmitted in an atypical X-linked (sex-linked) manner.

Clinical Features

Symptoms:
- It typically begins with sudden, painless, and unilateral visual loss. Later, the fellow eye becomes similarly affected and the condition becomes bilateral.
- Loss of color vision.

Signs: In early LHON:
- Disc may be hyperemic with blurred disc margins.
- Telangiectatic capillaries are seen in and around the optic disc but this occurs transiently. Subsequently, these telangiectatic vessels (*dilated and tortuous vessels*) regress and pseudoedema resolves. *These telangiectatic vessels do not leak on FA.*

In late stages: Temporal optic disc appears pale and severe optic atrophy, most pronounced in papillomacular bundle, supervenes **(Fig. 14.11)**.

Visual field defect: It consists of central or centrocecal scotoma.

Diagnosis: LHON can be differentiated from toxic and nutritional optic neuropathies by:
- Family history.
- Presence of telangiectatic vessels around optic disc during acute phase.
- No simultaneous involvement of both eyes.
- Laboratory study of point mutation in mitochondrial DNA.

Treatment: It is generally ineffective.

Prognosis: The prognosis is poor.

Optic neuropathies with Mendelian inheritance are listed in **Table 14.8.**

■ Toxic and Nutritional Optic Neuropathy

Nutritional deficiency states and certain toxins may cause optic neuropathy. Certain toxins have a direct effect on nerve fibers while some of them (tobacco and methyl alcohol) primarily affect retinal ganglion cells and cause secondary degeneration of nerve fibers.

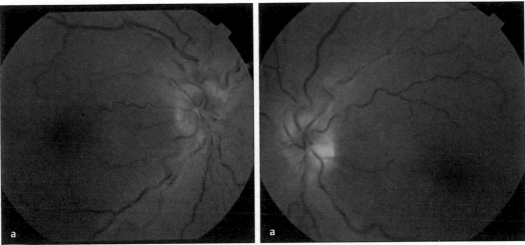

Fig. 14.11 (a, b) Leber hereditary optic neuropathy. Source: Levin A, Zanolli M, Capasso J, ed. Wills Eye Handbook of Ocular Genetics. 1st Edition. Thieme; 2017.

Table 14.8 Various optic neuropathies with mendelian inheritance

Optic neuropathies with mendelian inheritance	Inheritance	Age	Clinical features	Systemic features
Kjer syndrome (Kjer's autosomal dominant optic atrophy)	It is autosomal dominant.	It commences between 5–10 years of age.	Insidious visual loss Loss of color perception. Optic disc appears pale in temporal region.	These are absent in majority of cases.
Behr syndrome	It is autosomal recessive.	Early childhood	Visual loss Nystagmus Optic atrophy is diffuse.	Spastic gait Ataxia Mental deficiency (due to spino cerebellar degeneration with mild mental deficiency)
Wolfram syndrome	It is autosomal recessive.	Early childhood	It is characterized by diminished vision (<6/60) with diffuse and severe optic atrophy in early childhood.	These include: Diabetes insipidus Diabetes mellitus Deafness (**DIDMOAD** - **D**iabetes Insipidus, **D**iabetes **M**ellitus, **O**ptic **A**trophy, **D**eafness)

Tobacco (smoking or chewing) may result in optic neuropathy but its toxicity increases in heavy drinkers. Most patients neglect their diet and obtain their calories from alcohol instead. Poor nutrition and poor absorption of vitamin associated with alcohol consumption results in toxic or nutritional deficiency optic neuropathy (**tobacco–alcohol amblyopia**).

Tobacco–Alcohol Amblyopia

Pathogenesis of tobacco–alcohol amblyopia is explained in **Flowchart 14.7**.

■ Classification

On the basis of direction of degeneration:
- Ascending optic atrophy.
- Descending optic atrophy.

On the basis of ophthalmoscopic appearance:
- Primary optic atrophy.
- Secondary (postneuritic) optic atrophy.
- Consecutive optic atrophy.
- Glaucomatous optic atrophy.

Ascending Optic Atrophy

In ascending type of optic atrophy, degeneration of nerve fibers progresses from optic disc toward lateral geniculate body. The primary lesion is in retinal ganglion cells or in the optic disc. It occurs in:
- Glaucoma.
- Retinochoroiditis.
- Retinitis pigmentosa (RP).
- Central retinal artery occlusion (CRAO).

Descending (Retrograde) Optic Atrophy

In descending type of optic atrophy, degeneration of nerve fibers proceeds from LGB, optic tract, chiasma, or posterior portion of optic nerve toward optic disc. It occurs in:
- ICSOLs.
- Multiple sclerosis.
- Meningitis.

Primary Optic Atrophy

In primary optic atrophy, there is no ophthalmoscopic evidence of optic disc swelling (**Fig. 14.12a**). It is caused by the lesions affecting visual pathways from the retrolaminar portion of the optic nerve to the LGB. The classical cause of primary atrophy used to be tabes dorsalis but the disease has now become rare due to the availability of effective antisyphilitic treatment. It is associated with:
- Multiple sclerosis (MS).
- Diseases of CNS.
- RBN.
- Compression by tumors or aneurysms (in the orbit or cranium).

Secondary Optic Atrophy

It is preceded by optic disc swelling as in (**Fig. 14.12b**):
- Papillitis.
- Neuroretinitis.
- Papilloedema.
- ICSOL causing raised intra cranial pressure.

ICSOL will produce:
- *Primary optic atrophy* if it presses upon chiasma or optic nerve.
- *Secondary optic atrophy* if it causes papilloedema due to raised intracranial pressure.

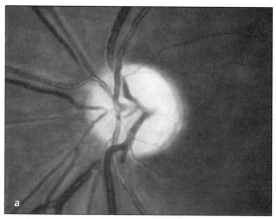 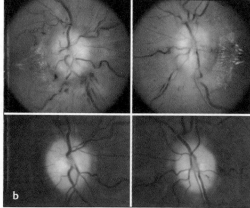

Fig. 14.12 (a) Primary optic atrophy. Source: Lang G, ed. Ophthalmology. A Pocket Textbook Atlas. 3rd Edition. Thieme; 2015. **(b)** Secondary optic atrophy. Source: Biousse V, Newman M, ed. Neuro-Ophthalmology Illustrated. 3rd Edition. Thieme; 2019.

- MS in 2/3rd cases causes RBN and produces *primary optic atrophy*. In 1/3rd cases, it causes papillitis, producing *secondary optic atrophy*. So, such a classification (primary or secondary) cannot indicate the actual cause of optic atrophy as evident from the above lesions.

Consecutive optic atrophy

It is caused by diseases of retina causing destruction of retinal ganglion cells as in:
- Pigmentary retinal dystrophy.
- CRAO.

Glaucomatous Optic Atrophy

It is caused by advanced glaucoma. Optic disc shows features of glaucomatous damage.

■ Etiology

The optic atrophy can follow:
- Papilloedema.
- Optic neuritis.
- Glaucoma.
- Ischemia.
- Trauma.
- Compression.
- Toxins.
- Secondary to retinal diseases.

■ Clinical Features

1. Visual acuity: loss of vision may be:
   - Sudden or gradual (depending on etiology).
   - Partial or total (depending upon degree of atrophy).

Findings in pupils are as follows:
- Size: Pupil is semidilated.
- Reaction: If optic atrophy is bilateral, both direct and consensual pupillary reactions are absent.
- If optic atrophy is unilateral, there is loss of ipsilateral direct reaction and contralateral consensual pupillary reaction.

For example, pupillary reactions in case of right eye optic atrophy will be as given in **Table 14.9**:

2. Optic disc: Its appearance varies with type of optic atrophy (**Table 14.10**).

Table 14.9 Pupillary reactions in case of right eye optic atrophy

	Right eye		Left eye	
	Direct reaction	Consensual reaction	Direct reaction	Consensual reaction
Unilateral optic atrophic (right)	–	+	+	–
Bilateral optic atrophy	–	–	–	–

Table 14.10 Optic disc findings in different type of optic atrophy

Optic disc	In primary optic atrophy	In secondary optic atrophy
Preceding disc oedema	–	+
Colour	Chalky white	Dirty grey
Margins	Sharply defined	Poorly delineated due to gliosis
Lamina cribrosa	Stippling is seen at bottom of physiological cup	Not visible
Physiological cup	Slight cupping is present. Cup is shallow and saucer shaped	Cup is obliterated
Note: (+) denotes presence and (–) denotes absence.		

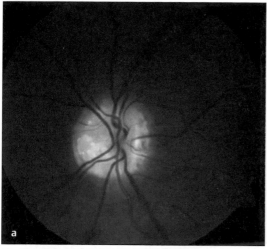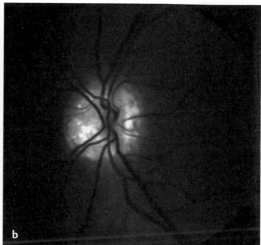

Fig. 14.17 (a, b) Optic disc drusen. Source: Lang G, ed. Ophthalmology. A Pocket Textbook Atlas. 3rd Edition. Thieme; 2015.

Complications

It can lead to serous macular detachment in 45% of cases. Sub retinal fluid (SRF) most likely originates from the vitreous cavity or the subarachnoid space that surrounds the optic nerve and *mistaken for central serous retinopathy (CSR)*. So, examine optic disc in all patients with suspected CSR. Optic pits are *not associated with brain malformations.*

Treatment

If serous macular detachment occurs, it is treated by:

Laser photocoagulation to block flow of SRF from disc to macula.

Internal gas temponade is used to displace SRF mechanically from beneath the macula.

Internal gas temponade is preferred over laser photocoagulation at the disc margin.

Optic Disc Drusen

It is composed of hyaline-like calcific material within the substance of the optic disc. It is usually bilateral and familial. Suggestive clinical signs of optic disc drusen are:

- Abnormal branching of retinal vessels from the center of the disc.

- Elevated disc.
- Surface vessels are not obscured despite disc elevation.
- Spontaneous venous pulsations are **present** in 80% of cases.
- Physiological optic cup is **absent.**
- Hyperemia is **absent (Fig. 14.17).**

Complications

Following are the probable complications in case of optic disc drusen:

- Choroidal (subretinal) neovascular membrane.
- CRAO.
- Central retinal vein occlusion (CRVO).

Differential Diagnosis

The appearance of disc may be confused with early papilloedema. On FA, optic disc drusen show progressive hyperfluorescence due to staining and no leakage of dye, while papilloedema shows increasing hyperfluorescence and late leakage.

Bergmeister Papilla

It is characterized by glial tissue projecting from the optic disc and derived from the avascular remnants of the hyaloid system.

The Afferent (Sensory) System

Introduction..421
Anatomy of Visual Pathway 421
Blood Supply of Visual Pathway 424
Lesions of Visual Pathway 424

■ Introduction

The images arising in each eye separately are appreciated as a single mental impression in the visual cortex. The vision achieved by the coordinated use of both eyes is known as binocular vision. The image of an object is built up of two separate halves with the object divided vertically. The image of the **right half of the object** is formed on the nasal retina of the right eye and the temporal retina of left eye which, in turn, is perceived by the left half of the visual cortex. Similarly, the image of **left half of the object** is formed on the temporal retina of the right eye and the nasal retina of left eye which, in turn, is perceived by the right half of the visual cortex. A composite picture of the whole object is built, therefore, by the activity of striate areas on both side of the visual cortex and the higher visual centers in the adjacent parastriate and peristriate areas.

■ Anatomy of Visual Pathway (AN30.5)

Visual sensations are perceived by rods and cones and conducted to the visual cortex through three sets of neurons:

- **First-order neurons** are bipolar cells of inner nuclear layer with their axons in the inner plexiform layer (IPL).
- **Second-order neurons** are ganglion cells in the retina, with their processes, which pass into the nerve fiber layer (NFL) and optic nerve to the lateral geniculate body (LGB).
- **Third-order neurons** transmit impulses through optic radiations to the visual center in occipital lobe.

Therefore, the visual pathway extends from retina to visual (occipital) cortex and consists of:

Retina – optic nerves – optic chiasma – optic tracts – lateral geniculate bodies – optic radiations – visual cortex (**Fig. 15.1**).

■ Arrangement of Nerve Fibers

Nerve fibers are arranged at the following places:
1. Within retina.
2. Within optic nerve head (ONH).

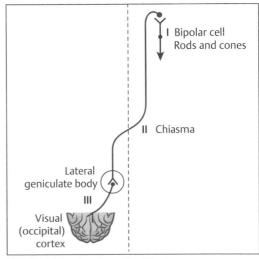

Fig. 15.1 Visual pathway **(outline).**

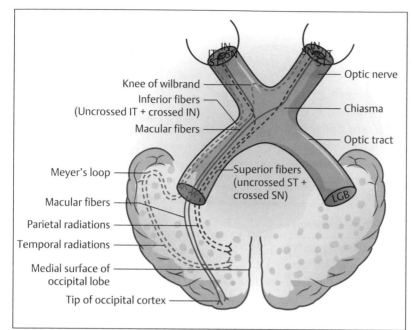

Fig. 15.5 Visual pathway. Abbreviations: IN, inferonasal; IT, inferotemporal; SN, superonasal; ST, superotemporal.

fissure. Visual fibers in optic radiations run behind the motor fibers in internal capsule (like other sensory tracts) and separate thereafter.

Inferior (ventral) **fibers from LGB** course **into temporal lobe** (**temporal radiations**). These fibers first loop forward into temporal lobe (called *Meyer's loop*) and then turn backward to the lower portion of visual cortex. Inferior "macular" fibers do not course as far anteriorly in the temporal lobe.

Superior (dorsal) **fibers from LGB** run backward in a direct course through **parietal lobe** to occipital cortex (**parietal radiations**).

In Occipital Cortex

Visual center (**striate cortex**) is located on the medial aspect of the occipital lobe, above and below the calcarine fissure. The part above calcarine fissure represents upper corresponding quadrants of both retinae (i.e., lower visual fields), while the part below calcarine fissure represents lower quadrants of both retinae (i.e., upper fields) (**Fig. 15.6**). The **anterior most part** of occipital cortex (striate cortex) subserves extreme nasal fibers, that is, temporal extremity of visual fields of

contralateral eye which is perceived monocularly (i.e., temporal crescent).

The **anterior part** (posterior to anterior most part) represents peripheral fibers. The **posterior tip** represents macular fibers, that is, central macular vision.

■ Blood Supply of Visual Pathway

Visual pathway is supplied by the ophthalmic artery which is a branch of internal carotid artery and Circle of Willis. Blood supply of different parts of visual pathway is listed in **Table 15.1** and depicted in **Fig. 15.7**.

■ Lesions of Visual Pathway (PY10.18)

Various field defects resulting from lesions in visual nervous pathway are as follows:

■ Anopia

It is the loss of vision in one (right or left) visual field (**Fig. 15.8**).

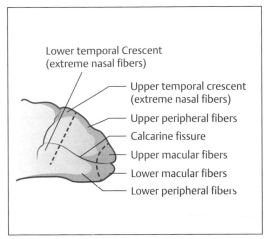

Fig. 15.6 Representation of occipital cortex (medial surface).

Table 15.1 Blood supply of parts of visual pathway

Part of visual pathway	Blood supply
Optic nerve: (Intraorbital, intracanalicular, and intracranial)	Branches of ophthalmic artery
Optic chiasma	Circle of Willis
Optic tract	Anterior choroidal artery (branch of middle cerebral artery)
Lateral geniculate body	Anterior choroidal and posterior cerebral arteries
Optic radiations	Branches of the MCA and PCA
Primary visual cortex	Calcarine branch of the PCA

Abbreviations: MCA, middle cerebral artery; PCA, posterior cerebral artery.

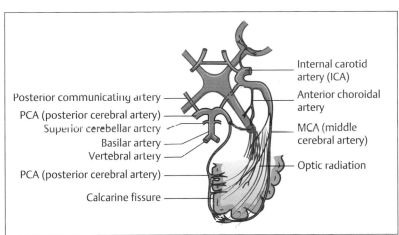

Fig. 15.7 Blood supply of visual pathway.

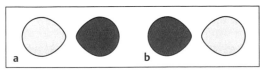

Fig. 15.8 (a) Right anopia. **(b)** Left anopia.

■ Hemianopia

It is the loss of vision in one half of visual field. It may be homonymous or heteronymous hemianopia.

Homonymous Hemianopia

It is the loss of vision in same halves (right or left) of both visual fields (**Fig. 15.9**). Homonymous hemianopia may be complete or incomplete.

- **Incomplete homonymous hemianopic defects** that are identical in size, shape, location, and slope of margins are called congruous defects. Field defects that are dissimilar in size, shape location, and slope of margins are called incongruous defects.

- Loss of direct pupillary reaction on the same side with loss of consensual pupillary reaction on the other side.
- Near or accommodation reflex is present.

Lesion of the proximal (posterior) part of optic nerve near chiasma results in ipsilateral blindness, with superotemporal quadrantanopia of opposite eye, due to the involvement of Knee of Wilbrand (**junctional scotoma**).

Field Defects in Lesions of Optic Chiasma

Important points to remember:
- Decussation of nasal fibers takes place in optic chiasma.
- Inferonasal (IN) fibers traverse the chiasm low and anteriorly.
- Superonasal (SN) fibers traverse the chiasm high and posteriorly.
- *Structures in relation to the optic chiasma are:*
  ◇ Pituitary gland.
  ◇ Cavernous sinus.
  ◇ Internal carotid arteries.
  ◇ 3rd ventricle.

Field defects in lesions of optic chiasma may be bitemporal and binasal hemianopia.

Bitemporal hemianopia (loss of vision in temporal half of both visual fields) is seen in:
- Pituitary adenoma or malignancy.
- Craniopharyngioma.
- Chronic chiasmal arachnoiditis.
- Fracture of the base of skull.

Binasal hemianopia (loss of vision in nasal half of both visual fields) is very rare and necessitates compression on each side of the chiasma. It is seen in:
- 3rd ventricular dilatation.
- Atheroma of carotids.
- Atheroma of posterior communicating arteries.

Optic chiasma is involved in the lesions of structures surrounding it.

1. **Pituitary gland** lies in sella turcica, a deep depression in the body of sphenoid bone.

A fold of duramater stretches between the anterior and posterior clinoids and forms the roof of sella called diaphragma sellae. Optic nerves and chiasma lie above the diaphragma sellae. Posteriorly, chiasma is continuous with optic tracts and forms the anterior wall of the 3rd ventricle (**Fig. 15.15**).

- **Pituitary adenoma (OP8.5)** is the most common cause of chiasmal compression. If it is confined to sella (intraseller tumors), the patient is visually asymptomatic and the visual field defects are absent. Therefore, absence of visual field defects does not exclude pituitary adenoma. Tumors less than 10 mm in diameter often remain intraseller. *If it is macroadenoma (> 10 mm)*, extrasellar extension with chiasmal compression takes place and visual field defects result. Visual field defect in a patient with pituitary tumor, therefore, indicates suprasellar extension (**Fig. 15.16**).

Expanding pituitary adenoma grows upward

↓

Compression of inferonasal fibers (lying low and anteriorly)

↓

Involvement of both superotemporal fields is first. The defect then progresses into *lower temporal fields* and **bitemporal hemianopia** results (**Fig. 15.17**)

As tumor growth is often asymmetrical, field loss is usually different on two sides.
- **Craniopharyngioma** arises from vestigial remnants of the Rathke pharyngeal pouch along the pituitary stalk. It compresses chiasma from *above and behind*. Therefore, superonasal

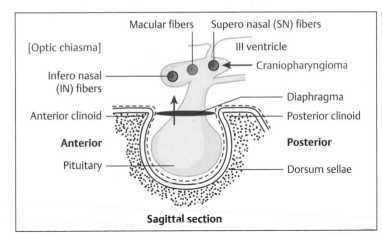

Macular fibers   Supero nasal (SN) fibers

[Optic chiasma]   III ventricle

Infero nasal   Craniopharyngioma
(IN) fibers

Anterior clinoid   Diaphragma

Anterior   Posterior clinoid

Pituitary   **Posterior**

                                           Dorsum sellae

Sagittal section

Fig. 15.15 Chiasma in relation to pituitary gland.

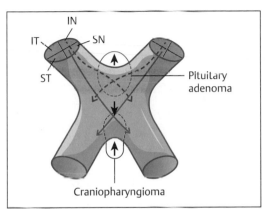

Fig. 15.16 Pituitary adenoma and craniopharyngioma affecting the decussating fibers. Abbreviations: IN, inferonasal; IT, inferotemporal; SN, superonasal; ST, superotemporal.

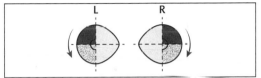

Fig. 15.17 Visual field defect in pituitary adenoma. Abbreviations: L, left; R, right.

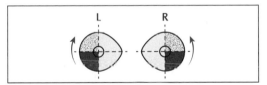

Fig. 15.18 Visual field defect in craniopharyngioma. Abbreviations: L, left; R, right.

fibers (high and posterior in chiasma) are involved first. **Inferotemporal field defects result initially,** which progress to superotemporal fields, resulting in bitemporal hemianopia (**Fig. 15.18**). So, if inferotemporal quadrants of visual field are affected more than superotemporal fields, a **pituitary adenoma is unlikely**.

2. In **chronic chiasmal arachnoiditis,** compression of chiasma by fibrous cicatricial bands results in bitemporal hemianopia.

3. **Fracture of the base of skull** also causes bitemporal hemianopia due to anteroposterior injury to the chiasma.

4. **3rd ventricle enlargement/dilatation** due to obstructive hydrocephalus and glioma of 3rd ventricle causes optic nerves to be pressed downward and outward against internal carotids, resulting in binasal hemianopia.

5. **Aneurysm of ICA** can compress optic nerve or chiasma. Internal carotid artery (ICA) curves posteriorly and upward from cavernous sinus and lies immediately below the optic nerves. ICA then ascends vertically alongside the lateral aspect of chiasma.

6. **Atheroma of carotids or posterior communicating arteries** destroys the

fibers to temporal halves of each retina, causing binasal hemianopia.

Field Defects in Lesions of Optic Tract

Each optic tract contains both visual and pupillo-motor fibers.

Visual fibers in optic tracts are uncrossed temporal fibers of same side and crossed nasal fibers of opposite side.

However, nerve fibers of corresponding retinal points are not closely aligned. So, *incongruous homonymous hemianopia results from optic tract lesions* (right homonymous hemianopia in left optic tract lesions).

Pupillomotor fibers in optic tract: Optic tract lesion results in afferent pupillary conduction defects. When light falls on involved hemiretina in patient with homonymous hemianopia, there is no pupillary light reaction, but when unaffected hemiretina is stimulated with light, normal pupillary light reflex is elicited. This is called **Wernicke hemianopic pupil**.

Optic tracts extend posteriorly around cerebral peduncles. The 3rd cranial nerve emerges from the midbrain on the medial aspect of cerebral peduncle. Therefore, owing to the proximity with cerebral peduncle, 3rd cranial nerve may be involved in the lesions of optic tract. For example,

Left optic tract lesion

↓

Involvement of left cerebral peduncle and left 3rd nerve

↓

- **Right homonymous hemianopia** *(due to involvement of left optic tract)*
- **Right hemiplegia** *(due to involvement of pyramidal tract in cerebral peduncle)*
- **Left 3rd nerve paralysis**.

Therefore, association of right homonymous hemianopia with right hemiplegia and left 3rd nerve paralysis indicates a left optic tract lesion involving left cerebral peduncle and left 3rd nerve.

As fibers in optic tracts are axons of retinal ganglion cells, so **optic atrophy may occur in optic tract lesions (Flowchart 15.1)**.

Atrophy of crossing nasal fibers in chiasmal compression leads to horizontal "bow-tie" pallor of both optic discs. As a rule, fixation point does not escape in tract hemianopia.

Causes of optic tract lesions are as follows:
- Syphilitic meningitis.
- Tuberculous meningitis.
- Tentorial meningioma.
- Temporal lobe glioma.

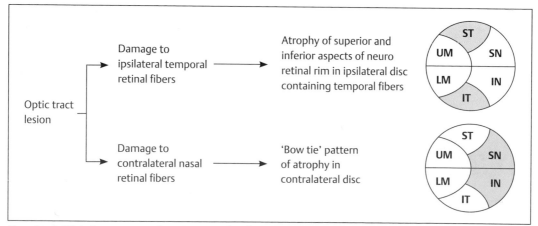

Flowchart 15.1 Appearance of optic nerve head in optic tract lesions. Abbreviations: IN, inferonasal; IT, inferotemporal; LM, lower motor; SN, superonasal; ST, superotemporal.

- Aneurysm of superior cerebellar or posterior cerebral arteries.

Field Defects in LGB

These are extremely rare. The lesions of LGB produce incongruous homonymous hemianopia with **sparing of pupillary reflexes** (as pupillomotor fibers leave the optic tract anterior to LGB).

Fields Defects in Lesions of Optic Radiations

Course of Optic Radiations

Visual fibers in optic radiations run behind the motor fibers in internal capsule. Thereafter, optic radiations separate into temporal radiations (coursing through temporal lobe) and parietal radiations (coursing through parietal lobe).

Lesions of Optic Radiations

1. **Lesion in posterior part of internal capsule:** In these lesions, there is involvement of sensory and/or motor fibers which leads to hemianesthesia with or without hemiplegia.
2. **Anterior temporal lobe lesions:** These lesions affect Meyer's loop formed by inferior fibers (ipsilateral IT and contralateral IN). These result in incongruous, contralateral, homonymous superior quadrantanopia ("**pie in the sky**"), sparing the fixation area *as inferior "macular" fibers do not cross as far anteriorly in the temporal lobe.*

   Other features of temporal lobe disease include paroxysmal olfactory and gustatory hallucinations due to involvement of the uncinate process of hippocampal gyrus.
3. **Parietal lobe lesions:** These lesions affect superior fibers of optic radiations (ipsilateral ST + contralateral SN fibers), resulting in contralateral homonymous inferior quadrantanopia ("**pie on the floor**").

Common Causes of Lesions of Optic Radiations

- Vascular occlusions.
- Cerebral tumors.
- Injury by fall on the back of head.

Features

- Optic radiations have a *dual blood supply* from middle cerebral artery (**MCA**) and posterior cerebral artery (**PCA**).
- As optic radiations are third-order neurons that originate in LGB (not from retinal ganglion cells), **so** *lesions of optic radiations* **do not produce optic atrophy.**
- As the radiations pass posteriorly, fibers from corresponding points lie close together; therefore, incomplete hemianopia due to lesions of posterior radiations are more congruous than those involving the anterior radiations.
- Pupillary reactions are normal as the fibers of light reflex leave the optic tracts to terminate in pretectal nuclei.

Field Defects in Lesions of Visual Cortex

Causes

Visual cortex is affected by:
- Vascular lesions in territory of PCA.
- Trauma: Fall on the back of head or gunshot injury.
- Cerebral tumors: Primary or metastatic.

Blood Supply of Medial Surface of Visual Cortex

The occipital lobe is supplied by PCA and MCA, both of which are seldom blocked at the same time. The tip of the occipital cortex (representing macular vision) is supplied by terminal branches of MCA and PCA (mainly by MCA). It is referred to as "**water shed area.**" The area anterior to the tip (representing peripheral visual fields) is supplied by only proximal (not terminal) branches of PCA. Therefore, **occlusion of** PCA tends to produce macular sparing congruous homonymous hemianopia (as ipsilateral macular visual cortex may be spared due to the blood supply provided by terminal branches of MCA) (**Fig. 15.19**).

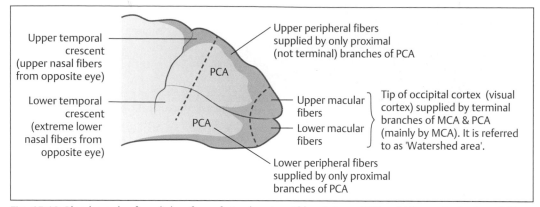

Fig. 15.19 Blood supply of medial surface of visual cortex. Abbreviations: MCA, middle cerebral artery; PCA, posterior cerebral artery.

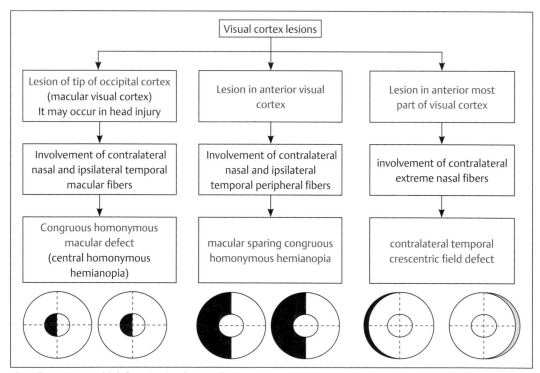

Flowchart 15.2 Field defects in visual cortex lesions.

Lesions of Visual Cortex

In visual cortex lesions:

- Pupillary light reflexes are normal.
- Optic atrophy does not occur because the fibers to visual cortex are **third**-order

neurons originating from LGB (not from retinal ganglion cells).

- Field defects in visual cortex lesions are depicted in **Flowchart 15.2**.

- Associated features of visual cortex disease (**cortical blindness**) are:
  - ◇ Denial of blindness (**Anton syndrome**): The patients afflicted with it are cortically blind but affirm that they are capable of seeing.
  - ◇ **Riddoch phenomenon:** It is characterized by the ability to perceive kinetic targets within the defective visual field *but static* visual targets are not appreciated. It is *typical of occipital lesion*, that is, patients with a damaged occipital lobe can still appreciate motion in the blind field.
  - ◇ Visual information from both occipital cortices is relayed to left angulate gyrus. The angulate gyrus of dominant hemisphere (commonly the left) subserves the ability to read. Involvement of

angulate gyrus of dominant cerebral hemisphere may result in **alexia** (word blindness and inability to read).

It is therefore mandatory to examine reading ability in the context of a right hemianopia (i.e., in left occipital lesion). Differences in the features of occipital lobe and optic tract lesions are listed in **Table 15.2**.

Table 15.2 Difference between occipital lobe and optic tract lesions

	Occipital lobe lesion	Optic tract lesion
Pupillary reaction	Normal	Abnormal
Field defect	Congruous	Incongruous
Macular involvement	Sparing	Involved
Optic atrophy	–	+

The Efferent (Motor) System

Extraocular Muscles 434

Ocular Movements...439

Nervous Control of Ocular Movements...442

Vestibular Pathway...444

Disorders of Ocular Motility 446

The efferent ocular motor pathway includes the cortical centers, intermediate gaze centers, cranial nerve nuclei, cranial nerves, and extraocular muscles (EOMs) which produce eye movements.

■ Extraocular Muscles

Ocular muscles may be extrinsic or intrinsic (**Flowchart 16.1**).

The extraocular muscles (EOMs) and their central nervous control subserve the motility and coordination to the eyes.

■ Anatomy of EOM

Origin

There are six EOMs. Five out of six extraocular muscles (except inferior oblique) originate at the orbital apex (**Fig. 16.1**). These EOMs are:

- Superior rectus (SR)
- Inferior rectus (IR)
- Medial rectus (MR)
- Lateral rectus (LR)

These arise from the annulus of Zinn, a fibrous ring around the optic foramen at the orbital apex.

- Superior oblique (**SO**) arises near the apex of the orbit, superomedial to the optic foramen.

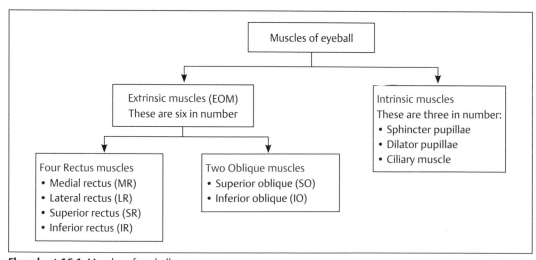

Flowchart 16.1 Muscles of eyeball.

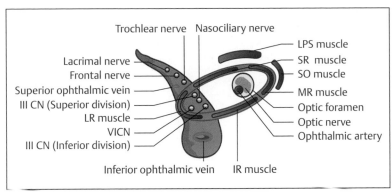

Fig. 16.1 Figure depicting origin of extraocular muscles at orbital apex (right superior fissure and annulus of Zinn). Abbreviations: CN, cranial nerve; IR, inferior rectus; LPS, levator palpabrae superioris; LR, lateral rectus; MR, medial rectus; O, inferior oblique; SO, superior oblique; SR, superior rectus.

- Inferior oblique (**IO**) arises anteriorly from the inferonasal angle of the orbit, just behind the orbital rim and lateral to the lacrimal fossa.

> SR and MR muscles are closely attached to the dural sheath of the optic nerve. That is why the pain occurs during elevation and adduction in patients with retrobulbar neuritis.

Insertion

Recti muscles are inserted into sclera via tendons anterior to the equator of globe (**Fig. 16.2**).

Table 16.1 shows that the MR tendon inserts closest to the limbus. Insertions get further away from limbus and make a spiral pattern (**spiral of Tillaux**).

Oblique muscles are inserted into sclera, posterior to the equator of globe (**Fig. 16.3**).

The **SO tendon** is inserted into the posterior upper temporal quadrant of the globe in a fan-shaped manner under the SR muscle. The insertion extends near the superotemporal vortex vein.

The **IO muscle** has almost no tendon at its insertion and inserts into the posterior lower temporal quadrant of the globe, close to the macula and inferotemporal vortex vein.

Nerve supply (Mnemonic-LR_6 $(SO_4)_3$)

The third, fourth, and sixth cranial nerves supply the EOMs in the following manner:

- **LR** is supplied by abducens (**6th**) nerve.
- **SO** is supplied by trochlear (**4th**) nerve.

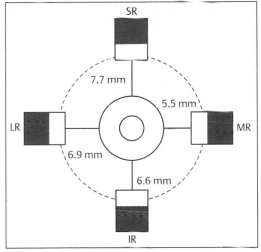

Fig. 16.2 Figure depicting insertion points of recti muscles.

Table 16.1	Insertion of recti muscles
Muscle	**Insertion**
MR	5.5 mm from nasal limbus
IR	6.6 mm from inferior limbus
LR	6.9 mm from temporal limbus
SR	7.7 mm from superior limbus
Abbreviations: MR, medial rectus; IR, inferior rectus; LR, lateral rectus; SR, superior rectus.	

- **SR** is supplied by *superior division* of oculomotor (**3rd**) nerve.
- **MR**, **IR**, and **IO** are supplied by the *inferior division* of the oculomotor (**3rd**) nerve.

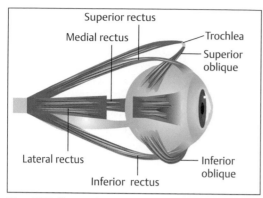

Fig. 16.3 Figure depicting insertion points of recti muscles.

Course of EOM (from Origin to Insertion)

Visual axis: It is the line passing from the object of fixation to the fovea through the nodal point of the eye.

Orbital axis: Medial orbital walls are approximately parallel to each other. The lateral and medial walls of the orbit are at an angle of 45° with each other. The orbital axis therefore forms an angle of 22.5° (≈**23°**) with both the lateral and medial walls (**Fig. 16.4a**).

Primary position of eye: The primary position is defined as the position when the eye and head are both directed straight ahead. In the primary position, the *visual axis forms an angle of* 23° *with the orbital axis* (**Fig. 16.4b**).

Horizontal Recti

Horizontal recti include MR and LR which arises from a common tendinous ring (the annulus of Zinn) and inserted into the sclera by a tendon. These rectus muscles move the eyes about the vertical axis (z-axis of Fick) (**Fig. 16.5**).

MR muscle: It courses anteriorly along the medial wall of the orbit.

- As MR muscle runs along the medial orbital wall, it can sustain damage during ethmoid sinus surgery.
- MR is the only rectus muscle that does not have a facial attachment to an oblique muscle. Thus, MR muscle is at a greatest risk of slippage during strabismus surgery.

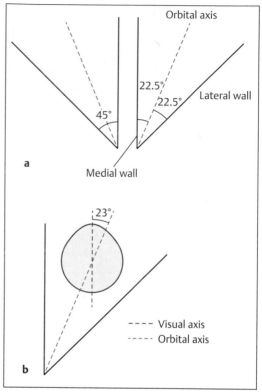

Fig. 16.4 (a) Orbital axis. **(b)** Primary position of eye.

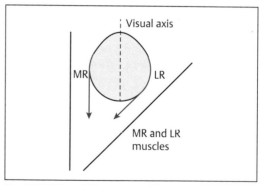

Fig. 16.5 MR and LR muscles. Abbreviations: LR, lateral rectus; MR, medial rectus.

LR muscle: It courses anteriorly along the lateral orbital wall.

Vertical Recti

Vertical recti (**SR** and **IR muscles**) run in line with the orbital axis, so they form an angle of **23°** with the visual axis in primary positions (**Fig. 16.6**).

Obliques

Obliques (**SO** and **IO muscles**) form an angle of 51° with the visual axis in primary position.

Actions of EOM

EOMs rotate the eye around the center of rotation *situated about 13 mm behind the cornea*. It lies, therefore, behind the nodal point of the eye on the visual axis. Ocular movements take place around three axes (termed as **axes of Fick**) passing through the center of rotation. These three axes are:

- Horizontal axis (x-axis of Fick): Movements around the horizontal axis are elevation or upward rotation and depression or downward rotation.
- Vertical axis (z-axis of Fick): Movements around the vertical axis are adduction or medial rotation and abduction or lateral rotation.

- Anteroposterior axis (y-axis of Fick): Movements around the anteroposterior axis are intorsion or incycloduction and extorsion or excycloduction (**Fig. 16.7**).

The actions of EOMs depend on the position of the globe at the time of muscle contraction and may be defined as primary or secondary. Primary action is the major effect of the EOM when the eye is in the primary position, while secondary actions are the additional actions which depend on the position of the eye.

These actions can be easily understood by the course of the respective EOMs and their relationship with the visual axis.

- **When visual axis lies in the muscle plane, the direction of movement is only upward and downward.**
- **If the muscle plane (line of muscle pull) is at a greater angle to the visual axis,**

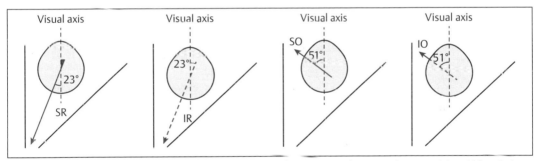

Fig. 16.6 Relation of vertical recti and oblique muscles in relation to visual axis in primary position. Abbreviations; IO, inferior oblique; IR, inferior rectus; SO, superior oblique; SR, superior rectus.

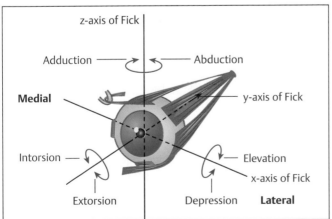

Fig. 16.7 Ocular movements around three axes.

■ Ductions

Various types of monocular movements are (**Fig. 16.12**):

- Adduction (inward movement).
- Abduction (outward movement).
- Elevation.
- Depression.
- Intorsion.
- Extorsion.

They are tested by occluding the fellow eye and asking the patient to follow the target in each direction of gaze.

■ Versions

These are the conjugate movements (in the same direction) of both eyes, that is, abduction of one eye is accompanied by adduction of the other (**Table 16.3**).

Torsional Movements of Both Eyes

These occur on tilting of the head to maintain upright images (known as righting reflexes).

On head tilt to right: Both eyes rotate to the left (**levocycloversion**), that is, intorsion of right eye and extorsion of left eye takes place (**Fig. 16.13a**).

On head tilt to left: Both eyes rotate to the right (**dextrocycloversion**), that is, intorsion of left eye and extorsion of right eye takes place (**Fig. 16.13b**).

Yoke muscles (contralateral synergists) are the pairs of muscles, one in each eye, that produce conjugate eye movements, for example, right SR and left IO are the yolk muscles in *dextroelevation* (**Table 16.4** and **Fig. 16.14**).

■ Vergences

These are the disjugate or disjunctive movements (in opposite directions) of both eyes (**Table 16.5**).

■ Positions of Gaze

There are six cardinal and nine diagnostic positions of gaze. The cardinal positions of gaze are the positions which allow examination of one EOM in each eye in their main field of action. These are:

- Dextroelevation.
- Dextroversion.
- Dextrodepression.
- Levoelevation.
- Levoversion.
- Levodepression.

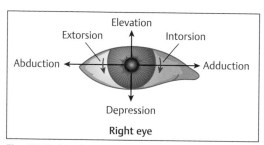

Fig. 16.12 Duction movements of an eye.

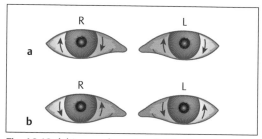

Fig. 16.13 **(a)** Levocycloversion. **(b)** Dextrocycloversion.

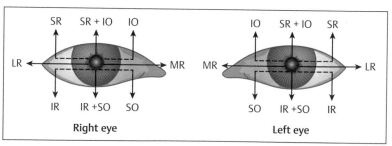

Fig. 16.14 Yoke muscle pairs in different eye movements.

Table 16.3 Conjugate movements (versions) of both eyes

Dextroelevation (right and upgaze)	**Elevation** (upgaze)	**Levoelevation** (left and upgaze)
It occurs due to simultaneous contraction of **right SR** muscle and **left IO** muscle.	It occurs due to simultaneous contraction of **both SR** muscles and **both IO** muscles.	It occurs due to simultaneous contraction of **right IO** muscle and **left SR** muscle.
Dextroversion (right gaze)	**Primary position**	**Levoversion** (left gaze)
It occurs due to simultaneous contraction of **right LR** muscle and **left MR** muscle.	It Is the position when the eyes and head are both directed straight ahead.	It occurs due to simultaneous contraction of **right MR** muscle and **left LR** muscle.
Dextrodepression (right and down gaze)	**Depression** (down gaze)	**Levodepression** (left and down gaze)
It occurs due to simultaneous contraction of **right IR** muscle and **left SO** muscle.	It occurs due to simultaneous contraction of **both IR** and **both SO** muscles.	It occurs due to simultaneous contraction of **right SO** and **left IR** muscles.

Abbreviations: IO, inferior oblique; IR, inferior rectus; LR, lateral rectus; MR, medial rectus; SO, superior oblique; SR, superior rectus.

Table 16.4 Yoke muscle pairs

Conjugate eye movements	Yoke muscle pairs
Dextroversion	RLR, LMR
Levoversion	LLR, RMR
Dextroelevation	RSR, LIO
Levoelevation	LSR, RIO
Dextrodepression	RIR, LSO
Levodepression	LIR, RSO

Abbreviations: LIO, left inferior oblique; LIR, left inferior rectus; LLR, left lateral rectus; LMR, left medial rectus; LSO, left superior oblique; LSR, left superior rectus; RIO, right inferior oblique; RIR, right inferior rectus; RLR, right lateral rectus; RMR, right medial rectus; RSO, right superior oblique; RSR, right superior rectus.

Table 16.5 Disjugate movements (vergences) of both the eyes

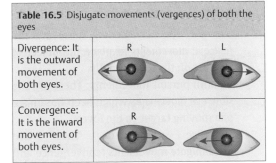

Divergence: It is the outward movement of both eyes.	
Convergence: It is the inward movement of both eyes.	

Important Terms
- Agonist is a muscle moving the eye in the direction of its action.
- Antagonist is the muscle which acts in the opposite direction to the agonist, for example, right LR is antagonist to right MR.
- Synergists are the muscles of the *same eye* that move the eye in the same direction, for example, right SR and right IO are synergists in elevation.

Diagnostic positions of gaze are the positions in which deviations are measured. These include six cardinal positions, primary position, elevation, and depression.

The vertical gaze center (**riMLF**) in midbrain receives input from:

- Frontal eye filed.
- Superior colliculus.
- Vestibular nuclei.

Each frontal eye field projects to contralateral PPRF and riMLF on each side. Vertical saccades require simultaneous activation of both frontal eye fields. POT junction projects to ipsilateral PPRF. *So, out of three conjugate eye movement pathways, two systems (voluntary saccades, and vestibular) have contralateral action, while one system (pursuit) has ipsilateral action.*

Internuclear Pathways

The horizontal gaze center (**PPRF**) sends projections to abducens (VI CN) nucleus. There is a significant percentage (60%) of neurons in abducens nucleus innervating ipsilateral lateral rectus (LR) muscle. The remaining 40% are interneurons that project via **MLF** to contralateral MR subnucleus in occulomotor (III CN) nuclear complex. **Flowchart 16.2** and **Fig. 16.18** depict that activation of right PPRF or abducens nucleus generates right (ipsilateral) horizontal gaze by stimulating right LR and left MR muscles. Damage to PPRF or abducens nucleus results in ipsilateral gaze palsy.

The vertical gaze centre (**riMLF**) contains neurons for both upward and downward saccades. Upward saccades fibers from riMLF pass through posterior commissure to III CN nuclei (SR and IO muscles) bilaterally. Downward saccades fibers from riMLF project to III CN nuclei (inferior rectus) and IV CN nuclei (superior oblique) bilaterally (**Flowchart 16.3**).

■ Vestibular Pathway

Vestibular eye movements maintain foveal fixation when the head moves in horizontal/vertical–sagittal or vertical coronal planes. For example, if the head turns 10 degree to the right, the eyes rotate 10 degrees to the left to maintain fixation. When the head is tilted towards the shoulder, the eyes rotate in the opposite direction to the head tilt. It is mainly induced by the vertical semicircular canals. The vestibulo-ocular reflexes (VORs) involve the activation of motor neurons that innervate the EOMs.

The function of these VORs is to maintain the orientation of eyes in space during head movements, so that the visual image remains stable on the retina. In absence of such compensatory eye movements, the visual image would shift wildly during movements of head and the visual orientation would be extremely difficult.

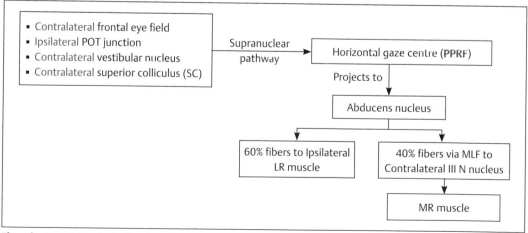

Flowchart 16.2 Control of horizontal eye movements. Abbreviations: LR, lateral rectus; MLF, medial longitudinal fasciculus; POT, Parietooccipitotemporal; PPRF, Paramedian pontine reticular formation..

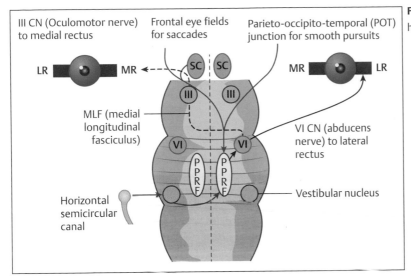

Fig. 16.18 Pathways for horizontal eye movements.

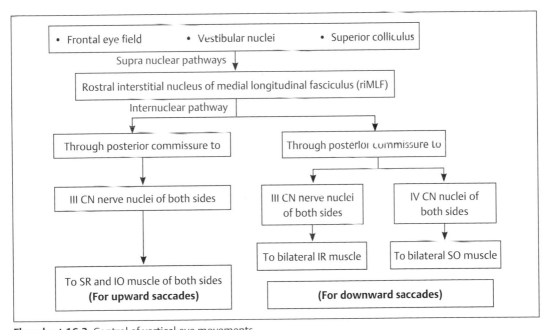

Flowchart 16.3 Control of vertical eye movements.

The latency for vestibular responses is about 10 msec (**Fig. 16.19**).

Fibers from the horizontal semicircular canal travel to vestibular nuclei via vestibular nerve and then send projections to each PPRF–excitatory projections travel to contralateral PPRF and inhibitory projections to ipsilateral PPRF. The projections then travel to VI CN nucleus and via MLF to the medial rectus subnucleus. So, excitatory projections are sent to contralateral LR muscle and ipsilateral MR muscle, while the inhibitory projections are sent to ipsilateral LR muscle and contralateral MR muscle. Information from right horizontal SCC sends excitatory information to the left horizontal gaze center (PPRF) and

For example, lesion of right MLF causes right INO which is characterized by:

a. Straight eyes in primary position.

b. Limitation of right adduction on left gaze.

c. Normal right gaze.

- **Combined lesion of MLF and PPRF on same side** (e.g., right) It results in loss of right horizontal gaze (one) and loss of adduction in right eye, that is, *right INO* **(half)– one-and a-half syndrome.** *Because of right INO, right eye cannot adduct. The abduction of left eye is the only horizontal movement left intact. It results in left eye exotropia and remains tonically abducted.* **Combined lesion of MLF and abducens nucleus on same side** also results in *one-and a-half syndrome.*

The combined lesion can occur in:

a. Multiple sclerosis.

b. Brain stem stroke.

c. Brain stem tumors.

■ Lesions of Cranial Nerve Nuclei and Respective Nerves

Eye movement abnormalities resulting from damage to the ocular motor nuclei and their respective cranial nerves are considered **infranuclear**.

Etiology

Damage to nuclei and nerves can be due to trauma, compression by tumors, demyelinating disease, vascular lesions, or inflammation. **III CN** may be affected at various sites through its course and present with distinct ocular and associated neurological signs and symptoms. III CN may be involved at the level of:

- Nucleus.
- Fascicle.
- Subarachnoid space.
- Cavernous sinus.
- Orbit.

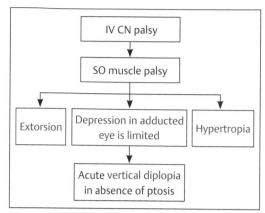

Flowchart 16.5 Important features of IV CN palsy. Abbreviation: CN, cranial nerve; SO, superior oblique muscle.

As the **trochlear nerve** exits the brainstem dorsally, so IVth nerve fasciculus is quite short. Therefore, isolated lesions that affect only nucleus or fascicle of IV CN are very rare and usually involve both the nucleus and fasciculus.

Damage within anterior medullary velum (anterior floor of IVth ventricle) causes damage to both IV CN fascicles at their decussation and results in bilateral SO palsy (**Flowchart 16.5**).

A lesion in and around the **6th nerve** nucleus involves the related structures. Damage to 6th nerve nucleus or caudal PPRF (horizontal gaze center) causes ipsilateral horizontal gaze palsy.

> Nuclear or fascicular involvement is unlikely among patients who have truly isolated VI CN palsy.

VI CN palsy at petrous apex results in **Gradenigo syndrome** which includes:

- VI nerve palsy.
- Ipsilateral facial pain (V CN).
- Ipsilateral facial palsy (VII CN).
- Ipsilateral hearing loss (VIII CN).

In the cavernous sinus, isolated 6th nerve palsy is rare. Lesions in cavernous sinus are associated with multiple CN palsies. Also, in the orbit 6th nerve palsy is associated with multiple CN palsies (III, IV).

Strabismus (Squint)

Terminology..449
Heterophoria and Heterotropia 450
Comitant Strabismus...452
Incomitant Strabismus 459
Adaptations in Strabismus 465
Clinical Evaluation of a Case of Strabismus..469

■ Terminology

Visual Axis

It is the line passing from the point of fixation to the fovea. It passes through the nodal point of the eye. In normal binocular vision, two visual axes intersect at the point of fixation.

Anatomical (Pupillary) Axis

It is the line passing from the posterior pole through the center of the cornea. *As fovea is temporal to the posterior pole of the eye*, the visual axis does not correspond to the anatomical axis of the eye (**Fig. 17.1**).

Angle Kappa

It is the angle between the visual and anatomical axes of the eye. It is usually **about 5 degrees**.

Normally, fovea is temporal to the posterior pole of the eye. A light thrown onto the cornea will therefore cause a reflex just nasal to the center of cornea. This is termed a positive angle kappa. *A large positive angle kappa* may produce the appearance of an *outward turn* of the eye and *simulate an exotropia*. When the fovea is situated nasal to the posterior pole (high myopia and ectopic fovea), corneal reflex is situated temporal to the center of cornea. It is termed negative angle kappa and may produce the appearance of an inward eye turn and simulate an esotropia.

So, an abnormal angle kappa is a common cause of pseudostrabismus.

Anisometropia

It is the difference in refraction between two eyes.

Primary Deviation

When the normal eye fixates, the deviation of squinting eye is called *primary deviation*.

Secondary Deviation

By covering the normal eye, the deviated eye is forced to fixate. When uncovered, the deviation shown by the normal eye is called *secondary deviation*.

Amblyopia

A condition of diminished visual form sense, which is not associated with any structural abnormality or disease of the media, fundus, or

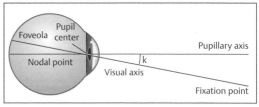

Fig. 17.1 Illustration depicting visual and anatomical axes.

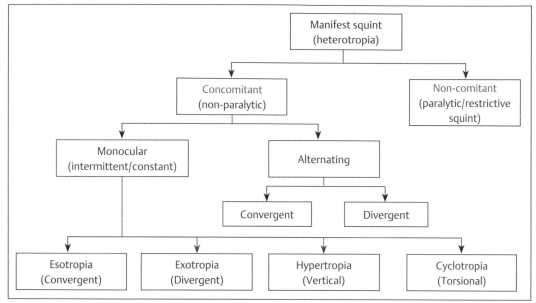

Flowchart 17.1 Classification of heterotropia.

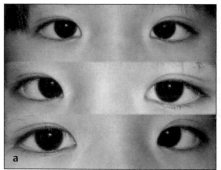

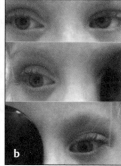

Fig. 17.2 (a) Pseudoesotropia. **(b)** Pseudoexotropia. Source: Pseudo-strabismus. In: Agarwal A, Jacob S, ed. Color atlas of ophthalmology. The quick-reference manual for diagnosis and treatment. 2nd edition. Thieme; 2009.

■ Pseudostrabismus (Apparent Squint)

In pseudostrabismus, eyes seem to have a squint in the absence of any deviation. Visual axes are, in fact, parallel.

1. Pseudoesotropia **(Fig. 17.2a):** It is the false impression of a convergent strabismus and is associated with:
   - Broad or prominent **epicanthal folds** which cover the normally visible nasal aspect of the globe.
   - Negative angle kappa.
2. Pseudoexotropia **(Fig. 17.2b):** It is the false impression of a divergent strabismus and is associated with:

- Hypertelorism: It is the condition of wide separation of two eyes.
- Large positive angle kappa.

■ Comitant Strabismus (OP9.2)

Comitant strabismus may be:

Intermittent	or	constant		
Monocular	or	alternating		
Convergent (esotropia)	or	divergent (exotropia)	or	hypertropia (vertical deviation)

In comitant strabismus, primary deviation is equal to secondary deviation and ocular deviation is equal in all directions of gaze.

■ Etiology

The following factors are contributory in the etiology of comitant strabismus:

- Genetics.
- Defective vision in one eye: It may result due to anisometropia or opacities in the media (corneal opacity or congenital cataract). It causes the affected eye to lose fixation and subsequently deviate.
- Muscular imbalance: The congenital or developmental defects of extraocular muscles (EOMs) may result in muscular imbalance. Initially, the fusional amplitudes maintain the alignment and heterophoria may precede the comitant strabismus.
- Imbalance between accommodation and convergence: In hypermetropia, the children accommodate continuously to see clearly, even for distance. It stimulates the excessive convergence, resulting in inward deviation. On the other hand, in high myopia, lack of accommodative impulse results in outward deviation.
- Defects in central mechanisms mediating fixation and fusional reflexes can lead to comitant strabismus.

■ Comitant Convergent Squint (Esotropia)

It is more common in hypermetropes and usually starts in childhood. It may be unilateral (monocular) or alternating. Esotropia could be accommodative or non-accommodative.

Accommodative Esotropia

Owing to the relatively late development of ciliary muscle, this type of esotropia rarely occurs before the age of 2 to 2½ years. To focus a near target, eyes accommodate and simultaneously converge to fixate bifoveally on the target. Accommodation and convergence have a fairly constant relationship to each other called **AC/A ratio** (accommodative convergence/accommodation). **AC/A ratio** is the amount of convergence in prism dioptres per dioptre (D) change in accommodation. Normal value of AC/A ratio is **3–5** prism dioptres. This means that 1D of accommodation is associated with 3 to 5 prism dioptre of accommodative convergence.

Accommodative esotropia is subdivided into **three types**:

- Refractive accommodative esotropia–normal AC/A ratio.
- Non-refractive accommodative esotropia–high AC/A ratio.
- Mixed (partially accommodative) esotropia.

Refractive Accommodative Esotropia

It is associated with uncorrected hypermetropia (usually between +2 and +7D). Excessive accommodation occurs due to uncorrected hypermetropia which, in turn, leads to excessive convergence. This manifests as convergent strabismus (esotropia). In this:

- AC/A ratio is normal.
- Ocular deviation at near ≥ at distance fixation.
- Asthenopic symptoms (OP9.3), intermittent diplopia (as evolution of esotropia is gradual), or closure of one eye when doing close work commonly occur during development of the disease.

Treatment

- Full correction of hypermetropia is done after cycloplegic refraction. Deviation is present if glasses are not worn (**Fig. 17.3**).

Nonrefractive Accommodative Esotropia

It results from abnormal synkinesis between accommodation and accommodative convergence. The effort to accommodate elicits an abnormally high accommodative convergence response, that is, **AC/A ratio** is **high**. This occurs independent of refractive error, although hypermetropia generally coexists. If the eyes are straight for distance and esotropic for near fixation, it means AC/A ratio is higher than normal.

Treatment

Eyes are straightened through *bifocals*. Bifocals are prescribed to relieve accommodation (and

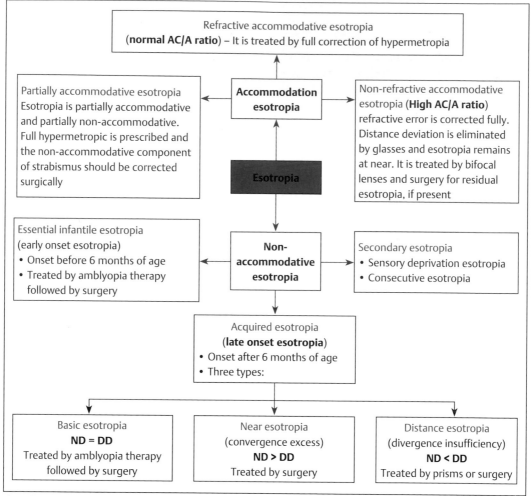

Flowchart 17.2 Outline of esotropia. Abbreviations: AC/A, accommodative-convergence over accommodation; ND, near deviation; DD, distant deviation.

Intermittent exotropia is more common and occurs at approximately 2 years of age with exophoria which breaks down to exotropia under conditions of fatigue or ill health. **Amblyopia is uncommon** in intermittent exotropia. Its subtypes are explained in **Table 17.2**.

Secondary Exotropia

It may be:

- Sensory exotropia as a result of primary sensory deficit.
- Consecutive exotropia arising iatrogenically after surgical overcorrection.

Sensory deprivation exotropia results from monocular visual impairment on account of acquired lesions. Common causes include:

- Anisometropia.
- Cataract.
- Opacities of media.
- Optic atrophy.
- Unilateral aphakia.

> **Exotropia** tends to occur in older children or adults. **Esotropia** tends to occur in infancy, but this is not invariable.

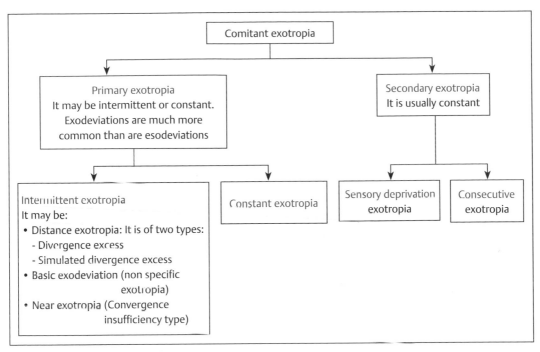

Flowchart 17.3 Classification of exotropia.

Table 17.2 Types of intermittent exotropia	
Type	**Features**
Distance exotropia (*divergence excess*)	Deviation for **distance** > deviation for **near** **Simulated divergence excess** is *associated with high AC/A ratio.* Initially, deviation for distance > deviation for near, as high AC/A ratio controls exodeviation for near. Deviations for near and distance are similar when near angle is remeasured with the patient looking through + 3D lenses or after occlusion of one eye for a time period. + 3D lens → accommodation relaxed → no accommodative convergence → near deviation and distant deviation are equal
Basic exotropia (*non-specific exotropia*)	Deviation for **distance** = deviation for **near**
Near exotropia (*convergence insufficiency*)	Deviation for **near** > deviation for **distance**
Abbreviation: AC/A, accommodative-convergence over accommodation.	

Consecutive exotropia results from surgical overcorrection of esotropia. Deviation is unilateral and constant.

■ Hypertropia (Vertical Deviation)

These may occur alone or in combination with horizontal deviation. The term right or left hypertropia is used depending on the eye which is up related to the other, for example, when right eye is fixing and left eye is higher than the right, it is called left hypertropia.

■ A- and V- Patterns

A horizontal deviation may increase or decrease with the eyes in upward or downward gaze, giving characteristic "A" and "V" patterns.

variation in the amount of deviation in different directions of gaze.

Etiology

- Nuclear lesions in midbrain.
  - ◇ Vascular cause: It includes hemorrhagic or thrombotic lesions of midbrain and may be associated with diabetes, hypertension, and arteriosclerosis.
  - ◇ Inflammation: It includes encephalitis and meningitis.
  - ◇ Toxins: It includes diphtheria, lead poisoning, and botulism.
  - ◇ Neoplasms: Brain tumors can produce ocular muscle palsies.
- Infranuclear lesions.

The ocular motor nerves (III, IV, and VI) may be involved in various pathological conditions as they traverse the cranial and orbital cavities. Therefore, these nerves may be involved at the level of fascicle, subarachnoid space, cavernous sinus, and orbit. The lesions involving the nerves may be inflammatory, vascular, pressure by tumors or aneurysm, and trauma. *In raised intracranial pressure, the most frequently involved nerve is abducens (VI) nerve.*

Different Types of Ocular Paralysis

There are six types of ocular paralysis, namely, IIIrd nerve palsy, total ophthalmoplegia, external ophthalmoplegia, internal ophthalmoplegia, double elevator palsy, and isolated muscle palsy–IVth and VIth nerve palsy.

IIIrd Nerve Palsy

Paralysis of IIIrd nerve may be complete, but often incomplete, and individual muscles may be selectively affected. Clinical features of complete IIIrd nerve palsy are listed in **Table 17.4**.

Total Ophthalmoplegia

It involves both extrinsic and intrinsic muscles of the eyeball. It results due to combined paralysis of IIIrd, IVth, and VIth nerves. It may be unilateral (in cavernous sinus thrombosis or lesions in superior orbital fissure) or bilateral (in lesions of the brain stem due to vascular or inflammatory causes). Clinical features include:

- Ptosis.
- No movement of eyeball in any direction.
- Fixed and dilated pupil.
- Total loss of accommodation.
- Slight proptosis.

External Ophthalmoplegia

It is due to paralysis of the extrinsic muscle of the eyeball (intraocular muscles are spared). It includes paralysis of six extraocular muscles and levator palpabrae superioris (LPS) muscle due to nuclear lesions sparing the Edinger–Westphal nucleus which supplies the intrinsic muscle. In external ophthalmoplegia, pupillary reactions and accommodation are normal.

Table 17.4 Clinical features of third nerve palsy	
III rd nerve palsy	**Clinical features**
Paralysis of LPS muscle	**Ptosis:** It prevents diplopia. On raising the lid, there is crossed diplopia.
Unopposed action of lateral rectus and superior oblique muscles	• **Eyeball** rotates outwards **(divergent squint)** and slightly downwards. • Restriction of **ocular movements** in all directions except outwards. • **Intorsion** of eye ball (because of intact SO muscle).
Paralysis of sphincter pupillae muscle	**Pupil** is **fixed** and **dilated**.
Paralysis of ciliary muscle	**Loss of accommodation.**
Loss of tone of paralyzed muscles	**Slight proptosis.**
Abbreviations: LPS, levator palpabrae superioris muscle; SO, superior oblique.	

Internal Ophthalmoplegia

It only involves intrinsic muscles (sphincter pupillae and ciliary muscle).

Double Elevator Palsy (Monocular Elevator Deficit)

It is characterized by paresis of superior rectus and inferior oblique muscle in the involved eye. Clinical features include:

- Inability to elevate one eye.
- Chin elevation to obtain fusion in downgaze.

Treatment involves the following:

- Base-up prism over the involved eye.
- Surgery must be considered if the chin elevation is required to maintain fusion.

Isolated Muscle Palsy—IVth and VIth Nerve Palsy

Trauma is the most common cause of isolated IVth nerve palsy, while VIth nerve palsy commonly occurs in raised intracranial tension due to its long intracranial course.

Clinical Features

The signs and symptoms of incomitant strabismus are as follows:

- Deviation of eye.
- Diplopia.
- Limitation of ocular movements.
- False projection (false orientation).
- Abnormal head posture.
- Vertigo.

Deviation

In incomitant strabismus, the affected eye gets deviated. The magnitude of deviation (angle of deviation) depends on the degree of paralysis and the direction in which the patient is looking. In incomitant strabismus:

- Secondary deviation (fixation with paretic eye) is always greater than primary deviation (fixation with normal eye). This can be explained by **Hering's law**.
- Angle of deviation is more if paralysis is severe.

- The eye deviates in the direction opposite to the field of action of paralyzed muscle due to unopposed action of ipsilateral antagonist of paralytic muscle, for example, the eye turns outward in medial rectus (MR) paralyses due to unopposed action of lateral rectus muscle.
- Angle of deviation is more if the patient is looking in the direction in which the paralyzed muscle acts, for example, in left lateral rectus (LR) muscle palsy, the deviation is more obvious on laevoversion (left gaze).

Clinical Application of Hering's Law in Paretic Squint

In case of paretic squint, amount of innervation flowing to both eyes is always determined by the fixating eye. Therefore, angle of deviation depends on which eye is used for fixation, for example, in case of right LR palsy, right eye is deviated inward due to unopposed action of right MR.

When left normal eye is used for fixation: When normal eye fixates, the deviation shown by the paralyzed eye is called **primary deviation**.

When paretic eye (right eye) is used for fixation: As right eye is deviated inward, excessive innervation is required to abduct the right eye. According to Hering's law, an equal amount of innervation flows to the normal MR of the left eye; hence, excessive adduction of the left eye takes place. This deviation of normal eye is known as **secondary deviation**. In paretic (incomitant) squint, secondary deviation is more than primary deviation.

Diplopia

Binocular diplopia occurs in the field of action of paralyzed muscle. The image seen by the squinting eye is the false image, while that seen by the sound eye is the true image. The false image is less distinct than the true image because true image falls upon the fovea. The diplopia may be homonymous (uncrossed) or heteronymous (crossed) (**Fig. 17.8**), for example:

If right eye deviates inward (**right esotropia**)	→	image is formed upon nasal retinal point	→	image is projected in the temporal field	→	right image is seen on the right of left image (homonymous diplopia)
If right eye deviates outward (**right exotropia**)	→	image is formed upon temporal retinal point	→	image is projected in the nasal field	→	left image is seen on the right of right image (heteronymous diplopia)

Depending upon the muscle involved, diplopia may be horizontal or vertical.

Limitation of Ocular Movement

Ocular movement is restricted in the direction of field of action of paralyzed muscle.

False Projection (False Orientation)

If a paralyzed eye attempts to fix an object, it is unable to locate the objects in space correctly. This is called false projection or false orientation, for example, in a patient with left LR palsy, the patient is asked to close his right eye and asked to fix an object situated on the left with his left eye. Due to left LR palsy, ocular movement is restricted in the direction of field of action of

paralyzed muscle, that is, to the left. So, the object will project to the nasal retina and the patient will point his finger more to the left of the object, that is, the object is projected too far in the direction of the action of paralyzed muscle.

Abnormal Head Posture

The patient adopts the abnormal head posture to lessen the diplopia and its unpleasant consequences. In horizontal muscle paralysis (LR or MR), the patient turns his face in the direction of the action of paralyzed muscle. In the paralysis of vertically acting muscles, in addition to face turn, the patient tilts his head which is associated with depression or elevation of chin.

The tilting of head and rotation of chin to compensate for defective vertical movements of the paralytic eye is known as **ocular torticollis.** It must be distinguished from true torticollis due to contraction of sternocleidomastoid muscle. In true torticollis, there is simple tilting of head without rotation of chin. SO (IVth cranial nerve [CN]) nerve palsy is the most common isolated vertical muscle palsy presenting with ocular torticollis.

Vertigo

It is partially due to diplopia and partially due to projection. It leads to nausea and vomiting. It occurs chiefly when the patient looks in the direction of the action of paralyzed muscle. It can be minimized by altering the position of head or by covering the affected eye.

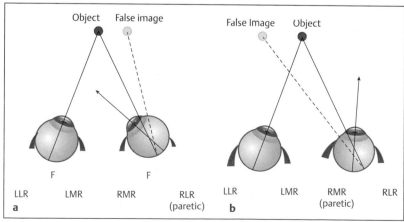

Fig. 17.8 (a) Right esotropia (object projects to nasal retina resulting in homonymous diplopia). **(b)** Right exotropia (object projects to temporal retina resulting in heteronymous diplopia). Abbreviations: LLR, left inferior rectus; LMR, left medial rectus; RLR, right lateral rectus; RMR, right medial rectus.

In congenital incomitant strabismus, these symptoms are not distressing due to poor vision in the affected eye or abnormal retinal correspondence (ARC).

Changes in Long Standing Paralysis

In long standing paralysis, the following changes takes place:
- The contracture of ipsilateral antagonist muscle.
- Overaction of contralateral synergist.
- Inhibitional palsy of contralateral antagonists, for example, in case of left LR palsy, the following changes are encountered:
  ◇ Contracture of left MR.
  ◇ Overaction of right MR muscle.
  ◇ Inhibitional palsy of right LR muscle.

Diagnosis of Paretic Muscle

The diagnosis of paretic muscle (oblique or vertical rectus) can be determined by a **three-step test**. The diagnostic scheme includes the following steps:

Step 1: Which one is the hypertropic eye in the primary position?

Hypertropia may be due to either weak depressor muscles (IR and SO) in hypertropic eye or weak elevators in hypotropic eye (SR and IO muscles). *Only overactions secondary to weak antagonists should be considered.* Thus, possible involvement has been reduced from eight to four muscles, two in each eye and all different.

Step 2: Examine the degree of diplopia in left and right gaze by asking the patient if the deviation increases in dextroversion or laevoversion?

In this step, see in which position (right or left gaze) the deviation is more, that is, the degree of diplopia in right and left gaze is examined.

As the deviation increases in the direction of action of paralyzed muscle, select two of the four muscles in each eye (isolated in step 1) which are likely to be affected.

At this point, it should be determined whether the muscles chosen are intortors or extortors. If one is an extortor and the other is an intortor, the error is in selection and the diagnostic steps must be checked.

Step 3: Bielschowsky head tilt test wherein the patient is asked whether the deviation increases with the head tilted to the right or left shoulder?

This step is used to determine torsional malfunction of vertical muscles. Tilt the patient's head toward each shoulder and see in which direction the vertical strabismus increases. On tilting the head toward one shoulder, the eye on the same side intorts and the other extorts, for example, if diplopia increases in left tilt, either a weak intortor in left eye or a weak extorter in right eye is responsible.

Field of action of vertical muscles in normal right eye are RSR, RIR, RIO, and RSO, whereas in normal left eye, they are LIO, LSO, LSR, and LIR. A few examples are mentioned below to help reach a diagnosis in case of paretic muscles of the eye.

Example 1

Let the right eye be hypertropic, and deviation increases on right gaze and left head tilt.

Step 1: Right hypertropia may be caused by weak depressor muscles in the right eye (**RIR, RSO**) or weak elevator muscles in the left eye (**LSR, LIO**). Thus, the possible involvement has been reduced to four.

Step 2: As the deviation increases on right gaze (dextroversion), the paretic muscles involved in dextroversion are **RIR** and **LIO**. Thus, the possible involvement has been reduced to two.

Step 3: As the right hypertropia increases on left tilt, left eye intorts and right eye extorts in left tilt. The paretic muscles selected in Step 2 are RIR and LIO (**both extortors**), so right eye extortor (**RIR**) **is the paretic muscle** as the right eye extorts.

Example 2

Let the right eye be hypertropic, and deviation increases on right gaze and right head tilt.

Step 1: Right hypertropia may be caused by weak depressor muscles in the right eye (**RIR, RSO**) or weak elevator muscles in the left eye (**LSR, LIO**). Thus, the possible involvement has been reduced to four.

Step 2– As the deviation increases on right gaze (dextroversion), the paretic muscles involved in dextroversion are **RIR** and **LIO**. Thus, the possible involvement has been reduced to two.

Step 3: As the right hypertropia increases on right tilt, right eye intorts and left eye extorts in right tilt. The paretic muscles selected in Step 2 are RIR and LIO (**both extortors**), so left eye extortor (**LIO**) **is the paretic muscle** as the left eye extorts.

Example 3

Let the right eye be hypertropic, and deviation increases on left gaze and left head tilt.

Step 1: Right hypertropia may be caused by weak depressor muscles in the right eye (**RIR, RSO**) or weak elevator muscles in the left eye (**LSR, LIO**). Thus, the possible involvement has been reduced to four.

Step 2: As the deviation increases on left gaze (laevoversion), the paretic muscles involved in laevoversion are **RSO** and **LSR**. Thus, the possible involvement has been reduced to two.

Step 3: As the right hypertropia increases on left tilt, left eye intorts and right eye extorts in left tilt. The paretic muscle selected in Step 2 are RSO and LSR (**both intortors**), so left eye intortor (**LSR**) **is the paretic muscle** as the left eye intorts.

Example 4

Let the right eye be hypertropic, and deviation increases on left gaze and right head tilt.

Step 1: Right hypertropia may be caused by weak depressor muscles in the right eye (**RIR, RSO**) or weak elevator muscles in the left eye

(**LSR, LIO**). Thus, the possible involvement has been reduced to four.

Step 2: As the deviation increases on left gaze (laevoversion), the paretic muscles involved in laevoversion are **RSO** and **LSR**. Thus, the possible involvement has been reduced to two.

Step 3: As the right hypertropia increases on right tilt, right eye intorts and left eye extorts in right tilt. The paretic muscles selected in Step 2 are RSO and LSR (**both intortors**), so right eye intortor (**RSO**) **is the paretic muscle** as the right eye intorts.

■ Restrictive Strabismus

Apart from nerve paralysis or muscle weakness, the ocular movements may be mechanically restricted. Characteristics features of restrictive type of strabismus include:

- Deviation in primary position is disproportionately less compared with the amount of limitation of ocular movement. It may even be paradoxical (e.g., exotropia in abduction deficit as in Duane retraction syndrome).
- Forced duction test is positive, that is, a restriction is encountered when the eye is moved in the direction of restrictive movement.

Etiology

Restrictive strabismus may be congenital or acquired. Congenital restrictive strabismus may be seen in congenital fibrosis of EOMs, Duane's retraction syndrome, Brown's syndrome, and strabismus fixus.

Acquired restrictive strabismus can be caused by:

- Trauma leading to blowout fracture of orbit with entrapment of EOM and soft tissues of the orbit.
- Edema and hemorrhage after trauma may cause a mechanical restriction of ocular movement. Also, scar tissue may cause

inability to relax and stretch the muscle, resulting in limitation of ocular movement.

- Inflammatory disease of the orbit as in dysthyroid eye disease and myositis.
- Tumors and space-occupying lesions may cause mechanical restriction of ocular movement.

Duane's Retraction Syndrome (DRS)

This condition is characterized by:

- Limitation of abduction and/or adduction, depending on the type. In type-I DRS, there is limitation of abduction and in type-II, adduction is limited. Type-III is characterized by limitation of adduction and abduction both.
- Retraction of the globe on adduction.
- Narrowing of the palpebral fissure on adduction, but widening of palpebral fissure on attempting abduction.

In DRS, aberrant innervation causes co-contraction of lateral and medial recti on adduction. In primary position, the eyes are straight (**Fig. 17.9**).

Treatment

When there is ocular deviation in primary position, surgery is indicated to eliminate any abnormal head posture.

Brown's Syndrome

This condition involves mechanical restriction, typically of SO tendon and is also known as

SO tendon sheath syndrome. This condition is characterized by a limitation of elevation in adduction (mimicking an IO palsy). The elevation in abduction is normal. The condition is confirmed by forced duction test which is positive on elevating the globe in adduction (**Fig. 17.10**).

Treatment

In severe cases with strabismus in primary position, surgical intervention (SO tenotomy) should be considered.

Strabismus Fixus

This is a congenital anomaly in which both eyes are fixed in convergent position (due to marked fibrosis of both medial recti) or in divergent position (due to marked fibrosis of both lateral recti).

Differentiating features of comitant and incomitant strabismus are listed in **Table 17.5**.

■ Adaptations in Strabismus

Binocular single vision (BSV) is the coordinated use of the two eyes to produce a single mental impression. The points on retina which are visually coordinated are called **corresponding retinal points**. If the binocular single vision is considered to be normal, there must be bifoveal fixation, that is, fovea of each eye is a corresponding retinal point. Points on nasal retina of one eye have corresponding points on the temporal retina of the other eye and vice versa.

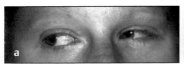
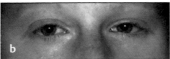
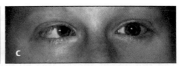

Fig. 17.9 (a–c) Duane's retraction syndrome (Type I). Source: Ancillary tests. In: Levin L, Arnold A, ed. Neuro-ophthalmology: The practical guide. 1st edition. Thieme; 2005.

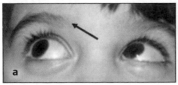
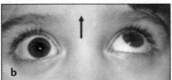
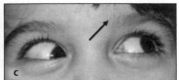

Fig. 17.10 (a–c) Congenital right brown syndrome. Source: The diagnosis of binocular diplopia. In: Biousse V, Newman N, ed. Neuro-ophthalmology illustrated. 3rd edition. Thieme; 2019.

Evaluation

The following points are taken into consideration for proper evaluation of amblyopia:

- Visual acuity: In absence of an organic lesion, a difference in best-corrected visual acuity of two Snellen's lines or more is indicative of amblyopia.
- Visual acuity with neutral density filters: In amblyopic eye, neutral density filters minimally degrade visual acuity or may even improve, while with organic lesions, neutral density filters decrease visual acuity significantly.
- Crowding phenomenon: It is present in amblyopics. Visual acuity in amblyopia is usually better while reading single letters than letters in a row.
- Cycloplegic refraction.
- Ophthalmoscopy to rule out pathology that might be causing deprivation.

Management

If amblyopia is not reversed within the first decade of life, then subnormal vision becomes permanent. Management protocols include the following:

- Correction of amblyogenic factor: Refractive error, congenital cataract, or complete ptosis, are treated at an early age to prevent visual deprivation.
- Occlusion therapy: Occlusion of normal eye (full time or part time) depends on the age of patient and the density of amblyopia. Occlusion of normal eye is done to encourage the use of amblyopic eye in treatment of amblyopia, but amblyopia in normal eye may be induced (iatrogenic amblyopia). So, monitor visual acuity regularly in both the eyes.
- If there is no improvement in amblyopia after 6 months of effective occlusion, occlusion therapy is stopped.
- Penalization: In penalization, vision in normal eye is blurred with atropine to encourage the use of amblyopic eye.

Best results are obtained in high hypermetropes with relatively mild amblyopia.

- Stimulation of amblyopic eye: It is done with CAM stimulator or pleoptic treatment.

Prognosis

It depends on the extent and duration of amblyopia and also the age at which therapy is initiated. If the amblyopia is severe before treatment is started, vision may not completely improve but treatment should be continued until no more improvement can be made. There is no treatment offered to adults with amblyopia. The key points of successful treatment are as follow:

- Younger age.
- Short course until intervention.
- Compliance with treatment.

■ Motor Adaptations to Strabismus

Motor adaptation involves the adoption of an abnormal head posture which is analyzed in terms of the following three components:

- Face turn (right or left).
- Head tilt (right or left).
- Chin elevation or depression.

Face Turn

It is the adoption to control a purely horizontal deviation. Face is turned in the direction of the action of paralyzed muscle, for example:

- In *left lateral rectus paralysis*, eye is deviated to the right and diplopia will occur in the left gaze, as field of action of left lateral rectus muscle is to the left. Therefore, the face will be turned to the left (in the direction of the action of paralyzed muscle).
- In *paresis of vertically acting muscles*, face is turned to avoid the side where the vertical deviation is greatest.

Head Tilt

Head tilt is adopted in the right or left shoulder to counter cyclotropia or vertical diplopia. When the head is tilted, it is physiological that torsion should occur to retain the upright position of the vertical meridian of the globe. Thus, *if the head is tilted to the left shoulder, the left eye will become intorted and the right eye extorted*. In addition, a tilt to one side will elevate the eye on the side of the tilt and depress the other eye. The torsion which causes difficulty may either be due to the defective action of the paralyzed muscle or the excessive action of the contralateral synergist. It should be remembered that the torsional power of the obliques is superior to that of the recti, **and frequently the head tilt is in consideration of this fact**, whether the oblique is the defective or the overacting muscle.

Chin Elevation or Depression

It is adopted to compensate the weakness of an elevator or depressor muscle in order to minimize the horizontal deviation in "A" or "V" pattern.

■ Head Posture in Different Ocular Paralysis

- Paralysis of **LR** muscle: **VIth nerve palsy:** LR palsy causes limitation of outward movement and hence the face is turned toward the paralyzed side to avoid the field of action of the LR muscle and diplopia.
- Paralysis of **MR** muscle: MR palsy causes limitation of inward movement and hence the face is turned toward the normal side to avoid the field of action of the MR muscle and diplopia.
- Paralysis of **SO** muscle: **IVth nerve palsy:**

  The SO muscle causes depression in the adducted position and is an intortor. So, the eye ball is deviated upward and inward with extorsion. Diplopia is more troublesome in downgaze. The compensatory head posture is adopted to avoid the field of action of the SO muscle, therefore:

  Face–is turned **toward the normal side** to avoid adduction.

  Chin–is **depressed** to avoid depression.

  Head–is tilted **toward the shoulder of the normal side** to avoid intorsion (as the affected eye extorts).

- Paralysis of **IO** muscle:

  IO muscle causes elevation in the adducted position and is an extortor. The compensatory head posture is adopted to avoid the field of action of the IO muscle, therefore:

  Face–is turned **toward the normal side** to avoid adduction.

  Chin–is **elevated** to avoid elevation.

  Head–is tilted **toward the shoulder of the paralyzed side** to avoid extorsion (as the affected eye intorts).

- Isolated SR palsy and IR palsy are uncommon, and the head tilt can be to either side in these cases, for example:

  SR muscle causes elevation in the abducted position and is an intortor. In right **SR** palsy, *the compensatory head posture is adopted to avoid the field of action of the SR muscle*, therefore/;

  Face–is turned **toward the paralyzed side (right)** to avoid abduction.

  Chin–is **elevated** to avoid elevation.

  Head– is tilted **toward the right shoulder (paralyzed side).** The head is tilted to the right shoulder because the palsy will have resulted in excessive action of left eye IO muscle (contralateral synergist). Alternatively, but rarely, the tilt may be toward the left shoulder because the defective secondary action (intorsion) of right SR muscle may have resulted in right extorsion, and this head tilt renders the right extorsion physiological.

  (*In case of oblique palsy, this possibility of variation does not exist*).

■ Clinical Evaluation of a Case of Strabismus

Below is the outline for evaluation of a case of strabismus.

- History.
- Examination.
  - ◇ Estimation of visual acuity.

Prism Bar Test

It combines the alternate cover test with prisms mounted in a prism bar which consists of a column of prisms of increasing strengths. The direction of deviation is established by the alternate cover test. The prism bar is placed in front of one eye, with the **apex pointing in the direction of deviation** (or **base opposite to the direction of deviation,** as light is bend toward the base of prism), for example, in convergent strabismus, fovea is displaced temporally, so prism is held base out (temporally), because it will bend the light toward the base or fovea.

The strengths of prisms are increased. As the strengths of prism approaches the extent of deviation, no movement of the eye is seen. The strengths of prisms at which no movement of the eye is seen give the objective angle of deviation.

In **Krimsky test**, the prisms are placed in front of the fixating eye until the corneal reflections are symmetrical. It reduces the problem of parallax.

Maddox Wing

Maddox wing dissociates the eye for near fixation and measures heterophoria. In this test, the patient looks through two slit holes in the eyepiece of an instrument (**Fig. 17.12**). The instrument is constructed in such a way that the right eye sees a white arrow pointing vertically upward and a red horizontal arrow, whereas the left eye sees a white horizontal row and a red vertical row of numbers. Both the arrows should be at zero.

- The number on the horizontal scale intersects with the *white arrow*, which gives the type and degree of horizontal deviation.
- The number on the vertical scale intersects with the *red arrow*, which gives the type and degree of vertical deviation.

Maddox Rod Test

A Maddox rod consists of 4 to 5 cylindrical red glass rods (**Fig. 17.13**) that convert the white spot of light into a red streak. The red streak of light appears perpendicular (at an angle of) to the long axis of rods. So, if the cylinder rods are placed

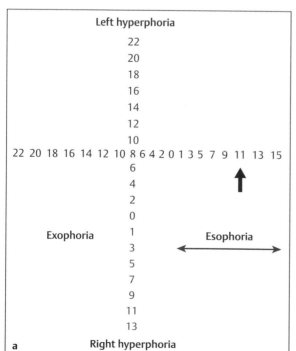

a

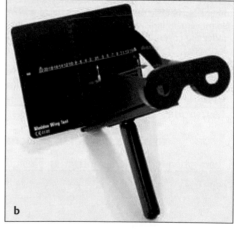

b

Fig. 17.12 (a, b) Eyepiece instrument used for Maddox Wing test.

with their axis horizontal, the red streak will be vertical and vice versa. The Maddox rod is placed horizontally in front of the right eye and the other eye is kept open. This dissociates the two eyes. The amount of dissociation is measured by the superimposition of two images using **prisms with the base placed opposite to the** direction of the deviation.

- If a spot light appears in the center of the vertical red line (with right eye), there is orthophoria.
- If a vertical red line (with right eye) is on the left of the spot light, there is exophoria.

- If a vertical red line (with right eye) is on the right of the spot light, there is esophoria (**Fig. 17.14**).

Vertical phorias can be tested by rotating the Maddox rod, so that the cylinders are vertical and the red line becomes horizontal. If line passes through the bright spot, there is no vertical deviation. If red line is either below or above the spot, the vertical deviation is present.

The degree of phoria can be read directly on a tangent scale. To measure phoria more accurately, a suitable prism is placed before one eye which brings the spot light in the center of the vertical red line. The test cannot differentiate a phoria from a tropia.

Determination of Type of Fixation

To test the type of fixation, the patient is asked to fixate on the star in a ophthalmoscope after closing the other eye.

- If the star falls on the fovea, it is called central fixation (*foveal fixation*).
- If the star falls on any area other than the fovea, it is called eccentric fixation (parafoveal, juxtafoveal, etc.).

Tests for Sensory Anomalies

Bagolini Striated Glasses Test

This test detects binocular single vision (BSV), ARC or suppression. Bagolini glasses are optically

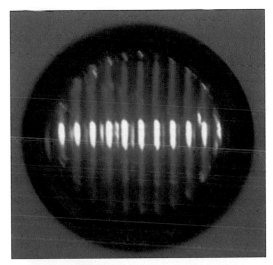

Fig. 17.13 Maddox rod.

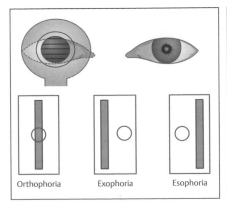

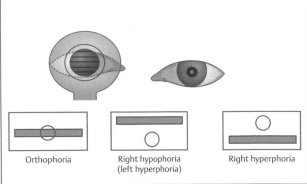

Fig. 17.14 Interpretation of the results of Maddow rod test.

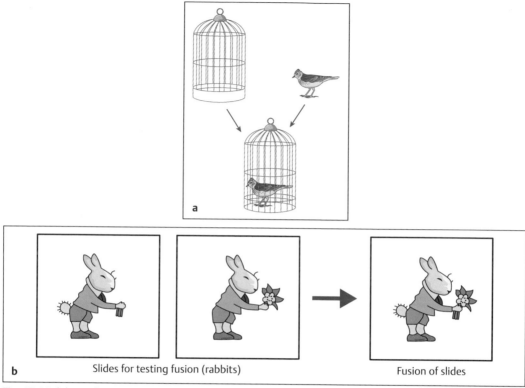

Fig. 17.18 (a) Simultaneous macular perception. **(b)** Fusion of slides.

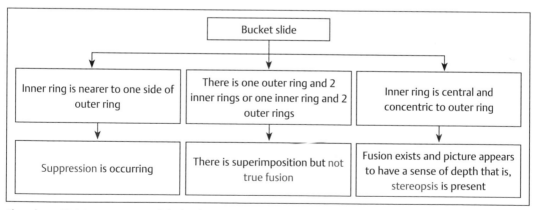

Flowchart 17.4 Interpretation of the bucket slide.

Motility Tests

Examination of Ocular Movements

In comitant strabismus: ocular movements are full in all directions. In acute comitant strabismus, the patient may complain of diplopia but the distance between images is the same in all directions. In case of long standing comitant strabismus, there is no complaint of diplopia.

In marked strabismus of long duration, the ocular movements may be defective due to contracture of the muscle, for example, in constant right convergent strabismus, the right MR muscle may develop contracture and restricts its abduction. This may mistakenly be diagnosed as right LR paresis. To confirm whether the defective eye movement is due to muscle weakness or physical restriction, a forced duction test is done.

Forced duction test: It is also referred to as *traction test* and is the most useful method for diagnosing the presence of mechanical restriction of ocular motility. It is performed under local anesthesia. The eye is then moved with a forceps applied to the conjunctiva near the limbus *in the direction opposite to that in which mechanical restriction is suspected*, for example, in case of restricted abduction, restricted abduction may be due to LR paralysis or contracture of MR muscle. To differentiate between the two, the eye is moved passively into abduction. Then, if no resistance is encountered, *paralysis of LR muscle* is the cause, and if *resistance* is encountered, contracture of MR muscle is the cause.

In children, the test must be performed under general anesthesia. The anesthesiologist is asked to avoid the use of succinylcholine chloride, since this drug may cause generalized tightness of the EOM which may simulate the mechanical restriction of the globe.

Examination of Near Point of Convergence

It is the nearest point of convergence at which the eyes can maintain binocular fixation. At this point, the patient reports diplopia and can be measured with the RAF (Royal Air Force) rule (**Fig. 17.19**). The RAF rule rests on the patient's cheek and the target is moved toward the patient's eyes. The normal near point of convergence should be nearer than 10 cm without effort.

Examination of Near Point of Accommodation

It is the nearest point of accommodation at which the eyes can maintain clear focus and can also be measured with the RAF rule. The near point recedes with age. At the age of 20 years, it is 8 cm, while at the age of 50 years, it recedes to 46 cm. The RAF rule rests on the patient's cheek and he fixates a line of print. The test card is slowly moved toward the patient and asked to report when he or she first notices the letters becoming

blurred. This distance denotes the near point of accommodation.

Estimation of Fusional Amplitudes

Fusional amplitudes measure the range of vergence movements and can be tested with synoptophore or prism bars.

Examination of Abnormal Head Posture

The compensatory head posture includes face turn, head tilt, and chin elevation or depression.

Testing for Diplopia

Diplopia may be due to paralysis of a muscle (incomitant strabismus), restrictive myopathy (contracture of muscle) in longstanding comitant strabismus. Diplopia charting is indicated in patients complaining of diplopia.

Diplopia Charting

The distance of separation of images and tilting of image is drawn in all the nine positions of gaze. The maximum separation of images is in the quadrant in which the muscle is restricted, that is, the field of action of the muscle. However, fine details regarding tilting of image cannot be recorded by this method.

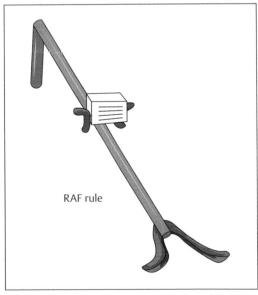

Fig. 17.19 RAF rule. Abbreviation: RAF, Royal Air Force.

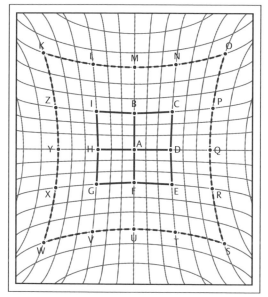

Fig. 17.21 Hess screen.

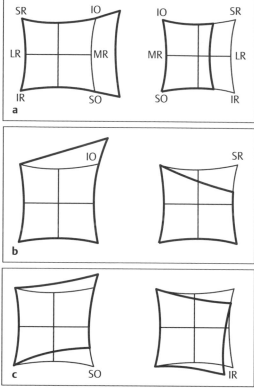

Fig. 17.22 (a) Hess charting in recent right lateral rectus palsy. **(b)** Hess charting in recent right superior rectus palsy. **(c)** Changes with time in Hess chart. Abbreviations: IO, inferior oblique; IR, inferior rectus; SO, superior oblique; SR, superior rectus.

restriction in the main direction of action of paretic muscle.

- The larger chart indicates the eye with overacting contralateral synergists. For example, in right LR palsy.
- The right chart is smaller than the left which shows marked underaction of right LR muscle.
- The left chart shows marked overaction of the left MR muscle.

Hess Charting in Right SR Palsy

If the paretic muscle recovers its function, both charts will revert to normal. However, if the paresis persists, the following changes take place:

- Contracture of ipsilateral antagonists (right IR)– It is reflected as overaction in the chart.
- Inhibitional palsy of the antagonist of contralateral synergist (left SO), which is reflected as underaction in the chart.

In investigating the diplopia, one determines the following:

- Whether the diplopia is uniocular or binocular?
- Whether the distance between the two images in the areas of diplopia remains the same or changes?
- Whether one image is inclined or both are erect?
- Whether the images are on the same level?
- Whether the diplopia is uncrossed or crossed?

Ocular Tumors

Introduction...481
Epibulbar Tumors..481
Intraocular Tumors...483

■ Introduction

Ocular tumors are a collection of cells that grow and multiply abnormally and form masses. These can appear on the eyelids, in the eye, and in the orbit. The tumors in the eye are usually secondary tumors, that is, metastatic from another part of the body (lung, breast, prostate, etc). Two types of primary tumors arise within the eye itself: retinoblastoma in children and melanoma in adults. **Ocular tumors** can be epibulbar or intraocular. All these tumors may be benign or malignant (**Flowchart 18.1**).

■ Epibulbar Tumors

Epibulbar tumors clinically manifest with a very wide spectrum and include several forms of epithelial, stromal, caruncular, and secondary tumors. These may be classified as given in **Flowchart 18.2**.

■ Congenital Tumors

These are not true tumors but choristomas (a mass of histologically normal tissue in an abnormal location) and include dermoids and dermolipomas.

Dermoid (OP2.1, 2.2)

It is a *congenital* tumor and consists of epidermoid epithelium containing sebaceous glands and hairs. It is located at the *limbus* (**Fig. 18.1**). It presents as yellowish, soft conjunctival mass in early childhood. Treatment includes simple excision if the tumor is small in size, but lamellar keratosclerotomy may be required if the tumor is large in size.

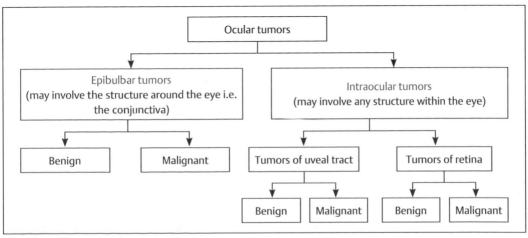

Flowchart 18.1 Types of ocular tumors.

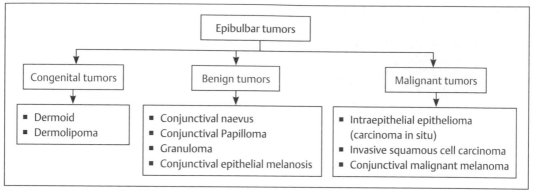

Flowchart 18.2 Types of epibulbar tumors.

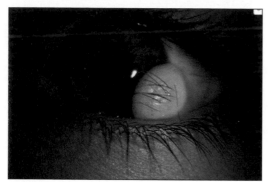

Fig. 18.1 Dermoid tumor. Source: Cornea, External Diseases, and Anterior Segment. In: Glass L, ed. Ophthalmology Q&A Review. 1st Edition. Thieme; 2019.

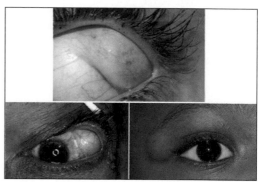

Fig. 18.2 Dermolipoma. Source: Selected orbital disorders. In: Leatherbarrow B, ed. Oculoplastic surgery. 3rd edition. Thieme; 2019.

Dermolipoma

It is a congenital tumor and consists of fibrous tissue and fat (fibro fatty tumors). It is commonly located at the outer canthus (**Fig. 18.2**). It presents as soft, yellowish subconjunctival mass in adult life. Treatment is generally avoided due to the possibility of complications.

Congenital epibulbar choristomas may have systemic association known as **Goldenhar syndrome** (Ocular auriculo vertebral anomalies) which is characterized by the following:

- **Ocular features:** Apart from dermoids, upper lid coloboma, microphthalmos, and disc anomalies have been reported.
- **Systemic features:** These include preauricular skin tags, vertebral anomalies, and hemifacial hypoplasia.

■ Benign Tumors

Benign tumors do not invade nearby tissue or spread to other parts of the body but they can be serious if they press on vital structures such as blood vessels or nerves. Therefore, at times, they require treatment, and at other times they do not.

Conjunctival Naevus (Conjunctival Mole)

It is congenital and tends to grow at puberty. It presents as elevated pigmented nodule in the first or second decade. It is located at the limbus or near plica semilunaris (**Fig. 18.3**). Naevi are mobile over underling sclera. Vast majority of naevi do not undergo malignant transformation. It is treated by simple excision which is performed for cosmetic purposes or on suspicion of malignancy.

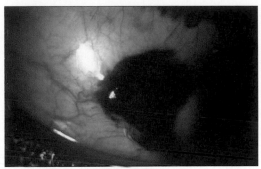

Fig. 18.3 Conjunctival naevus.

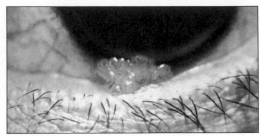

Fig. 18.4 Conjunctival papilloma.Source: Conjunctival papilloma. In: Lang G, ed. Ophthalmology. A pocket textbook atlas. 3rd edition. Thieme; 2015.

Conjunctival Papilloma

It is sessile or pedunculated and strongly associated with human papilloma virus infection. It is located at the limbus, near canthus or in the fornices (**Fig. 18.4**). Treatment includes excision performed with cryotherapy at the base and surrounding area, but recurrence rate is high.

Granuloma

It is a fibrovascular proliferation in response to conjunctival surgery, trauma, or foreign body incarceration, and consists of granulation tissue with inflammatory cells and blood vessels. It is treated by topical steroids but excision is carried out in resistant cases.

Conjunctival Epithelial Melanosis

It occurs due to the presence of excess melanin epithelial melanocytes in conjunctival basal layer. So, it is more common in darker-skinned individuals. *There is no melanocytic hyperplasia.* It is bilateral and appears during the first few years of life. It presents as patchy flat brownish pigmentation of conjunctiva and requires no treatment as it has no malignant potential.

■ Malignant Tumor

Bowen Intra Epithelial Epithelioma (Carcinoma in Situ)

It is a premalignant tumor of conjunctival epithelium. It has a chance of progression to invasive melanoma. It usually begins near the limbus. As it is superficial to basement membrane,

conjunctiva is freely movable over underlying episcleral tissue. It is treated by surgical excision with adjunctive cryotherapy or topical Mitomycin C or 5-FU to avoid recurrence.

Squamous Cell Carcinoma (Epithelioma)

It occurs at the epithelial transition zone. Therefore, it chiefly occurs at the limbus and the lid margin. It appears fleshy, and gelatinous with feeder vessels. Intraocular extension is uncommon (**Fig. 18.5**). It is treated by excision with cryotherapy of base. If recurrence takes place, enucleation or even exenteration may be necessary along with radiotherapy.

Malignant Melanoma

It is rare, usually pigmented, and often occurs in the 6th decade. It occurs typically at the limbus and spreads over the surface of the globe (**Fig. 18.6**). It rarely penetrates it. The main sites of metastasis are lymph nodes, liver, lung, and brain. It may require excision of globe or exenteration of orbit.

■ Intraocular Tumors

Intraocular tumors include tumors of uveal tract and retina (**Flowchart 18.3**).

■ Benign Tumors of Uvea

Uveal naevus is a benign tumor arising from the melanocytic cells. It occurs most commonly in the choroid but also occurs in the iris or ciliary body. Most naevi are likely to be congenital in nature but detectable clinically until after childhood.

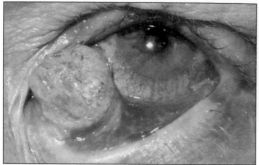

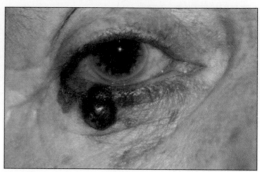

Fig. 18.5 Squamous cell carcinoma. Source: Welkoborsky H; Wiechens B, Hinni M, ed. Interdisciplinary management of orbital diseases: textbook and atlas. 1st edition. 2017.

Fig. 18.6 Malignant melanoma. Source: Melanoma. In: Leatherbarrow B, ed. Oculoplastic surgery. 3rd edition. Thieme; 2019.

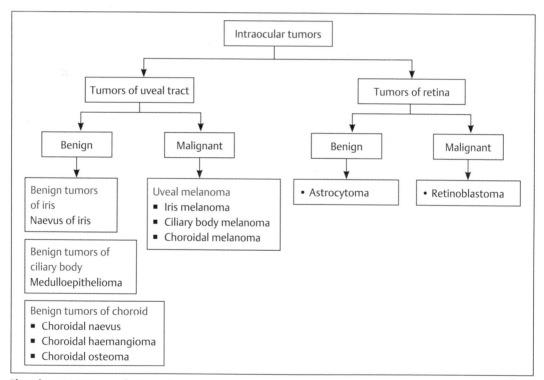

Flowchart 18.3 Types of intraocular tumors.

Most uveal naevi are asymptomatic; however, macular choroidal naevi can cause visual loss.

Naevus of Iris

It is a localized flat or elevated stromal lesion and can cause pupillary distortion, ectropion iridis, or both (**Fig. 18.7**). It is rarely associated with abnormal iris vasculature. Iris naevus must be differentiated from the multiple, small, yellow or brown, melanocytic iris lesions elevated above the iris surface (**Lisch nodules**). Lisch nodules appear to be nodular aggregates of dendritic melanocytes and not true naevi. *Lisch nodules are pathognomonic of neurofibromatosis, that*

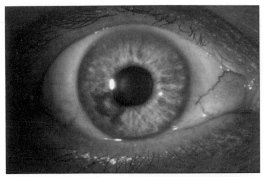

Fig. 18.7 Naevus of iris. Source: Biousse V, Newman N, ed. Neuro-ophthalmology illustrated. 3rd edition. 2019.

is, these are found on the iris of patient with neurofibromatosis.

Medulloepithelioma

It characteristically arises from the nonpigmented epithelium of ciliary body. Its characteristic features are:

- It is amelanotic tumor arising mainly in the ciliary body.
- The average age of affected individual is approximately 5 years. So, it affects infants and young children preferentially.
- It typically appears as brown to white lesions of extreme peripheral fundus and detectable only by indirect ophthalmoscope with scleral depression because of its peripheral location.
- Its common complication is the development of neovascular glaucoma.

Investigations

Medulloepithelioma can be detected by the following investigations:

- B-scan ultrasonography
- CT scan
- MRI

Choroidal Naevus

It appears as a small gray to brown choroidal tumor. Choroidal naevi are usually small (less than 2DD [disc diameter]) with indistinct margins. A lesion > 5DD must be considered malignant. They are usually associated with characteristic surface alterations such as drusen and pigment clumping in retinal pigment epithelium (RPE). It is asymptomatic but may cause blurred or distorted vision due to accumulation of serous subretinal fluid. It may result in localized serous detachment of RPE or neurosensory retina.

Investigations

Choroidal naevus can be detected by the following investigations:

- Ultrasonography (to measure the size and extent of choroidal naevus).
- Fluorescein angiography (FA) and indocyanine green (ICG) angiography to assess the presence of prominent blood vessels within the tumor. *Choroidal naevus is defined better by ICG angiography than by FA.*

Most benign choroidal naevi do not have blood vessels within the tumor, but choroidal melanomas do have blood vessels within the tumor.

Choroidal Hemangioma

It is a benign vascular tumor of choroid and occurs in two forms: circumscribed and diffuse.

Circumscribed choroidal hemangioma: These are reddish–orange, round to oval tumors and located in the posterior half of fundus. Such tumors almost never extend anterior to equator and are located within 2DD from the optic disc, foveola, or both. Circumscribed choroidal hemangioma results in degenerative changes in overlying RPE. Accumulation of serous subretinal fluid *or* degenerative changes in macular retina produce visual symptoms (blurred vision and metamorphopsia).

Diffuse choroidal hemangioma: It is usually a part of the Sturge–Weber syndrome. The choroid is thickened diffusely by the hemangiomatous vascular lesion, and the fundus on the affected side has a more saturated red appearance than the fundus on the uninvolved side. It is referred as *"tomato ketchup fundus."*

Choroidal hemangioma may cause elevated IOP (secondary glaucoma) and exudative retinal detachment.

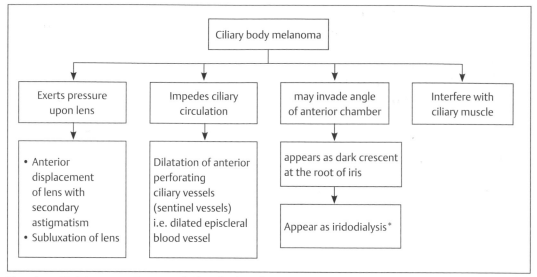

Flowchart 18.4 Important Features of Ciliary body melanoma.
Note: * On illumination with ophthalmoscope, if red reflex is present, it is iridodialysis, but if no red reflex is obtained, it is melanoma.

Choroidal Melanoma

It is most common among uveal melanomas. It appears as a dark brown, lens-shaped mass. As it grows, it stretches and eventually breaks through the overlying Bruch's membrane and RPE to form a nodular mass in the subretinal space, which is separated from the part in the choroid by a narrow neck. Thus, the tumor takes on a *mushroom-like configuration* which is *highly characteristic of choroidal melanoma* (**Fig. 18.9**). The neurosensory retina is detached at sides of the choroidal melanoma which is being filled with subretinal fluid. In some cases, the subretinal fluid is bloody.

Pathology

Choroidal melanoma is more likely to be *composed of epitheloid melanoma cells*. Therefore, the survival prognosis for choroidal melanomas is poor.

Investigations

Choroidal melanoma can be detected by the following investigations:
- B-scan ultrasonography.
- CT scan.
- MRI.

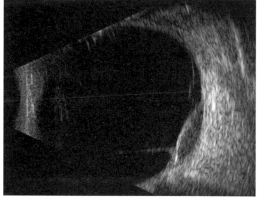

Fig. 18.9 B-scan: mushroom-like configuration of choroidal melanoma. Source: History. In: Singh K, Smiddy W, Lee A, ed. Ophthalmology Review: A Case-Study Approach. 2nd Edition. Thieme; 2018.

- Fluorescein angiography.
- ICG.
- Chest X-ray.

Choroidal melanomas that have erupted through the Bruch's membrane show the mushroom-like configuration on B-scan ultrasonography.

Clinical Course

The clinical course of choroidal malignant melanoma is divided into four stages:

- **Quiescent stage**: The choroidal malignant melanoma causes detachment of retina before the patient becomes symptomatic. The retina remains in contact with the tumor at the summit.
- **Stage of glaucoma**: The neoplastic cells in choroidal melanoma infiltrates trabecular meshwork, and compresses the vortex veins which lead to rise in IOP. Also, there is forward movement of lens iris diaphragm due to posterior pressure, leading to obstruction of trabecular meshwork. In case of tumor necrosis, macrophages engulf the melanin which further obstruct the angle of anterior chamber, leading to rise in IOP (**Flowchart 18.5**).
- **Stage of extra ocular extension**: It may spread to involve sclera and the orbit.
- **Stage of metastasis**: Distant metastasis occurs through hematogenous spread to the liver, and occasionally to the lungs, bone, skin, and brain.

Prognosis

Unfavorable pathological prognostic factor include:

- Large tumors.
- Extra scleral extension.
- Recurrence of tumor.

- Higher mitotic index of tumor.
- Closed vascular loop within tumors.
- Location– anterior tumors involving ciliary body grow relatively large by the time of presentation; hence, anterior tumors involving ciliary body have a worse prognosis.

Treatment

Many therapeutic options are available for choroidal melanomas but they must be managed by taking the following factors into consideration:

- Size and extent of tumor.
- Location of tumor.
- Effect on vision.
- State of fellow eye.
- Presence of extra scleral tumor extension.
- Presence of clinically detectable metastasis.

Treatment options for choroidal malignant melanoma are as follows:

- Enucleation.
- Exenteration.
- Radiation therapy.
- Thermo therapy.
- Photocoagulation.
- Chemotherapy.
- Local resection (choroidectomy).

Enucleation

It is most strongly indicated for large tumors, painful and blind eye, tumors invading the optic disc, and transscleral extension of tumor into the

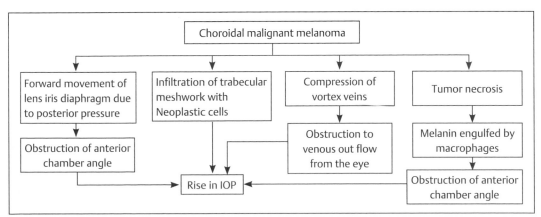

Flowchart 18.5 Stages of glaucoma. Abbreviation: IOP, intraocular pressure.

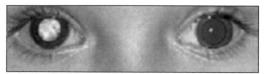

Fig. 18.10 Leukocoria. Source: Biousse V, Newman N, ed. Neuro-ophthalmologyillIustrated. 2nd edition. 2015.

- **Secondary glaucoma**: It is encountered less frequently.
- **Red eye** (due to tumor-induced uveitis), **iris nodules** (due to clumping of white tumor cells on the iris) which may be associated with pseudohypopyon, or **spontaneous hyphema** in retinoblastoma invading anterior segment.
- **Proptosis with bone invasion** due to orbital invasion in neglected cases.

Stages

If left untreated, retinoblastoma runs through the following four stages:

- *Quiescent stage*:It lasts from 6 months to a year. Discrete intraretinal tumors appear as white, round to oval elevated retinal masses. The tumors tend to attract retinal blood vessels which ramify prominently on a surface of lesion. Depending on the growth, retinoblastoma may be endophytic or exophytic.
- *Endophytic retinoblastoma* grows from the retina into the vitreous. There is no associated retinal detachment with an endophytic growth pattern. The child presents with white pupillary reflex (leukocoria or amaurotic cat's eye reflex). *Exophytic retinoblastoma* grows toward the RPE and choroid. It is frequently associated with nonrhegmatogenous retinal detachment.
- *Glaucomatous stage*: The tumor causes distension of globe or may involve the angle of anterior chamber, which results into the rise in IOP and secondary glaucoma. The child presents with red eye, excessive tearing, enlarged eyeball, corneal clouding, pain, and discoloration of iris in the involved

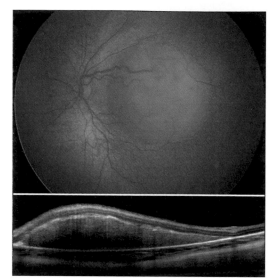

Fig. 18.11 Retinoblastoma. Source: Retinal tumors. In: Agarwal A, Kumar D, ed. Essentials of OCT in ocular disease. 1st edition. Thieme; 2015.

eye (usually caused by neovascularization of iris).

- *Stage of extraocular extension*: The retinoblastoma may invade the orbit and is followed by rapid fungation.
- *Stage of metastasis*: The metastatic spread may take place in regional lymph nodes (preauricular and cervical lymph nodes), cranial, and other bones. The direct extension of retinoblastoma to optic nerve involves the brain. Blood-borne metastasis is relatively uncommon. Metastasis in the liver is relatively rare.

Diagnosis

It includes detailed ocular examination and certain investigations.

Ocular Examination

A detailed and careful ocular examination of the child, including fundus examination by indirect ophthalmoscopy with scleral indentation, must be performed under general anesthesia. Without indentation, the preequatorial tumors may be missed. The fellow eye is also examined to rule out bilateral involvement (**Fig. 18.11**).

Investigations

- Ultrasonography: It provides information regarding tumor size and calcification within the tumor. B-scan ultrasonography of a calcified tumor with intralesional calcification shows the lesion to be strongly sonoreflective.
- CT scan: It also detects calcification because *retinoblastoma tumors are characteristically calcified in 75% cases. However, intralesional calcification is not always present in retinoblastoma*. It should be performed only if ultrasonography has not detected calcification due to significant radiation problems. It also detects the extent of tumor invasion.
- MRI: cannot detect calcification; hence, appears it to be less valuable than CT in assessing intralesional calcification. However, it is superior to CT for the purposes of studying orbital optic nerve and detection of extraocular extension or a pineal gland tumor (pinealoblastoma). It also differentiates the tumor from simulating conditions.
- Lumbar puncture and bone marrow aspiration– These may be needed in patients of retinoblastoma with metastasis.
- Bone scan– It is indicated in presence of metastatic disease. A bone scan can help show if the retinoblastoma has spread to the skull or other bones.

Differential Diagnosis

Several conditions mimic the picture of retinoblastoma and they are grouped under the term **pseudoglioma**. It must be differentiated from the following (**Table 18.1**):

- Causes of leukocoria.
- Causes of vitreous seeds.
- Causes of discrete retinal tumors.

Treatment

Treatment modalities for retinoblastoma include:

- Enucleation.
- Radiation therapy (external beam radiotherapy and plaque radiotherapy).
- Intravenous chemotherapy.
- Photocoagulation cryotherapy.

Factors influencing the management include:

- Size of tumor/tumors.
- Location of tumors.
- Laterality of diseases.
- Visual potential in the affected eye.
- Vision in unaffected eye (if the disease is unilateral).
- Associated ocular problems such as retinal detachment, vitreous hemorrhage, neovascularization of iris, and secondary glaucoma.

Treatment of small tumors (diameter up to 3 mm and thickness up to 2mm):

- *Cryotherapy* for anterior (preequatorial) tumors using the triple freeze–thaw technique.
- *Photocoagulation* for posterior tumors.

Treatment of medium-sized tumors (diameter up to 12 mm and thickness up to 6 mm):

- *Plaque radiotherapy*– For anterior tumors, it is performed using iodine-125 or ruthenium-106.

Table 18.1 Differential diagnosis of retinoblastoma

Causes of leukocoria	Causes of vitreous seeds	Causes of discrete retinal tumors
• Coats disease* • Persistent hyperplastic primary vitreous (PHPV) • Ocular toxocariasis • Retinopathy of prematurity • Norries disease • Congenital cataract	• Endophthalmitis • Uveitis with vitreous exudation • Retinitis	• Retinal astrocytoma • Retinoma (retinocytoma)– a benign variant of retinoblastoma

Note: *Coats disease is the disorder most frequently mistaken for retinoblastoma.

- *Chemotherapy*—The most commonly used chemotherapeutic regimen *consists of a combination of* carboplatin, etoposide, and vincristine (**CEV**). Intravenous CEV is given as a cyclic treatment every 3 to 4 weeks for six or more cycles. It reduces the size of intraocular retinoblastoma (**chemoreduction**). Cyclosporin may be added to this regimen in order to reduce the multidrug resistance that occurs in many retinoblastomas. Partially regressed tumors must be treated by local treatment such as cryotherapy, laser therapy, and plaque radiation therapy.

Retinoblastomas are sensitive to radiation but *external beam radiotherapy is avoided*, if possible, because of the high-risk of inducing second malignancy such as osteosarcoma (if radiotherapy is administered in the first 6 months of life) and radiation-related cataract (posterior subcapsular). External beam radiotherapy results in highly effective regression of vascularized retinal tumors. It is applicable to eyes with tumors involving the optic disc, eyes with diffuse vitreous seeding, and eyes with failed local treatments.

Treatment of large tumors:
- Chemotherapy (**chemoreduction**) to reduce the size of tumor.
- *Local treatments* such as cryotherapy, laser therapy or plaque radiation therapy following chemoreduction to avoid enucleation, or external beam radiotherapy.
- *Enucleation* is indicated in the following situations:
  ◊ Failed chemo reduction.
  ◊ Optic nerve invasion.
  ◊ Rubeosis.
  ◊ Vitreous hemorrhage.

◊ Poor visual prognosis.
◊ High risk of recurrence.

If enucleation is performed, it is imperative to obtain a long piece of optic nerve (10–15 mm) in every case. Any postoperative chemotherapy should be delayed for at least a week to allow healing.

Treatment of extraocular extension:
- *Enucleation.*
- *Chemotherapy* after enucleation. A course of CEV is given for 6 months.
- *External beam radiotherapy.*

Follow Up

If retinoblastoma has been treated conservatively (chemotherapy + local treatment), children must be reexamined every 2 to 4 weeks until the age of 3 years. Thereafter, the child should be examined at 6-month intervals until the age of 5 years and then annually until the age of 10 years. Although the chances of recurrence after three years are remote, the child is examined at frequent intervals for a much longer period.

Untreated children with retinoblastoma almost always die of intracranial extension or widely disseminated disease within 2 years of tumor detection.

Prognosis

The prognostic factors for tumor-related mortality in retinoblastoma are:
- Optic nerve invasion.
- Massive choroidal invasion.
- Transscleral tumor extension into the orbit.

The principle prognostic factors for failure to retain useful vision and preserve the eye include:
- Size of intra ocular tumors.
- Presence and extent of vitreous seeds.
- Presence and extent of retinal detachment.
- Location of tumors within the eye.

Ocular Injuries

Light Damage to the Eye..495

Chemical Injuries..496

Ocular Foreign Bodies...499

Blunt Trauma..503

Penetrating and Perforating Injuries..508

Injuries due to Physical Agents...511

The eye is protected by the lids and orbital margins from direct injury, but it can be injured by light, chemicals and mechanical trauma. Trauma involves ocular foreign bodies, blunt trauma, and penetrating and perforating injuries.

■ Light Damage to the Eye (OP9.5)

UV spectrum is subdivided into:

- UV-A: 400–320 nm (90% of UV [ultraviolet] radiations from sun).
- UV-B: 320–280 nm.
- UV-C: ≤ 280 nm.

The ozone layer (2–3 mm in thickness) is produced in the stratosphere by a photochemical reaction which filters out most of the destructive UV light. The depletion of ozone layer leads to an increase in UV-B radiation.

■ Biochemical Mechanism of UV Radiation Damage

For photodamage to occur, the tissue must contain a molecule that absorbs light. Tissue photo damage may occur in two ways:

1. **Molecular fragmentation:** The molecules containing alternate double bonds (proteins, enzymes, and nucleic acid) resonate with radiation of UV wavelength. The increased intensity of UV radiation breaks the molecular bonds and the new

molecules may induce inflammation or affect the immune system.

2. **Free radical generation:** Free radical light damage requires three components: light absorbing molecule, oxygen, and short-wavelength radiation (**Flowchart 19.1**).

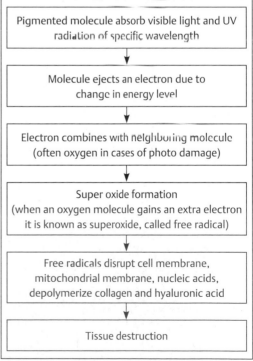

Flowchart 19.1 Mechanism of damage by light. Abbreviation: UV, ultraviolet.

Ocular Light Damage

Fortunately, the body contains protective free radical scavengers which include superoxide dismutase, vitamin C and E, glutathione peroxidase, and carotene. The shortage of free radical scavengers in premature infants, elderly, or nutritionally impaired persons may cause greater vulnerability to light damage. With age, many of the photoprotective mechanisms of the eye degrade. Excessive exposure to UV radiations can lead to cataract development and risk of macular degeneration.

The reduction of environmental exposure and use of absorptive lenses diminish the risk of light damage to the eye. Also, intake of antioxidant as dietary supplements may slow the development of cataracts and macular degeneration.

Lids

Acute sunburn reaction occurs in lids, which is essentially an UV-B-induced response. Clouds do not filter out UV radiation and therefore do not prevent sunburn. Malignant skin changes include basal cell carcinoma, squamous cell carcinoma, and malignant melanoma. Other features include epidermal keratoses and sebaceous hyperplasia.

Cornea

The most effective range of damaging wavelength is 260 to 290 nm, but as a result of absorption by the ozone layer, radiations of these wavelengths rarely penetrate to the Earth's surface. The cornea absorbs rays of wavelength <320 nm, that is, UV-B and UV-C. Apart from UV radiation, welding flashes, germicidal lamps, and sun lamps cause superficial punctate keratitis (SPK). Chronic exposure to UV radiations results in pterygium and spheroidal degeneration of cornea.

Lens

Short-wavelength radiations are cataractogenic (primarily cortical cataract). Infrared (IR) radiation also has an effect on lens. Lower wavelength of IR radiation closely matches the resonant frequency of water molecules. In glass blowers, lens water absorbs radiations from IR source, resulting in aggregation of insoluble lens proteins and glass blower's cataract.

Retina

Prolonged illumination from indirect ophthalmoscope with a focusing lens, operating microscope, or sun cause maculopathy. Oxygen with fluorescent lights in nursery may enhance damaging potential of oxygen (due to damaging free radicals) in premature infants, as immature retina is devoid of protective free radical scavengers. It may result in retinopathy of prematurity.

Light Protection

Eyes can be protected from light damage by taking the following measures:
- During surgery, light can be blocked by occuluder disc placed on cornea or bubble of air in anterior chamber.
- Intraocular lens (IOLs) with UV filters– These IOLs filter out all wavelengths of light <400 nm and prevent decrease in visual function such as color vision and contrast sensitivity.
- Use of photochromatic lenses: When shorter wavelength light (300–400 nm) interacts with glass photochromatic lenses, they darken ($Ag^+ \rightarrow$ elemental Ag).
- UV-absorbing lens.

■ Chemical Injuries

Chemical injuries may be due to alkalis or acids. It may be accidental or as a result of an assault.

■ Alkali Burns

Alkali burns are more common than acid burns since alkalis are more widely used at home and in the industries.

Most commonly involved alkalis are–
- Lime—usually fresh mortar or white wash $Ca(OH)_2$.
- Caustic potash (KOH).
- Caustic soda (NaOH).
- Ammonia (NH_4OH)—It is most harmful.

Ocular Damage

Alkali burns are more severe than acid burns because alkalis penetrate deeper into tissues and may involve various ocular tissues (**Table 19.1**). **Flowchart 19.2** explains the mode of damage of various eye structures by alkalis.

Table 19.1 Various ocular injuries incurred by alkalis

Ocular part affected	Lesions
Conjunctiva	Conjunctival congestion, edema, and necrosis, with formation of symblepharon.
Cornea	Corneal epithelial damage, opacification, and vascularization.
Uvea	Uveitis and ciliary epithelial damage.
Lens	Cataract.

Thus, alkalis cause extraocular as well as intraocular complications. Ammonia (NH4OH) and sodium hydroxide (NaOH) may produce severe damage due to rapid penetration.

■ Acid Burns

Acids *coagulate tissue proteins.* The coagulated surface proteins act as a protective barrier and prevent deep penetration of acids (*except hydrofluoric acid*). So, the main damage is restricted to lids, conjunctiva, and cornea. Therefore, acids produce limbal ischemia, symblepharon, corneal necrosis, and sloughing. Common acids involved are:

- Sulphuric acid (H_2SO_4)– used in industries and batteries in inverters.
- Hydrochloric acid (HCl).

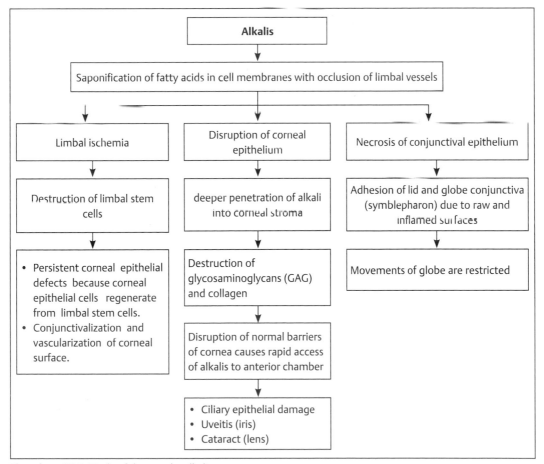

Flowchart 19.2 Mode of damage by alkalis.

- Blepharospasm.
- Conjunctival congestion.

Vertically oriented linear corneal abrasions indicate a FB under upper eyelid. Fluorescein staining is done to reveal the presence of corneal abrasion caused by FB. An infected FB can cause conjunctivitis. Retained FB carries a risk of secondary infection and corneal ulceration.

Iron FB often results in rust staining of the bed of corneal abrasion, but fades away with the time, leaving a corneal opacity.

Treatment

Treatment aims at removal of FB using slit-lamp under topical anesthesia. After removal of FB, antibiotic eye ointment is applied and eye is bandaged for a day. Protective glasses must be used to protect the eyes.

■ Intraocular Foreign Body (IOFB)

Penetrating injury may be associated with retention of FB in the eye (intraocular FB). Once the FB enters the eye, it may lodge in any of the structures it encounters (**Fig. 19.1**).

Types of FBs

IOFBs could be of three types.
- Foreign bodies producing inflammatory reactions:
  ◊ Iron and steel.
  ◊ Copper.
- Foreign bodies prone to result in infection:
  ◊ Stone.
  ◊ Organic FB.
  ◊ Spicules of wood.
- Inert FBs:
  ◊ Lead pellets.
  ◊ Glass.
  ◊ Gold.
  ◊ Platinum.
  ◊ Silver.

A piece of glass in anterior chamber is exceptionally difficult to observe because its refractive index is very close to that of aqueous.

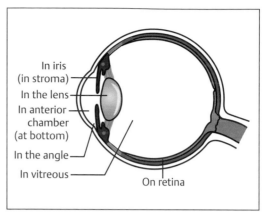

In iris (in stroma)
In the lens
In anterior chamber (at bottom)
In the angle
In vitreous
On retina

Fig. 19.1 Common sites of retention of IOFB. Abbreviation: IOFB, intraocular foreign body.

Modes of Damage to the Eye

An IOFB can cause damage the eye in three ways:
- By mechanical effects.
- By introduction of infection.
- By specific reactions of FB on intraocular tissues.

Mechanical Effects of IOFB in the Eye

A FB may enter the eye through either cornea or sclera. When it pierces the cornea, it may be retained in the anterior chamber or may be lodged in the iris stroma. It may pass into the lens, vitreous, or retina.

FB in the lens may gain access through the iris or pupil. When it passes through the iris, perforation leaves behind a hole in it at the site of impact. A hole in the iris is of great diagnostic significance since it rarely occurs, except due to perforation by a FB. A FB in the lens produces traumatic cataract.

FB in the vitreous: A FB may access the vitreous by various routes as depicted in **Fig. 19.2**.

FB in vitreous may cause either degenerative changes in vitreous gel, resulting in liquefaction of gel vitreous, or vitreous hemorrhage.

FB in the retina may get access through cornea or directly through scleral perforation. FB in retina may be surrounded by retinal hemorrhages and exudates and is eventually encapsulated by fibrous tissue. It may also cause pigmentary degeneration of retina, resulting in diminished vision. FB in retina can lead to retinal tears and eventual detachment.

Introduction of Infection by IOFB

Metallic FBs are often sterile owing to the heat generated during their transit through air. *Organic FBs (wood spicules) and stone* carry a higher risk of infection (endophthalmitis or panophthalmitis).

Reactions of IOFB on Ocular Tissues

Reactions of IOFBs on ocular tissues depend on its chemical nature. Metals like gold, silver, platinum, and glass produce no reaction (inert FB). Iron and copper produce specific degenerative effects, for example, iron causes siderosis and copper causes chalcosis. Lead pellets (shotgun pellets) and aluminum produce local irritative reactions, while zinc nickel and mercury FBs cause suppurative reaction.

Siderosis

Siderosis bulbi refer to the degenerative changes in the eye and brownish discoloration of ocular tissues induced by intraocular iron FB. **Flowchart 19.3** explains the mechanism of degenerative changes due to siderosis.

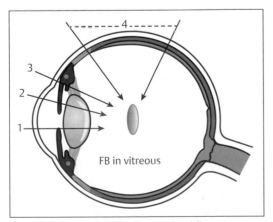

Fig. 19.2 Entry of FB in vitreous by different routes. 1, through pupillary area; 2, through iris substance; 3, through limbus; 4, through sclera. Abbreviation: FB, foreign body.

Clinical Features

1. Deposition of iron in lens epithelium: Oval patches of rusty deposit on anterior capsule of lens are the earliest manifestations of siderosis and are pathognomonic. These are arranged in a ring, corresponding with the edge of the dilated pupil, and result in development of cataract.

2. Deposition of iron in iris: Deposition of iron in sphincter pupillae leads to dilated pupils and causes initially greenish and later reddish–brown discoloration of iris (heterochromia iridis).

3. Deposition of iron in trabecular meshwork: It results in degenerative changes in trabecular meshwork, leading to rise of intraocular pressure (IOP) (secondary glaucoma).

4. Deposition of iron in retina: It causes pigmentary degeneration of retina associated with marked attenuation of blood vessels resembling retinitis pigmentosa and causing profound effect on vision.

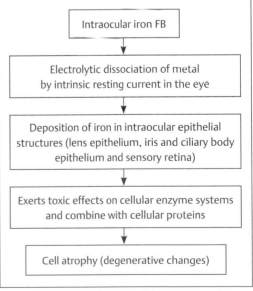

Flowchart 19.3 Mechanism of degenerative changes in siderosis.

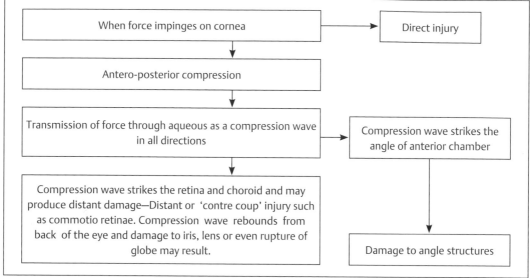

Flowchart 19.4 Mechanism of injury by blunt trauma.

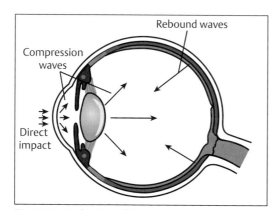

Fig. 19.4 Mechanism of injury by blunt trauma.

Cornea

Corneal Abrasion

Abrasion involves breach of corneal epithelium which stains with fluorescein dye.

Symptoms include pain, FB sensation, watering, photophobia, and blurring of vision (if over pupillary area).

Treatment involves patching of eye after applying ointment and topical cycloplegic drops to promote comfort.

Recurrent Corneal Erosion (Recurrent Traumatic Keratalgia)

It is more common following scratches, especially with body fingernails or paper. *In these cases,* epithelium is abnormally loosely attached to Bowman's membrane. Epithelium is torn off by upper lid generally upon awakening (due to abnormal adhesion of epithelium to underlying Bowman's membrane), resulting in manifestation of symptoms like acute pain, lacrimation, FB sensation, photophobia, and redness especially in the morning. The epithelial defect stains with fluorescein. The epithelial defect heals but recurs repeatedly.

Treatment
- Topical antibiotics.
- Hypertonic saline ointment at bed time to prevent recurrence.
- Topical lubricants.
- If attacks are repeated:
  ◊ Debridement is done.
  ◊ or Bandage soft contact lens are used.
  ◊ or Excimer laser phototherapeutic keratectomy is done.

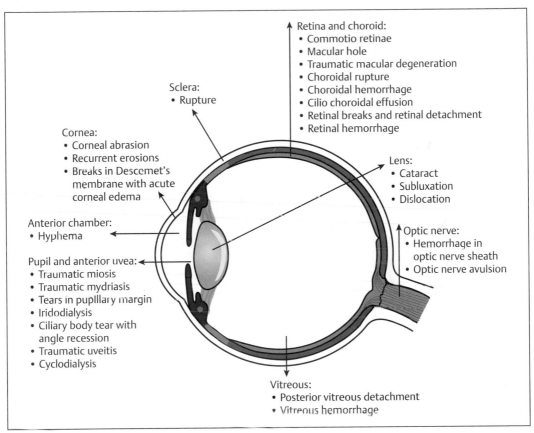

Sclera:
• Rupture

Retina and choroid:
• Commotio retinae
• Macular hole
• Traumatic macular degeneration
• Choroidal rupture
• Choroidal hemorrhage
• Cilio choroidal effusion
• Retinal breaks and retinal detachment
• Retinal hemorrhage

Cornea:
• Corneal abrasion
• Recurrent erosions
• Breaks in Descemet's membrane with acute corneal edema

Lens:
• Cataract
• Subluxation
• Dislocation

Anterior chamber:
• Hyphema

Optic nerve:
• Hemorrhage in optic nerve sheath
• Optic nerve avulsion

Pupil and anterior uvea:
• Traumatic miosis
• Traumatic mydriasis
• Tears in pupillary margin
• Iridodialysis
• Ciliary body tear with angle recession
• Traumatic uveitis
• Cyclodialysis

Vitreous:
• Posterior vitreous detachment
• Vitreous hemorrhage

Fig. 19.5 Injuries produced by blunt trauma.

Acute Corneal Edema

The forceps delivery may cause tears in Descemet's membrane, followed by acute corneal edema, and deep corneal opacities may develop. Blunt trauma may also cause dysfunction of corneal endothelium, folds in Descemet's membrane, and stromal edema which clear spontaneously.

Anterior Chamber

Hyphema (Blood in Anterior Chamber) (OP6.4)

The source of bleeding is tear in vascular iris or ciliary body. Hyphema may be mild or massive. It is usually associated with rise of IOP. If IOP remains high for >5 days, it may cause blood staining of cornea which simulates dislocation of clear lens in the anterior chamber. Rebleeding may occur up to a week after the original injury. *A total hyphema may be black or red. When black,* *it is called an "8-ball" or "black-ball" hyphema, indicating deoxygenated blood.* Symptoms include blurring of vision and redness of eye.

Treatment: To prevent blood staining of cornea:

• Lowering of IOP: Blunt trauma can cause elevation of IOP, so it is advisable to monitor IOP for a few days. If IOP is elevated, it must be treated appropriately by lowering it, so as to prevent secondary corneal blood staining.

• Paracentesis of anterior chamber to evacuate blood in case of massive hyphema and prevent blood staining of cornea.

To treat associated uveitis:

• Topical steroid drops.

• Topical atropine 1%.

• Oral prednisolone.

To prevent rebleed

- Bed rest for first 5 days.
- Avoid aspirin containing products.

Pupil and Anterior Uvea

Important manifestations in pupil and anterior uveal injury are:

- Contusion injury causes irritation of parasympathetic nerves, initially leading to traumatic miosis. Later on, paralysis of parasympathetic nerve fibers occurs, leading to traumatic mydriasis. Pupil remains moderately and permanently dilated.
- Iris pigment imprints on anterior lens capsule, which correspond to the size of miosed pupil, are called **Vossius' ring.**
- **Iridodialysis:** It is the tearing of iris root from its ciliary attachment. A dark biconvex area is visible near the limbus and the pupil is typically "**D-shaped.**" Large iridodialysis may lead to uniocular diplopia and glare (**Fig. 19.6**).
- **Damage to iris sphincter** (sphincter tear) results in radial iris tears at the pupillary margin.
- **Traumatic uveitis.**
- Damage to ciliary body can cause tear in ciliary body which splits the circular from radial (longitudinal) fibers. It results in *hyphema,* angle recession, *and* glaucoma.

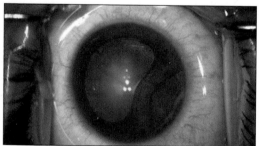

Fig. 19.6 Iridodialysis. Traumatic iridodialysis. Source: Goniosynechialysis and iris Reconstruction. In: Agarwal A, Narang P, ed. Video atlas of anterior segment repair and reconstruction: managing challenges in cornea, glaucoma, and lens surgery. 1st edition. Thieme; 2019.

Blunt trauma may also cause **cyclodialysis** (disinsertion of ciliary body from scleral spur), leading to hypotony.

Treatment depends on the type of injury (**Table 19.4**).

Lens

Blunt trauma may cause damage to the lens, resulting in the following listed manifestations:

Rupture of lens capsule usually at the posterior pole of the lens where it is thinnest. This causes accumulation of fluid, which marks out the *star-shaped cortical sutures* and lens fibers radiating from sutures (**Fig. 19.7**). This leads to the formation of a rosette-shaped cataract usually in the posterior cortex. This is also an effect of direct mechanical effect of injury to lens fibers.

Table 19.4 Type of injury and its treatment in blunt trauma (concussion injury)

Type of injury	Treatment
Angle recession	Monitor IOP and treat glaucoma.
Cyclodialysis	Hypotony is treated with: • Atropine B.I.D. to approximate ciliary body to sclera. • Steroids to decrease inflammation. • Laser photocoagulation.
Iridodialysis	• Cosmetic contact lens. • Surgical repair for monocular diplopia.
Iridocyclitis (uveitis)	Topical steroids.
Abbreviation: IOP, intraocular pressure.	

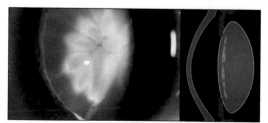

Fig. 19.7 Cataract in blunt trauma. Source: Traumatic cataract. In: Lang G, ed. Ophthalmology. A pocket textbook atlas. 3rd edition. Thieme; 2015.

Anterior subcapsular lens opacities: There appears a circular ring (**Vossius' ring**) of brown iris pigment on the anterior capsule, which is of pupillary size, owing to blunt trauma. This, in turn, causes anterior subcapsular lens opacities which underlie the Vossius' ring.

- Rupture of suspensory ligaments may cause subluxation of lens (if rupture is incomplete) or dislocation of lens (if rupture is complete). Subluxation of lens leads to variation in depth of anterior chamber, while the dislocation of lens causes tremulousness of iris on eye movements (**iridodonesis**).

Treatment depends on the type of lesion (**Table 19.5**).

Vitreous

Manifestations of injuries on vitreous by blunt trauma are as follows:

- **Posterior vitreous detachment** (PVD): It refers to dehiscence of posterior vitreous surface from retina.
- **Vitreous hemorrhage** (i.e., blood in vitreous cavity): Patients notice floaters and blurred vision. Red reflex may be poor or even absent.
- **Pigmentary opacities:** These are derived from uvea and are found floating in the anterior vitreous.

Retina and Choroid

Choroidal lesions following blunt trauma include:

- **Choroidal rupture:** It involves a tear in choroid, Bruch's membrane, and retinal pigment epithelium (RPE). It may be anterior rupture parallel to ora serrata, or posterior rupture temporal and concentric to optic nerve head. Choroidal rupture near macula may cause loss of central vision.
- Choroidal or suprachoroidal **hemorrhage**.
- **Ciliochoroidal effusion:** It is characterized by collection of fluid in suprachoroidal space. Besides blunt trauma, it may also occur after ocular surgery, uveitis, and hypotony.

Retinal lesions following blunt trauma include:

- **Commotio retinae (Berlin's edema):** Blunt trauma causes cloudy swelling of sensory retina at the posterior pole due to edema. "*Cherry red spot*" may be seen at fovea and may simulate central retinal artery occlusion (CRAO). In mild cases, the prognosis is good with spontaneous resolution. Severe involvement of macula may be associated with RPE degeneration, with pigmentary deposits at macula and intraretinal hemorrhage (**Fig. 19.8**).
- Retinal **hemorrhage**.
- **Macular lesions**.

Table 19.5 Treatment of different type of lenticular lesions in blunt trauma	
Type of lesion	**Treatment**
Traumatic cataract	It is managed on general lines.
Dislocation into anterior chamber	Extraction of lens with anterior vitrectomy as early as possible to prevent uveitis and glaucoma.
Dislocation into vitreous	Lens should be left there and spectacle correction of aphakia is done.
Subluxation of lens	Astigmatism in subluxation is usually impossible to correct and a correction for aphakic part of pupil may provide better visual results.

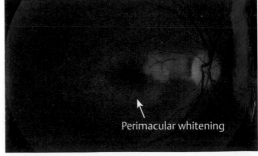

Perimacular whitening

Fig. 19.8 Commotio retinae. Source: What is seen with an ophthalmoscope. In: Biousse V, Newman N, ed. Neuro-ophthalmology illustrated. 2nd edition. Thieme; 2015.

- Macular degeneration.
- Macular hole.
- Retinal **breaks** and **retinal detachment** (RD).

Optic Nerve

Blunt trauma can cause damage to optic nerve (**traumatic optic neuropathy**). It is usually due to:

- Optic nerve sheath hematoma.
- Compression from orbital hemorrhage.
- Impingement of optic nerve in the fracture at the orbital apex.

Clinical features of injury to optic nerve includes:

- Decreased visual acuity.
- Initially, optic nerve head (ONH) and fundus are normal. The only finding being a relative afferent pupillary defect (**RAPD**).

RAPD may be absent if bilateral, symmetrical optic neuropathy is present. Later, most patients develop permanent visual impairment due to **optic atrophy**.

Avulsion of optic nerve is very rare with blunt trauma but occurs in gunshot wounds of orbit.

Globe Rupture in Blunt Trauma (Rupture of Sclera)

It may result from very severe blunt trauma. Rupture of sclera is an open-globe injury occurring from *inside outward*. Rupture is usually anterior in the vicinity of Schlemm's canal. Eyeball is least protected by orbital margin in the inferotemporal direction. The mechanism of injury to sclera following blunt trauma is explained in **Flowchart 19.5**.

In this condition, conjunctiva is often intact. Prolapse of intraocular structures such as iris, ciliary body, lens (subconjunctival dislocation of lens), and vitreous may occur. Intraocular hemorrhage may be profuse. There may be detachment of retina with or without subretinal or suprachoroidal hemorrhage.

Treatment

Prolapsed uvea (if covered by conjunctiva) is reposited or otherwise excised and scleral rupture is sutured. If rupture extends posterior to ciliary body, cryopexy should be done to prevent future retinal detachment. Vitreoretinal surgery may be required. Injuries to extraocular structures and orbit are dealt with in respective chapters.

■ Penetrating and Perforating Injuries

Laceration is a full-thickness **outside-to-inside wound** in ocular coats, which is caused by a sharp object. The globe opens at the site of impact. It can be subdivided into:

Penetrating injury: When the object transverses the coats only once, that is, it consists of a *single full-thickness* wound without an exit wound caused by sharp objects (such as knives, needles, arrows, scissors, etc.). It may be associated with intraocular retention of a FB.

Perforating injury: When the objects transverses the coats twice, that is, it consists of *two full-thickness wounds*—one entry and one exit

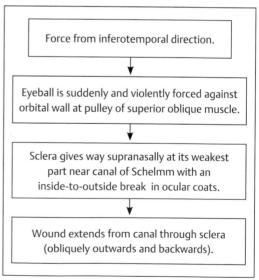

Flowchart 19.5 Mechanism of rupture of sclera.

wound. It is usually caused by bullet injuries or air gun pellets. The extent of damage caused by these FBs is determined by their kinetic energy.

■ Modes of Damage to the Eye

Penetrating injuries may damage the ocular structures in following manner:

- Mechanical effects of trauma.
- Introduction of infection.
- Sympathetic ophthalmitis.

Mechanical Effects of Penetrating/ Perforating Trauma

Wounds of lids: Horizontal cuts can damage levator palpebrae superioris (LPS) muscle, leading to ptosis. Severed LPS should be sutured and lid is repaired in layers. Injury near medial canthus may involve lacrimal canaliculi, which require intubation with silicone stent for 3 to 6 months and repair.

Wounds of conjunctiva are usually associated with subconjunctival hemorrhage. A wound of >3 mm should be sutured.

Wounds of cornea: These may be:

- Linear or lacerated.
- Small or large.
- Clean or infected.

Small corneal wounds generally do not require suturing as margins swell up after injury and become cloudy due to accumulation of fluid. Therefore, spontaneous closure of wound with restoration of anterior chamber takes place.

Large corneal wounds usually require suturing, especially if the anterior chamber is shallow or flat. Large peripheral corneal wounds may result in prolapse of iris, lens, and vitreous. *Iris prolapse* usually requires *iris abscission*. A recently prolapsed iris under conjunctiva may be reposited and wound is sutured with 10–0 nylon sutures. If *lens injury* is present, suture the corneal wound, remove the lens by *phacoemulsification and implant an IOL.*

If lens matter is present in the wound associated with *vitreous prolapse*, remove the lens matter followed by *anterior vitrectomy*.

Wounds of sclera: *Anterior scleral wounds* may be associated with iridociliary prolapse and vitreous incarceration. Reposit viable uveal tissue and cut prolapsed vitreous, and sclera is sutured. *Posterior scleral wounds* are frequently associated with retinal breaks. Suture the wound followed by prophylactic cryotherapy for retinal breaks.

Wounds of lens:

- If there exists a small wound in the anterior capsule, aqueous enters the lens, resulting in localized cloudiness and formation of a rosette-shaped cataract. The lens may become completely opaque.
- If the lens is damaged, lens matter in anterior chamber induces traumatic iridocyclitis and secondary glaucoma. To control inflammatory reaction, topical steroids, antibiotics, and cycloplegic are employed. Aspiration of lens matter is often necessary.
- If traumatic cataract is complicated by vitreous loss, remove the cataract, perform vitrectomy, and implant an IOL, if possible.

Introduction of Infections

Corneal wounds caused by organic matter often get infected by pyogenic organisms which may cause corneal abscess or rapid necrosis of entire cornea.

If pyogenic infection gets access into anterior chamber, it may cause:

- Purulent iridocyclitis with hypopyon.
- Endophthalmitis.
- Panophthalmitis.

Infected cases should be treated intensively with:

- Local antibiotics.
- Systemic antibiotics.
- Therapeutic keratoplasty (if there is danger of perforation of cornea).

Table 19.6 Ocular lesions caused by electrical injuries

Structure involved	Lesion
Cornea	Corneal opacities
Uvea	Uveitis
Lens	Cataract
Retina	Retinal hemorrhages
Optic nerve	Optic neuritis

■ Radiation Injuries

Radiations leading to ocular injuries can be UV, IR, and ionizing radiations.

Ultraviolet radiation: Exposure to an arc welding or reflected sunlight from snow, especially among mountain climbers, cause photophthalmia, superficial corneal ulceration, cataract, and snow blindness. Use of protective glasses prevents damage.

Treatment consists of topical cycloplegic, antibiotic ointment, and patching.

Infrared radiation: IR rays of sunlight are absorbed by the ocular pigment epithelium and cause photoretinitis (solar retinopathy).

Ionizing radiation: Ionizing radiation injuries to the eye are caused by radiations for the treatment of neoplasm in the vicinity of the eyes, such as tumors of nasopharynx. The radiations may cause damage to tissue or blood vessels, resulting in ischemic necrosis.

The common ocular lesions include:
- Loss of eyelashes.
- Radiation dermatitis.
- Dry eye syndrome.
- Keratitis.
- Necrosis of the conjunctiva and cornea.
- Radiation cataract.
- Radiation retinopathy.

Prophylaxis includes protection of the eye before exposure to radiation. Laser photocoagulation may be needed for proliferative radiation retinopathy. Radiation cataract is managed by surgery.

CHAPTER 20

The Lids

Anatomy..513

Edema of the Eyelids..518

Inflammation of the Lids..519

Inflammation of Lid Glands..522

Deformities of Eye Lashes..524

Disorder of Lid Margins and Palpebral Aperture...526

Tumors of Eyelids...539

Lid Injuries...543

Congenital Anomalies of Lids..543

■ Anatomy

The eyelids protect the eyes, spread the tear film over the eyeball, and help in drainage of the tears. The two eye lids meet at medial and lateral canthi. With open eyes, upper eye lid covers about ⅙th (2 mm) of the cornea and the lower eyelid just touches the limbus. Therefore, the palpebral aperture, with open eyes, measures approximately 10 mm (normal corneal diameter being 12 mm) vertically and 28 to 30 mm horizontally.

■ Lid Margin

The lids are covered anteriorly by skin and posteriorly by conjunctiva. The margin or free edge of the lid between anterior and posterior borders is called **intermarginal strip**. Other important features of lid margin are as follows:

- Anterior border is rounded.
- The sharp posterior border lies in contact with the globe.
- Intermarginal strip is covered by stratified squamous epithelium and divided into anterior and posterior part by a gray line. The eyelashes originate anterior to the gray line. The ducts of the Meibomian glands

open in a single row posterior to the gray line. The gray line is important as the lid is split at this level.

■ Structure of Eyelid

Eyelids contain muscle, glands, blood vessels, nerves and connective tissue. The eyelid is made up of several layers (superficial to deep) which are as follows (**Fig. 20.1**):

1. Skin.
2. Subcutaneous tissue.
3. Orbicularis oculi.
4. Fibrous layer (consisting of tarsal plate and orbital septum).
5. Lid retractors of upper and lower eyelids.
6. Retroseptal pad of fat.
7. Conjunctiva.

Skin

The skin of eyelids is the thinnest of the body, covered with finer hairs, and contain sebaceous and sweat glands. The upper eye lid skin crease (8–11 mm superior to the eyelid margin) is formed by the superficial insertion of levator aponeurotic fibers into the skin. At the margins, the eyelashes are arranged in two or more rows.

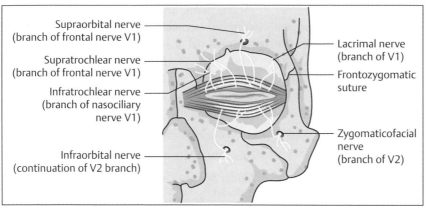

Fig. 20.3 Nerve supply of eyelids.

Supraorbital nerve (branch of frontal nerve V1)

Supratrochlear nerve (branch of frontal nerve V1)

Infratrochlear nerve (branch of nasociliary nerve V1)

Infraorbital nerve (continuation of V2 branch)

Lacrimal nerve (branch of V1)

Frontozygomatic suture

Zygomaticofacial nerve (branch of V2)

■ Nerve Supply

The eyelid is supplied by three cranial nerves (CNs) (III, V, and VII) and a sympathetic nerve (**Fig. 20.3**).

Sensory Nerve Supply

- The upper lid is supplied by the ophthalmic division of the trigeminal (V) nerve through the supraorbital nerve, supratrochlear nerve, and lacrimal nerve.
- The lower lid is supplied by the maxillary division of the trigeminal (V) nerve through the infraorbital (from V_2) and medial aspect from the infratrochlear nerve (V_1).

Motor Nerve Supply

- LPS is supplied by the 3rd nerve.
- Orbicularis oculi is supplied by the 7th nerve.
- Muller muscles are supplied by sympathetic nerves.

■ Lymphatic Drainage

The eyelids drain into preauricular and submandibular lymph nodes as depicted in **Fig. 20.4**.

■ Blood Supply

Arterial Supply

The internal and external carotid arteries contribute to lid arterial supply. Internal carotid artery gives off ophthalmic artery (medially) and

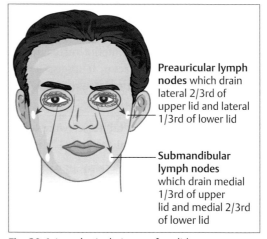

Preauricular lymph nodes which drain lateral 2/3rd of upper lid and lateral 1/3rd of lower lid

Submandibular lymph nodes which drain medial 1/3rd of upper lid and medial 2/3rd of lower lid

Fig. 20.4 Lymphatic drainage of eyelids.

lacrimal artery (laterally). Ophthalmic artery gives off supraorbital, supratrochlear, dorsal nasal, and two medial palpebral arteries, while lacrimal artery gives off two lateral palpebral arteries. External carotid artery gives off the following three arteries:

- *Facial* artery which continues as angular artery (it anastomoses with the dorsal nasal artery from the ophthalmic artery).
- *Superficial temporal* artery.
- *Infraorbital* artery (anastomose with vessels of the lower eyelid).

The two medial palpebral arteries arise as superior marginal vessel (supplying the upper lid) and inferior marginal vessel (supplying the lower lid), which pass horizontally as marginal arcades lying on the anterior tarsal surface 4 mm from the upper lid margin and 2 mm from the lower lid margin. In the upper lid, a peripheral arcade arises from the marginal arcade and lies on the anterior surface of the Muller muscle, just above the superior tarsal border. In the lower lid, no peripheral arcade exists. The two lateral palpebral arteries from the lacrimal artery pass medially to the upper and lower eyelids and anastomose with the marginal arcades (**Fig. 20.5**).

Venous Drainage

Each lid is drained by two plexuses: pretarsal plexus and post tarsal plexus. Pretarsal plexus drains into the subcutaneous vein, while the post tarsal plexus drains into the ophthalmic vein.

■ Glands of the Eyelids

There are five glands in the eyelids as described below (**Fig. 20.6**):

- Meibomian glands (tarsal glands): These are **modified sebaceous glands** located *in the tarsal plate*. There are approximately 30 glands in each lid, which are vertically directed and open by a single duct on the margin of the eyelids. Each gland consists of a central duct with multiple acini. The Meibomian glands synthesize lipids

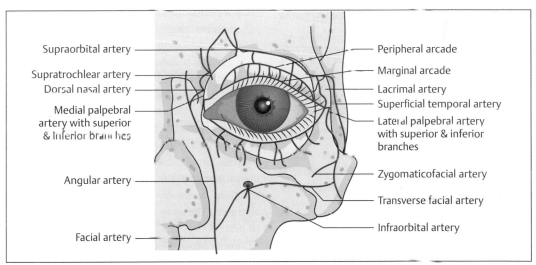

Fig. 20.5 Arterial blood supply of eyelids.

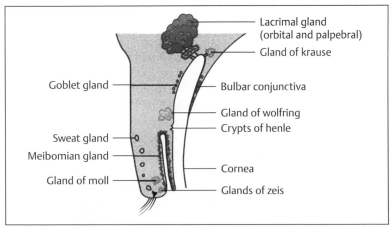

Fig. 20.6 Glands of eyelids.

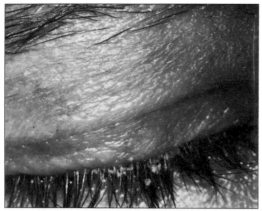

Fig. 20.7 Seborrheic blepharitis. Source: History. In: Singh K, Smiddy W, Lee A, ed. Opthalmology Review: A Case-Study Approach. 2nd Edition. Thieme; 2018.

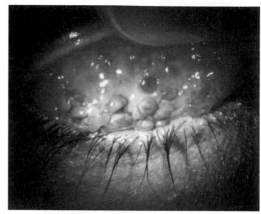

Fig. 20.8 Papillary conjunctivitis. Source: General Notes on the Causes, Symptoms, and Diagnosis of Cojunctivitis. In: Lang G, ed. Ophthalmology. A Pocket Textbook Atlas. 3rd Edition. Thieme; 2015.

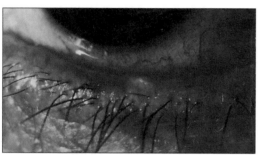

Fig. 20.9 Ulcerative blepharitis. Source: History. In: Singh K, Smiddy W, Lee A, ed. Ophthalmology Review: A Case-Study Approach. 2nd Edition. Thieme; 2018.

Sequelae

If infective blepharitis is not treated properly, it becomes chronic and causes (**Flowchart 20.1**).

- Madarosis: The lashes fall out and often not replaced. The condition is known as **madarosis**. Eyelashes may be replaced by small and distorted cilia.
- Trichiasis (misdirection of eyelashes).
- Tylosis (thickening of lid margin).
- Ectropion leading to epiphora.
- Eczema.
- Punctate epithelial erosions in the lower part of cornea (marginal keratitis).
- Recurrent styes.

Treatment

- Removal of scales after softening with luke-warm solution of 3% sodium bicarbonate.
- Application of antibiotic ointment at the lid margins after removing the scales (b.i.d or t.ds. for 2–3 weeks).
- Systemic tetracycline or doxycycline may be useful.
- Topical steroids are very effective in papillary conjunctivitis and marginal keratitis, as steroids control the hyper-sensitivity reaction.
- Tear substitutes as eyes with blepharitis show the associated tear film instability.
- Lid hygiene:
  ◇ Daily swabbing of lid margin after elimination of infection.
  ◇ Rubbing of lids is completely avoided.

Posterior Blepharitis

It is also called Meibomian blepharitis or meibomitis and caused by Meibomian gland dysfunction. Posterior blepharitis produces abnormal oil secretions. Bacterial lipases may result in the formation of free-fatty acids, increasing the melting point of the meibum.

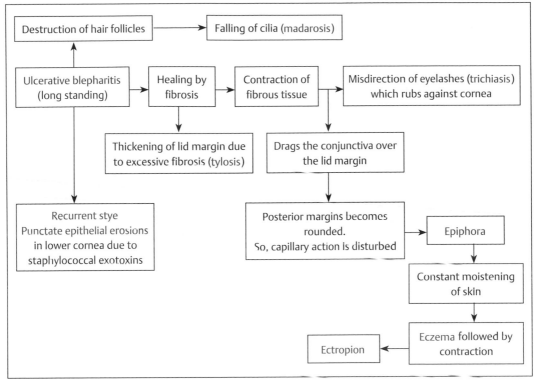

Flowchart 20.1 Sequelae of ulcerative blepharitis.

Thus, posterior blepharitis reduces Meibomian gland output, resulting in irritation of ocular surface, evaporation of tears, and instability of tear film.

Clinical Features

Oil droplets are seen at the Meibomian gland orifices. Pressure on the lid margin results in expression of Meibomian secretion that is turbid or toothpaste-like. In severe cases, expression is impossible due to inspissated secretions. Blockage of ducts may result in cystic dilatation of Meibomian ducts. The tear film is oily and foamy. The condition may result in papillary conjunctivitis and inferior corneal punctate epithelial erosions.

Treatment

Treatment modalities include:
- Warm compresses.
- Lid hygiene.
- Systemic tetracyclines.

- Topical antibiotics and steroids.
- Tear substitutes.

Systemic tetracyclines (doxycycline or minocycline) for 6 weeks are the mainstay of treatment. *Tetracyclines block the Staphylococcal lipase production.*

Parasitic Blepharitis

Etiology

The crab louse Phthirus pubis can cause blepharitis. It is adapted to living in pubic hairs and may be transferred to another hairy area such as chest, axillae, or eyelids in an infected person. The infestation of lashes (Pthiriasis palpebrum) is common in children living in poor hygienic conditions.

Clinical Features

It causes chronic irritation and itching of lids. The lice are anchored to the lashes with the claws.

> In patients with recurrent chalazion in old age, the histopathological examination (biopsy) must be done to rule out adenocarcinoma of Meibomian gland.

■ Molluscum Contagiosum

It is caused by a double-stranded DNA poxvirus. It presents as a small, multiple, white, and umbilicated swellings near the lid margin. It produces severe conjunctivitis and superficial keratitis (**Fig. 20.14**).

Treatment

The lesion should be incised and the substance resembling sebum is expressed.

The interior of the lesion is cauterized with tincture of iodine or pure carbolic acid.

■ Deformities of Eye Lashes

■ Trichiasis (OP2.1, 2.2, 2.3)

It is a condition in which cilia are misdirected backward and rub against the cornea (**Fig. 20.15**). It may occur in isolation or as a result of scarring of lid margin secondary to the following conditions:

- Trachoma (**Fig. 20.16**).
- Chronic blepharitis.
- Chemical burns.
- Injuries (mechanical or surgical).
- Pemphigoid.
- Herpes zoster ophthalmicus.
- Diphtheria.
- Stevens–Johnson syndrome.

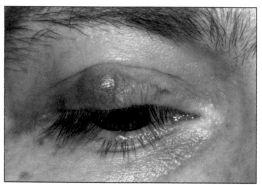

Fig. 20.13 Chalazion (meibomian cyst). G, ed. Ophthalmology. Source: Benign Eyelid And Periocular Tumors. In: Leatherbarrow B, ed. Oculoplastic Surgery. 3rd Edition. Thieme; 2019.

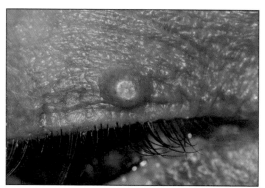

Fig. 20.14 Molluscum contagiosum. Source: Benign Eyelid and Periocular Tumors. In: Leatherbarrow B, ed. Oculoplastic Surgery. 3rd Edition. Thieme; 2019.

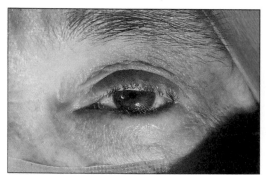

Fig. 20.15 Trichiasis. Source: History. In: Singh K, Smiddy W, Lee A, ed. Ophthalmology Review: A Case-Study Approach. 2nd Edition. Thieme; 2018.

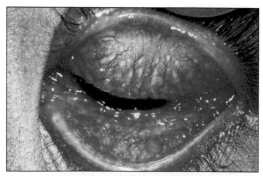

Fig. 20.16 Trachoma (stage II–III). Source: Trachoma. In: Lang G, ed. Ophthalmology. A Pocket Textbook Atlas. 3rd Edition. Thieme; 2015.

Clinical Features

Presenting symptoms include foreign body sensation, irritation, lacrimation, conjunctival congestion, pain, and photophobia.

There is posterior misdirection of lashes rubbing the cornea which cause punctate epithelial erosion, vascularization of cornea, and corneal ulceration.

Treatment

Following are the treatment modalities used for trichiasis:

- *Epilation* is a simple and temporary method of pulling out the misdirected eyelashes with forceps. It must be repeated every few weeks due to recurrences.
- *Electrolysis* is useful for few isolated lashes. In electrolysis, a fine needle is inserted into the root of eyelash and the follicle of eye lash is destroyed by passage of electric current of 2 mA. Then, the eye lash is removed. In diathermy, a current of 30 mA is applied for 10 seconds. The electrolysis is painful and tedious, therefore, local anesthesia can be injected into the lid margin.
- *Cryotherapy* is effective in eliminating many lashes. A cryoprobe at -20 degree C is applied after injecting local anesthesia, and the double freeze-thaw technique is applied. Cryotherapy may lead to depigmentation of the lid, skin necrosis, and damage to Meibomian gland which may affect the tear film.
- *Argon laser ablation* is useful for few scattered lashes and is less effective than cryotherapy.
- *Surgery* is undertaken if many cilia are displaced and resistant to other methods of treatment. The operative procedures are similar to that for entropion.

■ Distichiasis

In distichiasis, an extra row of lashes emerge at or is slightly behind the Meibomian gland orifices. These lashes are often directed posteriorly, rubbing the cornea. It may be congenital or acquired (associated with chemical injury Stevens–Johnson syndrome and ocular cicatricial pemphigoid). These are treated with cryotherapy or electrolysis (**Fig. 20.17**).

■ Madarosis

It is the decrease in number of eyelashes. The lashes that fall out are not replaced.

Etiology

Local:
- Chronic anterior lid margin disease.
- Burns.
- Radiotherapy or cryotherapy of lid tumors.

Skin disorders:
- Generalized alopecia.
- Psoriasis.

Systemic diseases:
- Hypothyroidism.
- Lepromatous leprosy.

Others:
- Iatrogenic.
- Trichotillomania (psychiatric disorder of hair removal).

■ Poliosis

It is a premature localized whitening of eyelashes and eyebrows (**Fig. 20.18**).

Etiology

- Chronic anterior blepharitis.
- Vogt–Koyanagi–Harada syndrome.
- Vitiligo.
- Tuberous sclerosis.

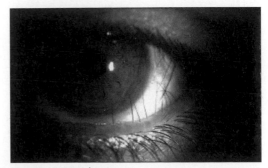

Fig. 20.17 Distichiasis.

■ Disorder of Lid Margins and Palpebral Aperture

Following are the common disorders of lid margins and palpebral aperture:

1. Drooping of upper lid (ptosis).
2. Lid retraction.
3. Abnormal position of lid margins:
   - Entropion.
   - Ectropion.
4. Miscellaneous disorder:
   - Symblepharon.
   - Ankyloblepharon.
   - Blepharophimosis.
   - Blepharochalasis.
   - Dermatochalasis.
   - Blepharospasm.
   - Lagophthalmos.

■ Ptosis (OP2.1, 2.2, 2.3)

Ptosis refers to drooping of the upper eyelid (**Fig. 20.19**). Normally, the upper eyelid covers the upper 2 mm of the cornea. If the upper eyelid covers more than 2 mm of cornea, it is labeled as drooping of the upper eyelid.

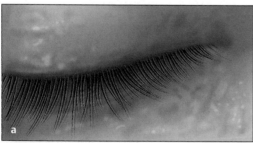

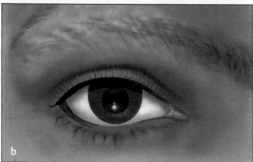

Fig. 20.18 (a, b) Poliosis.

Classification

Ptosis may be congenital or acquired, unilateral or bilateral, partial or complete, that is, ptosis may be of variable severity (mild, moderate, or severe).

Congenital ptosis is associated with imperfect differentiation of the LPS muscle; although, it may be associated with:

- Normal superior rectus function (simple congenital ptosis).
- Superior rectus weakness (as LPS with superior rectus is the last to be differentiated).
- Blepharophimosis syndrome.
- Synkinesis (synkinetic ptosis):
  ◇ Marcus Gunn jaw-winking syndrome.
  ◇ III nerve misdirection.

Acquired: Depending upon the cause, ptosis can be classified into:

- Neurogenic ptosis.
- Myogenic ptosis.
- Aponeurotic ptosis.
- Mechanical ptosis.

Neurogenic Ptosis

It is caused by innervational defects and includes:

- Oculomotor (III) nerve palsy: Ptosis may be due to involvement of entire III nerve or the superior division supplying the LPS muscle. In complete paralysis of the III nerve, if the lid is raised, diplopia results due to strabismus. Other features of third nerve palsy are provided in chapter 23.
- Horner's syndrome: It occurs due to involvement of oculosympathetic innervation and is characterized by:

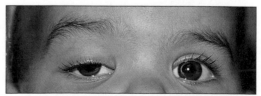

Fig. 20.19 Ptosis of the right upper lid. Source: History. In: Singh K, Smiddy W, Lee A, ed. Ophthalmology Review: A Case- Study Approach. 2nd Edition. Thieme; 2018.

◇ Ptosis (due to paralysis of Muller's muscle with preserved LPS function).

◇ Miosis (due to involvement of dilator pupillae).

◇ Anhydrosis (reduced ipsilateral sweating).

• Marcus Gunn jaw-winking syndrome: This form of synkinetic ptosis is typically unilateral and not hereditary. There is intermittent elevation of ptotic eyelid with contraction of the muscles of mastication (ipsilateral pterygoid muscle). It results in "winking" movement during jaw movements in relation to chewing or eating. It has been postulated that a branch of mandibular (II) division of V cranial nerve is misdirected to the LPS muscle.

• III nerve misdirection: Aberrant regeneration of III nerve palsy is frequent and results in bizarre movements of the upper lid on various eye movements. It may also be congenital.

Myogenic Ptosis

It is caused by the involvement of the LPS muscle itself or due to impaired transmission at the neuromuscular junction. It may be seen in the following mentioned conditions:

• *Simple congenital (myopathic) ptosis*: This simple congenital ptosis is due to a *developmental dystrophy of LPS muscle*. It is present at birth and remains stationary throughout life. The normal muscle fibers are replaced by fibrous tissue. Its characteristic features include the following:

• The ptotic lid is higher than the normal lid in down gaze due to poor relaxation of LPS muscle. In acquired ptosis, the affected lid is lower than the normal lid on down gaze.

• Upper lid crease is usually absent.

• LPS function is poor.

• Chin or eyebrows elevation is often present.

• It may be associated with an ipsilateral superior rectus weakness because of close embryonic association of LPS and superior rectus muscles.

> *If the ptosis is surgically corrected, the lid lag may worsen in down gaze.*

• *Blepharophimosis syndrome*: 6% of children with congenital ptosis may be associated with blepharophimosis syndrome. The palpebral apertures are horizontally shortened (blepharophimosis), resulting in telecanthus (a wide intercanthal distance, **Fig. 20.20**). It can be managed by canthoplasty.

• *Myasthenia gravis*: It is caused by a deficiency of acetylcholine which results in inability of the muscle fibers to respond to the nerve stimulation. The extraocular muscles (particularly the LPS muscle) are often the first to be affected. Its characteristic features include the following:

◇ Ptosis is often initially unilateral and becomes bilateral gradually.

◇ The symptoms are minimal early in the day but gradually worsen toward evening due to fatigue.

◇ The eyelid twitches or slowly falls on prolonged up gaze.

◇ The weakness of extraocular muscles causes convergence insufficiency and diplopia but pupillary muscles are seldom affected.

◇ The accompanying symptoms are difficulties in swallowing, chewing, talking, combing, breathing, and walking.

Diagnostic test for myasthenia gravis is **Tensilon test**. In this, IV injection of anticholinesterase (Tensilon) combines with cholinesterase and blocks its enzymatic action, resulting in accumulation of acetylcholine at the neuromuscular junction; thereby, providing a temporary but rapid improvement in muscle action.

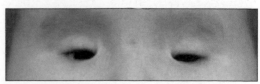

Fig. 20.20 Blepharophimosis syndrome. Source: Codner M, McCord, ed. Eyelid & periorbital surgery. 2nd edition. Thieme; 2016.

> *Ptosis repair in M. gravis patients may cause postoperative ocular exposure due to coexisting orbicularis muscle weakness or a poor Bell's phenomenon.*

- *Dystrophia myotonica* (myotonic dystrophy): In this condition, ptosis is associated with weakness of the facial muscles, resulting in mournful facial expression.
- *Progressive external ophthalmoplegia*: It presents in early adulthood with gradually developing ptosis. The other extraocular muscle soon becomes involved, resulting in diffuse ophthalmoplegia. The eyes gradually become fixed in primary position or turned slightly downward. Bell's phenomenon is absent. The pupillary reactions and power of accommodation remain unaffected.

Aponeurotic Ptosis

It is the most common form of acquired ptosis and develops secondary to involutional changes in the levator aponeurosis. The dehiscence or stretching of levator aponeurosis causes slowly progressive ptosis. Aponeurotic dehiscence may occur following ocular surgery or trauma. Its characteristic features include the following:

- LPS function is usually good in this form of ptosis.
- High upper lid crease (owing to loss of aponeurotic attachment).
- The eyelid above the tarsal plate appears to be unusually thin and the superior sulcus deepens.

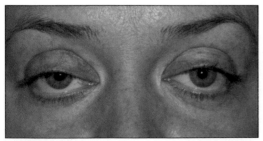

Fig. 20.21 Blepharochalasis. Source: Dermatochalsis. In: Leatherbarrow B, ed. Oculoplastic Surgery. 3rd Edition. Thieme; 2019.

Aponeurotic ptosis may be associated with the following conditions:

1. *Ptosis and blepharochalasis:* Ptosis may be associated with blepharochalasis. True blepharochalasis is hereditary in most instances and manifests in childhood with recurrent attacks of severe lid edema. Eventually, the levator aponeurosis becomes thinned and stretched. The orbital septum breaks down and orbital fat may prolapse into the eyelid. All of these factors cause the eyelid to droop (**Fig. 20.21**).
2. *Ptosis and normal pregnancy:* Ptosis may be associated with normal pregnancy which might be due to high-progesterone levels in late pregnancy and consequent increased interstitial fluid content of the tissues. It weakens the attachment of levator aponeurosis to the tarsus. The incipient levator disinsertions then become manifest due to the physical stress of parturition.
3. *Hyperthyroidism and ptosis:* Hyperthyroidism can lead to ptosis. Aponeurotic disinsertion secondary to inflammation is more likely.

Mechanical Ptosis

Mechanical ptosis is caused by increased weight of eyelid and scar tissue that interferes with eyelid mobility. It may be caused by tumors of upper lid, multiple chalazia, neurofibromatosis, severe lid edema, and scarring in trachoma and ocular pemphigoid.

Pseudoptosis

It is an apparent drooping of upper eye lid resulting from:

- Insufficient posterior support to the eye lid as in congenital anophthalmos, microphthalmos, phthisis bulbi, and following enucleation.
- Dermatochalasis in which a fold of skin overhangs a normally placed lid margin.

It may obstruct vision and require blepharoplasty (**Fig. 20.22**).

- Contralateral lid retraction.
- Ipsilateral hypotropia: There is a correlation between the position of eyelid and the direction of gaze. The persons with hypotropia may appear to have a unilateral ptosis. This pseudoptosis disappears when hypotropic eye assumes fixation on covering the normal eye.

Clinical Evaluation

A detailed history and proper clinical examination are necessary for thorough evaluation of a case of ptosis.

History

A thorough history is necessary and should include:

- Age at the onset of ptosis and its duration.
- History of its improvement or worsening since the onset.
- History of trauma.
- History of any eye surgery.
- History of associated systemic symptoms and diplopia
- Variability of ptosis during the day and fatigue.
- History of any medication.

Examination

- Assessment of visual acuity and refractive error: In ptosis, stimulus deprivation can

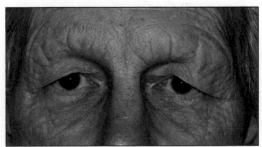

Fig. 20.22 Bilateral upper eyelid dermatochalasis. Source: Dermatochalsis. In: Leatherbarrow B, ed. Oculoplastic Surgery. 3rd Edition. Thieme; 2019.

cause amblyopia which should be looked for and treated.

- Examination of pupil must be done because miosis occurs in Horner's syndrome, while mydriasis happens in III nerve palsy.
- Look for blepharophimosis syndrome (telecanthus, epicanthus inversus. and shortening of lids).
- Look for upper lid crease which is the vertical distance between the lid margin and the lid crease in down gaze. Normal lid crease measures 8 to 10 mm. An absent lid crease is often accompanied by poor levator function, while a deeper upper lid sulcus on the side suggests levator disinsertion.
- Look for corneal sensations as there will be some exposure postoperatively.
- Look for strabismus: The patient should also be examined for strabismus since correction of strabismus may relieve the ptosis. Correction of an ipsilateral hypotropia (in superior rectus weakness with congenital ptosis) may improve the degree of ptosis. In case of horizontal strabismus with ptosis, surgery for both can be performed at the same sitting because the result of one rarely influences the result of the other.
- Look for Bell's phenomenon: To test for Bell's phenomenon, the examiner attempts to separate the lids while the patients close them tightly. The eyes are in upgaze with normal Bell's phenomenon. If Bell's phenomenon is absent, surgical correction of ptosis may be associated with increased incidence of exposure keratitis.
- Look for jaw-winking phenomenon.
- Look for fatigability (tested by asking the patient to look up without blinking for 30 seconds): The progressive drooping of upper lid or inability to maintain upgaze indicates myasthenia gravis.
- Assessment of the function of Muller's muscle: It is tested by applying 10% phenylephrine drops to the eye on the side of ptosis. It stimulates the sympathetically

innervated Muller's muscle. If the upper lid assumes a normal level 10 to 15 minutes after instillation of the drops, it means the normal functioning of Muller's muscle. Therefore, the resection and advancement of Muller's muscle and conjunctiva can relieve the ptosis.

- Assessment of margin reflex distance (**MRD**) (**Fig. 20.23**):

MRD is the distance between the central portion of the upper lid margin and the corneal light reflex, with the eye in primary position of gaze.

Vertical corneal diameter = approximately 12 mm

So, distance of upper limbus from pupillary reflex = 6.0 mm

Covering of cornea by upper lid = 2 mm

Therefore, normal MRD = 6 – 2 = 4 mm (with a variation of 1 mm)

MRD is the most important measurement in assessing the degree of ptosis (**Table 20.2**).

In unilateral ptosis, the difference between MRD of two eyes determines the degree of ptosis.

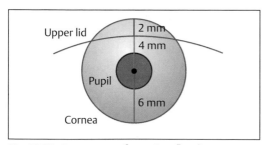

Fig. 20.23 Assessment of margin reflex distance.

The position of each of the eyelid margins should be noted when the eyes are up, down, and straight. In many cases of unilateral "congenital" ptosis, the eyelid covers the cornea by a similar amount in downward gaze. Sometimes, however, the lid of the ptotic eye is slightly higher than that of the normal eye on down gaze. The levator muscle, being congenitally dystrophic in congenital ptosis, may fail to relax by reciprocal innervation. This causes the lid to depress deficiently. *This is a useful diagnostic sign in differentiating congenital ptosis from acquired ptosis.* In acquired ptosis, the lid of the ptotic eye is usually slightly lower than that of the normal eye in the downward gaze.

- Palpebral fissure height: It is the distance between the upper and lower lid margins in the pupillary plane with the eyes in primary gaze.
- Levator function: The levator function must be assessed and is determined by measuring the lid excursion from down gaze to extreme up gaze (Berke's method). A thumb of one hand is placed firmly over the patient's brow, with the eyes in down gaze. It will fix the frontalis muscle. Place a scale opposite the lid margin and note the reading. Now, the patient is asked to look up as far as possible without moving the head. The amount of excursion is measured with the rule. Levator function can be graded as depicted in **Table 20.3**.

Management

Surgery is often the only option for the treatment of ptosis. However, in complete III nerve palsy, the elevation of ptotic lid leads to diplopia

Table 20.2 Assessment of degree of ptosis by measuring MRD		
Amount of ptosis	**MRD**	**Grading of ptosis**
Ptosis of ~2 mm	2	Mild ptosis
Ptosis of ~3 mm	1	Moderate ptosis
Ptosis of 4 mm or more	Less than 0	Severe ptosis
Abbreviation: MRD, margin reflex distance.		

Table 20.3 Grading of the levator function

Amount of excursion	Levator function
15 mm or more	Normal
8 mm or more	Good
5–7 mm	Fair
4 mm or less	Poor

because of ophthalmoplegia. Hence, the surgery is contraindicated.

Aim of Operation

The aim of any operation should be:

- To lift the ptotic lid *above the pupillary aperture* when the eyes are in primary position.
- *Height* of two lids should be equal.
- *Mobility of the lid* should be adequate when blinking.
- There should be a *normal lid fold*.
- There should be *no diplopia*.

When to Correct Ptosis Surgically

- Mild ptosis need to be corrected only if the patient desires good cosmesis.
- Severe, congenital ptosis may cause amblyopia and must be surgically repaired as soon as possible to preserve normal vision.
- Bilateral ptosis interfering with child's learning walk must be operated upon as early as possible.
- An acquired ptosis from a traumatic injury or III nerve palsy should not be operated for 6 to 9 months because often some levator function will return.

Contraindications for Ptosis Surgery

- Poor orbicularis muscle function.
- Loss of corneal sensations.
- Dry eyes.
- III nerve palsy causing total ophthalmoplegia.

Absence of Bell's phenomenon is not a contraindication for surgery in patients with congenital ptosis; however, extreme caution should be taken, as it may cause exposure keratitis during sleep.

Choice of Surgery for Ptosis

In general, there are three procedures for ptosis surgery:

- Tarso–Muller muscle resection (Fasanella–Servat operation): Indicated in Horner's syndrome and very mild congenital ptosis.
- Levator resection: Indicated in ptosis of any cause with levator function of at least 5 mm.
- Frontalis sling operation (brow suspension): Indicated in case of severe ptosis (>4 mm) with poor LPS (<4 mm) function, Marcus–Gunn jaw-winking syndrome, III nerve misdirection, and blepharophimosis syndrome. Brow suspension involves the suspension of tarsus from the frontalis muscle with a sling of fascia lata or prolene (a non-absorbable material).

Surgically, LPS aponeurosis can be approached through the skin (Everbusch's operation) or conjunctiva (Blaskovics' operation), but Muller muscle can be approached transconjunctivally (Fasanella–Servat operation). In case of severe ptosis with poor LPS function or unsatisfactory results from previous levator resection, brow suspension is done.

In severe unilateral ptosis, weakening of the opposite normal levator followed by bilateral sling operation can be considered for symmetric results. However, many surgeons prefer to leave the normal eyelid alone.

One drawback of all ptosis procedures is that perfect cosmetic and functional results cannot be expected in every case. The final result depends on the nature of ptosis and the type of operation selected.

In general, *levator resection is performed in ptosis cases with levator action of 4 mm or more, whereas frontalis sling operation is performed when the levator function is poor, that is, 3 mm or less.*

There is an **old rule of thumb** that the levator should be resected 2 mm or the tarsus resected 1 mm for each millimeter of desired elevation of the eyelid. In congenital ptosis, this always leads to an under correction. This may well be because

Muller's muscle is resected by an equal amount in the standard procedures, and a large amount of lifting power is thereby lost.

LPS resection of 10 to 13 mm is termed small; 14 to 17 mm is termed moderate; 18 to 22 mm is termed large; and 23 mm or more is the maximum resection.

The amount of resection can vary depending on the variations in levator function and the severity of ptosis (**Table 20.4**).

In treating **congenital ptosis**, it is wise to choose the larger resection because overcorrection is easier to treat than undercorrection when dealing with the congenital type. In treating **acquired ptosis**, the resection must be more conservative. Here, overcorrection is easy to obtain but may be disastrous.

■ Eyelid Retraction

The upper lid normally covers the 2 mm of cornea. When the upper lid margin is at or above the superior limbus, the lid retraction is suspected (**Fig. 20.24**).

Causes of lid retraction are:
- Congenital:
  ◇ Duane's retraction syndrome.
  ◇ Down's syndrome.
  ◇ Thyroid eye disease.
- Neurogenic:
  ◇ Contralateral unilateral ptosis.

◇ Facial palsy (due to unopposed LPS action).
◇ III nerve misdirection.
◇ Sympathomimetics drops.
◇ Parinaud syndrome (collier sign of midbrain).
- Mechanical:
  ◇ Surgical over correction of ptosis.
  ◇ Scarring of upper lid skin due to burn or trauma.
- Miscellaneous:
  ◇ Uremia.
  ◇ Prominent globe (pseudo-lid retraction).

■ Entropion (OP2.1, 2.2, 2.3)

It refers to the inward rolling of the lid margin toward the globe (**Fig. 20.25**).

Types

The entropion may be:
- Involutional (age-related).
- Spastic.
- Cicatricial.
- Congenital.

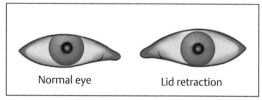

Normal eye   Lid retraction

Fig. 20.24 Eyelid retraction.

Table 20.4 Grading of ptosis with LPS function and surgical procedures		
Severity of ptosis	**Levator function**	**Surgical procedure**
Mild ptosis (1.5–2 mm)	Good (≥ 8 mm)	• Small (10–13) LPS resection • Fasanella-servat operation
Moderate ptosis (3 mm)	Good (≥ 8 mm) Fair (5–7 mm) Fair <5- rare	• Moderate (14–17 mm) LPS resection • Large (18–22 mm) LPS resection • Maximum (23 or more) LPS resection
Severe ptosis (4 mm or more)	Fair (5–7 mm) Poor (4 mm or less)	• Maximum (23 or more) LPS resection • Frontalis sling operation*

Note: * If LPS function is poor, maximum (23 or more) LPS resection is done as the first procedure but due to poor LPS function, the lids tend to fall from 1 to 3 mm in which case frontalis sling is done as a secondary procedure. Abbreviation: LPS, levator palpebrae superioris.

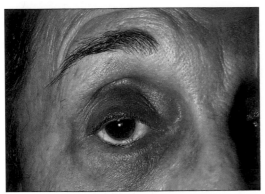

Fig. 20.25 Entropion. Source: History. In: Singh K, Smiddy W, Lee A, ed. Opthalmology Review: A Case-Study Approach. 2nd Edition. Thieme; 2018.

Involutional (age-related) Entropion

It mainly affects the lower lid because the upper lid has a broader and stable tarsus. The lower lid derives stability from the orbicularis oculi, lower lid retractors, tarsus and canthal ligaments.

Pathophysiology

Entropion occurs due to the combination of the following:

- *Horizontal lid laxity: Horizontal lid stability is provided by canthal ligaments and tarsal plate.* Laxity of medial and lateral canthal ligaments result in loss of horizontal lid support. Smaller tarsal plate allows for more horizontal lid laxity and orbicularis override. Females have smaller tarsal plates than males which explains, in part, why entropion is more prevalent in females.
- *Vertical lid instability: Vertical lid stability is provided by the lower lid retractors* which are analogous to levator aponeurosis and Muller's muscle in the upper lid. The capsule of palpebral head of retractors fuses with the septum at the inferior border of the tarsal plate. Loosening of these vertical stabilizing structures due to disinsertion, atrophy, or dehiscence of lower lid retractors allows the lid to rotate inwards.
- *Overriding of pretarsal by preseptal orbicularis oculi muscle:* The lower lid retractors have fine extensions to the orbicularis oculi and overlying skin. As these connections weaken or dehisce, the preseptal orbicularis can travel superior and override the pretarsal muscle. It tends to move the lower border anteriorly away from the globe and upper border toward the globe, resulting in the inward rolling of the lid margin.
- *Atrophy of orbital fat:* Orbital fat content decreases with age, producing enophthalmos. Greater spacing between the globe and eyelid creates lid laxity. Enophthalmos also allows for greater orbicularis override, resulting in entropion.

Treatment

- *Medical therapy*: It includes a temporary treatment with lubricants, taping, and soft bandage contact lens.
- *Surgical treatment:* The aim of surgery for involutional entropion is to correct the underlying problems involved in its pathogenesis. The surgery for involutional entropion may involve a combination of more than one procedure which includes:
  ◊ Resection and reconstruction of lateral canthal tendon.
  ◊ Wies procedure.
  ◊ Jones procedure.

Spastic Entropion

It comes about due to the spasm of orbicularis oculi which can be induced by local irritation or infection. Spastic entropion is almost always restricted to the lower lid. Spastic entropion is thought to be a subset of involutional entropion, and the spasm of orbicularis oculi can unmask the symptomatic involutional changes that allow the orbicularis to ride up in front of tarsal plate and approximate the lid margins and turn them inwards, resulting in temporary entropion. The condition is found particularly in old age and may be caused by tight bandaging. It is favored by narrowness of palpebral aperture (blepharophimosis).

Cicatricial Ectropion

It is caused by burns, trauma, and chronic inflammations of skin, resulting in scarring of the skin and underlying tissues which pulls the eyelid away from the globe.

Treatment

It includes:

- Localized areas with scarring can be released by **Z-plasty** or **V–Y operation**.
- Severe generalized scars require skin grafts.

Paralytic Ectropion

It is caused by:

- Facial nerve palsy.
- Parotid surgery.
- Head injury.
- Intracranial surgery.
- Tumors (acoustic neuroma).
- Middle ear disease.

Treatment

It includes temporary and permanent measures. *Temporary measures* are aimed at protecting the cornea, especially for temporary paralysis, and include:

- Lubricating drops.
- Ointments.
- Taping of eyelids during sleep.

Permanent measures are considered in permanent paralysis of facial nerve. The treatment is aimed at reducing the dimensions of palpebral aperture by one of the following procedures:

- *Medial canthoplasty*: The eyelids are sutured medial to lacrimal puncta and the fissure at inner canthus is shortened.
- *Lateral tarsorrhaphy*: The palpebral aperture is shortened by suturing the lids at the outer canthus. In this procedure, the lateral edges of upper and lower lid are freshened and then sutured (OP4.7).

Mechanical Ectropion

It is caused by tumor of lower eyelid which mechanically everts the lid.

Treatment

The treatment involves the removal of underlying cause.

Congenital Ectropion

It is a rare condition and more frequently associated with Down syndrome. It may involve both upper or lower eyelids and is due to a developmental vertical foreshortening of anterior lamellar tissue, resulting in eversion of lid margin.

Treatment

It often requires no treatment as the condition may resolve spontaneously or may need surgical intervention (full-thickness skin graft) for vertical lengthening of anterior lamellar tissue.

Grading

It can be divided into three grades:

Mild: The puncta is not apposed to the globe in up gaze.

Moderate: The puncta is not apposed even in primary gaze and there is eversion of the entire lid margin.

Severe: Palpebral conjunctiva fornix are exposed in severe cases.

Clinical Features

The puncta drains tears from the palpebral sac to the lacrimal sac. Due to eversion of lower punctum, the tears are not drained into the nose but overflow onto the cheek (epiphora). A long-standing ectropion can lead to chronic conjunctivitis due to exposure. Conjunctiva becomes dry and thickened. In severe cases, exposure keratitis may occur.

■ Symblepharon (OP3.7)

It is a partial or complete adhesion of the palpebral conjunctiva with the bulbar conjunctiva, resulting in adhesion between the eyelid and eyeball (**Fig. 20.27**). It results from:

- Burns (chemical or heat).
- Trauma.

- Conjunctival ulceration.
- Membranous conjunctivitis.
- Ocular surgeries.
- Ocular cicatricial pemphigoid.
- Stevens–Johnson syndrome.
- Diphtheria.

Types

The bends of fibrous tissue are formed between the lid and the globe which may be narrow or broad and may involve the fornices. Depending upon the site of adhesions, the symblepharon can be anterior, posterior, or total (**Table 20.5**).

Clinical Features

Characteristic clinical features of symblepharon are:

- Limitation of ocular movements.
- Diplopia due to restricted motility.
- Lagophthalmos (inability to close the lids efficiently).
- Cosmetic disfigurement.

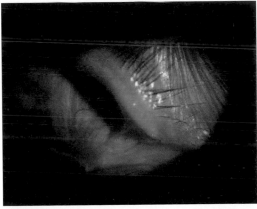

Fig. 20.27 Symblepharon.

Treatment

Once the bands are formed, they need excision and the raw surfaces should be covered with conjunctival, buccal mucosal, or amniotic membrane graft. A therapeutic bandage contact lens may be used to prevent the formation of adhesions between the raw surfaces.

Prevention

Symblepharon formation can be prevented by:

- Frequent use of a glass rod coated with lubricant and swept around the fornices.
- Therapeutic bandage contact lens.

■ Ankyloblepharon

It is the adhesion between the margins of the upper and lower eyelids.

It may be complete or partial and is usually associated with symblepharon.

It may be either congenital or may result following burns.

Treatment

The adhesions between the lid margins are excised and the lids are separated and kept apart during the healing process. If the angle of lid is also involved, epithelial grafts should be used to prevent the recurrence.

■ Blepharophimosis

It is the narrowing of palpebral fissure. It may be congenital or acquired. In acquired blepharophimosis, the presence of a vertical fold of skin at the lateral canthus (*epicanthus lateralis*) obscures it.

Table 20.5 Types of symblepharon	
Type of symblepharon	**Extent of adhesions**
Extent of adhesionsnn on	Bends are limited to anterior parts between lid and bulbar conjunctiva or cornea. Fornix is not involved.
Ends are limited to ant	The fornix is also involved, so the lid is completely adherent to the eyeball over a considerable area.
The lid is complete	The lid is completely adherent to the globe.

single or multiple, flesh-colored, and sessile or pedunculated.

Treatment

Treatment modalities involve the following:
- Electrocautery.
- Chemical cauterization.
- CO_2 laser ablation.
- Simple excision.

Hemangioma

Hemangiomas are found along the distribution of first and second divisions of trigeminal nerve. In the Sturge–Weber syndrome, hemangiomas of the lid and face are often associated with hemangioma of the choroid, leptomeninges, and glaucoma. It occurs in two forms: capillary hemangioma and cavernous hemangioma.

- *Capillary hemangioma*: It is common vascular lesion of childhood. It appears as a superficial, red, raised nodular mass which blanches with pressure. Initially, it grows followed by a period of stabilization. Small lesions undergo subsequent involution over several years. It may be confused with nevus flammeus, which is usually flatter, darker, and does not blanch with pressure (**Fig. 20.29**).
- *Cavernous hemangioma*: It usually appears during adulthood and does not normally undergo spontaneous regression. It is superficial and composed of dilated capillaries lying in the subcutaneous tissue. The lesions are dark blue, compressible, and increase in size on crying or lowering the head due to venous congestion.

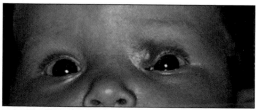

Fig. 20.29 Capillary hemangioma. Source: Selected Orbital Disorders. In: Leatherbarrow B, ed. Oculoplastic Surgery. 3rd Edition. Thieme; 2019.

Treatment

- *Small hemangioma* are left alone as spontaneous resolution occurs in most of the cases.
- *Large hemangioma* may interfere with vision and cause amblyopia or strabismus, requiring treatment. The treatment modalities include:
    - ◊ Intralesion injection of triamcinolone acetonide (40 mg) and betamethasone sodium phosphate (6 mg).
    - ◊ Systemic corticosteroids may be given on alternate days for large diffuse tumors.
    - ◊ Superficial radiotherapy (100–200 rad) monthly may be given for 6 months.
    - ◊ Surgical excision using a cutting diathermy may be needed in some cases.

Neurofibroma

It may be seen on the eyelid as a part of generalized neurofibromatosis (von Recklinghausen's disease). The disease involves eye, skin, and the central nervous system (CNS). The plexiform neurofibroma, characteristic of type I neurofibromatosis, often occurs as a diffuse infiltration of the eyelid and orbit. Multiple pedunculated growth of varying sizes may be seen on the skin of the eyelid. It may cause mechanical ptosis with an S-shaped curvature. Small multiple tumors are distributed along the hypertrophied nerves.

Xanthelasma

It is commonly located near the inner canthus. It usually affects elderly women. It presents as bilateral, symmetrical, soft, slightly raised, yellow plaques (**Fig. 20.30**). It is sometimes associated with diabetes and hypercholesterolemia. Recurrence is quite common.

Treatment

Treatment modalities include:
- Surgical excision.
- Laser ablation.
- Topical trichloroacetic acid.

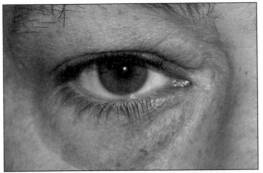

Fig. 20.30 Xanthelasma. Source: Benign Eyelid & Periocular Tumors. In: Leatherbarrow B, ed. Oculoplastic Surgery. 3rd Edition. Thieme; 2010.

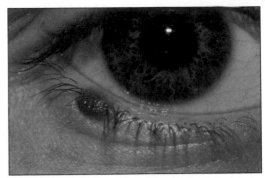

Fig. 20.31 Naevi. Source: Benign Eyelid & Periocular Tumors. In: Leatherbarrow B, ed. Oculoplastic Surgery. 3rd Edition. Thieme; 2010.

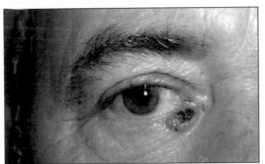

Fig. 20.32 Basal cell carcinoma. Source: Malignant Eyelid Tumors. In: Codner M, McCord C, ed. Eyelid & Periorbital Surgery. 2nd Edition. Thieme; 2016.

Naevi

These are derived from nevus cells or nevocytes which usually form nests of cells within the epidermis. These are usually pigmented, affect the lid margin, and involve both the skin and conjunctiva. It typically occurs during childhood as small and flat tan macules, and consists of nevus cells arranged in an alveolar manner (**Fig. 20.31**). It rarely undergoes malignant transformation.

Treatment

Treatment is generally not required unless cosmesis is desired. It may be removed by complete and extensive excision.

■ Malignant Tumors of Eyelid

These include carcinomas, sarcomas, and malignant melanomas.

Basal Cell Carcinoma (BCC)

It is the most common type of eyelid tumor (90%). Risk factors include people with fair skin and chronic exposure to sunlight. It rarely occurs before 40 years of age. BCC most often occurs in the lower eyelid and shows predilection for the medial canthus (**Fig. 20.32**). It commences as a small nodule which ulcerates in its central part. The edges of ulcer are raised and indurated. It spreads very slowly, extending under the skin in all directions and penetrating deeply like a rodent (hence the name "rodent" ulcer). Clinical types include nodular-ulcerative, sclerosing, and pigmented. Nodulo-ulcerative type is the most common presentation.

BCC of the eyelid is locally invasive and can invade the orbital bones. It rarely spreads to lymph nodes. Since its metastasis is rare, therefore the prognosis for this type of tumor is very good.

Treatment

The goal of therapy is the complete removal of tumor cells with preservation of unaffected eyelid and periorbital tissues. An incisional biopsy bilateral and give rise to appearance of convergent squint (pseudo-esotropia). It may disappear with the development of nose.

Small folds are treated by Y–V plasty, while large folds require a Mustarde Z-plasty.

◼ Telecanthus

Telecanthus is the increased distance between the medial canthi as a result of abnormally long medial canthal tendons. It should not be confused with hypertelorism in which there is wide separation of the orbits.

Treatment involves shortening and refixation of the medial canthal tendons to the anterior lacrimal crest or insertion of a transnasal suture.

◼ Cryptophthalmos

Crypto means hidden and ophthalmos means eyes. In this condition, lids fail to develop and the layer of skin passes from eyebrows to the cheek continuously, which hides and fuses with a microphthalmic eye.

◼ Microblepharon

Micro means (small) and blepharon means (lids). Microblepharon is characterized by small eyelids. It is often associated with microphthalmos or anophthalmos. It the lids are absent, the condition is called ablepharon.

◼ Coloboma of Lid

Coloboma of lid is due to either incomplete closure of the embryonic facial cleft or mechanical forces such as amniotic bands. It may be a unilateral or bilateral, and partial or full-thickness, lid defect. It may affect the upper or lower lid. Upper lid colobomas are situated at the inner side of the midline at the junction of the middle and inner thirds. Lower lid colobomas are situated at the junction of the middle and outer thirds (**Fig. 20.38**).

Treatment
- Small defects require primary closure.
- Large defects require skin grafts and rotation flaps.

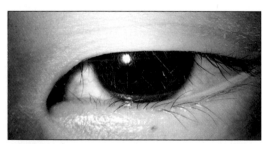

Fig. 20.37 Epicanthus. Source: Indications. In: Freitag S, Lefebvre D, Lee N, et al., ed. Ophthalmic Plastic Surgery: Tricks of the Trade. 1st Edition. Thieme; 2019.

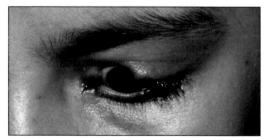

Fig. 20.38 Coloboma of lid. Source: Coloboma. In: Lang G, ed. Ophthalmology. A Pocket Textbook Atlas. 3rd Edition. Thieme; 2015.

CHAPTER 21

The Lacrimal Apparatus

Anatomy of Lacrimal Apparatus 545
Physiology 547
Watering Eye 550
Dacryocystitis 558
Dry Eye 559
Diseases of Lacrimal Gland 564

■ Anatomy of Lacrimal Apparatus

Lacrimal apparatus consists of tear-secreting glands and the lacrimal drainage system. Tear-secreting glands include lacrimal gland and accessory lacrimal glands (glands of Krause and Wolfring). Lacrimal drainage system includes puncta, canaliculi, lacrimal sac, and nasolacrimal duct (NLD).

■ Tear-secreting Glands

Tear-secreting glands comprise of lacrimal glands and accessory lacrimal glands.

Lacrimal Gland

In the orbit, it is *situated in* lacrimal fossa at the outer part of the orbital plate of frontal bone. The lateral aponeurosis of levator muscle tendon produces an indentation in the gland, so that the gland appears to be composed of two separate lobes: An orbital portion lying above the aponeurosis and a palpebral portion lying below the aponeurosis.

Ducts of Lacrimal Glands

About 10 to 12 ducts from both parts open in the lateral part of the upper fornix. The ducts from the orbital lobe pass through the palpebral lobe. *Thus, surgical removal of the palpebral lobe will abolish secretion from the entire lacrimal gland.*

Nerve Supply

Nerve supply to lacrimal gland involves *three components* (**Fig. 21.1**):

Sensory innervation: The principal **afferent pathway** for reflex lacrimal secretion comes from lacrimal nerve (branch of 1st division of **Vth CN**).

Parasympathetic innervation: It is secretomotor and forms the **efferent pathway** of the reflex lacrimal secretion mechanism. It originates from superior salivary nucleus in pons, and travels via VIIth nerve and the greater superficial petrosal nerve. The fibers synapse in the pterygopalatine ganglion. The postganglionic fibers are carried by zygomatic nerve (branch of IInd division of Vth nerve) and lacrimal nerve (branch of 1st division of Vth nerve).

Sympathetic innervation: It is **vasomotor** in function. Postganglionic sympathetic fibers originate in the superior cervical ganglion and travel along the plexus surrounding the internal carotid artery. They travel via deep petrosal nerve and zygomatic nerve to the lacrimal gland.

Blood Supply

It is supplied by *lacrimal artery* (a branch of ophthalmic artery).

Accessory Lacrimal Glands

These include glands of Krause and Wolfring. Glands of Krause are microscopic groups of

reflex tearing. Psychogenic reflex tearing can be abolished by blocking the pterygopalatine ganglion (efferent pathway).

While reflex secretion of lacrimal gland is controlled by the parasympathetic supply, sympathetic fibers may control the basic secretors in the lids and conjunctiva. Directly acting parasympathomimetic drugs such as pilocarpine produce an increase in lacrimal flow, whereas parasympatholytics such as atropine reduce tear flow.

After lesions of facial ganglion, regenerating salivary gland nerve fibers may be misdirected to the lacrimal gland. Therefore, mastication produces tearing as well as salivation–"**crocodile tears**."

Pre-ocular Tear Film

It *consists of three layers* (**Fig. 21.3**):
- Superficial lipid layer (outermost).
- Middle aqueous layer.
- Deep mucin layer (innermost).

Lipid (oily) Layer

It is secreted by Meibomian glands and glands of Zeiss.

The lipid layer is composed of phospholipids (polar lipids), cholesterol esters, and triglycerides (nonpolar). Blinking causes lid movement, leading to release of lipids from lid glands. So, thickness of layer can be increased by forced blinking and reduced by infrequent blinking.

Functions

- It reduces rate of evaporation of underlying aqueous layer.
- It forms a barrier along lid margins and prevents overflow of aqueous strip onto the skin.
- It acts as a surfactant, allowing spread of tear film.

Aqueous Layer

It is secreted by the main lacrimal gland and accessory lacrimal glands of Krause and Wolfring. It contains:

- Electrolytes: HCO_3^-, Cl^-, Na^+, K^+
- Glucose.
- Proteins: Albumin and globulins. Immunoglobulins (Ig) found in normal tear fluid are IgA, IgG, and IgM. **IgA** is dominant in tears; **IgE** increases in allergic conjunctivitis; and **IgG** is found in tears of patients with acute infections.
- Lactoferrin.
- Urea.
- Glycoproteins.
- Lysozyme enzyme, a high-molecular weight proteolytic enzyme is produced by lysosomes. It dissolves bacterial wall and considered to be the antibacterial substance

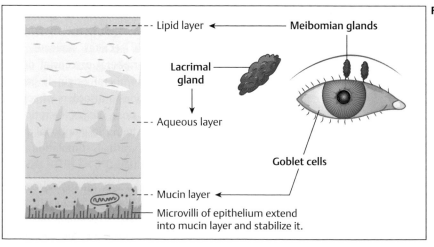

Fig. 21.3 Tear film.

Lipid layer ◄———— Meibomian glands

Lacrimal gland

Aqueous layer

Goblet cells

Mucin layer ◄———

Microvilli of epithelium extend into mucin layer and stabilize it.

in tears. The action of lysozyme depends on pH. The optimum pH for lysis lies between 6.0 and 7.4.

Functions

- It provides atmospheric O_2 to corneal epithelium which is essential for normal corneal metabolism.
- It has antibacterial function due to presence of IgA and lysozyme.
- It washes away debris.
- It provides a smooth optical surface to cornea.

Mucin Layer

Mucins are high-molecular weight glycoproteins secreted mainly by goblet cells of conjunctiva and also by glands of Manz.

Mucin layer is spread over and adsorbs on hydrophobic corneal epithelium through the act of blinking. Thus, it converts hydrophobic corneal epithelium into a hydrophilic one over which tear fluid spreads evenly (**Flowchart 21.1**).

Properties of Tear Film

Characteristic features of tear film are:
- *Thickness of tear film* is **8 μm**.
- *Average pH of tears* is **7.25** (slightly alkaline). Tear pH is lowest on awakening due to acid byproducts.

Prolonged lid closure during sleep creates anaerobic conditions and leads to acid byproducts. It results into low pH on awakening. As eyes are open, pH increases due to loss of .

When solutions having a pH <6.6 or >7.8 are instilled into conjunctival sac, subjective discomfort occurs.
- *Refractive index of tear film*– **1.336**.
- *Osmolality*– 309 mosm/L ($\equiv$ 0.9% NaCl).
- *Chemical composition is same as explained in aqueous layer*. Rate of tear secretion– It is about **1.2 μL/min**.

Functions of Tear Film

Tear film serves the following functions:
- *Optical function*: It maintains optically uniform corneal surface.
- *Mechanical function*: It flushes cellular debris and foreign matter.
- *Nutritional function*: It provides oxygen to cornea which is essential to normal corneal metabolism.
- *Antibacterial function:* Due to the presence of proteins such as IgA, lysozyme and lactoferrin tear film has antibacterial property.

■ Spread of Tear Film

Tear film is spread over the ocular surface through blinking. Shear forces produced by the moving lids play a vital role in maintenance of normal

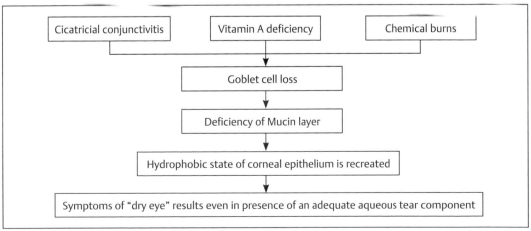

Flowchart 21.1 Mechanism of development of dry eye.

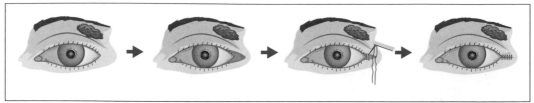

Fig. 21.6 Lateral canthoplasty.

Canaliculitis

Acute canaliculitis is usually due to herpes simplex infection. *Chronic canaliculitis* is usually caused by actinomyces israelii—an anaerobic Gram +ve bacterium. Its clinical features include:

- Mucopurulent discharge on pressure over canaliculus which is associated with chronic mucopurulent conjunctivitis refractory to conventional treatment.
- 'Pouting' punctum.
- Concretions within canaliculus which consist of sulfur granules.

Treatment of Canalicular Causes

Treatment of **canalicular obstruction** depends on the length of patent canaliculus.

- If **7 to 8 mm of patent normal canaliculus** is present between punctum and obstruction, canaliculodacryocystorhinostomy (CDCR) is the treatment. In CDCR, obstructed common canaliculus is resected and patent part of canaliculus is anastomosed with lacrimal sac which, in turn, is anastomosed into nose.
- When there is **<7 mm of patent canaliculus**, it is difficult to anastomose the remaining canaliculi to lacrimal sac, that is, CDCR is impossible. Therefore, an artificial tear drainage system is created by inserting a special tube (Lester Jones tube) between inner canthus and the nose through a dacryocystorhinostomy (DCR).
- If obstruction of common or individual canaliculi is partial, it may be treated by intubation. The silicone tubes are passed via puncta and sac into nose where they are tied and left in place for 3 to 6 months.

Trauma can cause canalicular laceration which is treated by approximating the ends of laceration under the operating microscope and bridged with a silicone tube which is left in situ for approximately 6 months.

In the treatment of **canaliculitis,** topical antibiotics are rarely curative. Canaliculotomy is performed which involves a linear incision into the conjunctival side of canaliculus. Concretions become evident following canaliculotomy.

Lacrimal Sac Causes

Functional blockage: This may occur due to lacrimal pump failure secondary to:

- Lower lid laxity with old age.
- Facial nerve (VII CN) palsy, resulting in weakness of orbicularis muscle.

Obstruction of sac: It may be due to:

- Chronic dacryocystitis leading to fibrosis and strictures commonly at the junction of lacrimal sac and NLD.
- Fungal growth.
- Neoplastic growth.
- Stones (dacryolithiasis).

Treatment of Lacrimal Sac Causes

- **Chronic dacryocystitis** leads to fibrosis and strictures commonly at the junction of the lacrimal sac and **NLD**, which is termed as acquired nasolacrimal duct obstruction. Dacryocystitis and dacryolithiasis are both treated by **DCR**.
- **Tumors of lacrimal sac** are rare. Tumors of epithelial cell origin are the most common and treated by complete excision followed by irradiation.

Nasolacrimal Duct (NLD) Causes

Obstruction of NLD may be congenital or due to inflammation.

Congenital Nasolacrimal Duct Obstruction (OP2.3)

The lower end of NLD (at the valve of Hasner) is the last portion of lacrimal drainage system to canalize, which usually opens spontaneously soon after birth. Congenital NLD obstruction is due to an imperforate membrane at the Hasner valve. It presents as:

- Wet looking eye or epiphora.
- Matting of eyelashes due to mucopurulent material on eyelashes.
- Reflux of mucoid or mucopurulent material from punctum when pressure is applied over the lacrimal sac.
- Recurrent conjunctivitis may be another sign.
- Preseptal cellulitis or acute dacryocystitis may rarely develop.

Congenital Dacryocele

Distention of sac with mucus may occur due to imperforate Hasner valve, which is known as **mucocele**. Pressure over sac leads to regurgitation of mucoid material from punctum in this case.

Congenital dacryocele is caused by both a distal and proximal obstruction of nasolacrimal apparatus. It presents with a bluish, cystic swelling just below the medial canthal area accompanied by epiphora. It results due to collection of amniotic fluid or mucus in the lacrimal sac (also called **amniontocele** or **encysted mucocele**). There is no regurgitation from punctum when pressure is applied over lacrimal sac.

Treatment of NLD Causes

Congenital NLD obstruction *is treated as follows:*

- Massage of lacrimal sac: Place index finger over common canaliculus to block the exit of material through puncta. Apply firm pressure in a downward fashion to increase hydrostatic pressure within lacrimal sac. It may rupture the membranous obstruction. Pressure is applied 10 to 12 times at one sitting and repeated four times a day.
- Topical antibiotics are instilled if mucopurulent discharge is present.

- Probing of lacrimal system: It should not be performed until the age of 6 months. If the block persists, probing is performed after the age of 6 months and can be repeated, if required. The procedure is performed under general anesthesia as follows (**Fig. 21.7**):
  ◊ Dilate the punctum with punctum dilator.
  ◊ Pass the probe of small size through dilated punctum along the canaliculus into sac.
  ◊ Turn the probe past the angulation.
  ◊ Advance the probe inferiorly until it perforates the membrane.
  ◊ After probing, instill steroid–antibiotic drops Q.I.D. × 1 to 2 weeks.

Success rate of probing is high and >90% are cured by the 1st probing, if performed within first year of life. Success rate decreases if probing is performed after the age of 18 months.

If 1st probing fails and epiphora persists even after 6 weeks, probing may be repeated. Failure is usually due to abnormal NLD anatomy.

- Intubation: If the repeated probing fails to relieve the obstruction, intubation with silicone tube is performed and left in situ for 6 months.
- **DCR**: If all the measures fail, DCR is performed after the age of 5 years. A DCR should not be performed earlier, as the bones are not adequately developed till then.

Nasal Causes

Nasal infections, inflammation, or tumors may result in epiphora.

■ Evaluation of a Case with Watering Eye

Evaluation of a case starts with history and then examination.

History

It is important to differentiate hypersecretion (lacrimation) from epiphora by a careful history (**Table 21.1**).

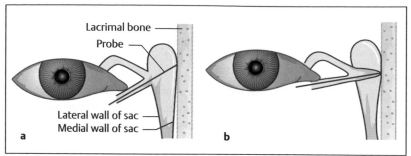

Lacrimal bone

Probe

Lateral wall of sac
Medial wall of sac

a

b

Fig. 21.9 (a) Hard stop in NLD obstruction. **(b)** Soft stop in common canalicular obstruction. Abbreviation: NLD, nasolacrimal duct.

Jones Test I

It differentiates watering due to partial obstruction of lacrimal passage from primary hypersecretion of tears. A drop of 2% fluorescein dye is instilled into the conjunctival sac and a cotton-tipped bud moistened with local anesthetic is inserted under the inferior turbinate at the NLD opening (which is situated approximately 3 cm from external nares). After 5 minutes:

- If fluorescein is recovered on bud from the nose, it indicates drainage system is patent (**Positive Jones test I**) and watering is due is due to primary hypersection. No further tests are necessary.
- If no dye is recovered from the nose (**Negative Jones test I**), it indicates partial obstruction or failure of lacrimal pump. *Jones test II is performed in this situation to identify the probable site of partial obstruction* (**Fig. 21.10**).

Jones Test II

It is performed if Jones test I is negative. Residual fluorescein in the conjunctival sac is washed out and topical anesthetic is instilled. The *lacrimal syringing is performed with saline* and a cotton bud is placed under the inferior turbinate.

If fluorescein stained saline is recovered from the nose (**Positive Jones test II**), it indicates that the dye has reached the lacrimal sac during Jones test I, that is, orbicularis, puncta, and canaliculi are functioning sufficiently to transport the fluorescein into the lacrimal sac. The dye was prevented from entering the nose by a partial obstruction in the NLD and syringing of lacrimal system forced the dye past the obstruction into the nose, that is, partial obstruction of the NLD is the cause of epiphora which can be treated by **DCR**.

If unstained saline is recovered from nose (**Negative Jones test II**), it indicates that dye did not enter the lacrimal sac during Jones test I, that is, the upper drainage system (puncta, canaliculi or common canaliculus) is faulty and implies a partial obstruction of the upper drainage system.

Diagnostic Imaging

Dacryocystography (DCG)

DCG is indicated to determine the exact site of obstruction or stenosis within the lacrimal drainage system Also, in the diagnosis of diverticula, filling defects are due to stones or tumors.

Procedure

- Lower punctum is dilated with punctum dilator.
- Radio-opaque dye, **lipiodol**, is injected into the canaliculus (1–2 mL).
- Postero–anterior and lateral radiographs are taken.
- Exposures are repeated after 30 minutes.

The test is usually performed on both sides simultaneously.

Interpretation

If the dye is retained in the lacrimal sac after 30 minutes, it indicates an anatomical obstruction.

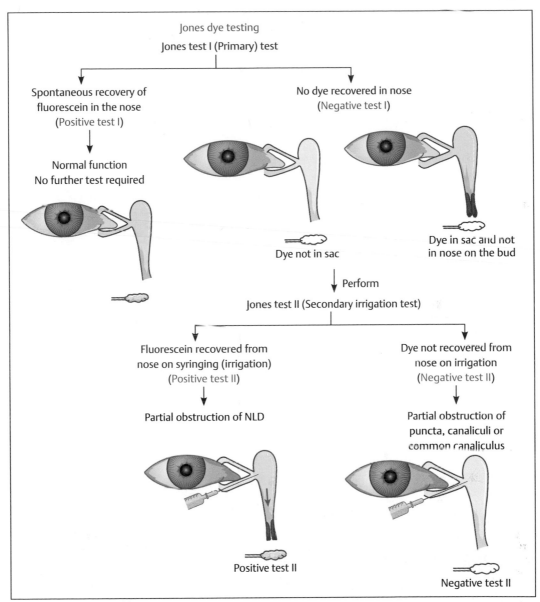

Fig. 21.10 Jones dye tests.

The commonest site of such an obstruction is the junction between the sac and NLD which is at the level of inferior orbital rim on an X-ray.

Radionucleotide Testing (Lacrimal Scintillography)

This involves labelling of tears with gamma-emitting radioactive substance—**Technetium 99m**—and assesses the tear drainage. It is an imaging technique to study the functional integrity of lacrimal passage. It does not provide detailed visualization of anatomical structures as in DCG.

Procedure

- A drop of technetium 99m is placed into the lateral conjunctival sac. Tears are thus labelled with this gamma-emitting substance.

- A gamma camera is used to record its transit to the nose. A sequence of images is recorded over 20 minutes.
- Images can be reviewed on a video screen or transferred to X-ray plates.

Dacryocystitis (OP2.1)

It is the inflammation of lacrimal sac. It may be congenital or acquired. Acquired dacryocystitis could be acute or chronic.

Congenital Dacryocystitis

It is due to incomplete canalization of lacrimal sac (congenital NLD obstruction), resulting in stasis of secretion in lacrimal sac (**Fig. 21.11**). The common organisms cultured are:

- Staphylococcus aureus.
- Hemophilus influenzae.
- Streptococci.
- Pneumococci.

It presents with epiphora, mucopurulent discharge from the eyes, and swelling on the sac area.

Complications

- Orbital cellulitis leading to even meningitis.
- Lacrimal fistulae.
- Lacrimal abscess.

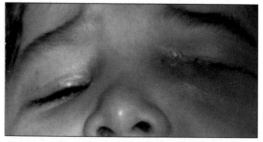

Fig. 21.11 Congenital dacryocystitis. Source: Lacrimal System Disorders. In: Agarwal A, Jacob S, ed. Color Atlas of Ophthalmology. The Quick-Reference Manual for Diagnosis and Treatment. 2nd Edition. Thieme; 2009.

Treatment

Treatment includes the following:

- Massage over the lacrimal sac.
- Antibiotic drops.
- Frequent expression of sac contents.
- Lacrimal irrigation with antibiotics.
- Probing of nasolacrimal duct is done between 3 to 6 months of age. During probing, care must be taken to avoid injuring the walls of the canaliculus and duct.
- If there is no marked improvement after repeated probing, balloon dilatation of the duct can be performed.
- Placement of a silicone tube for approximately 6 months can be considered if the above procedures fail.
- If the child is brought late, DCR operation must be performed after the age of 5 to 6 years. Till then, the child is kept on conservative treatment.

Acquired Dacryocystitis

It may be acute or chronic. It may be localized in the sac, extend to include a pericystitis, or progress to orbital cellulitis. When dacryocystitis is localized to the sac, a palpable painful mass is found at the inner canthus. Chronic dacryocystitis may be the end stage of acute dacryocystitis but it may present initially as a cause of NLD obstruction. In dacryocystitis with pericystitis, the infection around the sac is present and may spread to the anterior orbit. If the infection proceeds posterior to orbital septum, orbital cellulitis may occur.

Acute Dacryocystitis

It presents with pain near medial canthus and epiphora, and red and tender swelling over the sac area (**Fig. 21.12a**).

Acute dacryocystitis is treated by hot fomentation oral antibiotics; DCR is done after the acute infection has been controlled. Irrigation and probing should not be performed in acute dacryocystitis. If lacrimal abscess is formed,

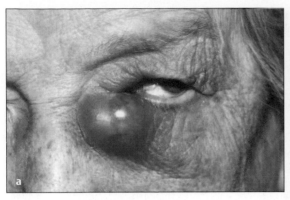

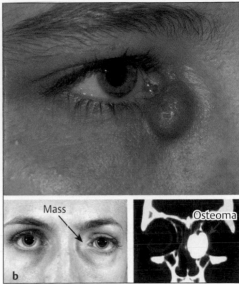

Fig. 21.12 (a) Acute dacryocystitis. Source: Lang G, ed. Ophthalmology. A Pocket Textbook Atlas. 3rd Edition. Thieme; 2015. **(b)** Chronic dacryocystitis. Source: External Examination. In: Leatherbarrow B, ed. Oculoplastic Surgery. 3rd Edition. Thieme; 2019.

incision and drainage may be considered if pus points. However, a persistent lacrimal sac–skin fistula may be formed.

Chronic Dacryocystitis

It is more common than acute form. It is commonly due to the stricture of nasal duct arising from mild-grade inflammation, which is usually of nasal origin (**Fig. 21.12b**). Obstruction of the lower end of NLD may be caused by:

- Nasal polyps.
- Hypertrophied inferior turbinate bone.
- Marked deviation of nasal septum.

The stagnation of secretions and tears within the lacrimal sac due to NLD obstruction leads to infection and dacryocystitis. It may also be associated with ethmoidal infections.

Causative Organisms

The bacteria causing infection include *staphylococci*, *streptococci*, and *pneumococci*. These may cause hypopyon ulcer in an abraded cornea and panophthalmitis, if an intraocular surgery is undertaken. *Hence, because of the risk of panophthalmitis, it is often wise to postpone intraocular surgery till lacrimal infection has been treated.*

Presentation

The patient presents with epiphora. It may be associated with chronic or recurrent unilateral conjunctivitis. Other signs include a painless swelling over the sac area (**mucocele**) near the medial canthus, and reflux of mucopurulent discharge through the puncta on pressing over the sac.

Sequlae

Untreated chronic dacryocystitis never undergoes spontaneous resolution. If left untreated, the sac ultimately become atonic and acute infection may lead to formation of lacrimal abscess.

Treatment

It is treated with **DCR**. In case of marked fibrosis of lacrimal sac, dacryocystectomy (**DCT**) is performed.

■ Dry Eye (OP4.4)

Dry eye is an ocular surface disease which occurs due to inadequate tear secretion or instability of tear film. Tear film has three layers:

- **Lipid layer** secreted by *Meibomian glands*.
- **Aqueous layer** secreted by *lacrimal glands*.

- **Mucous layer** secreted by *conjunctival goblet cells.*

So, abnormalities in one or more of the tear components result in ocular surface disease (**dry eye**).

Three factors are required for effective spread of tear film over the ocular surface:
- Normal blinking.
- Contact between ocular surface and eyelids.
- Normal corneal epithelium.

So, impaired lid functioning or blinking and irregularity of corneal surface can result in dry eye.

■ Etiology

Dry eye can result from:
- **Aqueous tear deficiency:** The condition caused by the deficiency of aqueous component of tear is also called as **kerato conjunctivitis sicca** (**KCS**). It may be associated with:
  - ◊ Absence of lacrimal gland (congenital or surgical removal).
  - ◊ Destruction of lacrimal gland tissue by tumor or inflammation.
  - ◊ Reflex hyposecretion ⟶ Sensory—in refractive surgery, diabetes, and neurotrophic keratitis. Motor—in VIIth cranial nerve damage.

Sjogren syndrome: It is an autoimmune disorder and affects middle-aged women after menopause. It is characterized by lymphocytic infiltration of lacrimal, salivary, and other exocrine glands, resulting in xerostomia and dry eyes. It can be seen alone (primary Sjogren syndrome) or in association with other autoimmune diseases such as rheumatoid arthritis or systemic lupus erythematosus (secondary Sjogren syndrome). Classical triad consists of:
- Dry eyes.
- Dry mouth.
- Parotid gland enlargement.

- ◊ Sjogren syndrome: It is an autoimmune disorder associated with destruction of lacrimal and salivary glands.
- ◊ Lacrimal gland obstruction in trachoma, chemical injury, cicatricial pemphigoid, and Stevens-Johnson syndrome.
- **Mucin deficiency:** It results from goblet cell dysfunction (**Flowchart 21.2**). Goblet cell loss occurs with:
  - ◊ Cicatrizing conjunctivitis.
  - ◊ Vitamin A deficiency.
  - ◊ Drugs such as sulfonamides.
  - ◊ Chemical burns.
  - ◊ Stevens–Johnson syndrome.
- **Lipid deficiency:** It results from Meibomian gland deficiency. It can occur with chronic blepharitis and acne rosacea. Lipid layer prevents evaporation of aqueous layer. Its deficiency results in evaporative dry eye.
- **Impaired lid function:** Normal blinking maintains tear film and moistens the ocular surface. Abnormality of normal blinking process can adversely affect the tear film stability as in prolonged reading, watching TV, prolonged use of computer monitor, and lid paralysis.

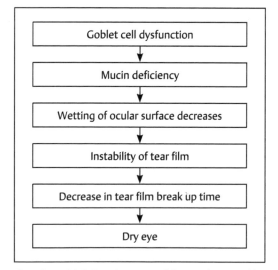

Flowchart 21.2 Development of dry eye due to goblet cell dysfunction.

- **Irregular corneal surface:** Superficial epithelial cells of cornea and conjunctiva produce transmembrane mucins which form glycocalyx and convert the corneal epithelial from a hydrophobic to hydrophilic surface.
- Damage to epithelial cells will prevent normal tear film adherence. The tear film becomes thin and retracts in the area of epithelial irregularity.
- **Other causes:**
  ◊ Drugs that decrease tear production are:
  a. Atropine.
  b. β-blockers.
  c. Antihistaminics.
  d. Hypnotics, e.g. nitrazepam.
  e. Tranquilizers, e.g. diazepam.
  ◊ Contact lenses: Use of contact lenses also contribute to the development of dry eyes. Contact lenses decrease the corneal sensation, a factor which may be necessary for the tear secretion. Soft contact lenses cause the reflex hyposecretion of aqueous layer of tear film, while rigid lenses disrupt the lipid layer, enhancing the evaporation of the tear film.

■ Clinical Features

Dry eyes present with symptoms like dryness, burning, grittiness, and stringy discharge. Symptoms of KCS are exacerbated in conditions associated with increased tear evaporation as in air conditioner, prolonged reading (due to reduced blinking), central heating, and wind.

Clinical signs of dry eye presentation are listed in **Table 21.2**.

■ Diagnostic Tests

The aim of the tests is to ascertain the following:
- Tear secretion: It is assessed by Schirmer's test.
- Stability of tear film: It is diagnosed by tear film break up time (BUT).
- Ocular surface diseases (density of goblet cells): It is assessed by corneal staining and conjunctival impression cytology.

Assessment of Tear Secretion (Schirmer's Test)

Tear secretion may be divided into basal secretion and reflex secretion. Aqueous tear secretion is assessed by *Schirmer's test which may be performed without or after instillation of topical anesthesia*. Schirmer's test performed without topical anesthesia (**Schirmer's test I**) measures basic + reflex secretions, while Schirmer's test performed after instillation of topical anesthesia (**Schirmer's test II**) measures basic secretion. However, topical anesthesia cannot abolish all sensory and psychological stimuli for reflex secretion. The difference between the results of both tests is a measurement of reflex secretion, that is,

Schirmer's test I − Schirmer's test II = Reflex secretion

Table 21.2 Presenting signs of dry eye	
Conjunctiva	• Redness. • Conjunctiva may lose its normal lustre.
Corneal	• Epithelial erosions staining with fluorescein. • Filamentary keratitis (filaments stain with rose Bengal). • Mucous plaques are usually seen associated with corneal filaments.
Tear film	In dry eyes, the mucin layer becomes contaminated with lipid, and the tear film shows the mucus debris and strings of mucoid discharge that move with each blink. The marginal tear meniscus become thin or absent in dry eyes (in normal eyes it is ~1 mm in height). In meibomian gland dysfunction, froth occurs in the tear film or along the eyelid margin.

Procedure

The test is performed by measuring the amount of wetting of a special filter paper (Whatmann no 41 filter paper) which is 5 mm wide and 35 mm long.

Schirmer's test I

- The filter paper is folded 5 mm at one end.
- Place the filter paper in lower conjunctival sac at the junction of outer 1/3rd and medial 2/3rd of lower eyelid.
- Remove filter paper after 5 minutes.
- Measure the amount of wetting from the fold; less than 10 mm of wetting after 5 minutes without anesthesia is considered abnormal (**Fig. 21.13**).

Schirmer's test II

- Instill topical anesthesia into conjunctival sac and the amount of wetting is measured after 2 minutes. Less than 5 mm wetting is considered abnormal (hyposecretion).

Assessment of Stability of Tear Film (tear film BUT)

- Instill 2% fluorescein in lower fornix.
- Ask the patient to blink.
- Examine the tear film at slit lamp using cobalt blue light.

Appearance of black spots or lines in fluorescein-stained film indicates the formation of dry areas. Tear film **BUT** is the interval between the last blink and the appearance of first dry spot. It is abnormal in aqueous tear deficiency and Meibomian gland disorders.

A normal BUT is more than 10 seconds and BUT of less than 10 seconds is considered abnormal.

Assessment of Ocular Surface Diseases

It is assessed by *corneal staining* and *conjunctival impression cytology*. Fluorescein stains damaged corneal and conjunctival epithelium. Rose Bengal dye has an affinity for dead or devitalized epithelial cells that have lost or altered mucus layer. This test is useful in KCS. The staining of cornea and conjunctiva in interpalpebral area is common in aqueous tear deficiency. Impression cytology is a sophisticated diagnostic strategy for confirming dry eye states. Conjunctival impression cytology is performed to determine goblet cell density of bulbar or palpebral conjunctiva. In dry eye states, there is a decrease in goblet cell counts.

■ Differential Diagnosis

Symptoms of dry eye may mimic to:
- Chronic blepharoconjunctivitis due to staphylococcus.
- Allergic conjunctivitis.
- Rosacea keratoconjunctivitis.

Therefore, these conditions must be eliminated.

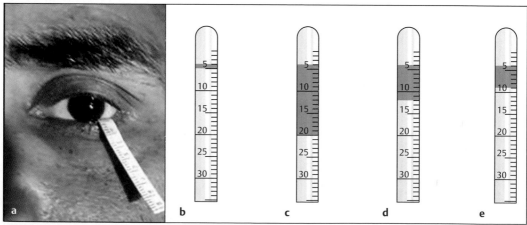

Fig. 21.13 (a) Procedure of Schirmer test. **(b)** Schirmer tear test strip. **(c)** Normal tear production (>15 mm). **(d)** Moderate insufficiency of tears (5–10 mm). **(e)** Insufficient tear production (<5 mm).

■ Treatment

The choice of treatment depends on the severity of the disease and involves:

- Patient education.
- Tear substitutes.
- Mucolytic agents.
- Anti-inflammatory agents.
- Treatment of underlying cause.

Supportive Measures

- Use of ophthalmic solutions *without preservatives* should be ensured in patients with severe dry eye syndrome as preservatives can aggravate ocular surface disorders.
- Avoidance of medications like atropine, antihistaminics, and hypnotics, as these decrease lacrimal secretion.
- Avoidance of contact lenses as they decrease tear production, possibly due to decreased corneal sensations.
- Emphasis must be given on the importance of blinking while reading.
- Caution must be taken against laser refractive surgery.

Tear Substitutes

Almost all tear substitutes are based on replacement of the aqueous phase of tear film.

Characteristics of ideal tear substitute are:

- It should form a stable tear film over the ocular surface.
- It should lower the surface tension of tear film and aid in the formulation of a hydrophilic layer.
- It should not react with tear proteins, that is, it should not encourage aggregate formation or denaturation.
- It should not compromise the integrity of the superficial lipid layer.
- It should not disturb the corneal metabolism.
- It should not be toxic with frequent use.
- It should have a sufficiently long-retention time.

The various tear substitutes that increase the wettability of hydrophobic corneal surface, stability of precorneal tear film, and conjunctival retention time include:

- Cellulose derivatives: These are appropriate for mild cases, for example, hydroxypropylmethylcellulose (HPMC) and carboxymethylcellulose.
- Carbomers: These are longer lasting but preservative limits the frequency.
- Polyvinyl alcohol: It is a water-soluble polymer which increases the persistence of tear film without increasing its viscosity.
- Sodium hyaluronate: It may be useful in promoting conjunctival and corneal epithelial healing and is free of ocular adverse effects in the concentration of 0.1%.

Mucolytic Agents

Acetylcysteine 5% drops: It is believed to exert its action on disulphide linkages in mucus, thereby lowering its viscosity. It has a limited shelf life, so that it can only be used for up to 2 weeks.

Anti-inflammatory Agents

Topical cyclosporine: It reduces T cell-mediated inflammation of lacrimal tissue, increasing the number of goblet cells.

Treatment of Underlying Cause

Chronic blepharitis which is frequently associated with ocular surface disorders and is treated with eyelid hygiene and topical antibiotics. Autoimmune disorders associated with KCS must be treated in consultation with a rheumatologist.

Other Options

- Punctal occlusion to reduce drainage, so that little secretion of natural tears is preserved and effect of artificial tears is prolonged.
- Reduction of room temperature to minimize the evaporation of tears.
- Room humidifiers give relief by increasing the humidity of indoor environment.
- Tarsorrhaphy diminishes surface evaporation (OP4.7).
- Submandibular gland transplantation into conjunctival sac may be attempted.

■ Diseases of Lacrimal Gland

Diseases of lacrimal gland include dacryoadenitis, dacryops, Mikulicz syndrome, and tumors of lacrimal gland.

■ Dacryoadenitis

It is the inflammation of lacrimal gland. It may be acute or chronic. **Acute dacryoadenitis** occurs in infections (mumps, influenza, and infectious mononucleosis), while **chronic dacryoadenitis** is associated with granulomatous diseases such as sarcoidosis and tuberculosis.

Presentation

Acute dacryoadenitis presents with a painful swelling and redness in the lateral part of the upper eyelid (**Fig. 21.14**). Chronic dacryoadenitis presents with painless and nontender swelling of lacrimal gland.

Signs

- S-shaped swelling of upper lid margin at the lateral aspect.
- Tenderness over lacrimal gland fossa.
- Mild downward and inward movement of eyeball in acute orbital dacryoadenitis.
- Injection of the palpebral portion of lacrimal gland and adjacent conjunctiva.

Bursting of the lacrimal abscess may result in permanent fistula.

Treatment

Acute dacryoadenitis is managed by:
- Hot compression.
- Systemic and local antibiotics.
- Systemic nonsteroidal anti-inflammatory drugs (NSAIDs).
- Lacrimal gland abscess needs surgical drainage.

Chronic dacryoadenitis is managed by:
- Systemic corticosteroids for sarcoidosis.
- Antitubercular treatment (ATT) for tubercular chronic dacryoadenitis.

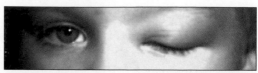

Fig. 21.14 Dacryoadenitis. Source: Orbital Complications of Other Cause. In: Welkoborsky H, Wiechens B, Hinni M, ed. Interdisciplinary Management of Orbital Diseases: Textbook and Atlas. 1st Edition. Thieme; 2017.

■ Dacryops

It is a ductal cyst of lacrimal gland. The blockage of one of the lacrimal ducts leads to retention of lacrimal secretion, resulting in cystic swelling in upper fornix. The treatment involves simple aspiration.

Mikulicz Syndrome

It is characterized by symmetrical enlargement of lacrimal and salivary glands.

Tumors of Lacrimal Gland (OP2.7)

Pleomorphic adenoma

The most common epithelial tumor of the lacrimal gland is *pleomorphic adenoma* (benign mixed-cell tumor). It is derived from the ducts and secretory elements. It presents in middle age with a painless, slowly progressive swelling in the superolateral part of the orbit. Treatment involves complete removal of tumor.

Lacrimal Gland Carcinoma

It occurs in elderly with a painful swelling of short duration. The eyeball is displaced inferonasally (down and in) due to mass in the lacrimal area. Posterior extension may involve superior orbital fissure, resulting in proptosis, periorbital edema, ophthalmoplegia, optic disc swelling, and choroidal folds.

Invasion of bone and calcification in the tumor is commonly observed. Treatment involves excision of tumors and adjacent tissues. Extensive tumors may require orbital exenteration. Radio therapy is combined with local resection.

22 The Orbit

Anatomy of the Orbit 565
Clinical Features and Investigations in Orbital Diseases 569
Proptosis 570
Orbital Inflammation 573
Cavernous Sinus Thrombosis 578
Graves' Ophthalmopathy 578
Orbital Tumors 582
Orbital Injuries 587

■ Anatomy of the Orbit

The orbit is a pear-shaped bony cavity which contains the eyeball, extraocular muscles, nerves, vessels, and connective tissue to support all orbital structures. Anteriorly, the orbit is limited by the orbital septum which separates the orbit from the eyelid. The orbit is formed by seven bones (**Fig. 22.1**):

- Ethmoid bone.
- Frontal bone.
- Lacrimal bone.
- Maxillary bone.
- Palatine bone.
- Sphenoid bone.
- Zygomatic bone.

■ Walls and Relations of the Orbit

The average volume of bony orbit is approximately 30 ml. It has four walls which converge posteriorly toward the apex and optic canal.

Orbital Roof

It slopes backward and downward toward the apex. It separates the orbit from frontal sinus anteriorly and anterior cranial fossa posteriorly. It is formed by two bones: orbital plate of frontal bone (main) and lesser wing of the sphenoid bone (small contribution at the apex of the orbit).

Applied Aspect

- Lacrimal gland fossa is located in the superotemporal aspect of roof. So, *globe will be displaced inferonasally in the lacrimal gland tumor.*
- A defect in orbital roof results in transmission of cerebrospinal fluid (CSF) pulsation to the orbit which may cause pulsatile proptosis.

Lateral Orbital Wall

It is formed by two bones: Zygomatic bones (anteriorly) and greater wing of the sphenoid bone (posteriorly).

Applied Aspect

Lateral wall only protects the posterior half of the globe; so, anterior half of the globe is vulnerable to lateral trauma.

Orbital Floor

It is the shortest of the orbital walls. It is formed by three bones: maxillary bone (main), zygomatic bone (forms anterolateral portion), and palatine bone (lies at posterior extent of the floor).

dural sheaths and sclera. In the lower part of the orbit, Tenon's capsule is condensed and forms a hammock on which the eyeball rests, which is called the suspensory ligament of Lockwood.

Blood Supply of the Orbit

Arterial supply: Mainly ophthalmic artery.

Venous drainage: Orbit is drained by superior and inferior ophthalmic veins into the cavernous sinus (**Fig. 22.3**).

Lymphatics: There are no lymphatics in the orbit.

Surgical Spaces of the Orbit

From the surgical point of view, there are four self-contained spaces. The inflammatory processes tend to remain within the space affected.

Therefore, each space must be opened separately. These spaces are as follows (**Fig. 22.4**):

- Subperiosteal space is a potential space between the bones of orbital wall and the periorbita.
- Peripheral space is the space between periorbita and extraocular muscles joined by fascial connections.
- Central space is cone-shaped space enclosed by the muscles (muscular cone) and their inter muscular septa.
- Tenon's space is a space around the globe between sclera and Tenon's capsule.

Applied Aspect

The **peripheral space** is the site for peribulbar anesthesia, and proptosis produced due to tumors in this space is eccentric. The **central space** is

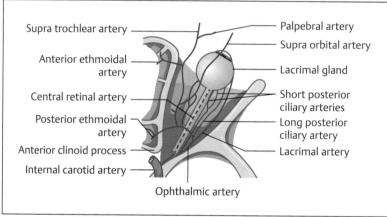

Fig. 22.3 Blood supply of orbit.

Supra trochlear artery — Palpebral artery
— Supra orbital artery
Anterior ethmoidal artery —
— Lacrimal gland
Central retinal artery —
— Short posterior ciliary arteries
Posterior ethmoidal artery —
— Long posterior ciliary artery
Anterior clinoid process —
— Lacrimal artery
Internal carotid artery —
Ophthalmic artery

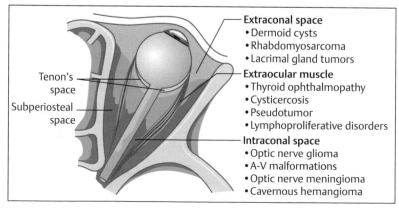

Fig. 22.4 Surgical spaces of orbit.

Extraconal space
• Dermoid cysts
• Rhabdomyosarcoma
• Lacrimal gland tumors
Extraocular muscle
• Thyroid ophthalmopathy
• Cysticercosis
• Pseudotumor
• Lymphoproliferative disorders
Intraconal space
• Optic nerve glioma
• A-V malformations
• Optic nerve meningioma
• Cavernous hemangioma

Tenon's space
Subperiosteal space

the site for retrobulbar anesthesia, and proptosis produced due to tumors in this space is axial.

Clinical Features and Investigations in Orbital Diseases (OP2.7, 2.8)

The main features of orbital diseases are pain, proptosis, diplopia, visual impairment, and enophthalmos. Investigations of orbital lesions are listed in **Flowchart 22.1**.

Plain X-rays highlight bony disorders and are taken in different views (**Table 22.1**).

Computerized Tomography Scan (CT Scan)

Its main advantage is its ability to take combination of axial, coronal, oblique, and sagittal sections of the orbit, which enables a space-occupying lesion within the orbit to visualize in three dimensions.

Its main disadvantage is its inability to distinguish between pathological soft tissue masses.

Orbital Ultrasonography

B-scan ultrasonography produces a two-dimensional picture of orbital structures. It requires a probe functioning at lower speed (generally 5 mHz) for greater penetration into the orbit. It gives clear delineation of soft tissues and is less useful in the evaluation of bony lesions.

Magnetic Resonance Imaging

It generates images without the use of ionizing radiation. It images soft tissues not only within the orbit but also within the globe. It is contra-indicated in the presence of magnetic foreign body or patients with pacemaker.

> CT scan is better for viewing bony lesions, while MRI (magnetic resonance imaging) is better for soft tissues.

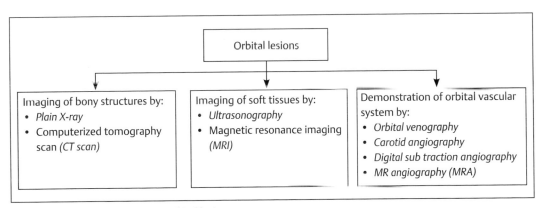

Flowchart 22.1 Investigations in orbital lesions

Different X-ray views	Structure to be visualized
Caldwell view	To visualize orbital details.
Waters view (position is similar to that adopted when drinking water, i.e., X-ray with slightly elevated chin)	It delineates the floor of the orbit and the sinuses; therefore, useful in detecting orbital floor fractures.
Rhese view	To visualize optic foramen and superior orbital fissure.
Lateral view	To study for intracranial lesions.
Posteroanterior view	To visualize calcification or hyperostosis due to meningiomas.

Table 22.1 Structures visualized in various views of X-rays

- Associated symptoms: History of visual loss, pain, and diplopia is taken.

Examination

It includes the following:
- Inspection.
- Palpation.
- Auscultation.
- Visual acuity.
- Ocular movements.
- Pupillary reactions.
- Fundus examination.
- Measurement of proptosis.
- Examination of paranasal sinuses.
- Systemic examination.

Inspection

Objectives of inspection are:
- Rule out the possibility of pseudoproptosis and enophthalmos of opposite eye (**Table 22.4**).
- Ascertain the laterality (unilateral or bilateral) of proptosis.
- Ascertain the type of proptosis (axial or eccentric).
- Look for pulsations of the eye which are caused by:
  ◊ A defect in orbital roof through which CSF pulsation is transmitted to the orbit. It may be congenital (as in neurofibromatosis) or acquired (as in trauma).
  ◊ Arteriovenous (AV) communication: Dilated corkscrew epibulbar vessels may be found in AV malformations.

Look for increase in proptosis on Valsalva maneuver or on bending forward. These maneuvers may increase the proptosis in vascular lesions such as orbital varices.

Palpation

Observe the following points during palpation:
- Compressibility: Push the normal and then the proptosed eye gently back into the orbit with the fingers. If resistance is felt during retropulsion, it suggests the presence of a tumor or thyroid ophthalmopathy.
- Orbital thrill: Orbital bruits are vibrations resulting from turbulent blood flow. Although usually heard with the stethoscope, such sounds may occasionally also be palpated as a thrill.
- Presence of mass.
- Orbital rim: Feel whether the finger can be insinuated between orbital rim and globe? Palpation of orbital rim may reveal erosion or a mass.
- Regional lymph nodes.

Auscultation

A bruit is detected by auscultating the orbit with the bell of a stethoscope. It is present with pulsations in the carotid-cavernous fistula. *Both pulsation and bruit can be diminished or abolished by compressing the ipsilateral carotid artery in the neck.*

Visual Acuity

Visual acuity may be impaired in orbital lesions due to:
- Optic nerve compression.
- Exposure keratopathy.
- Choroidal folds involving posterior pole changing the refractive status.

Table 22.4 Causes of pseudoproptosis and enophthalmos	
Causes of pseudoproptosis	**Causes of enophthalmos**
Enlargement of ipsilateral eye from: • Buphthalmos • High-axial myopia	Structural abnormalities as in: • Blowout fracture of orbital floor, causing herniation of soft tissues into the maxillary sinus • Microphthalmos
Retraction of upper eyelid on ipsilateral side	Atrophy of orbital contents as in postirradiation for malignant tumors or sclero derma
Craniofacial dysostosis	Resolved orbital cellulitis followed by fibrosis and mechanical retraction

The retrobulbar lesion can compress the optic nerve in the absence of significant proptosis. A marked impairment of vision with minimal proptosis is suggestive of optic nerve glioma in children.

Ocular Movements

The restricted ocular movements may be caused by:

- Thyroid ophthalmopathy involves inferior rectus muscle, causing its fibrosis and restriction of elevation.
- Restrictive myopathy.
- Blowout fracture.
- Neurological lesion.

Forced duction test is conducted to differentiate the defective ocular movements due to fibrosis from a neurological lesion. The muscle of the involved eye to be tested is grasped with toothed forceps under topical anesthesia. The difficulty in moving the globe (in the field of action of muscle) with the forceps indicates fibrotic contracture as in thyroid ophthalmopathy. In case of palsy due to neurological lesion (III nerve palsy), no resistance will be encountered.

Pupillary Reactions

The pupillary reactions may be slow reacting or absent which indicates the optic nerve involvement.

Fundus Examination

During fundus examination, one should look for:

- *Optic disc*: The optic disc may show edema or pallor.
- *Choroidal folds*: These may occur in orbital tumors or thyroid.
- *Venous engorgement*.

Measurement of Proptosis

The normal distance between the lateral orbital rim and the apex of cornea is usually less than 20 mm. A difference of >2 mm between the two eyes or a reading of ≥21 mm is regarded as abnormal. The amount of proptosis is measured by **Hertel's exophthalmometer** or with a **plastic rule** placed on the bone at lateral canthus (**Fig. 22.6**).

Examination of Paranasal Sinuses

Paranasal sinuses are examined to exclude mass or mucocele projecting into the orbit.

Systemic Examination

It is performed to rule out the systemic cause of proptosis, such as thyroid disorder, leukemia, neuroblastoma, and primary tumors of breast, lungs and gastrointestinal tract (GIT).

Investigations

Investigations include:

Laboratory tests: Serum T3, T4, thyroid stimulating hormone (TSH) estimation, total leucocyte count (TLC), differential leucocyte count (DLC), and erythrocyte sedimentation rate (ESR).

Histopathological examination:
- Fine needle aspiration biopsy.
- Excisional biopsy.

Imaging investigations
- Noninvasive investigations:
  ◇ Plain X-ray.
  ◇ CT scan.
  ◇ Ultrasonography.
  ◇ MRI.
- Invasive procedures:
  ◇ Venography.
  ◇ Arteriography.

■ Orbital Inflammation

Orbital inflammation is the third most common orbital disease after Grave's ophthalmopathy and lymphoproliferative diseases. The orbital inflammation is most commonly unilateral with symptoms and clinical findings depending on the site involved as well as the degree of inflammation,

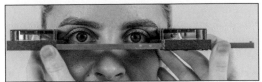

Fig. 22.6 Hertel's exophthalmometer. Source: Lang G, ed. Ophthalmology. A pocket textbook atlas. 3rd edition. Thieme; 2015.

- Lid swelling.
- Redness.
- Optic nerve dysfunction (if the inflammation involves the posterior orbit).

The severe prolonged inflammation eventually leads to fibrosis of orbital tissues, resulting in the "**frozen orbit**."

Investigations

Following investigations help in diagnosing idiopathic orbital inflammation:

- Ultrasonography.
- CT scan.
- Biopsy in persistent cases.

> On CT, both thyroid ophthalmopathy and myositis cause thickening of extraocular muscle, but in pseudotumor, thickening of extraocular muscle occurs with its tendinous insertions; whereas in thyroid eye disease, muscle enlargement is confined to the belly, sparing their tendinous portion.

Treatment

- *Systemic steroid*: Oral prednisolone is initially given at a dose of 1 to 2 mg/kg/day, subsequently being tapered and discontinued over several weeks.
- *Radiotherapy* may be considered if there has been no improvement after 2 weeks of adequate steroid therapy.
- Cytotoxic drugs (methotrexate and azathioprine) may be given as supplementary treatment or in resistant cases.

■ Tolosa–Hunt Syndrome

The Tolosa–Hunt syndrome is an idiopathic condition characterized by nonspecific granulomatous inflammation of orbital apex/superior orbital fissure or cavernous sinus in which a mass of granulation material is found around the carotid artery. It is a diagnosis of exclusion and should not be made without arteriography or venography.

Clinical Features

- Ipsilateral pain (periorbital or hemicranial).
- Ophthalmoplegia due to one or more ocular motor pareses.

- Diplopia.
- Proptosis: it is usually mild.
- Involvement of ophthalmic (I) division of trigeminal nerve, resulting in sensory loss along its distribution.

Investigations

Following investigations help in diagnosing Tolosa–Hunt syndrome:

- CT/MRI.
- Arteriography.
- Venography.

Full investigations are performed in Tolosa–Hunt syndrome because vascular causes, neoplasms and others make the differential diagnosis of the disease and the disease is a diagnosis of exclusion.

Treatment

It is characterized by remissions and recurrences and treated with systemic steroids and immunosuppressants.

■ Periostitis

It is the inflammation of periorbita and usually affects the orbital margin. However, deeper parts of the orbit may be involved. Trauma, tuberculosis, and syphilis could be the probable causes of periostitis.

Clinical Features

Periostitis of orbital margin presents with painful swelling and tenderness of underlying bone. Tuberculosis lesion usually results in a fistula formation. The periostitis of deeper parts of orbit is characterized by deep-seated pain and proptosis. The involvement of the orbital apex causes the **orbital apex syndrome** which is characterized by:

- Ocular motor palsies (III, IV, and VI) resulting in *ophthalmoplegia*.
- *Trigeminal anesthesia* and *neuralgia* due to involvement of 1st division of V nerve.
- *Amaurosis* due to the involvement of optic nerve.

Treatment

- Antibiotics.
- Evacuation of pus by incision into the abscess.
- Removal of any carious bone.
- Exploratory orbitotomy in deep-seated periostitis.

If it is left untreated, the disease may cause meningitis or cerebral abscess.

■ Fungal Orbital Cellulitis

It is a fatal fungal infection of the orbit and typically affects patients with diabetic ketoacidosis or immunosuppression. The most common causative fungi are Mucor (**Mucor mycosis**) and Aspergillus (**aspergillosis**). Spread of infection is explained in **Flowchart 22.2**.

Symptoms include pain, visual impairment, proptosis, and diplopia. The signs are less acute with slower progression. The infarction on septic necrosis is responsible for the classic **black eschar**

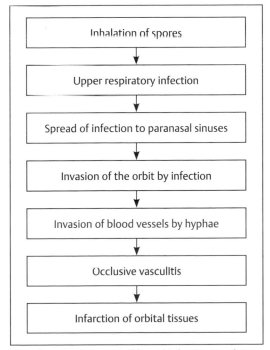

which may be seen on nasal septum, turbinates, palate and eyelids.

Complications include retinal vascular occlusion and cerebrovascular occlusion. Diagnosis can be confirmed by biopsy of necrotic tissue. Treatment involves the following considerations:

- Correction of diabetic ketoacidosis.
- Intravenous antifungal (Amphotericin B, 5 mg/kg).
- Excision of necrotic tissue.
- Exenteration in unresponsive cases.

■ Parasitic Diseases of the Orbit: Cysticercosis

Cysticercosis is caused by the pork tapeworm, Taenia solium. The larval form of Taenia solium is called **cysticercus cellulosae**. The tapeworm lives in the small intestine and the larvae of the worm penetrates the intestine, travels through the blood stream, and may develop into cysticerci in the muscles, brain, or eyes. Orbital cysticercosis presents with proptosis, restricted ocular motility, and recurrent inflammation.

Investigations

To diagnose orbital cysticercosis, CT scan and orbital ultrasonography are helpful. Demonstration of cystic lesion with a central hyperechoic, highly reflective scolex is diagnostic feature of cysticercosis.

Treatment

- Intramuscular cysticerci do not require treatment.
- Albendazole (15 mg/kg/day) is given twice daily for 8 to15 days

  or

- Praziquantel (50 mg/kg/day) is given thrice daily for 15 days.
- Systemic corticosteroids are administered simultaneously to counter the inflammatory response of local tissues.

Intraocular and intracranial cysticercosis must be ruled out before starting cysticidal therapy.

Flowchart 22.2 Spread of fungal infection to orbit.

The flowchart shows: Inhalation of spores → Upper respiratory infection → Spread of infection to paranasal sinuses → Invasion of the orbit by infection → Invasion of blood vessels by hyphae → Occlusive vasculitis → Infarction of orbital tissues

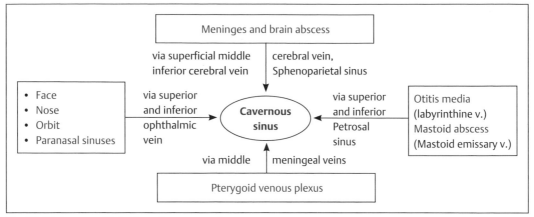

Fig. 22.10 Sources of infection of cavernous sinus.

Table 22.5 Ocular features of cavernous sinus thrombosis

Pain	Severe supraorbital pain (owing to the involvement of 1st division of trigeminal nerve)
Visual acuity	Reduced
Position of globe	Proptosis (often bilateral)
Ocular movement	Reduced due to involvement of III, IV, and VI nerves in cavernous sinus
Conjunctiva	Congestion and chemosis
Cornea	Anesthetic
Pupil	Dilated
Fundus	Retinal veins engorgement and disc edema indicate implication of orbital veins and tissues

Table 22.6 Classification of thyroid ophthalmopathy

Grade	Symptom and sign
0	No symptoms and signs
1	Only signs (of lid retraction and mild exophthalmos) but no symptoms
2	Soft tissue involvement Symptoms- Lacrimation, photophobia Signs- Lid retraction, lid lag, chemosis and exophthalmos
3	Marked exophthalmos
4	Restrictive myopathy involving extra ocular muscle (EOM) associated with diplopia
5	Exposure keratitis due to corneal involvement
6	Visual impairment or loss due to optic neuropathy

Pathogenesis

Thyroid ophthalmopathy involves an autoimmune reaction in which the antibody reacts against thyroid gland cells and orbital fibroblasts (**Flowchart 22.3**).

Clinical Features

Graves' ophthalmopathy is generally associated with hyperthyroidism (90%). It can also, though less commonly, occur in euthyroid and hypothyroid patients. Graves' ophthalmopathy includes ocular features and systemic features of hyperthyroidism.

Systemic features of hyperthyroidism include:
- Tachycardia.
- Palpitations.
- Tremors.
- Increased basal metabolic rate lead to heat production, weight loss, and warm and sweaty skin.

Ocular features include symptoms like:
- Retrobulbar discomfort.
- Red eyes.
- Puffy lids.
- Lacrimation.
- Photophobia.
- Tear insufficiency with grittiness.

Signs of Graves' Ophthalmopathy

Lid signs: These include:
- Retraction of upper lid (**Dalrymple sign**) in primary gaze. Increased thyroid hormones

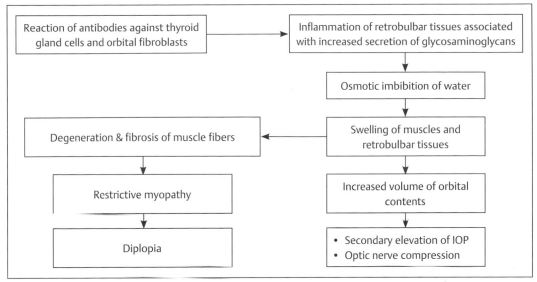

Reaction of antibodies against thyroid gland cells and orbital fibroblasts	→ Inflammation of retrobulbar tissues associated with increased secretion of glycosaminoglycans

Osmotic imbibition of water

↓

Degeneration & fibrosis of muscle fibers ← Swelling of muscles and retrobulbar tissues

↓

Restrictive myopathy

Increased volume of orbital contents

↓

Diplopia

- Secondary elevation of IOP
- Optic nerve compression

Flowchart 22.3 Pathogenesis of Graves' ophthalmopathy.

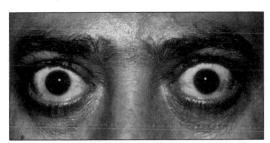

Fig. 22.11 Dalrymple sign (lid retraction). Source: Orbital involvement in autoimmune disorders: graves's disease. In: Lang G, ed. Ophthalmology. A pocket textbook atlas. 3rd edition. Thieme; 2015.

overstimulates sympathetic nervous system, leading to overaction of Muller muscle and resulting in lid retraction (**Fig. 22.11**).

- Lid lag (**von Graefe sign**): Upper lid lags behind the globe on down gaze.
- Puffy edematous eye lids (**Enroth sign**).
- Infrequent and incomplete closure of lids (**Stellwag sign**).
- Difficult eversion of upper eye lid (**Gifford sign**).

Defects of ocular movement: Ocular motility is restricted initially by inflammatory edema and later by fibrosis (restrictive myopathy). It leads to diplopia. *The most commonly involved muscle is inferior rectus.* The fibrotic contracture of inferior rectus muscle causes elevation defect which is the most common motility defect. It is followed by fibrosis of medial rectus (abduction defect), fibrosis of superior rectus (depression defect), and fibrosis of lateral rectus (adduction defect). There may be convergence deficiency (**Mobius sign**).

Exophthalmos: It is *axial*, unilateral or bilateral and frequently permanent. It is due to edema and lymphocytic infiltration of orbital contents, particularly the extra ocular muscles. Severe exophthalmos along with lid retraction and tear insufficiency may lead to exposure keratopathy, corneal ulceration, and infection.

Optic neuropathy: Retrobulbar edema and infiltration may cause the compression of optic nerve or its blood supply at the orbital apex. It may lead to severe visual impairment. The optic disc may be normal, swollen or, rarely, atrophic.

■ Diagnosis

It is based on the examination and investigations. Classical signs of the diseases include: eyelid retraction, exophthalmos and restrictive myopathy. Investigations include thyroid function test. Testing for THS receptors antibodies, ultrasonography, CT

Table 22.8 Types of vascular tumors of the orbit

Features	Capillary hemangioma	Cavernous hemangioma
Age of onset	It is congenital and presents during first 6 months of life. These show rapid growth followed by spontaneous involution over months to years.	Although it is congenital, it typically presents in adults (20–40 years).
Sex	Females > males	Females > males
Location	Usually extraconal, more common in *superonasal quadrant* of upper lid or may be posterior to orbital septum.	Usually intraconal, more commonly in *temporal quadrant*.
Histology	It is composed of varying-sized small vascular channels without true encapsulation.	It is a slowly progressive tumor of large, endothelial-lined channels separated by fibrous septae. It is usually well-encapsulated.
Symptoms	Superficial lesions cause ptosis and sometime associated with astigmatism and amblyopia. Deep lesions cause proptosis and displacement of globe.	It produces proptosis and motility restriction. The lesions may enlarge during pregnancy.
Signs	Superficial cutaneous lesions are bright-red and also known as "strawberry naevus." Deep-seated capillary hemangioma causes bluish discoloration.	• Axial proptosis. • Choroidal folds in case of large lesions. • Decreased vision due to optic nerve compression.
Diagnosis	It is confirmed by orbital ultrasonography and MRI.	By ultrasonography, MRI and contrast-enhanced CT.
Treatment	As they are benign and many lesions undergo spontaneous involution, treatment consists of simple observation. If vision is threatened, it is treated by the steroid injection of triamcinolone acetonide 40 mg/ml and betamethasone 4 mg/ml into the lesion. If necessary, injections may be repeated after ~2 months. If the lesion is small and well circumscribed it can be surgically excised.	Surgical excision is required because the lesion gradually enlarges. Being encapsulated it is relatively easy to remove the cavernous hemangioma, unlike capillary hemangioma.

Abbreviations: CT, computerizd tomography; MRI, magnetic resonance imaging.

as nerve sheaths, Schwann cells, axons, and endoneural fibroblasts, give rise to tumors. These may be divided into:

- Ectodermal tumors of nerve.
- Optic nerve glioma.
- Mesodermal tumors of the sheath of the nerve–meningiomas.

Optic Nerve Glioma

It is a tumor derived from the astrocytes of the optic nerve (**Fig. 22.14**). It typically affects children during the first decade of life. It is an intraconal tumor. It may be either a solitary manifestation

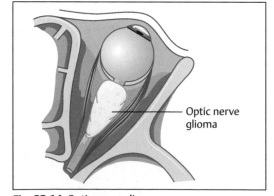

Fig. 22.14 Optic nerve glioma.

or may be associated with neurofibromatosis in 30% of the cases. Clinical features include slowly progressive loss of vision, unilateral, painless, and axial proptosis, and swollen optic nerve head initially which becomes atrophic subsequently. It may spread intracranially to involve chiasma and hypothalamus.

Diagnosis is conducted by CT scan and MRI. On orbital imaging, the lesion typically appears as intraconal fusiform enlargement of the optic nerve.

Treatment

- If vision is good: No treatment is required but simple observation is needed.
- If vision is poor and proptosis is significant: Surgical excision with preservation of globe is required for the tumors confined to the orbit.
- For tumors with intracranial extension: Radiotherapy and chemotherapy are the treatment modalities.

Prognosis

Prognosis for vision is poor. For lesions confined to the optic nerve, the prognosis for life is good. For lesions with intracranial extension, the prognosis is poor.

Optic Nerve Sheath Meningioma

It is a benign tumor arising from meningothelial cells of arachnoid, surrounding the intraorbital portion of the optic nerve. It typically affects middle aged adults (20–60 years). Females are more commonly affected than males. It is an intraconal tumor (**Fig. 22.15**). It presents with visual loss (gradual and unilateral). It causes chronic disc swelling followed by optic atrophy. In many cases, opticociliary shunt vessels are found which regress as optic atrophy supervenes. Restriction of ocular movements, particularly in upgaze, is common. Proptosis usually develops after the onset of visual loss due to intraconal spread.

> In tumors outside the dural sheath, the proptosis develops long before the optic nerve compression.

Diagnosis is confirmed by CT scan and MRI. If vision remains good, treatment consists of observation. Surgical excision is required with aggressive tumors (i.e., blindness with significant proptosis). Prognosis for life is good but visual prognosis is typically poor.

Plexiform Neurofibroma

It is the most common benign peripheral nerve tumor of orbit and eyelid. It is invasive and not encapsulated. It occurs almost exclusively in association with neurofibromatosis type 1. It affects children in the first decade of life.

Involvement of upper eyelid causes "**S**" shaped contour of eyelid with mechanical ptosis (**Fig. 22.16**). The tumor feels like a "**bag of worms**" on palpation. It may be associated with optic nerve glioma and pulsatile proptosis due

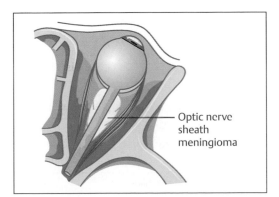

Fig. 22.15 Optic nerve sheath meningioma.

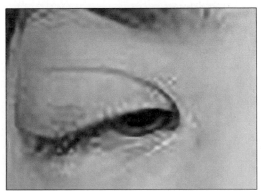

Fig. 22.16 S-shaped contour of eyelid.

to the absence of greater wing of sphenoid bone. Treatment involves surgery which is difficult.

Mesenchymal Tumors

Rhabdomyosarcoma

It is the most common primary *mesenchymal tumor* in children. It is a *highly malignant neoplasm* and *arises from* pluripotent mesenchymal precursors which normally differentiate into striated muscle. *It does not arise from the striated muscle.* It occurs during the *first decade* of life (average 7–8 years). Males are more affected than females. It most frequently involves the superonasal quadrant or retrobulbar muscle cone (**Fig. 22.17**).

Symptoms may be acute or subacute and are characterized by rapidly progressive exophthalmos, eyelid edema, and ptosis. It may cause bony erosion.

Diagnosis is conducted by CT scan, MRI, and ultrasonography. The most common sites of metastases are lung and bone. Excision biopsy may be performed through anterior orbitotomy. It should be differentiated from orbital cellulitis, metastatic neuroblastoma, and myeloid sarcoma, owing to its rapid progression. It is treated by local radiotherapy and chemotherapy with vincristine, actinomycin D, and cyclophosphamide. If the local treatment fails, orbital exenteration may be needed. Patients with orbital tumors have 95% cure rate and there is *more favorable prognosis because of near absence of orbital lymphatics.*

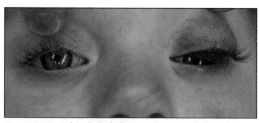

Fig. 22.17 Orbital rhabdomyosarcoma (left). Source: Orbital lesions. In: Burnstine M, Desner S, Samimi D et al., ed. Ophthalmic plastic surgery of the upper face: eyelid ptosis, dermatochalasis, and eyebrow ptosis. 1st edition. Thieme; 2019.

Lymphoid Tumors

Malignant Orbital Lymphoma (Lymphosarcoma)

It is a low-grade malignancy which arises in lymph nodes or an extranodal site such as the orbit. It presents usually in old age (50–70 years). Most lesions are located in the anterosuperior and lateral orbits. A palpebral mass may be present in the anterior orbit. It frequently involves the lacrimal gland. Symptoms include exophthalmos, diplopia, lid edema, and ptosis.

It can be diagnosed by investigations such as peripheral blood picture, chest X-ray, bone marrow aspiration, and thoracoabdominal CT lymphatic angiogram.

When the disease is confined to the orbit, radiotherapy is the best treatment. For disseminated disease, treatment is by chemotherapy.

■ Secondary Orbital Tumors

Tumors may invade the orbit from adjacent structures such as:
- Retinoblastoma and malignant melanoma from the eyeball.
- Squamous cell carcinoma and adenocarcinoma from eyelids.
- Squamous cell carcinoma of maxillary sinus from sinuses.
- Meningioma from brain.

Malignant tumors of paranasal sinuses may invade the orbit. Maxillary carcinoma is the most common sinus tumor to invade the orbit. *Maxillary carcinoma* causes facial pain and swelling, upward displacement of globe, diplopia, epiphora, epistaxis, and nasal discharge. Ethmoidal carcinoma causes lateral displacement of globe.

Nasopharyngeal carcinoma may spread to the orbit through the infraorbital fissure. The Vth and VIth nerves are most frequently involved, with rare involvement of III, IV, and optic nerves. Proptosis is a late finding. Treatment includes radiotherapy.

■ Metastatic Orbital Tumors

Metastases reach the orbit via hematogenous spread and are much less common than metastases to the choroid. In adults, most metastases are carcinomas. In children, metastases are more likely to be carcinomas and embryonal tumors of neural origin.

Adult Metastatic Tumors (Metastatic Carcinoma)

The most common *primary sites* of metastatic carcinoma to the orbit (in order of frequency) are:

1. Breast.
2. Bronchus.
3. Prostate.
4. Skin melanoma.
5. GIT.
6. Kidney.

The **clinical symptoms** include the following:
- Proptosis.
- Axial displacement of globe.
- Ptosis.
- Diplopia.
- Pain.
- Chemosis.

In females, the common source of orbital metastasis is breast carcinoma, while in man, it is bronchogenic carcinoma. Scirrhous cell breast carcinoma and gastric carcinoma cause orbital fibrosis, resulting in enophthalmos. In prostatic metastases, pain is more common because of bony involvement and occurs most commonly in elder patients.

Investigations helpful for diagnosis are CT scan and fine needle aspiration biopsy.

Treatment

It includes:
- Local radiotherapy combined with chemotherapy.
- Orchiectomy may be needed for prostatic carcinoma.
- Hormonal therapy may be indicated for breast carcinoma.

Prognosis is generally poor as orbital metastasis reflects more widespread systemic diseases.

Childhood Metastatic Tumors

Neuroblastoma arises from primitive neuroblasts of sympathetic chain. The primary tumor may be in the abdomen followed by the thorax and pelvis. It presents in early childhood (<7 years). Orbital metastatic causes bilateral abrupt onset of proptosis associated with lid ecchymosis.

Myeloid sarcoma may occur as a manifestation of acute myeloid leukemia and is composed of malignant cells of myeloid origin. It exhibits a characteristic green color, so formerly it was referred to as chloroma. It presents with rapid onset of unilateral/bilateral proptosis associated with ecchymosis and lid edema.

■ Orbital Injuries

The orbital fat surrounded by connective tissue fascia completely fills the spaces between the muscles, nerves, and vascular elements. These fat lobules provide a cushion to protect these delicate structures from injury during ocular movement. Blunt trauma involving the orbit usually results in hemorrhage or fracture of orbital bones.

■ Orbital Hemorrhage (Retrobulbar Hemorrhage)

Blunt or surgical trauma may cause bleeding in the orbit behind the globe. Accumulation of blood behind the globe may produce a compartment syndrome, **orbital compartment syndrome** which is characterized by (**Fig. 22.18**):
- Compression of optic nerve and decreased vision.
- Proptosis (protrusion of eyeball).
- Resistance to retropulsion of globe.
- Restricted ocular motility.
- Raised intraocular pressure (IOP).
- Pain.
- Diffuse subconjunctival hemorrhage.
- Lid ecchymosis.
- Tense eyelids that are very difficult to open.

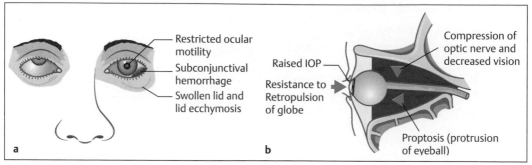

Fig. 22.18 (a, b) Features of orbital compartment syndrome. Abbreviation: IOP, intraocular pressure.

Treatment

Following points are important while treating orbital hemorrhage:

- Aggressive decompression: Orbital pressure must be relieved immediately by performing *lateral canthotomy* (a full-thickness incision is made from lateral canthus posterolaterally to the lateral orbital rim). It allows globe to proptose forward and decrease compartment syndrome.
- Reduction of IOP.
- Canthoplasty (repair of eyelid) is done approximately 1 week later.

■ Orbital Fractures (OP 9.5)

Blunt trauma may cause fractures of orbital walls and fractures of orbital margin.

Fracture of orbital margin: It is diagnosed by unevenness of margin and may involve:

- Inferior orbital rim (maxilla).
- Superotemporal rim (zygomaticofrontal suture).

Fractures of orbital walls: Blowout fractures of orbit occur when orbital walls are pressed indirectly. These result from blunt trauma caused by a large object such as fist, cricket ball, or football (**Fig. 22.19**, **Flowchart 22.4**).

Thus, blowout fractures most frequently involve floor of the orbit and medial orbital wall. Bones of lateral wall and the roof are usually able to withstand such trauma.

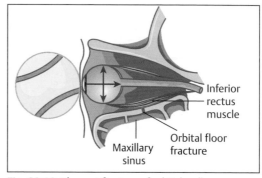

Fig. 22.19 Blowout fracture of orbital wall.

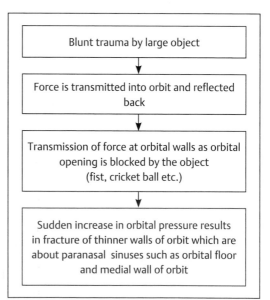

Flowchart 22.4 Mechanism of development of blowout fractures of orbit.

Blow-out Fracture of Orbital Floor

It is the *most common* blowout fracture of the orbit. Orbital floor consists of three bones—zygomatic, maxillary, and palatine. The *posteromedial portion of maxillary bone is relatively weak* and may be involved in "blowout" fracture. The orbital floor is traversed by infraorbital canal and forms the roof of the maxillary sinus.

Clinical features include diplopia, enophthalmos (sunken globe), infraorbital nerve hypoesthesia, orbital and lid emphysema, periocular ecchymosis, and edema (**Flowchart 22.5**).

Diagnosis

CT scan of orbit: Both axial and coronal views are obtained. Coronal section is useful in determining the herniation of orbit contents into maxillary sinus and entrapment of inferior rectus to be localized accurately. Entrapment can be confirmed by forced duction test under topical anesthesia. The eye is grasped at limbus and rotated in deficient direction of gaze. Limitation of passive eye movement confirms muscle entrapment.

CT scan is a better imaging modality for bony structures of orbit than plain X-ray or MRI.

Treatment

- Instruct the patients not to blow nose.
- Antibiotics: If fracture involves maxillary sinus and patient has a history of chronic sinusitis, diabetes, or is otherwise immunocompromised.
- Surgical intervention: Surgery is indicated when:
- Large fractures involving ≥½ of orbital floor.
- Persistent diplopia due to muscle entrapment.
- Entrapment of orbital contents with enophthalmos >2 mm.

Surgical repair is approached through eyelid (lower) and includes:

- Elevation of periosteum from orbital floor.
- Orbital contents are removed from atrum and release of entrapped inferior rectus muscle.
- Placement of an implant—teflon or silicon—to repair the defect in floor and suture of periosteum.

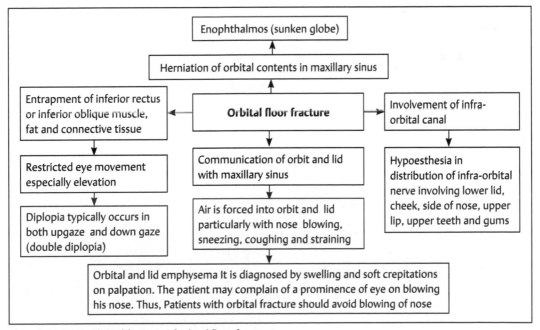

Flowchart 22.5 Clinical features of orbital floor fracture.

Blow out Fracture of Medial Wall

Medial wall of orbit is formed by four bones: ethmoid, lacrimal, maxillary, and sphenoid. Lamina papyracea, which forms part of medial wall and covers the ethmoid sinus, is paper thin and perforated by nerve and blood vessels. *This bone can be involved in blowout fractures of the orbit.* Medial wall orbit fractures are mostly associated with floor fractures.

Clinical Features

It includes the following:

- Periorbital hematoma.
- Defective abduction, if medial rectus muscle is entrapped in fracture.
- Severe epistaxis, if damage to anterior ethmoidal artery occurs.
- Orbital and lid emphysema, due to communication with sinus, typically develops on blowing the nose.

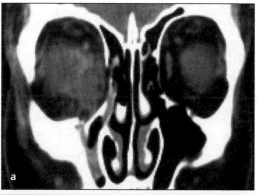

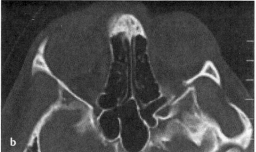

Fig. 22.20 (a, b) Fracture of lateral wall. Source: Orbital trauma. In: Agarwal A, Jacob S, ed. Color atlas of ophthalmology. The quick-reference manual for diagnosis and treatment. 2nd edition. Thieme; 2009.

It is diagnosed accurately by CT scan of orbit. Treatment involves release of entrapped tissue and repair of bony defect.

Fracture of Orbital Roof

The roof of orbit is formed by two bones: orbital plate of frontal bone and lesser wing of sphenoid bone. Roof is located subjacent to anterior cranial fossa and frontal sinus. The orbital roof fractures may involve frontal sinus, cribriform plate, and brain.

Clinical Features

- Periocular hematoma (black eye) associated with subconjunctival hemorrhage without a visible posterior limit.
- May present with CSF rhinorrhea.
- Large fractures may be associated with transmission of CSF pulsations to the orbit. Pulsations of globe unassociated with a bruit. It is best defected on applanation tonometry.

> If pulsations of globe (or pulsatile proptosis) is associated with a bruit which can be heard on auscultation over eye, AV fistula (e.g., carotid-cavernous fistula) is the underlying pathology.

Fracture of Lateral Wall

It is rare because lateral wall of orbit is more solid than other walls (**Fig. 22.20**).

Fracture of Base of Skull

It may involve one or both optic foramen and may cause injury to optic nerve, resulting in optic atrophy and pulsating exophthalmos. Basal skull fracture may give rise to characteristic bilateral ring hematomas– **"Panda eyes"** (**Fig. 22.21**).

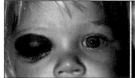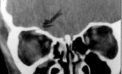

Fig. 22.21 Ring hematomas in case of fracture of base of skull. Source: Periorbital and eyelid anatomy. In: Codner M, McCord C, ed. Eyelid & periorbital surgery. 2nd edition. Thieme; 2016.

Ocular Manifestations in Neurological Disorders

Pupil Anomalies...591

Disorders of Cranial Nerves..595

Nystagmus...607

Vascular Disorders 612

Demyelinating Disease 618

Intracranial Infections 621

Intracranial Space-Occupying Lesions (ICSOL) 623

Trauma and the Brain (Head Injury)..626

Hereditary and Degenerative Diseases...628

Headache 630

■ Pupil Anomalies

Pupil regulates the amount of light, increases the depth of focus, and reduces various optical aberrations. It is regulated by two muscles–sphincter pupillae (supplied by parasympathetic system) and dilator pupillae (supplied by sympathetic system).

Normally, pupils constrict equally. Retina and optic nerve provide the afferent signals, while the oculomotor nerve provides the efferent component to both direct and consensual light reactions. Pupillary disorders may involve:

- *The afferent pathways.*
- *The efferent pathways*: It may be parasympathetic or sympathetic. Disorders of parasympathetic system include III nerve palsy, while the interruption of sympathetic nerve supply to the eye causes Horner's syndrome.

■ Afferent Pupillary Defect

It may be absolute or relative. The relative afferent pupillary defect is the most common abnormal pupillary finding which was described by

R. Marcus Gunn. Kestenbaum named the findings after Marcus Gunn and Levatin introduced the "swinging flash light test."

Absolute Afferent Pupillary Defect (Amaurotic Pupil)

It is caused by complete optic nerve lesion, so there is no light perception in involved eye, that is, the involved eye is completely blind. Characteristic features of absolute afferent pupillary defect are as follows:

- Both pupils are equal in size in diffuse illumination.
- Near reflex is normal in both eyes.

Characteristic reactions are listed in **Table 23.1**.

Relative Afferent Pupillary Defect (Marcus Gunn Pupil)

Relative afferent pupillary defect (RAPD) is caused by an incomplete optic nerve lesion or severe retinal disease. It is never caused by a dense cataract. The causes include:

- Unilateral optic neuropathy: Traumatic and ischemic (arteritic and nonarteritic).

- Optic neuritis.
- Glaucoma: Normally, glaucoma is a bilateral disease; if one optic nerve has particularly severe damage, a RAPD can be seen.
- Compressive damage to optic nerve as in optic nerve tumor or thyroid orbitopathy.
- Radiation optic nerve damage.

Due to incomplete optic nerve lesion, pupils respond weakly to the stimulation of involved eye and briskly to that of normal eye (**Table 23.2**).

Swinging flash light test: In this test, each eye is stimulated in rapid succession. The light source is alternatively switched from one eye to the other and back. This compares the direct and consensual pupillary constriction of each eye to look for a difference in the afferent conduction between them, which is called a RAPD. It relies on a comparison between the two eyes and is looking for (and can only detect) an asymmetrical abnormality in the afferent pathway (**Fig. 23.1**).

■ Efferent Pupillary Defect

The physiology behind a normal pupillary constriction is a balance between sympathetic and parasympathetic systems. The sphincter pupillae encompass the pupil and is innervated by parasympathetic system which leads to pupillary constriction.

The dilatation is controlled by the dilator pupillae (in the peripheral 2/3rd of iris), which is innervated by sympathetic system.

Etiology

- Brain stem lesions.
- III nerve lesion (fascicular).
- Ciliary ganglion lesion.
- Iris damage.

Characteristic features of efferent pupillary defect are:

There is no response of involved eye, while there is constriction and dilatation in normal eye, so **anisocoria** prevails. In **normal eye**, direct and consensual light reflexes are present. In **involved eye**, direct and consensual light reflexes are absent. Near reflex is also absent. Pupil is fixed and dilated.

In **afferent** (sensory) nerve lesions, the pupils are equal in size.

In **efferent** (motor) nerve lesions, or the iris itself, **anisocoria** (asymmetrical pupil diameter) is the finding.

Table 23.1 Reactions of pupils in absolute afferent pupillary defect

Features	Involved eye	Normal eye	Remark
Stimulation of involved eye	Direct light reflex is absent	Consensual light reflex is absent	So, neither pupil reacts
Stimulation of normal eye	Consensual light reflex is present	Direct light reflex is present	Both pupils react normally

Table 23.2 Reactions of pupils in relative afferent pupillary defect

Features	Involved eye	Normal eye	Remark
Stimulation of involved eye	Direct light reflex is present but sluggish	Consensual light reflex is present but sluggish	On stimulation of normal eye, both pupils constrict, but when the light is swung to the involved eye, both pupils dilate instead of constriction
Stimulation of normal eye	Consensual light reflex is present and brisk	Direct light reflex is present and brisk	

■ Horner's Syndrome (Oculosympathetic Paresis) (AN31.3)

Horner's syndrome results from damage to sympathetic innervation of the eye and is characterized by miosis, partial ptosis, loss of hemifacial sweating as well as enophthalmos.

Etiology

It is caused by an interruption of the sympathetic nerve supply to the eye. Causes of Horner's syndrome are depicted in **Fig. 23.2**.

Clinical Features

The classical signs of Horner's syndrome are as follows:

- A constricted pupil (due to unopposed action of sphincter pupillae with resultant anisocoria, **Table 23.3**).
- Mild ptosis (due to weakness of Muller muscle).
- Absence of facial sweating (anhydrosis), if the lesion is below the superior cervical

ganglion because the sudomotor fibers supplying the skin of the face run along the external carotid artery.

- Slight enophthalmos.
- Pupillary reactions are normal to light and near.

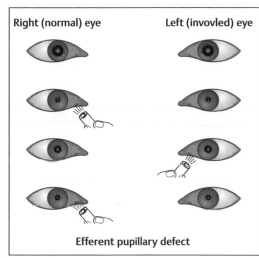

Fig. 23.1 Swinging flash light test.

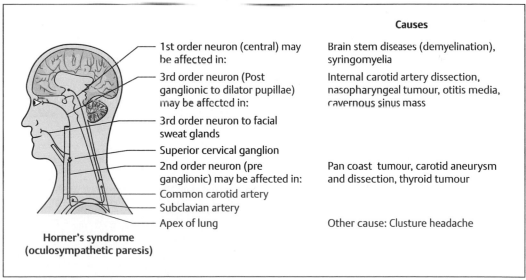

Fig. 23.2 Causes of Horner's syndrome.

■ Pupillary Light-Near Dissociation

The term pupillary light-near dissociation refers to any situation in which pupillary near reaction is present and the light reaction is absent. It is seen in Argyll Robertson (AR) pupil and Adie's tonic pupil. It is possible to distinguish between the two types of pupil. The accommodation response in AR pupils is brisk and immediate. The near response in tonic pupils is slow and prolonged.

Etiology

Light-near dissociation may be unilateral or bilateral and the causes are as listed in **Table 23.4**.

Argyll Robertson (AR) Pupil

It is a bilateral small pupil which responds to accommodation reflex but does not react to light. So, the pupil shows light-near dissociation and does not respond to both direct and consensual reactions.

Etiology

It is caused by neurosyphilis and attributed to a dorsal midbrain lesion. Neurosyphilis leading to accommodation reflex present (ARP) causes damage in the area of pretectal to the internuncial neuron. The pupillary near reflex pathway is more ventral than pupillary light reflex pathway, which is why the lesion interrupts the light reflex pathway but spares the near reflex pathway. It results in light-near dissociation. Characteristic features of AR pupil are as follows:

- Involvement is usually bilateral but asymmetrical.
- The pupils are small in size (**<2 mm**) and irregular in shape.
- The light reflex is absent but near reflex is present (**ARP**).
- The pupils are difficult to pharmacologically dilate. They dilate poorly with mydriatics like atropine.

Table 23.3 Distinguishing features of Horner's syndrome and physiological anisocoria

Test	Response of normal pupil	Response of Horner pupil	Remark
• Instillation of a drop of 4% cocaine	*Dilates*	*Does not dilate*	Cocaine blocks the reuptake of noradrenaline secreted at postganglionic nerve endings. In Horner's syndrome, cocaine has no effect as no noradrenaline is secreted.
• Instillation of a drop of apraclonidine 0.5–1%	*Unaffected*	*Dilates*	Alpha-1 receptors are upregulated in the denervated dilator pupillae.
• Instillation of a drop of phenylephrine 1%	*Does not dilate*	*Dilates in postganglionic lesion **but** will not dilate in central or preganglionic lesions.*	There is denervation hypersensitivity of dilator pupillae in postganglionic Horner's syndrome.

Table 23.4 Causes of unilateral and bilateral light-near dissociation

Unilateral light-near dissociation	Bilateral light-near dissociation
• Afferent conduction defect • Adie's pupil • HZO • Aberrant III nerve regeneration	• Neurosyphilis • Parinaud (dorsal midbrain) syndrome • Encephalitis • Myotonic dystrophy • Diabetic neuropathy • Alcoholic midbrain degeneration.

Abbreviation: HZO, Herpes zoster ophthalmicus.

Adie's Tonic Pupil

Etiology

It is due to damage to the ciliary ganglion or postganglionic parasympathetic fibers, following a viral illness, for example, herpes zoster ophthalmicus (HZO). Characteristic features of Adie's tonic pupil are:

- It typically affects younger women (third or fourth decade) and is unilateral in 80% cases.
- Pupil is large and there exists a difference in the size of the pupils (anisocoria). There is abolition of light reflex with retention of near reflex (i.e., light-near dissociation). The near reflex is slow and tonic, that is, once the pupil has constricted, it remains small for an abnormally long time (**tonic pupil**).
- On slit lamp examination, vermiform movements of the pupillary border are typically seen.

Pharmacological Testing

It helps in the diagnosis of Adie's tonic pupil. There is cholinergic supersensitivity of the denervated muscle. In 80 to 90% of patients with Adie's tonic pupil, 0.125% Pilocarpine causes denervation super sensitivity (i.e., Adie's tonic pupil constricts with 0.125% Pilocarpine, while normal pupil does not). The concentration is too weak to cause constriction of the normal pupil (*0.125% pilocarpine is prepared by diluting one part 1% Pilocarpine with 7 parts balanced salt solution*).

Adie's syndrome is applied when both pupil and associated hyporeflexia are present. The association includes diminished deep tendon reflexes of the knee and ankle– **Holmes–Adie syndrome**.

Wernicke's Hemianopic Pupil

It is caused by division of the optic tract which results in a contralateral homonymous hemianopia. The pupils fail to react light when a narrow pencil of light is shone onto the nonseeing part of the retina (i.e., temporal retina of affected side and nasal retina of opposite side), but they do react if it falls onto the seeing retinal areas (i.e., nasal retina of affected side and temporal retina of opposite side).

■ Abnormalities of Size

The pupil may be small (miotic) or large (mydriatic) (**Table 23.5**).

■ Disorders of Cranial Nerves

The cranial nerve (CN) palsies are of neuro-ophthalmological significance. These may be:

- **Nuclear** ocular motor palsies that occur at the level of ocular motor nucleus.
- **Fascicular** nerve palsies, which are caused by lesions of the fascicle of nerve, travel through the brain stem from the nerve nucleus to its exit into the subarachnoid space.
- Isolated and multiple **cranial nerve** palsies.

Nuclear and fascicular nerve palsies are often associated with other neurological signs because of many structures located nearby. Damage to nuclei and nerves results in specific deficits,

Table 23.5 Causes of miotic and mydriatic pupil	
Miotic (<2 mm) pupil	**Mydriatic (>5 mm) pupil**
- Horner's syndrome (due to sympathetic paralysis) - Uveitis - Sympathetic denervation - Drugs: Parasympathomimetics (e.g., pilocarpine) - Morphine - Argyll Robertson pupil	- Third CN palsy (due to parasympathetic paralysis) - Traumatic iris damage - Drugs: Sympathomimetics, parasympatholytics (e.g., atropine) - Adie's pupil - Iris rubeosis - Uncal herniation (due to stretch)
Abbreviation: CN, cranial nerve.	

Table 23.6 Characteristic features of lesion of third CN at various sites of involvement

Site of involvement	Features
Nucleus (nuclear IIIrd CN palsy) (due to infarction or tumors)	Unilateral III nerve palsy with contralateral SR paresis (sparing ipsilateral SR muscle) and bilateral partial ptosis suggests nuclear lesion.
	As a *central caudal nucleus* innervates both LPS muscles; so, nuclear III CN palsy causes bilateral ptosis. **A unilateral ptosis excludes a nuclear lesion.**
	Rostral nuclear lesion spares central caudal subnucleus for LPS muscle and results in bilateral III nerve palsy without ptosis.
Fascicular IIIrd CN palsy	As fascicles have already left IIIrd CN nucleus, so ocular manifestations are present only on one side.
• Involvement of IIIrd CN fascicle as it passes through red nucleus	It is called **Benedikt syndrome** and is characterized by: • Ipsilateral IIIrd nerve palsy, and • Contralateral hemitremor (extrapyramidal sign)
• Involvement of IIIrd CN fascicle as it passes through cerebral peduncle	It is called **Weber syndrome** and is characterized by: • Ipsilateral IIIrd nerve palsy, and • Contralateral hemiparesis as cerebral peduncle contains corticospinal tract.
IIIrd CN palsy in subarachnoid space	Aneurysm of posterior communicating artery at its junction with internal carotid artery compresses IIIrd CN, resulting in acute, isolated, painful IIIrd nerve palsy with pupillary involvement. In a truly isolated IIIrd nerve palsy, the presumed location is subarachnoid space.
Intracavernous IIIrd CN palsy	Because of proximity to other CN, intracavernous IIIrd CN palsy is usually associated with involvement of IVth, VIth CN, 1st division of trigeminal nerve (V1), and oculosympathetic paralysis (Horner's syndrome). Pupil is usually spared (90%).
Intra orbital IIIrd CN palsy	It is characterized by: • Drooping of eyelid (**Ptosis**) • Binocular crossed diplopia as eye is abducted in primary position (exotropia). • Enlarged pupil. • Difficulty in focusing due to involvement of accommodation. • Elevation is limited due to SR and IO muscles weakness. So, eye is deviated down and out (hypotropia and exotropia). • Intorsion of eye at rest due to weakness of extorters (IO and IR muscles).

Abbreviations: CN, cranial nerve; IO, inferior oblique; IR, inferior rectus; LPS, levator palpebrae superioris; SR, superior rectus.

to both IVth CN fascicle at their decussation and results in bilateral superior oblique (SO) palsy. **So, when bilateral IVth CN palsy occurs, the site of injury is likely in the anterior medullary velum**.

In cavernous sinus, IVth nerve palsy occurs in association with other CN palsies (IIIrd, Vth, and VIth) and oculosympathetic paralysis.

Since 1st division of 5th CN (trigeminal nerve) is also involved, pain may be a prominent feature. Most common cause of an isolated IVth CN palsy

is trauma. Clinical features of trochlear nerve palsy are mentioned in **Flowchart 23.3**.

■ Abducens Nerve (VIth CN) and its Lesions (AN31.5)

Abducens nucleus is located at the midlevel of pons, just ventral to the floor of 4th ventricle. It is closely related to the following:

- Paramedian pontine reticular formation (PPRF) (horizontal gaze center).
- MLF.

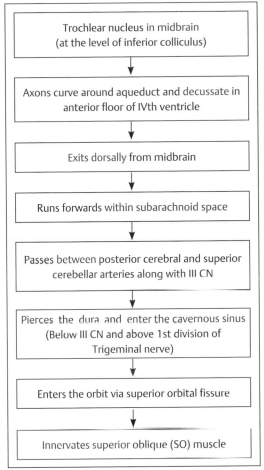

Flowchart 23.2 Course of IV nerve.

- 1st order sympathetic fibers.
- Spinal tract of trigeminal nerve (Vth CN).
- Facial nerve (VIIth CN): Fasciculus of VIIth CN (facial nerve) wraps around the VIth nerve nucleus. **So, isolated 6th nerve palsy is never nuclear in origin**.

It contains two types of neurons:

- 60% project directly to LR muscle via abducens nerve.
- 40% are interneurons which project via MLF to contralateral MR subnucleus and cause adduction of contralateral eye.

Course of VIth cranial nerve is explained in **Flowchart 23.4** and depicted in **Fig. 23.5**.

Lesions of VIth CN

VIth CN lesions may involve the nerve at the level of nucleus, fascicle, cavernous sinus, and orbit.

Nuclear VIth CN Palsy

A lesion in and around the 6th nerve nucleus involves the related structures. Damage to the 6th nerve nucleus or caudal PPRF (horizontal gaze center) causes ipsilateral horizontal gaze palsy. **Associated deficits** with ipsilateral horizontal gaze palsy (nuclear VIth CN palsy) may be:

- Ipsilateral lower motor neuron (LMN) facial nerve palsy (due to damage to facial nerve fasciculus).

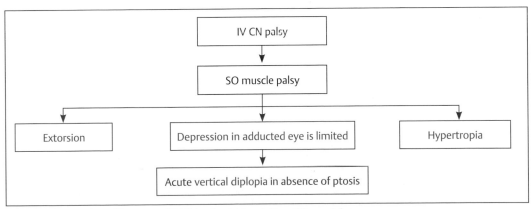

Flowchart 23.3 Clinical features of IV CN palsy. Abbreviation: CN, cranial nerve.

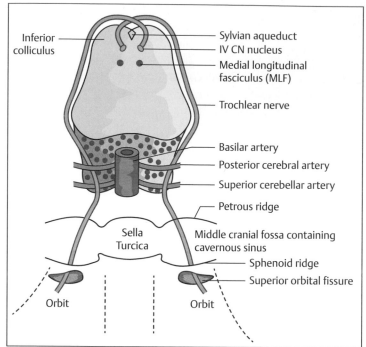

Fig. 23.4 Course of fourth cranial nerve.

Inferior colliculus

Sylvian aqueduct

IV CN nucleus

Medial longitudinal fasciculus (MLF)

Trochlear nerve

Basilar artery

Posterior cerebral artery

Superior cerebellar artery

Petrous ridge

Sella Turcica

Middle cranial fossa containing cavernous sinus

Sphenoid ridge

Superior orbital fissure

Orbit

Orbit

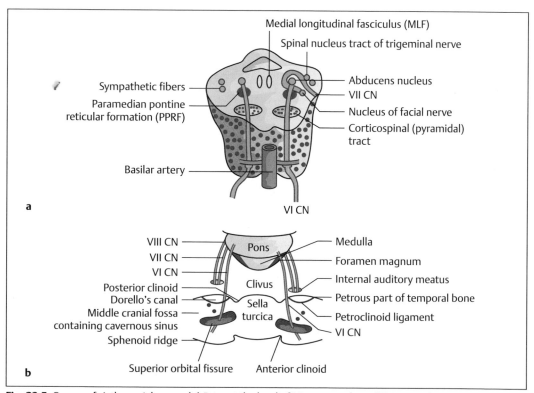

Medial longitudinal fasciculus (MLF)

Spinal nucleus tract of trigeminal nerve

Sympathetic fibers

Paramedian pontine reticular formation (PPRF)

Abducens nucleus

VII CN

Nucleus of facial nerve

Corticospinal (pyramidal) tract

Basilar artery

a

VI CN

VIII CN

Pons

Medulla

VII CN

Foramen magnum

VI CN

Internal auditory meatus

Posterior clinoid

Clivus

Dorello's canal

Sella turcica

Petrous part of temporal bone

Middle cranial fossa containing cavernous sinus

Petroclinoid ligament

Sphenoid ridge

VI CN

b

Superior orbital fissure

Anterior clinoid

Fig. 23.5 Course of sixth cranial nerve. **(a)** Pons at the level of VI nerve nucleus. **(b)** Occipital view.

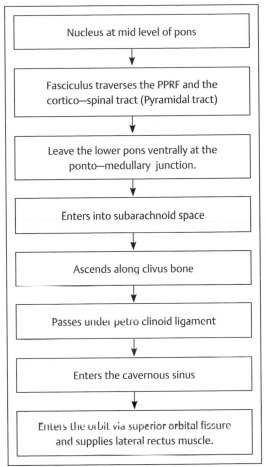

```
┌─────────────────────────────────────┐
│      Nucleus at mid level of pons    │
└─────────────────────────────────────┘
                  │
                  ▼
┌─────────────────────────────────────┐
│  Fasciculus traverses the PPRF and the │
│  cortico–spinal tract (Pyramidal tract)│
└─────────────────────────────────────┘
                  │
                  ▼
┌─────────────────────────────────────┐
│   Leave the lower pons ventrally at the │
│      ponto–medullary junction.        │
└─────────────────────────────────────┘
                  │
                  ▼
┌─────────────────────────────────────┐
│      Enters into subarachnoid space   │
└─────────────────────────────────────┘
                  │
                  ▼
┌─────────────────────────────────────┐
│      Ascends along clivus bone        │
└─────────────────────────────────────┘
                  │
                  ▼
┌─────────────────────────────────────┐
│  Passes under petro clinoid ligament  │
└─────────────────────────────────────┘
                  │
                  ▼
┌─────────────────────────────────────┐
│      Enters the cavernous sinus       │
└─────────────────────────────────────┘
                  │
                  ▼
┌─────────────────────────────────────┐
│ Enters the orbit via superior orbital fissure │
│   and supplies lateral rectus muscle. │
└─────────────────────────────────────┘
```

Flowchart 23.4 Course of the VI CN. Abbreviation: CN, cranial nerve.

- Ipsilateral preganglionic Horner's syndrome (due to damage to 1st order sympathetic fibers traveling the pons).
- Ipsilateral facial analgesia (due to damage to spinal tract of Vth CN).
- Ipsilateral internuclear ophthalmoplegia (INO), due to involvement of ipsilateral medial longitudinal fasciculus. So, ipsilateral eye cannot adduct or abduct, while contralateral eye can only abduct. It is called **one-and-a-half syndrome**.

Fascicular VIth CN Palsy

- VIth nerve fasciculus, involving pyramidal tract, results in VIth nerve palsy with

contralateral hemiplegia, since pyramidal tracts decussate in medulla to control contralateral voluntary movements (**Raymond's syndrome**).
- Lesions involving VIth nerve fasciculus, VIIth nerve fasciculus, and pyramidal tract results in **Millard–Gubler syndrome**.

So, patients who have truly isolated VIth CN palsy, nuclear or fascicular involvement is unlikely.

VIth CN palsy at petrous apex results in **Gradenigo syndrome** which includes:
- VIth nerve palsy.
- Ipsilateral facial pain (Vth CN).
- Ipsilateral facial palsy (VIIth CN).
- Ipsilateral hearing loss (VIIIth CN).

Intracavernous VIth CN Palsy

In cavernous sinus, isolated VIth nerve palsy is rare. Lesions in cavernous sinus are associated with multiple CN palsies. VIth CN is more prone to damage than other nerves because VIth CN is most medially situated and runs through the middle of sinus in close relation to internal carotid artery while other CNs (IIIrd, IVth, 1st division of Vth CN) are protected within the wall of sinus.

Intraorbital VIth CN Palsy

VIth nerve palsy is associated with multiple CN palsies (IIIrd, IVth,).

■ Trigeminal (V) Nerve and Its Lesion

It is the *largest* and *mixed* (sensory and motor) CN.

Trigeminal nucleus extends through the whole of the midbrain, pons and medulla, and into the high cervical spinal cord. It consists of *sensory nuclei* (mesencephalic, principal sensory, and spinal nuclei of trigeminal nerve) and one *motor nucleus* (motor nucleus of the trigeminal nerve) in the upper pons, medial to the principal sensory nucleus (**Fig. 23.6**).

Course of Trigeminal Nerve

At the level of pons, the sensory root emerges from the sensory nuclei, and the motor nucleus continues to form the motor root (ventromedial

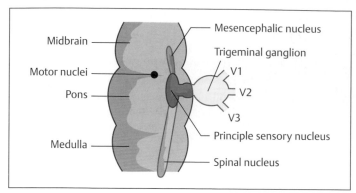

Fig. 23.6 Nucleus and ganglion of trigeminal nerve.

to the sensory root). In middle cranial fossa, the sensory root expands into the trigeminal ganglion, located lateral to the cavernous sinus in a depression of temporal bone known as the **trigeminal cave**. The trigeminal ganglion (**Gasserian ganglion**) gives rise to three divisions (**Fig. 23.7**):

- Ophthalmic nerve (V1)– It exits via the superior orbital fissure and enters into the orbit. It carries sensory information from the scalp and forehead, upper eye lid, conjunctiva and cornea of the eye, nose (including the tip of nose except alae nasi), nasal mucosa, frontal sinuses, lacrimal gland, and parts of meninges. In the orbit, it divides into three branches: frontal, lacrimal, and nasociliary.
- Maxillary nerve (V2)– It leaves the skull via the foramen rotundum and supplies the face. It carries sensory information from the lower eye lid and cheek, nares and upper lip, upper teeth and gums, palate, roof of pharynx, and sinuses (maxillary, ethmoid, and sphenoid).
- Mandibular nerve (V3)– The motor root passes inferior to the sensory root (from the Gasserian ganglion) at the level of ganglion and both exit the skull via the foramen ovale. After leaving the skull, both roots unite to form a single trunk as the mandibular nerve. It has mixed sensory and motor fibers. It carries sensory information from the lower lip, lower teeth and gums,

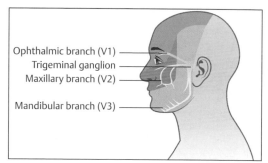

Fig. 23.7 Divisions of trigeminal nerve.

chin and jaw, except the angle of mandible, parts of external ear and meninges. The motor fibers supply the muscles of mastication.

Ophthalmic and maxillary nerves are **purely sensory,** while the mandibular nerve has **both sensory** and **motor** functions.

Applied Aspect (Disorders of Trigeminal Nerve)

- **Corneal reflex**—The corneal reflex is the involuntary blinking of the eye lids (**Flowchart 23.5**).

Afferent limb: In the corneal reflex, the ophthalmic nerve acts as the afferent limb, which is stimulated by tactile, thermal, or painful stimulation of the cornea.

Efferent limb: In the corneal reflex, the facial nerve is the efferent limb causing contraction of the orbicularis oculi muscle.

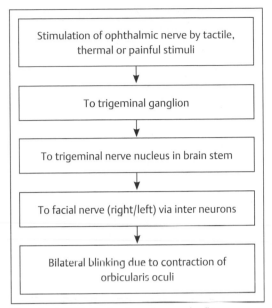

Flowchart 23.5 Mechanism of corneal reflex.

If the corneal reflex is absent, it is a sign of damage to the trigeminal/ophthalmic nerve or facial nerve.

- **Trigeminal neuralgia** (Tic Douloureux)

Neuralgia is pain in the distribution of a nerve. Trigeminal neuralgia affects the sensory branches of the Vth cranial nerve.

It is usually idiopathic but may be due to:
- Demyelination of the nerve (multiple sclerosis).
- Petrous ridge compression.
- Post traumatic neuralgia.
- Intracranial tumors.
- Viral infections.

Clinically, it is characterized by pain in the distribution of one or more branches of the trigeminal nerve. The pain has the following clinical characteristics:
- Sudden.
- Unilateral.
- Intermittent paroxysmal.
- Sharp shooting.
- Rarely crosses the midline.
- Short duration.

- Mask-like face.
- Lancinating shock like pain elicited by slight touching.

Its treatment includes:
- Medical treatment.
- Surgical treatment.

Medical treatment includes:
- Oral carbamazepine 100 to 200 mg four times a day as first-line treatment.
- Baclofen and lamotrigine as second-line treatment.
- Others:
  ◇ Clonazepam.
  ◇ Oxcarbazepine.
  ◇ Gabapentin.
  ◇ Topiramate.

Surgical treatment: When drug fails to relieve the pain, surgery is indicated which includes:
- Percutaneous stereotactic radiofrequency thermal lesioning (**RFL**) of the trigeminal ganglion and/or root. This procedure selectively destroys nerve fibers associated with pain.
- Posterior fossa exploration and microvascular decompression (**MVD**) of the trigeminal root.
- Gamma knife radiation (**GKR**) to the trigeminal root entry zone.

■ Facial (VIIth) Nerve and Its Lesions

It is a mixed nerve. The **sensory component** arises from the nucleus solitarius (located in medulla) and carries taste sensations from the anterior 2/3rd of the tongue. The **motor component** arises from the facial nucleus at the level of pons and innervates the muscles of facial expression. The **parasympathetic component** arises from the superior salivary nucleus and acts as preganglionic secretomotor component. It supplies lacrimal glands, and submandibular and sublingual salivary glands.

Course of Facial Nerve

The course of the facial nerve can be divided into two parts: *intracranial and extracranial.*

Intracranial Part

The nerve arises in the pons, as large motor and small sensory roots, and emerges from the brain stem between the pons and medulla. The nerve travels through the internal acoustic meatus in the petrous part of temporal bone. The roots leave the internal acoustic meatus and enter the facial canal ("Z"-shaped structure). Within the facial canal (**Fig. 23.8**):

- The two roots fuse to form the facial nerve.
- The nerve forms the geniculate ganglion.
- The nerve gives rise to three branches:
  ◊ The greater petrosal nerve (para-sympathetic fibers to glands).
  ◊ The nerve to stapedius (motor fibers to stapedius muscle).
  ◊ The chorda tympani (special sensory fibers to the anterior 2/3rd of tongue).

The facial nerve exits the facial canal via the stylomastoid foramen (located posterior to the styloid process of temporal bone).

Extracranial Part

After exiting the skull via the stylomastoid foramen, the facial nerve continues anteriorly and inferiorly into the parotid gland (*parotid gland is innervated by the glossopharyngeal nerve, not facial nerve*) and supplies the muscles of facial expression by splitting into five terminal branches (**Fig. 23.9**):

- Temporal branch.
- Zygomatic branch.
- Buccal branch.
- Marginal mandibular branch.
- Cervical branch.

Applied Aspect (Disorders of Facial Nerve)

Central connections of facial nerve nucleus: All voluntary movements depend upon excitation of LMN by upper motor neuron (UMN).

UMN controls LMN through two different pathways: pyramidal tract and extrapyramidal tract.

LMN functions as the final common pathway between the central nervous system (CNS) and skeletal muscles.

- The upper part of facial nucleus receives bilateral supranuclear (cortical) innervation.
- The lower part of facial nucleus receives contralateral supranuclear (cortical) innervation (**Fig. 23.10**).

Function of forehead is preserved in supranuclear lesions

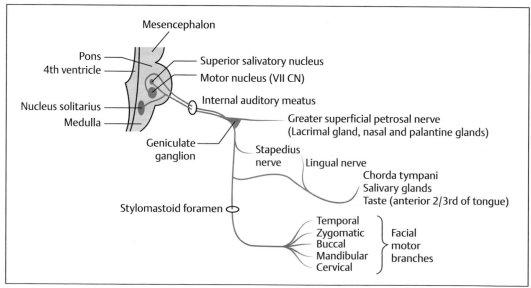

Fig. 23.8 Course of facial nerve (central and peripheral).

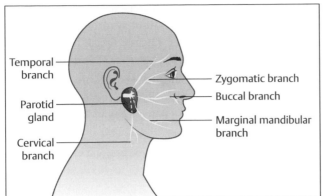

Fig. 23.9 Terminal branches of facial nerve.

Temporal branch

Parotid gland

Cervical branch

Zygomatic branch

Buccal branch

Marginal mandibular branch

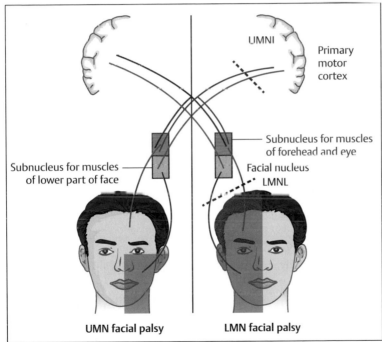

Fig. 23.10 Disorders of facial nerves (UMN and LMN). Abbreviations: LMN, lower motor neuron; UMN, upper motor neuron.

UMNI

Primary motor cortex

Subnucleus for muscles of forehead and eye

Subnucleus for muscles of lower part of face

Facial nucleus

LMNL

UMN facial palsy

LMN facial palsy

The facial nerve has a wide range of functions. Thus, damage to the nerve can produce a varied set of symptoms, depending on the site of the lesion.

Facial nerve lesions may be supranuclear, nuclear, or peripheral type. Peripheral lesions occur due to the following reasons:

- Injury at internal acoustic meatus.
- Injury distal to geniculate ganglion.
- Injury at stylomastoid foramen.

Features of supranuclear type lesions (upper motor neuron lesion [**UMNL**]) are:

- Paralysis of the lower part of face contralateral (opposite side) to the lesion.
- Partial paralysis of the upper part of face.
- Normal taste and saliva secretion.
- Stapedius is not paralyzed.

Physiological Nystagmus

It may be:

- End-gaze nystagmus (at extremes of gaze).
- Optokinetic nystagmus.
- Vestibular nystagmus: may be caloric nystagmus or rotational nystagmus.

End-Gaze Nystagmus

It is found in extreme positions of gaze and there is no nystagmus in the primary position. It is a jerk nystagmus with fast phase in the direction of gaze.

Optokinetic Nystagmus (OKN)

It is physiological nystagmus commonly known as rail-road nystagmus. It is a jerk nystagmus induced by moving repetitive targets across the visual fields or when a person in a mobile vehicle looks at an outside object. In the slow phase (pursuit movement), the eyes follow the target and are controlled by the ipsilateral parieto-occipito temporal (POT) junction. The fast phase (saccadic movements) occurs in the opposite direction, as the eyes fixate on the next target and are controlled by the contralateral frontal eye field in the frontal lobe (see **Fig. 16.18**). For example, if the OKN drum is moved from right to left, slow phase is to the left and controlled by the left (ipsilateral) POT region, while the fast phase is to the right and controlled by the left (contralateral) frontal lobe. It is useful for detecting malingerers and visual acuity testing in small children.

Vestibular Nystagmus

It may be physiological as well as pathological nystagmus.

Physiological Vestibular Nystagmus

Each SSC of membranous labyrinth contains endolymph which may move toward or away from its ampulla. Horizontal SCC are oriented 30° above horizon with ampulla anteriorly located. Anterior SCC are oriented in vertical plane and directed outward and forward at 45°. Posterior SCC are oriented in vertical plane and directed outward and backward at 45°. The nystagmus varies according to the SCC stimulated. Thus, for maximal effect of rotational forces on horizontal SCC, head is inclined forward 30°. When head is tilted forward at 30° angle, horizontal SCC of both sides are at horizontal plane. For maximal effect of caloric testing (irrigating the ear with cold or warm water), head is inclined backward 60°.

Vestibular nystagmus may be caloric nystagmus or rotational nystagmus. Movement of endolymph in a SCC may be caused by cold or warm water (**caloric nystagmus**). SCC can also be stimulated by rotation, with the head in a suitable position (**rotational nystagmus**). Movement of endolymph toward ampulla results in stimulation of that ampulla. Movement of endolymph away from ampulla results in inhibition of that ampulla.

Caloric nystagmus: Vestibular nystagmus may be elicited by caloric stimulation with head tilted back 60° as described below. On irrigation of external ear (say left) with warm water, endolymph rises toward ampulla. Left SCC is stimulated, sending impulse to the left vestibular nucleus. It results in excitation of right PPRF, leading to slow eye movement to the right and fast phase to the left. *So, warm water causes fast phase to the same side.*

On irrigation of external ear (say left) with cold water, endolymph moves away from ampulla. Thus, inhibition of left SCC and vestibular tone from right SCC dominates, which sends impulse to the right vestibular nucleus. It results in excitation of left PPRF, leading to slow eye movement to the left and fast phase to the right. *So, cold water causes fast phase to the opposite side.*

It can be remembered by the mnemonic **"COWS,"** wherein **C** = cold, **O** = opposite, **W** = warm, and **S** = same

(The direction of nystagmus refers to the fast phase)

Bilateral Simultaneous Caloric Stimulation

When **cold** water is poured into both ears simultaneously, vertical nystagmus results in fast phase **upwards**. When **warm** water is poured into both ears, vertical nystagmus results in fast phase **downward**. *If tympanic membrane is perforated, oxygen piped through ice should be used instead of water.*

It can be remembered by the mnemonic **"CUWD,"** wherein **C** = cold, **U** = upward, **W** = warm, **D** = downward.

Rotational nystagmus: It is performed with the head tilted forward at 30°. On rotation of head to the left, the endolymph moves toward the left ampulla and away from the right ampulla because of inertia. It results in stimulation of left horizontal SCC. If the head is rotated to the right, endolymph moves toward the right ampulla and away from the left ampulla because of inertia. It results in stimulation of right horizontal SCC (**Flowchart 23.6**).

So, direction of fast component during rotation is same as that of rotation. This test should not be performed if the neck is unstable.

Pathological Nystagmus

It may be early onset or acquired nystagmus.

Early onset nystagmus (congenital nystagmus)

It is an early onset nystagmus rather than truly congenital and usually develops because of the inability to develop normal fixation. It can occur secondary to poor vision early in life or due to ocular motor disturbance. Early onset nystagmus is commonly pendular but may be jerky.

Characteristics of congenital nystagmus are:
- Both eyes have similar amplitude.

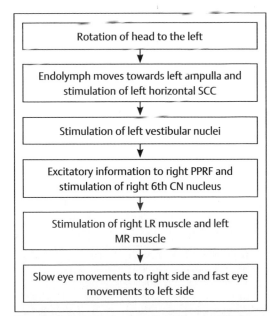

Flowchart 23.6 Mechanism of rotational nystagmus.

- There is no oscillopsia (illusion of environmental movement).
- It is not present during sleep, that is, it is abolished in sleep.
- It may be dampened by convergence.
- It is increased by fixation effort.
- There is usually a null point
- Plane of the nystagmus, usually horizontal, remains unchanged in all positions of gaze including vertical gaze.

> Patients may be helped by base-out prism glasses that induce convergence during distance fixation, as the nystagmus is dampened by convergence.

Sensory Deficit Nystagmus

The basic cause in this form is the inadequate image formation on the fovea in early life, for example, congenital cataract, optic nerve hypoplasia, and macular hypoplasia. It is always bilateral, pendular and horizontal. If a child loses vision before 2 years, he will invariably develop nystagmus. After 6 years, the child usually does not develop nystagmus.

Motor Defect Nystagmus

The primary defect is in the efferent mechanism. The family history is common and no ocular abnormalities are present. The child presents with nystagmus approximately 2 to 3 months after birth which persists throughout life. The nystagmus is pendular in primary position and may convert to jerk nystagmus on the side gaze.

Spasmus Nutans

Nystagmus in infancy may be acquired after the period at which fixation develops. Spasmus nutans develops between 3 and 18 months of life and disappears by 3 to 4 years of age. It is characterized by the triad of nystagmus, head nodding and head turn. Characteristics of nystagmus are:
- Pendular.
- Horizontal, vertical or torsional.
- Low amplitude.
- High frequency.
- Generally unilateral or may be binocular with asymmetry.

Gliomas may mimic spasmus nutans; therefore, spasmus nutans requires high-resolution CT scan to exclude afferent visual pathway pathology.

Acquired Nystagmus

Nystagmus that develops at any time beyond early infancy is called acquired nystagmus and is often associated with other neurological abnormalities. Anything that impacts the parts of the brain that control eye movements can result in nystagmus. The main effect of acquired nystagmus is the sense that things are always moving (oscillopsia). It includes periodic alternating nystagmus, vestibular nystagmus, upbeat nystagmus, down beat nystagmus, see-saw nystagmus, gaze-paretic nystagmus, ataxic nystagmus, bruns nystagmus, and convergence-retraction nystagmus.

Periodic Alternating Nystagmus

It is a conjugate, horizontal, jerk nystagmus which periodically reverses its direction. The nystagmus with the fast phase beats in one direction for a period of 1 to 2 minutes with an intervening null phase. Then, nystagmus begins to beat in the opposite direction for 1 to 2 minutes and the process repeats itself. It can be congenital or may be caused by cerebellar disease.

Pathological Vestibular Nystagmus

Vestibular nystagmus can also occur as pathologic nystagmus. It may be central or peripheral (**Table 23.7**).

Vestibular nystagmus with interstitial keratitis is known as **Cogan syndrome**.

Up Beat Nystagmus

The fast phase is upward in this vertical nystagmus. It is seen in:

- Lesions of posterior fossa.
- Vermis of cerebellum.
- Drug toxicity (phenytoin).

If it is present in primary gaze, the lesion typically involves the brain stem or anterior vermis of cerebellum. If present only in up gaze, it is most likely due to drug toxicity. It often worsens in upgaze, so *base up prisms in reading glasses* can be used to force the eyes downward.

Down Beat Nystagmus

The fast phase is downward in the vertical nystagmus. It is seen in lesions at the foramen magnum (lesions at cervicomedullary junction) such as the Arnold–Chiari malformation, syringomyelia, and multiple sclerosis. Oscillopsia is usually prominent. It often worsens in downgaze (convergence), so *base down prisms in reading glasses* can be used to force the eyes upward.

See-Saw Nystagmus

It is a pendular nystagmus characterized by conjugate rotatory component (intorsion of one eye and extorsion of the other) and disconjugate vertical component (elevation of one eye and depression of the other), that is, one eye elevates and intorts, while the other eye depresses and extorts simultaneously, followed by reversal of cycle, so the eye moves like a see-saw. It is seen in parachiasmal diseases (often with bitemporal hemianopia) involving chiasma or IIIrd ventricle or both.

Gaze-Paretic Nystagmus (Muscle Paretic Nystagmus)

It is a jerk nystagmus and occurs in motility defects in the direction of paresis. It disappears completely in total gaze paralysis and is absent in primary position. It is not visually disabling

Table 23.7 Distinguishing features between central and peripheral vestibular nystagmus

Central vestibular nystagmus	Peripheral vestibular nystagmus
• It is seen in lesions of vestibular nucleus in the brain stem and not dampened by fixation.	• It is seen in lesions of vestibular apparatus such as labyrinthitis, trauma, and ischemia.
• Deafness or tinnitus is usually absent in central vestibular nystagmus.	• Deafness or tinnitus is often present in peripheral vestibular nystagmus.

and is associated with brain stem disorders at the pontine level.

Brun's Nystagmus

It is a combination of gaze-paretic and vestibular nystagmus and is characteristic of cerebellopontine angle tumors such as acoustic neuroma.

Convergence-Retraction Nystagmus

It is a jerk nystagmus and caused by co-contraction of EOM, often the medial recti, especially on attempted upgaze. The convergence movement is associated with retraction of globe. It is seen in:

- Lesions of pretectal area: Pineal gland tumor (pinealoma).
- Midbrain abnormalities involving aqueduct of Sylvius (**Sylvian aqueduct syndrome** or **Parinaud syndrome**).

Sylvian Aqueduct Syndrome

Vertical gaze center (rostral interstitial nucleus of MLF) lies in the midbrain, just dorsal to red nucleus. From vertical gaze center, impulses pass to the subnuclei of eye muscles controlling vertical eye movements. The causes include:

- Aqueduct stenosis.
- Pinealoma.
- Midbrain vascular accidents (basilar artery stroke).

Features of Sylvian aqueduct syndrome include:

- Supranuclear upgaze palsy (eyes are straight in primary position and downgaze is normal), so upward gaze is limited.
- Eyelid retraction (Collier's sign).
- On attempting vertical gaze, convergence like eye movements accompanied by globe retraction take place (convergence-retraction nystagmus).
- Pupils are bilaterally mid dilated, which react poorly to light but constrict better to convergence (light-near dissociation).

Latent Nystagmus

It is seen only when one eye is covered. With both eyes open, there is no nystagmus. It is a jerk nystagmus with the fast phase in the direction of the uncovered eye. Visual acuity is diminished due to nystagmus when each eye is tested separately, but improves when both eyes are open, that is, *binocular vision is better than monocular vision*. It is often associated with infantile esotropia.

> Sometimes, nystagmus is present even without covering the eye (manifest nystagmus) but worsens on covering one eye, that is, amplitude of nystagmus increases (manifest-latent nystagmus).

Gaze-Evoked Nystagmus

In this type, nystagmus is present only in peripheral gazes and absent in the primary position of gaze. It is a jerk nystagmus with the fast phase in the direction of gaze. Its frequency is low (3–8 beats/sec) and caused by:

- Alcohol intoxication.
- Barbiturates (sedatives).
- Cerebellar disease.
- Brainstem disease.

Rebound Nystagmus

In rebound nystagmus, the fast phase is in the direction of gaze, but fatigue occurs with sustained gaze and the fast phase changes direction. It is seen in cerebellar lesions.

Nystagmus Blockage Syndrome

It is a specific form of nystagmus which disappears when the fixating eye is in adduction and manifests with straight eyes. So, the patient demonstrates esotropia to dampen the nystagmus. If face turn is large, muscle surgery may be considered as a treatment.

Miners' Nystagmus

It is essentially rotatory and very rapid. It occurs in coal miners. The patient complains of defective vision which is worse at night. Fixation difficulties in dim illumination may be an etiological factor. It may be eliminated by improvement in miners' lamps and lighting of mines.

Nystagmoid Movements

These resemble the nystagmus and include the following:

Ocular flutter: These are horizontal saccadic oscillations with no intersaccadic interval. In ocular flutter, oscillations are purely horizontal.

Opsoclonus: In opsoclonus, the oscillations are in multiple directions. It often follows the viral encephalitis.

Ocular dysmetria: When gaze is shifted from one point to another in space, there is inability to fixate the target accurately, and the eyes may either overshoot or undershoot the target.

Ocular bobbing: In ocular bobbing, there is rapid downward conjugate eye movements with slow return to primary position. It may be caused by pontine lesions, cerebellar lesions compressing pons, and metabolic encephalopathy.

Oculopalatal myoclonus: It is a disorder in which oscillation of eyes are associated with movements of masticatory muscles, tongue and facial muscles. It may be caused by brain stem damage or brain stem encephalitis.

■ Management of Nystagmus

It includes:
- *Careful history*:
  ◇ Age of onset.
  ◇ Oscillopsia.
  ◇ Drug/alcohol use.
  ◇ Associated symptoms.
  ◇ Occupational history.
  ◇ Family history.
- *Ocular examination*: Look for eye movements, visual fields and ocular albinism.
- *Neurological examination* (to rule out diseases of CNS): Neuroimaging by CT or MRI should be done.
- *Correction of* refractive error with spectacles, prisms and contact lenses must be performed.
- Amblyopia must be treated with occlusion or penalization.
- Medications such as baclofen (for periodic alternating nystagmus) and gabapentin (for acquired pendular nystagmus) may be helpful.

- Retrobulbar injections of botulinum toxin has only temporary effect.
- *Surgery*: It is done in cases with null point to reduce nystagmus and eliminate abnormal head posture.

■ Vascular Disorders

The **circle of Willis** is the part of the cerebral circulation which involves circulatory anastomosis between vertebrobasilar artery (posterior circulation) and internal carotid artery (ICA, anterior circulation). The posterior communicating artery is given off as a branch of ICA before its division into anterior and middle cerebral arteries (ACA and MCA). The anterior communicating artery connects the two anterior cerebral arteries. The posterior cerebral arteries (PCA) arise from the basilar artery which is formed by the left and right vertebral arteries. The vertebral arteries arise from the subclavian arteries. The circle of Willis is composed of the following arteries:
- Right and left ACA.
- Anterior communicating artery.
- Right and left ICA.
- Right and left PCA.
- Right and left posterior communicating artery.

The MCAs, supplying the brain, are not considered part of the circle.

Vascular disorders can affect visual pathway (sensory), oculomotor system (motor pathway) of the eye, and CNS.

■ Mechanism of Vascular Lesion

Vascular lesions could occur due to the following causes:
- Aneurysms, carotid–cavernous fistulas and arteriovenous (AV) malformations produce damage to the eye and brain.
- Occlusion of vessels.
- Intracerebral hemorrhage.

The blood supply to the eye is provided by branches of the ophthalmic artery which is a branch of **ICA**.

The blood supply to the brain is provided by anterior circulation (from the ICA and its branches) and posterior circulation (vertebrobasilar system).

The **carotid arteries** supply the eye and the anterior portion of the brain, which includes most of the cerebrum. The **vertebral arteries**, merging to form the basilar artery, feed the posterior portion of the brain (occipital cortex, cerebellum and brain stem). Hence, patients with **carotid artery disease** present with ipsilateral visual changes, while the **vascular diseases affecting the posterior circulation** result in binocular visual loss or abnormal extraocular movements.

The two basic types of neurovascular conditions affecting blood vessels in the brain are ischemic (due to occlusion) and hemorrhagic (due to leakage of blood from aneurysms and blood vessels).

Intracranial Aneurysms

Aneurysms most commonly arise at the bifurcation of vessels and are usually congenital or developmental. Aneurysms affect the circle of Willis and originate from the branches of ICA, usually at the posterior communicating artery, ophthalmic artery, or within the cavernous sinus.

Sites of Aneurysms Formation

Manifestations of the aneurysm depend on its location and its size. Aneurysms of ≥25 mm are almost always symptomatic. Aneurysms that have ophthalmological manifestations affect the following portions of the circle of Willis (**Fig. 23.12**):

1. Junction of ICA and posterior communicating artery: These cause IIIrd CN palsy producing motor (IIIrd CN) signs and symptoms.
2. Junction of ICA and ophthalmic artery: These cause compression of optic nerve and/or chiasma, producing sensory (optic nerve and chiasma) symptoms and signs.
3. Intracavernous carotid artery: These cause EOM palsy, facial sensory loss over Vth CN and, rarely, optic nerve compression.

Fate of Aneurysm

Aneurysms may either exert *mechanical pressure* on neighboring structures or *rupture. Therefore, ocular manifestations occur due to either of the above two reasons.*

Aneurysms of Circle of Willis

- *Neuro-ophthalmic manifestations due to mechanical pressure: ICA–ophthalmic artery*

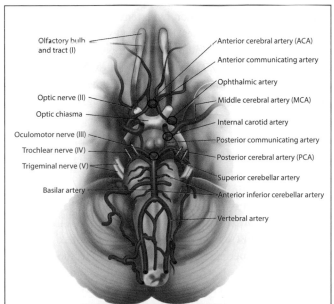

Olfactory bulb and tract (I)
Optic nerve (II)
Optic chiasma
Oculomotor nerve (III)
Trochlear nerve (IV)
Trigeminal nerve (V)
Basilar artery

Anterior cerebral artery (ACA)
Anterior communicating artery
Ophthalmic artery
Middle cerebral artery (MCA)
Internal carotid artery
Posterior communicating artery
Posterior cerebral artery (PCA)
Superior cerebellar artery
Anterior inferior cerebellar artery
Vertebral artery

Fig. 23.12 Circle of Willis with sites of aneurysms (*black circle*) and nerves in relation.

Ocular examination may be completely normal, or an embolus may be visible within a retinal arteriole. The emboli may be composed of calcium, platelets and fibrin, or cholesterol material (**Hollenhorst plaques**). Auscultation over a partial stenosis give rise to a bruit which is best heard with the bell of stethoscope. Auscultation of a bruit in the neck indicates the need for carotid magnetic resonance arteriography or carotid Doppler imaging.

> *Prolonged monocular transient visual loss (TVL) occurs in patients with hypertension and blood dyscrasias. Binocular TVL may be seen with classic migraine, occipital ischemia, and tumor of occipital lobe.*

Treatment

General measures include cessation of smoking, control of diabetes, hypertension and hyper-lipidemia, control of obesity by losing weight with diet and exercise. Specific measures include the following:

- Antiplatelet therapy by aspirin.
- Carotid endarterectomy in patients with symptomatic stenosis.
- Cardiac surgery in case of valvular heart disease.
- Calcium-channel blockers if the occlusion is vasospastic.

Carotid Artery Occlusive Disease

The ischemia due to occlusion can either be temporary, resulting in TIA, or permanent, resulting in thromboembolic stroke.

Etiology

Atherosclerosis is the leading cause of the disease, while embolism is another major cause.

Occlusion of ACA: The ACA branches off the ICA and supplies the anterior medial portions of the frontal and parietal lobes and is least commonly affected by stroke (**Fig. 23.13**). ACA stroke causes contralateral leg weakness and sensory loss. Behavioural abnormalities and incontinence also may occur.

Occlusion of MCA: *The MCA is the most common site of occlusion.* The MCA feeds the frontal, temporal and parietal lobes as well as the brain's deep structures—basal ganglia and internal capsule. Ischemia of MCA causes reversible neurological deficit (cerebral TIAs) in the territory supplied by MCA, which tend to be longer in duration than ocular TIAs. If the defect persists, the term stroke should be used. Depending upon the severity of occlusion, signs and symptoms may vary.

Occlusion of the main stem affects the entire territory of brain supplied by the MCA. MCA strokes *affect the face and arm more severely than the leg.* The hallmarks of an MCA stroke are facial asymmetry, arm weakness, and speech deficits. Complete MCA strokes typically cause varied symptoms, as listed in **Table 23.9**.

> Occlusion of **ACA** affects **lower limbs**; Occlusion of **MCA** affects **upper limbs**.

Vertebro-Basilar Insufficiency (VBI)

Posterior circulation (vertebrobasilar blood flow) supplies blood to brain stem, cerebellum, thalamus, and occipital cortex.

Reduction in vertebrobasilar blood flow causes ischemia of the brain stem and occipital cortex,

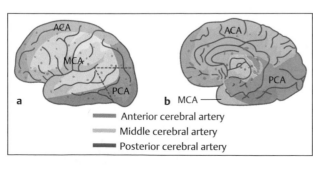

Fig. 23.13 Anterior, middle, and posterior cerebral arteries. **(a)** Lateral surface of brain. **(b)** Medial surface of brain.

Table 23.9 Ischemia of middle cerebral artery–signs and symptoms with respect to the area supplied

Area supplied by MCA	Sign and symptoms due to Ischemia of MCA
• Portion of frontal lobe	• Hemiparesis or hemiplegia of contralateral side affecting the lower part of the face, arm and hand while largely **sparing the leg**.
• Areas of speech (Broca's area in frontal lobe and Wernicke's area in temporal lobe of dominant hemisphere)	• Aphasia/speech impairments as a result of a dominant hemisphere lesion (usually the left brain). If TIA is due to right MCA (nondominant side), left transient motor or sensory loss results without aphasia.
• Portion of parietal lobe	• Contralateral sensory loss.
• Inferior optic radiations in temporal lobe	• Visual agnosia with contralateral homonymous hemianopia, preferably the upper quadrants of the field due to damage to the inferior optic radiations.

Abbreviations: MCA, middle cerebral artery; TIA, transient ischemic attack.

producing neurological and visual disturbances which may be transient or persistent. VBI is also called beauty parlor syndrome (**BPS**). Risk factors for VBI include hypertension, smoking, diabetes, obesity, and hyperlipidemia.

Clinical Features

The symptoms due to VBI vary according to which portions of the brain experience significantly decreased blood flow.

- The **midbrain infarction** (stroke) results in nystagmus, Weber's syndrome (oculomotor nerve dysfunction and contralateral hemiplegia) and Benedict's syndrome with contralateral cerebellar signs.
- **Pontine stroke** produces horizontal conjugate gaze palsy to the side of lesion, facial nerve palsy (VII nerve palsy), contralateral hemiparesis, and cerebellar signs. Isolated VIth nerve palsy without neurological signs may also be caused by a fascicular lesion. The infarction of MLF in the pons may result in unilateral internuclear ophthalmoplegia (INO).
- Vertigo is the most common neurological symptom. The vertigo due to VBI can be brought on by head turning, which could occlude the contralateral vertebral artery and result in decrease blood flow to the brain. Vertigo may be accompanied by ataxia, dysarthria, dysphasia, and **drop attacks** (sudden episodes of falling to the

ground without loss of consciousness due to weakness of the quadriceps. The patient may suddenly become weak at the knee and crumple).

- Hemiparesis and hemisensory disturbances:
  ◊ The **occlusion of PCA**: PCA arises from the top of the basilar artery and feeds the medial occipital lobe and inferior and medial temporal lobes. So, a stroke affecting PCA distribution usually causes isolated, macular sparing homonymous hemianopia and, therefore, is the hallmark of occipital stroke (while an MCA stroke also may cause this symptom, in that case, the visual deficit stems from damage to the visual pathways rather than direct occipital-lobe injury). Ipsilateral macular visual cortex may be spared because of the blood supply provided by the terminal branches of MCA. Transient visual symptoms due to PCA hypoperfusion are encountered less commonly. Other neurological deficits associated with hemianopia include alexia without agraphia, in which patient cannot recognize simple words but able to write words.
  ◊ **Obstruction of posterior inferior cerebellar artery** results in infarction of a wedge-shaped area on the lateral aspect of medulla. It may lead to

◇ Bladder dysfunction (urinary incontinence).

- *Ocular manifestations:* Manifestations of MS in the eye include both the afferent and efferent pathways. It manifests as:
  ◇ Optic neuritis.
  ◇ Retinal periphlebitis with sheathing.
  ◇ Paralysis of EOMs.
  ◇ Diplopia.
  ◇ *Gaze paresis.*
  ◇ Bilateral internuclear ophthalmoplegia.
  ◇ **RAPD.**
  ◇ Visual field defects due to patches of demyelination in the visual pathway.

Paralysis of EOMs. Of the individual nerves, *VIth CN is more often affected* than IIIrd nerve. **Total IIIrd nerve paralysis is never seen.** External ophthalmoplegia is partial but internal ophthalmoplegia is unknown.

- *Other clinical findings* include:
  ◇ Uhthoff's phenomenon (worsening of symptoms in higher temperature).
  ◇ Lhermitte's sign (an electrical sensation running down the back when the neck is flexed). The sign suggests a lesion of the dorsal columns of the cervical cord or caudal medulla.
  ◇ Trigeminal neuralgia.

Diagnosis

It includes:
- Detailed neurological examination.
- Laboratory tests include:
  ◇ Cerebrospinal fluid (CSF) analysis shows elevated IgG and oligoclonal (IgG) bands.
  ◇ Venereal disease research laboratory (VDRL), rapid plasma reagin (RPR), and fluorescent treponemal antibody absorption (FTA-ABS) for syphilis.
  ◇ Serum angiotensin-converting enzyme (ACE) for sarcoidosis.
  ◇ Erythrocyte sedimentation rate (ESR) and C-reactive protein (CRP) for inflammatory disorders.
  ◇ Antinuclear antibody (ANA) for SLE.

◇ Tuberculin skin tests or Quantiferon-TB for tuberculosis.
- Chest X-ray.
- MRI of head and spine: It reveals multiple periventricular lesions. CT scan is not effective in visualizing lesions of brain stem, cerebellum and optic nerve.
- VEP: It shows slowed conduction through pathways where myelin has been damaged.
- Visual field charting: Diffuse depression of sensitivity in the entire central field is the most common. Focal defects are frequently accompanied by the generalized depression.

Prognosis

MS can have severe debilitating effects within 20 to 25 years of onset. Visual prognosis following the first episode of optic neuritis is typically good. However, recurrent episodes are associated with less favorable prognosis.

Treatment

There is no cure for MS. Management involves intravenous methyl prednisolone, followed by oral prednisolone in tapering doses. In patients with progressive MS interferon and intravenous immunoglobulins are generally used as disease-modifying agents.

■ Neuromyelitis Optica (Devic's Disease)

In Devic's disease, inflammation involves the optic nerve and spinal cord. There is no involvement of other CNs. It is sudden in onset and a visual defect usually precedes the signs of myelitis. Its etiology is unknown.

Clinical Features

It is characterized by bilateral optic neuritis associated with acute transverse myelitis (*acute*– sudden onset; *transverse*– involvement across one level of the spinal cord; *myelitis*– inflammation of the spinal cord). Acute transverse myelitis is characterized by acute or subacute motor, sensory and autonomic spinal cord dysfunction, with progressive quadriplegia and anesthesia.

Treatment

Being a rare disease, there are no large-scale studies of treatment for neuromyelitis optica (NMO). Its acute attack can be treated with intravenous steroids (1 g methylprednisolone/day IV in combination with a proton pump inhibitor for 5 consecutive days), followed by tapering oral steroids. If the steroids are not effective, plasmapheresis is often used.

As NMO takes a relapsing course in most cases, a long-term immunosuppressive treatment with azathioprine, rituximab, cyclophosphamide, and methotrexate should be initiated.

Prognosis

The disease may be fatal in 25 to 50% of the pupil with loss of life most commonly due to respiratory failure. However, the life expectancy various from person to person.

■ Diffuse Sclerosis (Schilder's Disease)

It is a rare progressive demyelinating disorder and a variant of MS. It usually begins in childhood and the progressive demyelination involves the entire white matter of cerebral hemisphere and brain stem with no remissions.

Clinical Features

These include dementia, aphasia, seizures, personality changes, apathy, loss of memory, tremors, balance stability, incontinence, muscle weakness, headache, and vomiting.

Ocular manifestations include visual impairment due to destruction of optic radiation and visual centers, optic neuritis or retrobulbar neuritis due to demyelination of optic nerve, and ophthalmoplegia due to ocular motor palsies and nystagmus.

Prognosis

Death usually occurs within 1 year of onset.

■ Acute Disseminated Encephalomyelitis

It is a rare autoimmune disease marked by demyelination in the brain and spinal cord. It is often triggered after the viral infection (measles, mumps, influenza, chickenpox, infectious mononucleosis) or following the vaccination for rabies. It is characterized by bilateral optic neuritis at presentation.

■ Intracranial Infections

Ocular involvement in CNS infections is not infrequent and must be established. The CNS infections include meningitis, encephalitis, and brain abscess. The bacteria, viruses, fungi, nematodes, and parasites can all cause intracranial infections.

Most of the CNS infections share four cardinal manifestations, that is, headache, fever, altered mental status, and focal neurological signs.

■ Meningitis

It is an acute inflammation of meninges of CNS (brain and spinal cord). If the brain parenchyma is also involved, the condition is known as meningoencephalitis. It may be acute, chronic, or basal meningitis.

Etiology

It is caused by infection with bacteria, virus, fungi, protozoans, and nematodes.

Clinical Features

Systemic symptoms include fever, headache, stiffness of neck, nausea, vomiting, and seizures. Characteristic signs of meningitis are:

- **Neck rigidity** (resistance to passive neck flexion) is pathognomonic for most forms of meningitis.
- **Positive Kernig sign:** Kernig sign is assessed with patient lying supine, with hip and knee flexed to 90°. In *positive Kernig sign*, the pain limits passive extension of the flexed knee.

- **Positive Brudzinski sign:** Brudzinski sign is positive if flexion of neck causes involuntary flexion of knee and hip.

Ocular manifestations include:

- **Papillitis**: Meningitis causes optic neuritis due to descending infective perineuritis and reduced visual acuity.
- **Bilateral primary optic atrophy**: Meningitis causes chronic chiasmal arachnoiditis, resulting in bilateral primary optic atrophy and visual field defects.
- **Cranial nerve palsies**: Basilar meningitis causes cranial nerve palsies and binocular diplopia.
- **Miliary choroidal tubercles** in tuberculous meningitis (TBM).

Investigations

Blood analysis is done which includes total leucocyte count (TLC) (increased), differential leucocyte count (DLC) (neutrophilia) and culture and sensitivity. CSF analysis is done which reveals the following:

- Glucose content: Decreased in bacterial infections and normal in viral infections.
- Protein content: Increased in bacterial infection.
- Cells: increased in polymorphs (neutrophils) in bacterial meningitis; increased in lymphocytes in tubercular, viral and fungal infections.
- Gram staining: To identify the organism.
- India ink stain: To detect cryptococcal infection.

Neuroimaging with the help of MRI and CT. MRI is preferred to CT to detect cerebral edema and areas of ischemia.

Treatment

Treatment involves administration of IV antibiotic (third generation cephalosporins and vancomycin) and mannitol (to decrease raised intracranial pressure).

■ Encephalitis

It is the inflammation affecting the brain parenchyma. The most common cause is a viral infection.

Ocular manifestations include:

- Cranial nerve palsies: Ptosis is the commonest feature and diplopia is an early symptom.
- Pupils are usually normal.
- Papilloedema is rare.

■ Brain Abscess

These abscesses are similar to space-occupying lesions, leading to focal neurological signs which depend upon the location of abscess. Headache is the most common symptom. MRI scans are done to image these lesions and treated by neurosurgical drainage under antibiotic coverage.

Neurosyphilis

Ocular involvement is frequent with neurosyphilis (CNS invasion by Treponema pallidum) and manifests as:

- Cranial nerve palsies.
- AR pupil.
- Opticochiasmatic arachnoiditis.
- Tabes dorsalis: This is a syphilitic demyelination of posterior column and dorsal root ganglion, leading to:
  - ◊ Loss of pain and temperature sensations.
  - ◊ Loss of joint position.
  - ◊ Paresthesia.
  - ◊ Ataxic gates.
- Optic nerve involvement, resulting in optic atrophy.

General paralysis of insane (paralytic dementia or progressive paralysis): It is seen in tertiary syphilis and causes lesions in the posterior tracts of the cord. The clinical features are identical with those in tabes.

■ Intracranial Space-Occupying Lesions (ICSOL)

ICSOLs may be categorized into primary and secondary tumors.

Primary tumors: These begin in the brain and do not usually metastasize. In adults, 2/3rd of primary brain tumor are *supratentorial*, but in children, 2/3rd of brain tumors are *infratentorial*. These include:

- Gliomas.
- Meningiomas.
- Schwannomas.
- Pituitary adenomas.
- Craniopharyngioma.
- Acoustic neuromas.

Secondary tumors: These tumors are metastatic from malignancies elsewhere. The most common primary tumor being lung cancer, followed by breast cancer, carcinoma of the colon, and malignant melanoma (**Flowchart 23.7**).

■ Clinical Features

These tumors produce symptoms which may be either nonlocalizing or localizing.

Nonlocalizing Symptoms

(Nonspecific mechanical effects): These are due to blockage of CSF circulation, resulting in raised intracranial pressure (ICP). These are headache, vomiting, seizures, papilloedema, dizziness, VIth nerve palsy resulting in diplopia and alterations in respiratory rhythm, pulse rate and blood pressure. If epilepsy starts in middle age or beyond, space-occupying lesion of the brain is one of the possible diagnoses.

Headache

It may be associated with projectile vomiting. It is episodic initially which becomes continuous due to sustained raised ICP. Headache due to raised ICP is precipitated by straining, sneezing or coughing and may disturb sound sleep. *The classic brain tumor headache is worst in the morning and worse on bending or Valsalva maneuver. Headache is more common in posterior fossa tumors and rapidly growing tumors.*

Papilloedema

Tumors of anterior fossa tend to produce papilloedema later than those in the posterior fossa. Thus, tumors of midbrain, parieto-occipital region, and cerebellum produce papilloedema more rapidly. Cerebellar tumors are always accompanied by papilloedema.

Localizing Signs

Focal neurological signs and symptoms: These are due to compression of neighboring structures

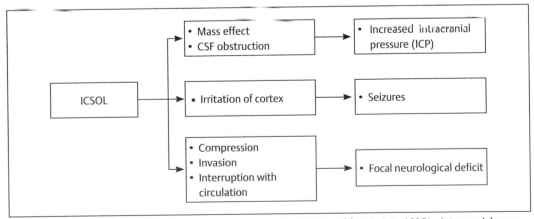

Flowchart 23.7 Mechanisms leading to symptoms due to ICSOLs. Abbreviation: ICSOL, intracranial space occupying lesion, CSP, cerebrospinal fluid.

such as field defects and ocular paresis. These depend upon the site of lesion and possess localizing value.

Tumors of Frontal Lobe

Tumors of frontal lobe, particularly meningioma of olfactory groove, are associated with **Foster–Kennedy syndrome** (pressure atrophy of optic nerve on the side of lesion and papilloedema on the other side due to raised ICP). The tumor compresses the optic nerve on the same side, causing optic atrophy. The atrophy occurs before the tumor takes up a significant amount of intracranial space. Then as the tumor grows, increased ICP develops and the other nerve shows papilloedema.

These can cause anosmia. This is especially insignificant if it is unilateral. There may be change in personality. Dysphasia can occur if Broca's area is involved. Hemiparesis or fits may affect the contralateral side.

Tumors of Temporal Lobe

Tumors of temporal lobe cause the following symptoms:

- Pressure on optic radiations (inferior fibers in Meyer's loop) lead to contralateral, usually incongruous upper quadrant anopia
- Irritation of visuopsychic area leads to visual hallucinations.
- Downward pressure at tentorial ridge leads to involvement of IIIrd nerve and Vth nerve.

Tumors of Parietal Lobe

Due to parietal lobe tumors there is involvement of upper fibers of optic radiations, leading to contralateral lower homonymous quadrant anopia. It also exerts pressure on POT junction, leading to conjugate deviation of the eyes. Other features include abnormal optokinetic nystagmus and visual and auditory hallucinations. There may be hemisensory loss, decreased two-point discrimination, and astereognosis (the inability to recognize a familiar object placed in the hand). The patient may systematically ignore one side of their body, which is known as sensory inattention.

If you ask them to draw a clock face, they omit the half contralateral to the lesion. Dysphasia may occur.

Tumors of Occipital Lobe

Occipital lobe tumors produce macular sparing and much more congruous visual field defects (**Fig. 23.14a**). Anteriorly situated tumors may produce contralateral temporal crescentric field defect, because the anterior most part of visual cortex represents extreme nasal fibers from opposite eye (**Fig. 23.14b**). Pupillary light reflexes are normal and optic atrophy does not occur in occipital cortex lesions.

Visual information from both occipital cortices is relayed to left angulate gyrus. The angulate gyrus of dominant hemisphere (commonly the left) subserves the ability to write. Involvement of angulate gyrus of dominant cerebral hemisphere may result in **alexia** (word blindness and inability to read) as well as **agraphia** (inability to write). *It is therefore mandatory to examine reading ability in the context of right hemianopia (i.e., in left occipital lesion).*

Tumors of Posterior Fossa (Brain Stem, Cerebellum, and IVth Ventricle)

The posterior fossa is a small region of the brain cradled on all sides by the bone and limited above by the tentorium. The brain stem, cerebellum, and IVth ventricle occupy this region of the brain.

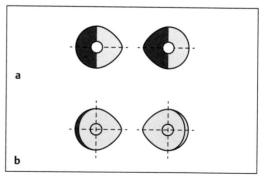

Fig. 23.14 (a) Macular sparing congruous homonymous hemianopia. **(b)** Contralateral temporal crescentric field defect.

Expansion of a mass in this infratentorial area may result in brain stem or cerebellar dysfunction, often associated with blockage of IVth ventricle and hydrocephalus. The different tumors arising in the posterior fossa are either medulloblastomas, cerebellar astrocytomas, brain stem gliomas or ependymomas. Because tumors do not respect discrete compartmental landmarks, those that arise in the thalamus or suprasellar region can extend inferiorly into the posterior fossa. Similarly, lesions that arise from the spinal cord can extend up into the medullary area and cause symptoms of brain stem dysfunction.

The clinical presentation associated with posterior fossa tumors is essentially similar in adults and children; symptoms usually include increased ICP, focal neurological deficits secondary to compromise of brain stem or cerebellar tissue, and meningeal irritation. The clinical triad of increased ICP (headache, vomiting, and blurred or double vision) is the hallmark of an infratentorial tumor. Vomiting, which occurs in the morning and is associated with relief of head pain, is a footprint of posterior fossa tumors that have obstructed the IVth ventricle.

Cerebellar deficits occur in most patients with posterior fossa tumors. Midline lesion causes *truncal and gait ataxia*, while *limb ataxia* occurs more frequently in lesions that involve the lateral cerebellar hemispheres, most commonly cerebellar astrocytomas.

Other focal neurologic deficits may occur in patients with posterior symptoms. *Ocular motor deficits are relatively frequent and tend to be of localizing value, except for a VIth nerve palsy,* which may be present secondary to diffuse increased ICP. Abducent nerve palsy is not a useful localizing sign, as it has a long and tortuous intracranial path that makes it vulnerable.

Epileptic seizures rarely occur in children or adults with subtentorial tumors, except in patients with infiltrating masses that extend into the subcortical areas, and in patients with lesions that have disseminated into the nervous system.

Alterations in consciousness may occur but tend to be a late finding. Acute hemorrhage in posterior fossa tumor may result in acute coma.

Infants and young children with posterior fossa tumors may have increasing head circumference due to their open sutures and fontanelles.

Horner's syndrome is not a good localizing lesion; as the path of the sympathetic nerves is long, and fibers do not cross the midline, it is a good lateralizing sign. The lesion may also be outside the skull.

If the headache is unilateral, this is often a good indicator of the side of the lesion.

Tumors of Midbrain

Midbrain is composed of the tectum, tegmentum, and cerebral peduncle. These structures are found in a dorsoventral sequence. The **tectum** lies dorsally to the cerebral aqueduct and has four round swellings: colliculi (two superior and two inferior colliculi). The superior colliculi help to integrate the visual pathways, and the inferior colliculus acts as an integration center for auditory pathways. The **tegmentum** is located in front of the tectum. It consists of fiber tracts and red nucleus, periaqueductal gray, and substantia nigra. The substantia nigra is a prominent area of the midbrain. The substantia nigra nuclei are involved in the control of voluntary movement.

The major cranial nerve nuclei within the midbrain are mesencephalic nuclei of trigeminal nerves, trochlear nuclei, and oculomotor nuclei. The oculomotor nerve immerges from the midbrain rostral to the pons.

The midbrain serves important functions in motor movement, particularly movements of the eye, and in auditory and visual processing.

All tumors of the midbrain exert pressure on the optic tracts, resulting in homonymous hemianopia. The localizing signs of tumor depend upon the site of involvement as follows:
- *Tumors of the upper part of midbrain:* The most characteristic sign is retraction of upper lid, followed by ptosis and loss of

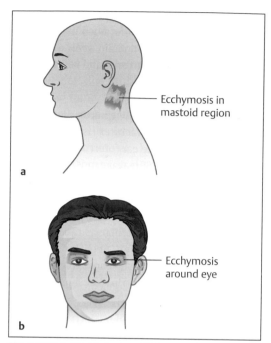

Fig. 23.16 (a) Battle's sign. **(b)** Raccoon's eyes.

visible, is a diagnostic sign of fracture base of skull. Pupillary reactions are inconsistent. A RAPD is most common on the side of lesion. The injury may cause visual field defects. Presence of papilloedema suggests hemorrhage into optic nerve sheath.

Complications

The possible complications could be carotid–cavernous fistula, cavernous sinus thrombosis, CSF fistula, basal meningitis, and panhypopituitarism.

Investigations

Investigations for establishing diagnosis are X-ray, CT and MRI scans. The gold standard for the radiographic detection of skull base fractures is CT.

■ Hereditary and Degenerative Diseases

A neurodegenerative disease is a neurological disorder due to progressive dying and loss of neurons in the CNS and often accompanied by gliosis and intracellular inclusions, while a genetic disorder may be hereditary or non-hereditary and is caused by one or more abnormalities in the genome.

■ Alzheimer Disease

It is a common cause of dementia in patients over 65 years. It was first described by Professor Alois Alzheimer in Germany in 1907. It may occur in two forms:

- *Early onset*—It has a genetic predisposition (autosomal dominant) with mutation in four different genes:
  - ◇ APP gene on chromosome 21.
  - ◇ Presenilin–1 (PS-1) on chromosome 14.
  - ◇ Presenilin-2 (PS-2) on chromosome 2.
  - ◇ Apo E gene on chromosome 19.
- *Late onset*: Inheritance is not clear in this form.

Pathology

Macroscopically, there is atrophy of cerebral cortex and hippocampus. *Microscopically*, the hallmarks of Alzheimer's disease are extraneural amyloid plaques and intraneural neurofibrillary tangles which consist of abnormally twisted microtubules inside the nerve cells.

Clinical Features

The initial symptoms involve forgetfulness, that is, inability to retrieve information acquired in the past. Both short-term and long-term memory are affected, but especially the former. Consequent increase in cognitive problems renders the patient confused. The patient develops apraxia and fails to carry out even routine tasks. Later symptoms are impairment of judgment, vision and speech.

Treatment

There is no definitive treatment and supportive therapy is the mainstay. Therapy includes administration of anticholinestrases—donepezil, rivastigmine, and galantamine—which may help some patients.

■ Parkinson Disease

It is a degenerative disease usually affecting people over the age of 50 years.

Etiology

It is mainly caused by damage to substantia nigra in the midbrain. The loss of neurons in substantia nigra result in depletion of dopamine. Dopamine is an inhibitory neurotransmitter and its depletion results in loss of control over movements.

Clinical Features

It is a clinical syndrome of motor disturbance, and severity of motor syndrome is proportional to the dopamine deficiency. The typical symptoms include systemic and ocular manifestations. Systemic features include tremors of the limb at rest, deterioration in hand writing, dementia, loss of facial expression, voice disorders, sleep disturbances, bradykinesia (slowing of voluntary movements), akinesia, rigidity (stiffness and resistance to limb movement caused by increased muscle tone), and postural instability in later stages leading to impaired balance and frequent falls. Gait and posture disturbances like festinating gait is seen commonly (rapid shuffling steps and a forward-flexed posture when walking).

Ocular features include blepharoclonus (fluttering of eyelids) when closed, blepharospasm (involuntary eye closure), infrequent blinking, limitation of upgaze, lid retraction (widened palpebral aperture), deficient ocular pursuit (eye tracking), and saccadic movements (fast automatic movements of both eyes in the same direction).

Treatment

There is no cure for Parkinson disease and the treatment is symptomatic and supportive. **Dopamine supplementation** is the main treatment of Parkinson disease.

- **Levodopa** (a metabolic precursor of dopamine) **combined with carbidopa** is given because dopamine cannot cross the BBB. *Carbidopa is a peripheral dopa decarboxylase inhibitor which helps to prevent the metabolism of Levodopa before it reaches the dopaminergic neurons in brain. Therefore, the side effects are reduced and bioavailability is increased.*
- **Several dopamine agonists** such as bromocriptine, pergolide, pramipexole, ropinirole, and cabergoline can be used alone or in combination with levodopa.
- Other drugs such as amantadine and anticholinergics may be useful as treatment of motor symptoms.

If the medical treatment fails, motor symptoms can be treated with surgery. The targeted area includes thalamus and globus pallidus. So, thalamotomy or pallidotomy should be considered in selected cases which are now performed using "gamma-knife."

■ Chronic Progressive External Ophthalmoplegia (CPEO)

It is due to myopathy of EOMs. CPEO is the most frequent manifestation of mitochondrial myopathies. EOMs are affected preferentially because their fraction of mitochondrial volume is several times greater than that of other skeletal muscle. There is no defined treatment to ameliorate the muscle weakness of CPEO.

Clinical Features

Ptosis is an early or only manifestation. It is bilateral and slowly progressive. Involvement of bilateral muscles in the course of time occurs. The intraocular muscles of the iris and ciliary body are not affected, hence pupil is spared. There is no response to cholinergic drugs. Ophthalmoplegia is the late or only manifestation. Downward gaze is preserved till late. There is no remission or acute exacerbation and no evidence of thyroid or myotonic dystrophy.

■ Wilson Disease (Hepatolenticular Degeneration)

It is an autosomal recessive disorder that prevents the body from expelling excess copper. Copper is classical migraine include blurred vision, scintillating scotomata, visual field defect, photophobia, and flashing lights. The aura develops gradually over 5 to 20 minutes, lasting for < 60 minutes and is accompanied or followed by a headache. *Sensory aura is the second most common*, for example, tingling may begin in one hand and then ascend the arm to the elbow and ipsilateral side of face (cheiro-oral distribution). Sometimes, auditory, olfactory, or gustatory hallucinations may occur as migraine aura. Rare aura includes mild hemiparesis, aphasia, vertigo, and/or confusion.

Other forms of migraine are:
- *Retinal migraine:* It involves sudden monocular visual loss for less than an hour and associated with headache.
- *Ophthalmoplegic migraine:* It typically starts before the age of 10 years and it is characterized by headache, followed by transient cranial nerve palsy (usually IIIrd).
- *Basilar migraine:* It is associated with symptoms related to vertebrobasilar arterial insufficiency such as bilateral blurring of vision, vertigo, tinnitus, dysarthria, diplopia, and formed visual hallucinations.
- *Familial hemiplegic migraine:* It is characterized by a failure of full recovery of neurological features after an attack of migraine subsides, that is, the neurological deficits outlasts the headache.
- *Childhood periodic syndromes* that involve cyclical vomiting (occasional intense periods of vomiting), abdominal migraine (abdominal pain, usually accompanied by nausea), and benign paroxysmal vertigo of childhood (occasional attacks of vertigo). They may be precursors or associated with migraine.
- *Complicated migraine* describes migraine headaches and/or auras, which are unusually long or unusually frequent, or associated with a seizure or brain lesion.

Pathophysiology

Classical vascular theory: It was believed that the *aura phase* is produced by constriction of intracerebral blood vessel and the *headache phase* is produced by subsequent rebound vasodilatation. Extracranial vessels become distended and pulsatile during an attack.

Neurovascular theory: Migraine is primarily a neurogenic process with secondary changes in cerebral perfusion. The complex series of neural and vascular events initiate migraine. The pathogenesis is divided into 3 phases:
- Brainstem generation.
- Vasomotor activation (both intra and extra-cranial) in which arteries may constrict or dilate.
- Trigeminal activation: The trigeminal nucleus caudalis in medulla is activated which is the pain processing center of head and face (**Flowchart 23.8**).

Clinical Presentation

Following are the four possible phases to migraine: prodromal, aura, pain, and postdrome, although not all phases are necessarily experienced.

Prodromal or Premonitory Symptoms

It occurs hours or days before the headache in approximately 60% of patients. These are:
- Increased sensitivity to light, sound and odors.
- Mental and mood changes.
- Lethargy.
- Excessive thirst and polyuria.
- Craving for certain foods.
- Anorexia.
- Diarrhea/constipation.

Aura Phase

It is a complex of symptoms that may precede or accompany the headache and can be visual, sensory, motor, or combination of these (**Table 23.10**).

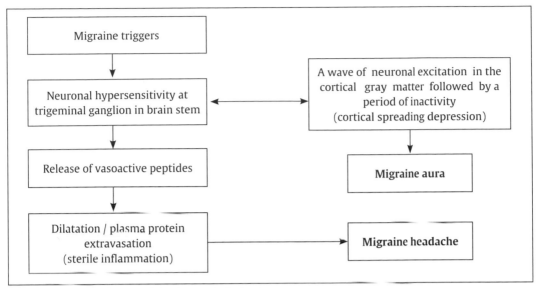

Flowchart 23.8 Mechanism of development of migraine.
Note: Both serotonin and norepinephrine mediate a broad spectrum of depressive symptoms.

Visual symptoms	Sensory symptoms	Motor symptoms
Positive symptoms: • Scintillating scotoma (highly characteristic of migraine) • Photopsia (flashes of light) • Micropsia, macropsia Negative symptoms: • Negative scotoma • Central scotoma • Homonymous hemlanopia • Altitudinal visual defects	Tingling: Numbness usually occurs after the tingling has passed with a loss of position sense Auditory, olfactory, gustatory hallucinations may occur	• Mild hemiparesis • Aphasla • Vertigo

Table 23.10 Visual, sensory and motor symptoms in the aura phase of migraine

Pain Phase (Headache Phase)

Classically, the headache is unilateral, throbbing, and moderate to severe in intensity, aggravated by physical activity, and neck pain is commonly associated with it.

The headache is frequently accompanied by nausea, vomiting, fatigue and sensitivity to light, sound and smell. Rarely, an aura occurs without a subsequent headache. This is known as acephalgic migraine.

Postdrome

It is defined as the constellation of symptoms occurring once the acute headache has settled.

Some people feel unusually refreshed or euphoric after an attack, whereas other note depression and malaise. For some individuals, this can vary each time.

Differential Diagnosis

Other conditions that can cause similar symptoms to a migraine headache are listed below along with their differentiating features which help to rule out their diagnosis:
- *Giant cell arteritis (temporal arteries):*
  - ◊ Age more than 55 years.
  - ◊ Scalp tenderness.
  - ◊ Jaw claudication.

CHAPTER 24

Ocular Manifestations of Systemic Diseases

Connective Tissue Disorders..636

Spondyloarthropathies..639

Endocrine/Metabolic Disorders...640

Eye in Infectious Diseases..641

Eye in Parasitic Diseases..646

Hematological Diseases..647

Muscular Disorders 648

Eye in Inherited Disorders...649

Nutritional Deficiencies 650

Numerous systemic diseases have ocular manifestations. Occasionally, the eye findings may be the first indication of underlying systemic diseases leading to diagnosis. The systemic diseases involving the eye include:

- Connective tissue/Collagen disorders.
- Spondyloarthropathies.
- Endocrine/Metabolic disorders.
- Eye in infectious diseases.
- Eye in parasitic diseases.
- Hematological diseases.
- Muscular disorders.
- Inherited disorders.

■ Connective Tissue Disorders

Various connective tissue disorders causing ocular manifestations are rheumatoid arthritis, systemic lupus erythematosus (SLE), giant cell arteritis, sarcoidosis, Vogt–Koyanagi–Harada (VKH) syndrome, Wegener's granulomatosis, Ehlers–Danlos syndrome, Marfan syndrome, and Pseudoxanthoma elasticum.

■ Rheumatoid Arthritis

It is an autoimmune, inflammatory polyarthropathy. It is more common in females than males. Clinical features are described in **Table 24.1**.

■ Systemic Lupus Erythematosus

It is an autoimmune disease of the body's connective tissues. It occurs between the ages of 15 and 40 years. Systemic Lupus Erythematosus (SLE) can affect joints, skin, kidneys, heart, lungs, blood vessels, and blood. Clinical features are described in **Table 24.2**.

Table 24.1 Systemic and ocular features of rheumatoid arthritis	
Systemic features	**Ocular manifestations**
• Joints swelling, usually of hands typically, involving the proximal interphalangeal (IP) joints and sparing the distal IP joints. • Ulnar deviation of metacarpophalangeal (MP) joints secondary to the chronic inflammation.	• Dry eyes (keratoconjunctivitis sicca) • Episcleritis • Scleritis • Ulcerative keratitis (corneal ulcer) • Uveitis

Table 24.2 Systemic and ocular features of systemic lupus erythematosus

Systemic features	Ocular manifestations

• **Joints**—painful, swollen joints.
• **Skin:**
  ◊ "Butterfly-shaped" facial rash over the cheeks below the eyes and across the bridge of the nose.
  ◊ Alopecia (hair loss).
• **Kidneys**—inflammation of kidneys (nephritis).
• **Heart**—pericarditis, myocarditis, and endocarditis.
• **Lungs**—pleurisy and shrinking lungs.
• **Blood vessels**—inflammation (vasculitis) with arterial and venous occlusion. Raynaud's phenomenon (fingers turn white and/or blue in the cold).
• **Blood**—anemia, leucopenia, and thrombocytopenia.
	• Keratoconjunctivitis sicca (dry eye)
	• Scleritis
	• Peripheral ulcerative keratitis
	• Retinal vasculitis
	• Optic neuropathy

Table 24.3 Systemic and ocular features of giant cell arteritis

Systemic features	Ocular manifestations
• Scalp tenderness • Headache • Jaw claudication (pain in jaw when chewing). • Polymyalgia rheumatica (pain and stiffness in proximal muscle groups, typically the shoulders).	• Anterior ischemic optic neuropathy (AION) resulting in blurred vision. • Extraocular muscle palsies resulting in diplopia.

Table 24.4 Systemic and ocular features of sarcoidosis

Systemic features	Ocular manifestations

• **Lungs** bilateral hilar lymphadenopathy, alveolitis, and *noncaseating granuloma in lungs is the characteristic lesion of sarcoidosis* and fibrosis.
• **Skin**—erythema nodosum, granuloma, and lupus pernio.
• **Liver**—cholestasis, fibrosis, cirrhosis, portal hypertension, and the Budd chiari syndrome have been seen.
	• Anterior uveitis is most common.
	• Other manifestations are:
	  ◊ Lacrimal gland granuloma.
	  ◊ Conjunctival nodule.

Investigations

To ascertain diagnosis, following investigations are performed:

- Complete blood count (CBC).
- ESR (raised).
- Urine analysis.
- Antinuclear antibody (ANA) test.
- Ultrasonography.
- X-ray chest.

■ Giant Cell Arteritis

It is systemic granulomatous vasculitis affecting medium- and large-sized vessels. It presents usually in 7th to 8th decades. Clinical features are described in **Table 24.3**.

■ Sarcoidosis

It is a multisystem disorder characterized by noncaseating granuloma. The most affected organ is the lungs, liver, spleen, skin, parotid glands, phalangeal bones, and eyes. Sarcoidosis presents in one of the following ways (**Table 24.4**):

- Lofgren's syndrome—acute triad of erythema nodosum, joint pains, and bilateral hilar adenopathy.
- Heerfordt syndrome (**uveoparotid fever**)— it is characterized by uveitis, parotid gland

Table 24.11 Systemic and ocular features of Reiter syndrome

Systemic features	Ocular manifestations
• Arthritis • Urethritis • Cystitis, cervicitis, orchitis and prostatitis • Mucocutaneous lesions (mouth ulcer)	• Conjunctivitis • Acute anterior uveitis • Keratitis • Episcleritis and scleritis • Retinal vasculitis

Table 24.12 Systemic and ocular features of diabetes mellitus

Systemic features	Ocular manifestations

• **Vascular**—atherosclerosis of lower limb arteries may result in ischemia and *gangrene* of feet and toes.
• **Neurological**—*peripheral neuropathy* affects the feet and may give rise to ulcer pressure points in the soles.
  ◊ *Cranial nerve palsies* as a result of small vessel involvement, so the **pupil is spared in IIIrd nerve palsy** (*Compressive lesions such as posterior communicating artery aneurysm have pupillary involvement.*)
• **Renal**—*nephropathy* which may eventually result in renal failure.
• **Cutaneous**—bacterial and fungal infections.
  ◊ Necrobiosis lipoidica (waxy plaques with irregular margins and shiny centers involving the shins).
	Diabetes can involve every structure of the eye.
	• **Lid**—recurrent stye.
	• **Conjunctiva**—conjunctivitis.
	• **Cornea**—keratitis.
	• **Iris**—uveitis and rubeosis iridis.
	• **Lens**—cataract.
	• **Retina**—diabetic retinopathy.
	• **Vitreous**—intraocular and vitreous hemorrhage due to new vessel formation.
	• **Glaucoma** (IOP)—neovascular glaucoma due to rubeosis.
	  ◊ Hypotony in diabetic coma.
	• **Optic nerve**—retrobulbar neuritis (often bilateral).
	• **Extra ocular muscles**—paralysis (diplopia).
	• **Vision**—transient refractive changes
	  ◊ Weakness of accommodation.
	  ◊ (diabetes mellitus involving nerve supply of ciliary muscle causes peripheral neuritis and the ciliary muscle becomes weakened).
	  ◊ Amaurosis.

Abbreviation: IOP, intraocular pressure.

Endocrine/Metabolic Disorders

Endocrine disorders involve the body's over production or under production of certain hormones while metabolic disorders affect the body's ability to process certain nutrients and vitamins. Diabetes mellitus, hyperthyroidism, hypothyroidism, and hypoparathyroidism are some common endocrine disorders, while homocystinuria and Cushing's syndrome are metabolic disorders.

Diabetes Mellitus

Ocular manifestations in diabetes mellitus depend much more on the duration and not the severity of the disease, commonly occurring in long-standing diabetes mellitus (**Table 24.12**). Diabetes lowers the resistance of patient to pyogenic infection.

Hyperthyroidism (Thyrotoxicosis)

Graves' disease, an autoimmune disorder, is the most common type of hyperthyroidism. IgG antibodies bind to TSH receptors in the thyroid gland and stimulate the secretion of thyroid hormones (**Table 24.13**).

Hypoparathyroidism

It is due to the deficiency of parathyroid hormone. It is characterized by hypocalcaemia and

Table 24.13 Systemic and ocular features of hyperthyroidism

Systemic features	Ocular manifestations

Systemic features of hyperthyroidism include:
• Tachycardia
• Palpitations
• Tremors
• Increased basal metabolic rate leading to heat production, weight loss, and warm and sweaty skin.
	Ocular features include:
	Symptoms—
	• Retrobulbar discomfort.
	• Red eyes.
	• Puffy lids.
	• Lacrimation.
	• Photophobia.
	• Tear insufficiency with grittiness.
	Signs—
	Lid signs—these include:
	• Retraction of upper lid in primary gaze (**Dalrymple sign**).
	• Lid lag—upper lid lags behind the globe on down gaze (**Von Graefe's sign**).
	• Puffy edematous eye lids (**Enroth sign**).
	• Infrequent blinking with staring look (**Stellwag's sign**).
	Joffroy's sign—loss of forehead corrugation when looking up.
	• Defects of ocular movement:
	  ◊ Restrictive myopathy leads to diplopia.
	  ◊ Convergence deficiency (**Moebius sign**).
	Exophthalmos—it is *axial* and may lead to exposure keratopathy, corneal ulceration, and infection.
	Optic neuropathy—retrobulbar edema and infiltration may cause severe visual impairment.

Table 24.14 Systemic and ocular features of homocystinuria

Systemic features	Ocular manifestations
• Mental retardation. • Thromboembolic episodes. • Arachnodactyly (infrequent).	• Bilateral subluxation of the lens (**inferiorly and nasally**). • Acute secondary glaucoma due to subluxation of lens in anterior chamber. • Retinal detachment and myopia may occur.

hyperphosphatemia. Systemic features include tetany and seizures. Cataract (bilateral), fasciculation, and disc edema could be seen as an ocular manifestation.

Homocystinuria

It is the disorder of methionine (amino acid) metabolism. It is caused by deficiency of cystathionine β-synthetase, leading to accumulation of homocysteine and methionine. This condition carries a thrombotic tendency. It has autosomal recessive inheritance (**Table 24.14**).

Cushing's Syndrome

It is caused by prolonged elevation of plasma glucocorticoids. Glucocorticoids are secreted by adrenal cortex. Cushing's disease is caused by hyper secretion of adrenocorticotrophic hormone (ACTH) by basophil cells of pituitary gland which, in turn, increases the secretion of glucocorticoids by adrenal cortex. Clinical features are described in **Table 24.15**.

Eye in Infectious Diseases

The infective diseases may be:

Bacterial:
• TB.
• Leprosy.

Viral:
• H. simplex.
• H. zoster.

Table 24.15 Systemic and ocular features of Cushing's syndrome

Systemic features	Ocular manifestations
• **Obesity**—it may be generalized or involve the trunk, abdomen, and neck ('buffalo hump'). • Swollen face (moon face). • Hyperpigmentation of skin may develop. • **Other features**—depression, osteoporosis, poor wound healing, hypertension, and pathological fractures.	• Hypertensive retinopathy • Papilloedema

Table 24.16 Systemic and ocular features of tuberculosis

Systemic features	Ocular manifestations
• Fever (evening rise) • Malaise • Granuloma of lung • Weight loss • Cough • Lymphadenopathy	**Adnexal manifestations:** • Lupus vulgaris • Eyelid tuberculous granulomas manifestations **Anterior segment manifestations:** • Conjunctivitis • Conjunctival granuloma • Tubercular scleritis • Interstitial keratitis • Phlyctenular keratoconjunctivitis • Iridocyclitis (chronic granulomatous, anterior and intermediate uveitis) **Posterior segment manifestations—** • Choroidal tubercles • Choroidal tuberculoma • Serpiginous like choroiditis • Retinal vasculitis • Eale's disease • Papilloedema • Optic neuritis papillitis, retrobulbar neuritis (RBN), and neuroretinitis

• AIDS.
• Cytomegalovirus.
• Rubella.

Fungal:
• Candida.
• Cryptococcus.

Spirochaetal:
• Syphilis.

■ Tuberculosis (TB)

TB primarily involves the lung. Other organs including the eye may be involved secondarily. Primary infection of the eye is rare. TB can affect all the ocular structures except lens. Active TB may not be associated with ocular involvement. Secondary ocular involvement occurs as a result of hematogenous spread or as a hypersensitive response to tubercular proteins. The hallmark of extrapulmonary TB is caseating granuloma and necrosis. Clinical features are listed in **Table 24.16**.

■ Leprosy (Hansen Disease)

It is a chronic granulomatous infection. The organism, Mycobacterium leprae, has the affinity for skin, peripheral nerves, and anterior segment of the eye. Tuberculoid leprosy is restricted to the skin and peripheral nerves. The eye is involved in lepromatous leprosy. Ocular involvement in leprosy is 70 to 75%. Lepromatous leprosy is a generalized infection involving skin, peripheral nerve, upper respiratory tract (URT), testes, and eyes. Clinical features are listed in **Table 24.17**.

Table 24.17 Systemic and ocular features of leprosy

Systemic features	Ocular manifestations
Skin—skin lesions appear as areas of impaired sensations or as macules (hypopigmented or erythematous). Thickening of cutaneous sensory nerves. **Nose**—**saddle-shaped,** nasal deformity due to destruction of nasal cartilage. **Peripheral nerves:** • Motor neuropathy claw hand (due to ulnar nerve palsy). • Sensory peripheral neuropathy may result in shortening and loss of digits. • Autonomic neuropathy. It leads to dry, cracked, and infection-prone skin.	**Lids**—madarosis and trichiasis. **Lacrimal system**—dacryocystitis, and chronic dacryoadenitis leading to keratoconjunctivitis sicca (KCS). **Sclera**—episcleritis and scleritis. **Conjunctiva**—conjunctivitis. **Cornea**—keratitis, thickened corneal nerves, corneal anesthesia, and superficial stromal keratitis. **Iris**—anterior uveitis. **VII nerve paresis**—lagophthalmos due to facial nerve involvement (zygomatic branch) and lower lid ectropion.

■ Syphilis

It is caused by the spirochaete, Treponema pallidum. It may be primary, secondary, or tertiary syphilis. Clinical features are listed in **Table 24.18**.

■ Herpes Simplex

It is caused by herpes simplex virus (HSV–HSV1 and HSV2), a DNA virus. Clinical features are listed in **Table 24.19**.

■ Herpes Zoster

It is caused by varicella-zoster virus (VZV). VZV causes chickenpox (varicella) and shingles (herpes zoster). Clinical features are listed in **Table 24.20**.

■ Cytomegalovirus

It is a β herpes virus. Clinical features are listed in **Table 24.21**.

■ Rubella (German Measles)

It is caused by Rubella virus. It is transmitted from an infected mother to the fetus through placenta, usually during the first trimester of pregnancy. Risk to fetus is closely related to the stage of gestation at the time of maternal infection. Clinical features are listed in **Table 24.22**.

■ Measles (Rubeola)

It is caused by a myxovirus, a RNA virus. Clinical features of measles are listed in **Table 24.23**.

■ Mumps

It is caused by paramyxovirus. Systemically, it presents as bilateral parotitis, epididymo-orchitis in adults and meningitis, while ocular manifestations include conjunctivitis and dacryoadenitis (bilateral), but episcleritis and peripheral keratitis are infrequent.

■ Acquired Immune Deficiency Syndrome

It is caused by human immunodeficiency virus (HIV), an RNA virus belonging to retrovirus family.

Acquired immune deficiency syndrome (AIDS) is transmitted by sexual intercourse, contaminated/infected blood, and transplacental or via breast milk. CD4+T (helper) lymphocytes are vital to the initiation of immune response to pathogens. HIV targets CD4+T lymphocytes. The disease is characterized by a deficiency of CD4+T lymphocytes, leading to progressive immune deficiency. Regular estimation of CD4+T count is, therefore, a useful measure of disease progression.

Diagnosis

For making provisional diagnosis when blood test may not be available, WHO has recommended clinical diagnostic criteria of AIDS which is based on the presence of any two major and at least one minor systemic sign.

Table 24.18 Systemic and ocular features of syphilis

Systemic features	Ocular manifestations
Primary—chancre (painless ulcer at the site of infection). The most common site is the penis in males and the vulva in females.	**Primary**—conjunctival chancre.
Secondary—it begins a few weeks to months after the chancre heals. It is characterized by: • Rashes on palms and soles. • Lymphadenopathy. • Condyloma latum in the anal region.	**Secondary:** • Eye lid rash. • Madarosis. • Dacryoadenitis. • Dacryocystitis. • Orbital periostitis. Anterior segment: • Conjunctivitis. • Interstitial keratitis. • Episcleritis. • Scleritis. • Uveitis. Posterior segment: • Chorioretinitis. • Neuroretinitis. • Retinal vasculitis. Neuro ophthalmological: • Optic neuritis. • Cranial nerve palsies.
Tertiary—it occurs in approximately 40% of untreated cases and is characterized by: • **Neurosyphilis**—tabes dorsalis, general paresis of insane, and syphilitic meningitis. • **Cardiovascular syphilis**—aortitis with aortic regurgitation and aneurysms, and gummas (destructive lesions of bones, skin, or liver). • **Congenital syphilis:** ◊ Hutchinson's teeth. ◊ VIII nerve deafness. ◊ Interstitial keratitis.	**Tertiary:** • Lens subluxation. • Horners syndrome. • Argyll Robertson pupil. • Optic atrophy (**R**elative **A**fferent **P**upillary **D**efect). • Cranial nerve palsies. • Ptosis. • Nystagmus. • Visual field defects. • Gummas of ocular structures.

Table 24.19 Systemic and ocular features of herpes simplex

Systemic features	Ocular manifestations
• **Primary infection:** Primary infections are often subclinical and cause mild fever, malaise, and upper respiratory tract symptoms. • **Recurrent infection** (reactivation of infection): The pattern of disease depends on the site of reactivation which may be remote from the site of primary disease.	• Primary infections in children may develop blepharoconjunctivitis and corneal micro dendrites in few cases. • The corneal lesions of recurrent herpes are characteristic and include: ◊ Dendritic ulcer: the ends of the ulcer have characteristic terminal buds; the enlargement of ulcer may produce the geographical configuration. ◊ Reduced corneal sensations. ◊ Disciform keratitis. ◊ Stromal necrotic keratitis. ◊ Metaherpetic ulceration.

Table 24.20 Systemic and ocular features of herpes zoster

Systemic features	Ocular manifestations
Symptoms: • Fever • Headache • Malaise • Unilateral skin rash in the area supplied by a single sensory nerve and vesicles appear within 24 hours.	The trigeminal nerve (Vth), especially the ophthalmic division (V1), is commonly involved in herpes zoster; the ocular manifestations of herpes zoster ophthalmicus (HZO) are: • Lid margin vesicles. • Conjunctivitis. • Episcleritis. • Scleritis and sclerokeratitis. • Cornea Epithelial keratitis (dendritic lesions have tapered ends without terminal bulbs): ◇ Nummular keratitis—stromal keratitis. ◇ Disciform keratitis. • Anterior uveitis. • *Trabeculitis* may cause secondary glaucoma. • It may cause acute retinal necrosis (ARN) and anterior segment ischemia. • Optic neuritis is a rare and late complication. • HZO affecting 3rd, 4th, and 6th CN results in extraocular muscle palsy, while facial N (7th CN) involvement results in facial palsy (**Bell's palsy**).

Abbreviation: CN, cranial nerve.

Table 24.21 Systemic and ocular features of cytomegalovirus

Systemic features	Ocular manifestations
In newborns and immunocompromised adults, it causes: • Fever • Hepatitis • Pneumonitis • Encephalitis	• Microphthalmos. • Necrotizing chorioretinitis. It is more severe and associated with retinal necrosis and retinal hemorrhages, especially in AIDS patients. • Optic atrophy.

Table 24.22 Systemic and ocular features of Rubella

Systemic features	Ocular manifestations
• Microcephaly • Mental retardation • Congenital heart disease • Deafness (sensorineural) • Hepatosplenomegaly	• Microphthalmos • Cataract • Glaucoma • Anterior uveitis • Iris atrophy • Keratitis • Retinopathy (**salt and pepper**)

Table 24.23 Systemic and ocular features of measles

Systemic features	Ocular manifestations
• Rash (erythematous and maculopapular) • **Koplik's spot** on buccal mucosa • Fever • Encephalitis • Middle ear infection • Diarrhea • Precipitates malnutrition	• Keratoconjunctivitis • Keratitis • Xerophthalmia • Optic neuritis

Table 24.31 Systemic and ocular features of myeloid leukemia

Systemic features	Ocular manifestations
• Hepatosplenomegaly • Bleeding • Infection • Vascular occlusion • Weakness and fatigue	• Retinal hemorrhages • Retinal edema • Neovascularization in retina • Orbital chloroma causing proptosis.

Table 24.32 Systemic and ocular features of polycythemia

Systemic features	Ocular manifestations
• Headache • Dizziness • Signs of cerebrovascular insufficiency • Red skin of nose, lips and cheeks • Bleeding from nose and gums	• Amaurosis fugax • Retinal hemorrhages • Papilloedema • Central retinal vein occlusion

Table 24.33 Systemic and ocular features of sickle cell disease

Systemic features	Ocular manifestations
• Anemia • Jaundice • Pain in back, chest, and extremities • Acute chest syndrome • Stroke • Painless hematuria • Leg ulcers	• Comma-shaped conjunctival vessels. • Atrophy and neovascularization of iris. • Black sunburst chorioretinal scars. • Sea-fan neovascularization of retina. • Retinal capillary occlusion

Table 24.34 Systemic and ocular features of multiple myeloma

Systemic features	Ocular manifestations
• Pallor • Fatigue • Dyspnea on exertion • Anemia • Purpura • Pathological fractures • Multiple osteolytic lesions • Hyperglobulinemia and classical punched-out lesions in skull, vertebrae, and ribs.	• Proptosis • Blood sludging • Infiltration of uvea, optic nerve, and lacrimal gland • Choroidal tumor • Hemorrhages and exudates in retina • Roths spots • Vascular occlusion

cells in the blood) is elevated. Systemic and ocular features of polycythemia are mentioned in **Table 24.32**.

■ Sickle-cell Disease

It is an inherited group of disorders in which red blood cells contort into a sickle shape and breakdown, leaving a shortage of healthy red blood cells. Systemic and ocular features of sickle cell disease are mentioned in **Table 24.33**.

■ Multiple Myeloma

Multiple myeloma is a cancer of plasma cell. Plasma cells are found in the bone marrow and are an important part of the immune system. In multiple myeloma, the overgrowth of plasma cells in the bone marrow can crowd out normal blood, forming cells and leading to low-blood counts that can cause anemia (low red blood cells), thrombocytopenia (low platelets), and leukopenia (low white blood cells). Systemic and ocular features of multiple myeloma are mentioned in **Table 24.34**.

■ Muscular Disorders

Muscular disorders may be congenital or acquired.

■ Myasthenia Gravis

It is an autoimmune disease in which acetylcholine receptors in striated muscle are destroyed by antibodies. It leads to impairment of neuromuscular conduction, resulting in weakness and fatigue of skeletal muscle (not of cardiac and involuntary muscles) (**Table 24.35**).

Table 24.35 Systemic and ocular features of myasthenia gravis

Systemic features	Ocular manifestations
Voluntary muscle weakness which worsen after exercise or in the evening. It affects limbs, facial expression, speaking (dysarthria), swallowing (dysphagia), and mastication; difficulty with breathing is rare but serious.	• Ptosis after exertion. • Diplopia after exercise or in the evening.

■ Myotonic Dystrophy

It is characterized by delayed muscular relaxation after cessation of voluntary effort (**Table 24.36**). It is inherited as autosomal dominant with gene locus on 19q 13.3.

■ Kearns–Sayre Syndrome

It is characterized by abnormal mitochondria associated with mitochondrial DNA deletions. It is characterized by the classical triad of retinitis pigmentosa, progressive external ophthalmoplegia, and heart block (**Table 24.37**).

■ Eye in Inherited Disorders

■ Down Syndrome (Trisomy 21)

It is a genetic chromosome 21 disorder, causing developmental and intellectual problems. Down syndrome is a genetic disorder caused when abnormal cell division results in extra genetic material from chromosome 21. Its systemic and ocular features are mentioned in **Table 24.38**.

■ Sturge–Weber Syndrome

It is a congenital phakomatoses and involves the face, leptomeninges, and eyes (**Table 24.39**).

Table 24.36 Systemic and ocular features of myotonic dystrophy

Systemic features	Ocular manifestations
• Difficulty in releasing grip. • Muscle wasting and weakness. • Bilateral facial wasting with hollow cheeks (mournful facial expression). • Swallowing difficulties due to involvement of pharyngeal muscles. • Slurred speech due to involvement of tongue. • Frontal baldness • Testicular atrophy • Cardiomyopathy • Low intelligence	• Ptosis • External ophthalmoplegia • Early-onset cataract (Christmas-tree cataract) • Pigmentary retinopathy • Pupillary light near dissociation • Low IOP
Abbreviation: IOP, intraocular pressure.	

■ Neurofibromatosis

It primarily affects the cell growth of neural tissues. It is of two types: neurofibromatosis-1 (von-Recklinghausen disease) and neurofibromatosis-2. Clinical features are listed in **Table 24.40**.

■ Albinism

It is a genetically determined disorder of melanin synthesis which may involve the eyes alone (ocular albinism) or eyes, skin, and hair (oculocutaneous albinism) (**Table 24.41**).

Table 24.37 Systemic and ocular features of Kearns–Sayre syndrome

Systemic features	Ocular manifestations
• Cardiac conduction defects resulting in heart block. • Ataxia • Deafness • Short stature • Hypoparathyroidism	• Bilateral ptosis with insidious onset • Progressive external ophthalmoplegia • Pigmentary retinopathy • Pendular nystagmus

Table 24.38 Systemic and ocular features of Down syndrome

Systemic features	Ocular manifestations
• Mental retardation • Brachycephaly with flattening of occiput • Protruding tongue • Broad short hands	• Upward slanting palpebral fissures • Epicanthic folds • Keratoconus • Cataract

Table 24.39 Systemic and ocular features of Sturge–Weber syndrome

Systemic features	Ocular manifestations
Face: • Facial naevus flammeus (**port wine stain**) distributed over the area corresponding to one or more branches of Vth nerve. **Leptomeninges:** • Angiomas of ipsilateral parietal or occipital meninges.	• Arteriovenous malformations of episclera. • Choroidal hemangioma. • Glaucoma (ipsilateral). • Iris heterochromia.

Table 24.40 Systemic and ocular features of neurofibromatosis

Systemic features	Ocular manifestations
• **Café-au-lait spots**: these are light-brown macules commonly found on the trunk. • **Subcutaneous neurofibromas** along the course of peripheral or autonomic nerves but do not occur on purely motor nerves. • Absence of greater wing of sphenoid bone.	**Orbital involvement:** • Optic nerve glioma • Spheno-orbital encephalocele due to absence of greater wing of sphenoid bone and resulting in pulsating proptosis. **Eyelid neurofibromas:** • These frequently cause a mechanical ptosis. **Iris lesions:** • Lisch nodules. **Fundus lesions:** • Choroidal naevi. • Retinal astrocytomas.

Table 24.41 Systemic and ocular features of albinism

Systemic features	Ocular manifestations
• Hypopigmented skin and hair	• Nystagmus. • Translucent iris giving rise to a pink-eyed appearance. • Large choroidal vessels are seen due to lack of pigment in fundus. • Foveal hypoplasia.

■ Von Hippel–Lindau Disease

Von Hippel-Lindau disease (VHL) is a hereditary condition associated with tumors arising in multiple organs (brain, kidneys, pancreas, adrenal glands, and reproductive tract). It is characterized by angiomatosis of the central nervous system, kidneys, and also retinal angiomas.

■ Nutritional Deficiencies

■ Vitamin A

It is a fat-soluble vitamin and consists of retinol (preformed vitamin), retinal, retinoic acids, and carotene (pro-vitamin). Some of the carotene is converted to retinol in the intestinal mucosa.

1 IU of vitamin A = 0.3 mcg of retinol

Sources

The richest animal sources of vitamin A (retinol) are livers like beef liver and cod liver oil, egg, fish, meat, and milk.

Plant foods containing vitamin A are yellow–orange fruits (papaya, mango, and pumpkins), green leafy vegetables (spinach and amaranth), some roots (carrot), vegetables rich in carotenoids, specifically β-carotene, provide provitamin A precursors.

Daily Requirement

Daily requirement of retinol (pure vitamin A) is:

Infants	350 µg
1 to 6 years	400 µg
7 to 12 years	600 µg
Adults and pregnancy	600 µg
Requirement of carotene is four times higher than retinol.	

Absorption

Approximately 80 to 90% of ingested vitamin A is absorbed. It is passed along with fat through the lymphatic system into the blood stream. Absorption is poor in case of diarrhea, jaundice, and abdominal disorder, and increases if taken with fat. Unabsorbed vitamin A is excreted within 1 or 2 days in feces. The absorption of retinol requires the presence of bile salts.

Transport, Storage and Excretion

It is transported via chylomicrons from intestinal cells to the liver and from the liver to target tissue. The liver has enormous capacity to store it in the form of retinolpalmitate. Under normal conditions a well-fed person has sufficient vitamin A reserves to meet his need for 6 to 9 months or more. Vitamin A is not readily excreted

Functions

Vitamin A plays a critical role in:
- Vision in dim light (vitamin A is a part of rhodopsin and visual pigment).
- Maintaining the integrity and normal functioning of glandular and epithelial

tissues which lines intestinal, respiratory, and urinary tracts as well as skin and eyes.

- Supports skeletal growth.
- Fertility (male and female).
- Embryogenesis.
- Hematopoiesis.
- Retinal and retinoic acid function as steroid hormones. They regulate the protein synthesis and are thus involved in cell growth and differentiation.
- Synthesis of certain glycoproteins.
- Essential for the maintenance of proper immune system.
- Carotenoids function as antioxidants and reduce the risk of cancers.

Vitamin A Deficiency

It is common in poorer countries and is the leading cause of preventable childhood blindness. Each year, millions of children in the developing countries suffer from night blindness or go blind due to hypovitaminosis A.

- Normal serum retinol level is 1 to 3 µmol/l (28 to 86 µg/dL).
- Plasma vitamin level of ≤0.35 µmol/L (10 µg/dl) indicates vitamin A deficiency.

The major causes of vitamin A deficiency are inadequate intake, iron deficiency (it can affect vitamin A uptake), excess alcohol consumption (it can deplete vitamin A), fat malabsorption, and liver disorders. The signs of deficiency are more accentuated in the presence of protein-energy malnutrition (PEM) and gastrointestinal disorders (malabsorption). Vitamin A deficiency may become severe after a precipitating illness such as measles, respiratory tract infections (due to increased metabolic absorption), or diarrhea (due to decreased absorption). Loss of functionality due to vitamin A deficiency is highlighted in **Table 24.42**.

Rhodopsin, the eye pigment responsible for sensing dim light, is composed of retinal (an active form of vitamin A) and opsin (a protein). Vitamin A deficiency has been associated with the loss of goblet cells in the conjunctiva. Goblet cells are responsible for secretion of mucus, and their absence results in xerophthalmia, a condition where the eyes fail to produce tears (**Flowchart 24.1**).

Xerophthalmia (Xeros: Dry; Ophthalmia: Eye)

Xerosis (dry lusterless condition of conjunctiva) occurs in two forms:

- **Parenchymatous xerosis**—It is a cicatricial degeneration of all layers of conjunctiva as a sequel to local disease such as trachoma,

Table 24.42 Functions of vitamin A and features of its deficiency	
Function of vitamin A	**Deficiency of vitamin A**

• Vision (night vision).
• Epithelial cell integrity against infections which line intestinal, respiratory and urinary tracts as well as skin and eyes.
• Immune response (mucosal cells function as a barrier and defence against infections).
• Hematopoiesis.
• Skeletal growth.
• Fertility (male and female).
• Embryogenesis.
• Antioxidants.
	• Night blindness and xerophthalmia:
	  ◊ The skin becomes keratinized, scaly, and toad like (phrynoderma), and the mucus secretion is suppressed.
	  ◊ Alteration in mucosa of renal pelvis and urinary bladder, and formation of renal and vesical calculi.
	  ◊ Collections of keratin in the conjunctiva (Bitot's spots).
	  ◊ Diarrhea.
	• Impaired immune function; deficiency leads to decreased resistance to infections:
	  ◊ Squamous metaplasia of respiratory mucosa and more prone to respiration infections.
	• Impaired hematopoiesis and leads to anemia.
	• Decreased bone development and growth rate.
	• Atrophy of germinal epithelium leading to infertility.
	• Birth defects.
	• Risk of cancers (lung, oral, and prostate cancers).
	• Age-related macular degeneration (ARMD).

Cryotherapy and Lasers in Ophthalmology

Cryotherapy 654
Lasers in Opthalmology 655

■ Cryotherapy

Cryotherapy or cryopexy involves the application of intense cold by a cryoprobe in certain eye diseases. It is used:

- As a **pain treatment** that produces tissue injury by localized freezing temperature but it can leave numbness or tingling as a side effect of cryotherapy treatment.
- To treat localized areas in some **cancers** such as prostate cancer.
- To treat abnormal **skin** cells but can cause redness and irritation of the skin, as side effects, which are generally temporary.

■ Cryounit

It is made of the following:

- A *cryoprobe* is made of silver, a highly conducting metal. Cryoprobes are available in different sizes for different indications (**Table 25.1**).
- A *cryomachine* to which the cryoprobe is attached.
- *Coolant*: Liquid nitrogen, nitrous oxide, or carbon dioxide, is used as a cooling agent.

Table 25.1 Indications for use of different sizes of cryoprobes

Size of probe	Indications
1 mm	Intravitreal pathology (straight)
1.5 mm	Cataract extraction (straight or curved)
2.5 mm	Retina (straight or curved)
3.5–4 mm	Cyclocryopexy in glaucoma (straight)

Temperature produced (−20 to −80) depends upon the size of the cryoprobe tip, duration of freezing process, and gas used.

■ Mode of Action

Cryotherapy produces different actions on tissues in different disease conditions:

- *Tissue necrosis* as in cyclocryopexy in glaucoma.
- *Tissue adhesion* as in retinal detachment.
- *Vascular occlusion* as in Coat's disease.
- *Ice crystal formation* as in cataract extraction.

■ Indications

Cryotherapy is used in the following eye problems:

- **Lids:** In lids, it is used for trichiasis, Molluscum contagiosum, hemangioma, and basal cell carcinoma.
- **Conjunctiva:** It is used for giant papillae of vernal keratoconjunctivitis.
- **Lens:** It is used for intracapsular cataract extraction but, nowadays, its use in cataract surgery is limited because of extracapsular cataract extraction.
- **Glaucoma:** In absolute and neovascular glaucomas, the cyclodestruction is done with cryo application to the ciliary body, which destroys the ciliary epithelium and reduces the aqueous formation and intraocular pressure (IOP). For cyclocryotherapy, the tip of cryoprobe is placed 1.5 mm from the limbus on bulbar conjunctiva. The tip of probe at −80°C

overlies the pars plicata and is applied for 60 seconds. 3 to 4 cryo applications per quadrant are given. If IOP is not controlled even after first cyclocryopexy, it can be repeated after 1 month.

- **Retina:** Cryotherapy is used in more anteriorly placed lesions in retina or in opaque media. Posteriorly placed retinal lesions are treated with laser photocoagulation. In retina, cryopexy is used for the following problems:
  - ◊ For prophylactic treatment of retinal degeneration and retinal breaks.
  - ◊ Retinal detachment.
  - ◊ Retinopathy of prematurity (ROP) to prevent neovascularization.
  - ◊ Cryodestruction of hemangioma and small-sized retinoblastoma.

■ Lasers in Opthalmology

LASER is an acronym for "*Light Amplification by Stimulated Emission of Radiation.*"

■ Properties of Laser Light

The properties of laser light that make it useful to ophthalmologist are as follows:

- Monochromaticity means that laser light is only a single-color light and emits only one wavelength. To prove the monochromaticity of laser light, we can use prism. When white light is passed through prism, it breaks into component colors (VIBGYOR) but if we a pass beam of laser light through the prism, then the beam is only changed in direction and not separated into different colors.
- Coherence means that the light waves are in phase which improve focusing. Laser light is much more coherent than ordinary light. The incoherent waves have no relationship to each other and do not have the same wavelength.
- Collimation is the process by which a beam of radiant electromagnetic energy is lined

up to minimize divergence or convergence. A collimated beam is a bundle of parallel rays. Laser light does not spread out or diverge and stays together in a beam. Divergence is more in ordinary light in comparison with laser light. Usually a laser generates a beam of less than 0.001 rad which means that a beam from the laser will spread to less than 1 foot diameter circle at a distance of 1000 feet from the laser.

- Ability to be concentrated in a short-time interval.
- Ability to produce nonlinear effects.

The combination of these properties makes laser light focus 100 times better than ordinary light (**Table 25.2**).

■ Production of Laser Beam

The production of laser beam involves three basic components:

- Laser medium: Solid, liquid, or gas.
- Exciting methods (for exciting atoms or molecules in the medium): Light and electricity.
- Optical cavity (laser tube) around the medium which acts as a resonator.

■ Delivery System

The laser can be delivered to the eye by:

- *Slit-lamp biomicroscope*: It is most common and the delivery is transpupillary.

Table 25.2 Laser versus incandescent light

Laser	Incandescent Light
Stimulated emission	Spontaneous emission
Monochromatic	Polychromatic
Highly energized	Poorly energized
Parallelism (directional)	Highly divergence (multidirectional)
Coherent	Not coherent
Can be sharply focused	Cannot be sharply focused

with each other and form light and dark fringe patterns on the retina. A rough estimate of visual acuity can be made by changing the distance between two beams, resulting in the alteration of fringe pattern.

Wavefront Analysis

Lasers are used in the measurement of complex optical aberrations of the eye using wavefront analysis.

Therapeutic Uses

Lasers can be used for various structures of the eye, for example (**Fig. 25.1**):

- Lids and adnexae: Lid tumors.
  - ◊ Blepharoplasty (carbon dioxide laser).
  - ◊ Xanthalesma (green laser).
- Laser in lacrimal surgery: Laser dacryo-cystorhinostomy (DCR).

- Laser in cornea: For long-time treatment of myopia.
- Laser in pupillary area: For coreoplasty, photomydriasis, and sphincterotomy.
- Laser in glaucoma: For trabeculoplasty, iridotomy, iridoplasty, cyclophotocoagulation, and goniopuncture.
- Laser in lens: For capsulotomy and phacoemulsification.
- Laser in vitreous: For vitreous membranes and traction bands.
- Laser in retina: For diabetic retinopathy, retinal vascular disorders, clinical significant macular edema (CSME), central serous chorioretinopathy (CSR), retinal breaks, retinal detachment, age-related macular degeneration (ARMD), Eale's disease, Coat's disease, retinopathy of prematurity, and retinal tumors.

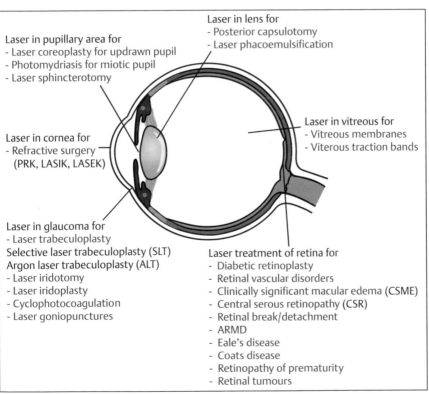

Laser in lens for
- Posterior capsulotomy
- Laser phacoemulsification

Laser in pupillary area for
- Laser coreoplasty for updrawn pupil
- Photomydriasis for miotic pupil
- Laser sphincterotomy

Laser in cornea for
- Refractive surgery (PRK, LASIK, LASEK)

Laser in vitreous for
- Vitreous membranes
- Viterous traction bands

Laser in glaucoma for
- Laser trabeculoplasty
Selective laser trabeculoplasty (SLT)
Argon laser trabeculoplasty (ALT)
- Laser iridotomy
- Laser iridoplasty
- Cyclophotocoagulation
- Laser goniopunctures

Laser treatment of retina for
- Diabetic retinoplasty
- Retinal vascular disorders
- Clinically significant macular edema (CSME)
- Central serous retinopathy (CSR)
- Retinal break/detachment
- ARMD
- Eale's disease
- Coats disease
- Retinopathy of prematurity
- Retinal tumours

Fig. 25.1 Lasers in anterior and posterior segments.

■ Femto Laser-Assisted in Situ Keratomileusis (OP1.4)

Hundred percent blade-free Laser-Assisted in Situ Keratomileusis (LASIK) surgery or intralase femtosecond LASIK laser is better and safer for creating the corneal flap. In case of blade-free LASIK, surgeons use a computerized laser for creating the corneal flap, which generates accuracy of micron level. This is used instead of the mechanical microkeratome, the older technique. Advantages of femtosecond laser are:

- Flaps are more accurate and uniform in thickness.
- Centration of flap is easier.
- Better adherence to underlying stroma.
- Patients are more comfortable.

■ Photodynamic Therapy (PDT)

It is the photochemical reaction following visible/infrared light, particularly after administration of exogenous photosensitizer. It involves i.v. injection of a light-sensitive dye followed by application of low-energy laser (**Flowchart 25.1**). Commonly used photosensitizers are:

- Hematoporphyrin.
- Benzoporphyrin derivatives such as verteporfin.

Indications

- Choroidal neovascular membrane (CNV).
- Choroidal hemangioma.
- Neovascular or wet ARMD.

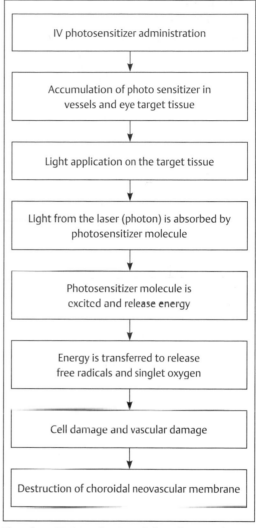

Flowchart 25.1 Mechanism of photodynamic therapy.

Eye Surgery

Lid Surgery 660
Lacrimal Sac Surgery..667
Strabismus (Squint) Surgery...670
Corneal and Refractive Surgery 676
Cataract Surgery...686
Surgical Treatment of Glaucoma 700
Vitreoretinal Surgery 701
Surgery on the Eyeball...706

▰ Lid Surgery

▰ Entropion

Treatment of entropion includes medical and surgical therapy. *Medical therapy*: It includes a temporary treatment with lubricants, taping and soft bandage contact lens. The aim of surgery for involutional entropion is to correct the underlying problems involved in its pathogenesis. The surgery for involutional entropion may involve a combination of more than one procedure.

- Horizontal lid laxity is corrected with resection and reconstruction of lateral canthal tendon and preferred over purely tarsal resection performed in central eyelid, as the evidence suggests that the dysfunction resides in the canthal tendon and its attachment rather than in the tarsal plate itself.
- Orbicularis muscle dysfunction is corrected by creating a fibrous barrier between the skin and the deeper eye lid structures at the junction of the pretarsal and preseptal orbicularis. This can be achieved through full-thickness horizontal lid splitting at this level and the insertion of everting sutures

(**Wies procedure**). The stimulation of fibrosis through the use of sutures creates a barrier between preseptal and pretarsal orbicularis, preventing the overriding of preseptal over pretarsal orbicularis (**Fig. 26.1**).

- Vertical lid instability is best corrected by reattachment or tightening of the lower eyelid retractors (**Jones procedure**). The capsulo-palpebral fascia is advanced or reattached to the inferior tarsal border via a transcutaneous approach (**Fig. 26.2**).

Spastic Entropion

It is due to the spasm of orbicularis oculi which can be induced by local irritation or infection. Spastic entropion is almost always restricted to the lower lid. Spastic entropion is thought to be a subset of involution entropion, as the spasm of orbicularis oculi can unmask the symptomatic involutional changes that allow the orbicularis to ride up in front of tarsal plate and approximate the lid margins and turn them inward, resulting in temporary entropion. The condition is found particularly in old age and may be caused by tight bandaging. It is favored by narrowness of palpebral aperture (blepharophimosis).

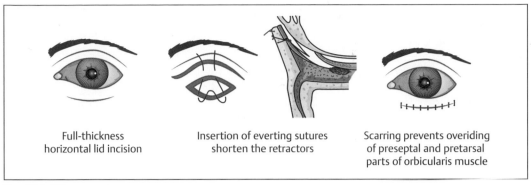

Fig. 26.1 Wies procedure.

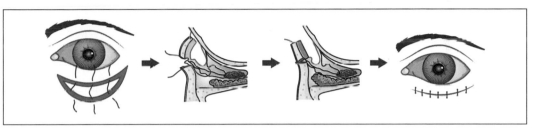

Fig. 26.2 Jones procedure.

Treatment

The cause for the spastic entropion must be identified and treated:

- If it is due to blepharitis, it is treated by eyelid hygiene, antibiotics and corticosteroids.
- If it is due to bandaging, it can be cured by removing the bandage.
- If the entropion persists, small amounts of botulinum toxin (BOTOX, 5U) may be injected into the pretarsal plate orbicularis and overriding is prevented by weakening it.
- Patients with cicatricial entropion secondary to ocular cicatricial pemphigoid may benefit from systemic chemotherapy, usually dapsone.

Cicatricial Entropion

Cicatricial entropion can be distinguished from involutional entropion by:

- The patient's *history*.

- *Digital traction* on eye lid: It will correct the abnormal margin position in involution entropion but not in cicatricial entropion.
- *Inspection of posterior aspect of eye lid* reveals scarring of tarsal conjunctiva in cases of cicatricial entropion.

Treatment

Medical treatment– Bandage contact lenses keep the lashes away from the cornea.

Surgical treatment: The repair of cicatricial entropion will depend on the degree of scarring and entropion, etiology of cicatricial changes, and status of tarsal plate. The basic principles governing the various operations are restoration of the normal direction of lashes and tarsal rotation.

Mild case can be treated with a transverse tarsotomy (**tarsal fracture**) and anterior rotation of lid margin (**Fig. 26.3**).

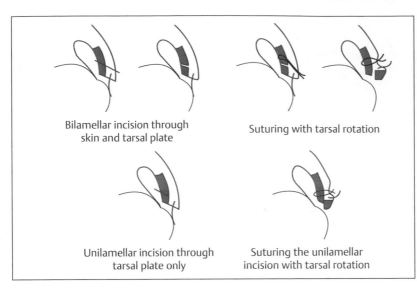

Fig. 26.3 Tarsal fracture.

Bilamellar incision through
skin and tarsal plate

Suturing with tarsal rotation

Unilamellar incision through
tarsal plate only

Suturing the unilamellar
incision with tarsal rotation

More extensive scarring may require the replacement of conjunctiva by a mucous membrane (e.g., buccal mucosa). Assess the status of tarsal plate in all cases of cicatricial entropion. If it is distorted, excision of the distorted portion of the tarsal plate is replaced by a cartilage (ear cartilage), hard palate grafts and chondromucosal grafts.

■ Ectropion

Treatment

The treatment depends predominantly on the location of ectropion.

- If the ectropion is generalized, it is treated with **horizontal lid shortening** by excision of a full-thickness pentagon of the lid. It corrects the ectropion completely. It can be performed at any point on the lower lid, but the preferred site is usually in the lateral third (**Fig. 26.4a**).
- Medial ectropion (involving punctal area) can be treated with **medial tarsoconjunctival diamond excision**. A diamond-shaped segment of tarsus and conjunctiva is resected directly below the punctum (edge of the diamond is placed 2 mm below the lid margin to protect the canaliculi). A suture is placed untied which rotates the medial lid margin and punctum inward (**Fig. 26.4b**).

If the medial ectropion with punctal eversion is associated with predominantly medial horizontal lid laxity, medial diamond excision is done with horizontal lid shortening (**Lazy-T procedure**) (**Fig. 26.4c**).

- If the ectropion is severe and more marked over the lateral half of the lower lid, a **Kuhnt–Szymanowski procedure** *modified by Bryon Smith* is performed. This procedure involves shortening of the eyelid with elevation of temporal margin. In this procedure, a tarsoconjunctival excision is made from the middle part of the lower lid. A line is drawn 3 mm inferior to the lid margin, following the contour of the lower lid. An incision is made 2 to 3 mm inferior to the lid margin. A skin flap is prepared and an appropriate triangular piece of skin is resected at the outer canthus. The wound is closed and the lid margin is mobilized upward and outward to cover the skin incision (**Fig. 26.4d**).

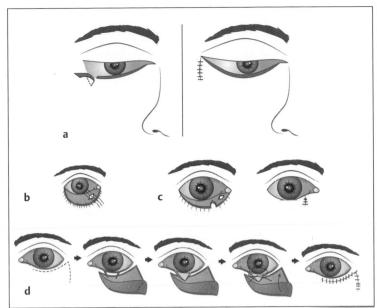

Fig. 26.4 (a) Horizontal lid shortening. **(b)** Medial tarso-conjunctival diamond excision. **(c)** Lazy-T procedure. **(d)** Kuhnt–Szymanowski procedure.

Cicatricial Ectropion

It is caused by burns, trauma and chronic inflammations of skin, resulting in scarring of the skin and underlying tissues which pulls the eyelid away from the globe.

Treatment

Localized areas with scarring can be released by **Z-plasty** or **V–Y operation**.

Z-plasty: The three stages of **Z-plasty** include:
- Incisions making triangular flaps.
- Flaps are moved into their new positions.
- Flaps are interlocked and wound is closed.

The middle line of the "Z"-shaped incision is made along the line of greatest tension or contraction, and the triangular flaps are raised on the opposite sides of two ends and transposed (**Fig. 26.5a**).

V–Y plasty: A "V"-shaped incision with its apex away from the lid margin is made to release the scarred tissue. The skin is undermined and sutured in a "Y"-shaped manner (**Fig. 26.5b**).

Severe generalized scars require skin grafts. Scars are excised and the surrounding skin is released from the underlying adhesions before the application of a skin graft. The sources of skin graft are the upper lid and behind the ear or inner upper arm.

■ Ptosis

The management of ptosis is variable according to the cause. In neurogenic ptosis, the patient should be reviewed periodically for any spontaneous recovery. In complete paralysis of III nerve, surgery is usually contraindicated, as elevation of the ptotic eye leads to diplopia due to ophthalmoplegia. The proper choice of operation for the various types and degrees of ptosis is performed.

Age for Surgery

The ideal time for surgery is when a sufficiently accurate preoperative examination can be made. If ptosis is partial, 4 to 5 years of age is probably an ideal age. If the lid covers the visual axis due to ptosis, a temporary placement of nonabsorbable sutures (for lid elevation by brow suspension) may be indicated as soon as possible to avoid sensory deprivation amblyopia. At the age of 4 to 5 years, sutures are removed to re-evaluate the ptosis and to do a more definitive operation.

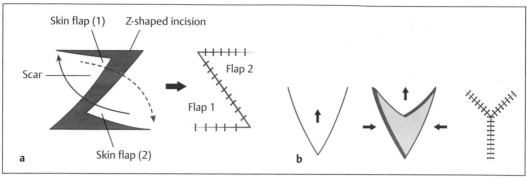

Fig. 26.5 (a) Z-plasty. **(b)** V–Y plasty.

Table 26.1 Determination of the amount of ptosis

Amount of ptosis	Droop of eyelid
Mild	If the eyelid droops 2 mm or less (≤**2 mm**) from its normal level.
Moderate	If the eyelid droops **3 mm**.
Severe	If the eyelid droops 4mm or more (≥**4 mm**).

Type of Surgery

It is determined by amount of ptosis, levator function and associated anomalies (e.g., Marcus–Gunn phenomenon).

- **Amount of ptosis: Table 26.1** highlights the amount of ptosis as per the eyelid droop.
- **Levator function:** It is termed good if it is 8 mm or more (≥**8 mm**), fair if it is **5 to 7 mm** and poor if it is 4 mm or less (≤**4 mm**).

Levator Palpebrae Superioris (LPS) Resection

A definitive preoperative determination of the amount of levator to be resected is required. A millimeter caliper is used at surgery to measure the resection.

A resection of: **10–13 mm** is termed small
14–17 mm is termed as moderate.
18–22 mm is termed as large
and LPS resection of **23 mm or more** (≥ **23 mm**) is termed as maximum.

The result of any resection can be enhanced slightly by advancement on the anterior surface of tarsus in skin-approach resection or tarsal resection when the conjunctival approach is used. A tarsal resection should not amount to more than half of its vertical width.

In treating **"congenital" ptosis**, it is well to choose the large resection because overcorrection is easier to treat than undercorrection. In treating **"acquired" ptosis**, the levator resection must be more conservative because more postoperative lift is expected after the surgical correction of these cases, that is, overcorrection is easy to obtain but may be disastrous.

Standard Ptosis Procedures

A basic set of procedures includes:

- Vertical lid shortening (Fasanella–Servat operation).
- LPS resection (conjunctival/skin approach).
- Aponeurosis advancement and tucking.
- Brow-suspension ptosis repair.

Fasanella–Servat Operation

It is chiefly a tarsal resection. The amount of LPS tendon excised is so small that no lifting effect could be expected from it. It is rather a *tarsectomy* and shortening of Müller's muscle and conjunctiva only.

Indication: Mild ptosis (1.5–2 mm) with good LPS function.

Procedure: Following are the steps involved to carry out Fasanella–Servat operation (**Fig. 26.6**):

1. Upper lid is everted. Two curved hemostats are applied grasping the conjunctiva, tarsus. Müller's muscle and LPS.
2. Upper tarsus is excised by 4 to 5 mm.
3. The running suture is placed. A small skin incision is made in the lid crease immediately above the lateral canthus. The two ends of suture are made through the skin incision and tied. The knot is buried beneath the skin surface.

LPS Resection

The muscle can be resected either through the conjunctival approach (Blaskovics operation) or skin approach (Everbusch's operation).

The steps involved in Blaskovics operation are as follows:

- Upper lid is doubly everted over Desmarre lid retractor.
- An incision is made at the upper border of tarsal plate through conjunctiva.
- Conjunctiva is reflected by sutures.
- Levator aponeurosis is identified and undermined with scissors.
- A ptosis clamp is inserted and LPS aponeurosis is freed from its attachments.
- 1 to 2 mm of upper border of tarsal plate is excised.

- The amount of LPS to be resected is measured with a caliper and three double-armed 5–0 vicryl sutures are passed through the aponeurosis.
- The aponeurosis is cut distal to the sutures.
- The cut end is anchored to the upper border of tarsal plate.
- The sutures are merged through the muscle and skin in a line to make the lid fold.
- The conjunctiva is closed with continuous suture.

Since the sutures used are tied exteriorly, they can be removed early in the event of overcorrection. *For this reason, it should be employed in most reoperations for undercorrection of congenital ptosis, in which overcorrection is a true hazard.*

Everbusch's operation (***skin approach*** *levator resection*).

Advantages:

- It should be used when ptosis is congenital and severe. LPS is better exposed through skin approach and is recommended in patients who require larger LPS resections.
- The suture can be fixed somewhat lower on the tarsus. The resulting advancement enhances the elevating effect of resection appreciably.

The steps involved in Everbusch's operation are as follows:

- A skin incision is made in the future lid fold.
- The dissection is carried under the orbicularis muscle to expose the orbital septum.
- A vertical incision is made in the orbital septum and the levator aponeurosis is exposed.
- Conjunctiva is separated from the Müller muscle and aponeurosis.

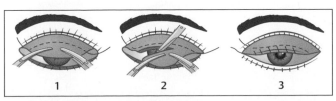

Fig. 26.6 Steps involved in Fasanella–Servat operation.

- A ptosis clamp is placed, grasping the aponeurosis.
- The amount of LPS aponeurosis to be resected is measured with a caliper, and three double-armed sutures are passed through the aponeurosis.
- The aponeurosis is cut distal to the sutures and anchored to the upper tarsal border. The sutures are tied.

Levator Advancement

Procedure: The steps involved in levator advancement are as follows:
- A skin incision is made along the lid fold.
- The levator aponeurosis is identified and detached.
- The lower edge of aponeurosis is attached to the anterior surface of tarsus.
- The skin incision is closed.

Levator Aponeurosis Tuck (Tucking/Levator Plication)

In this procedure, the levator, instead of being resected, is double-breasted over itself. It is done in mild to moderate ptosis with good or fair levator function. In severe ptosis, the results are poor as compared with LPS resection (**Fig. 26.7**).
- The levator aponeurosis is approached by a lid crease incision.
- Three mattress sutures are placed. Upper bites are placed in the aponeurosis and the lower bites engage the tarsus.
- Sutures are tied, and the skin incision is closed.

Frontalis (Brow) Suspension

Indication: It is used for severe ptosis (>4 mm) with very poor levator function (<4 mm).

Procedure: The steps involved in frontalis suspension are as follows: The tarsal plate is suspended from the frontalis muscle with a sling consisting of autologous fascia lata or nonabsorbable sutures (prolene). The best material available is autologous fascia lata. For most brow suspension procedures, a strip, which is 6 to 7 cm in length, should be sufficient.

Two incisions at the lid margin are considered appropriate for young children as it prevents postoperative bending of the eyelid. Three incisions are made approximately 4 mm from the lid margin. Two incisions are made 5 mm above the medial and lateral portions of the brow. The third brow incision is made midway between the two brow incisions, 15 to 16 mm above them. One fascia lata strip or suture (supramid or prolene) is passed through the openings in the lid and then upward, emerging with two ends in each of the openings above the brow. The end of each strip is carried beneath the brow to the central brow incision, and a ligature is fixed deep in the upper brow incision. The brow incisions are closed and the lid incisions are not sutured. The frost suture is placed in the lower lid and taped to the forehead for corneal protection (**Fig. 26.8**).

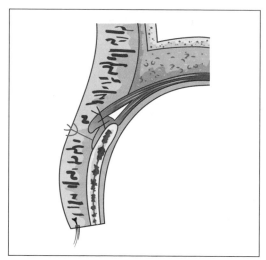

Fig. 26.7 Aponeurosis tuck.

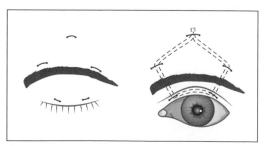

Fig. 26.8 Frontalis (brow) suspension.

Choice of Operation

Congenital Ptosis

Table 26.2 highlights the choice of cooperation for the treatment of congenital ptosis.

Acquired Ptosis

In acquired ptosis, laterality, severity, LPS function, and the cause of ptosis is taken into account.

Neurogenic ptosis

In all neurogenic ptosis, the patient should be reviewed periodically for any spontaneous recovery and stabilization of ptosis.

- In *complete III nerve paralysis*, surgery should not be done, since raising the eyelid produces a troublesome diplopia due to strabismus.
- Neurogenic ptosis due to *Horner's syndrome* is ideally suited for the Fasanella–Servat operation, since LPS function is normal in these cases and lid motility remains unimpaired.

Myogenic Ptosis

In myogenic ptosis, treatment of the primary disorder should be undertaken first, followed by crutch spectacles to help lift the lid.

Aponeurotic Ptosis

It is due to weakness or disinsertion of the LPS aponeurosis from the anterior tarsal surface. Treatment of aponeurotic ptosis consists of reinsertion of levator aponeurosis into the anterior tarsal surface with appropriate resection of LPS.

Mechanical ptosis

In mechanical ptosis, the treatment is that of the cause.

■ Lacrimal Sac Surgery

■ Dacryocystorhinostomy (DCR)

DCR involves anastomosis between lacrimal sac and nasal mucosa of middle nasal meatus to

Table 26.2 Choice of operation in congenital ptosis

Degree	LPS function	Operative procedure
Mild (1.5–2 mm)	Always good LPS function	Fasanella-Servat operation or Small (10–13 mm) LPS resection
Moderate (3 mm) LPS function is good or fair. In moderate ptosis LPS function of <5 mm is extremely rare.	If LPS function is good (≥8 mm) If LPS function is fair (5–7 mm) If LPS function of <5 mm is encountered	Moderate (14–17 mm) LPS resection. Larger (18–22 mm) LPS resection. Maximum (≥23 mm) LPS resection by skin approach should be done.
Severe (≥4 mm) Sometimes, this type of ptosis has a fair LPS function but usually LPS function is poor.	If LPS function is fair (5–7 mm) If, as is usual, LPS function is poor (≤4 mm)	Maximum (≥23 mm) LPS resection by skin approach should be done. The levator muscles should be well advanced on the anterior surfaces of the tarsi. Bilateral fascia lata brow suspension is done if the ptosis is bilateral. If ptosis is unilateral, a maximum (≥23 mm) LPS resection by skin approach should be done. The levator muscle should be well advanced on the anterior surfaces of the tarsus. The alternative that has usually been done is a unilateral brow suspension procedure.

Abbreviation: LPS, levator palpebrae superioris.

bypass the obstructed nasolacrimal duct (NLD). It is indicated for the obstruction beyond the opening of the canaliculus. DCR can be performed by:

- Conventional external DCR.
- Endonasal DCR.
- Transcanalicular laser DCR.

Endonasal DCR is cosmetically superior to external DCR. Differentiating features of external and endoscopic DCR are listed in **Table 26.3**.

Conventional External DCR

Indications

DCR is indicated in chronic dacryocystitis and mucocele of the lacrimal sac.

Preoperative Requisites

The following information needs to be in hand before going in for conventional external DCR:

- Hemoglobin levels.
- Bleeding and clotting times.
- Blood pressure measurement.
- Random blood sugars.
- ENT evaluation.
- Additional general anesthesia investigations when required.

Procedure

- *Nasal packing*: It is done to keep the mucosa taut and reduce bleeding. Instill 4% topical lignocaine in the ipsilateral nostril, followed by insertion of nasal pack (roller gauze soaked in 2% lignocaine-adrenaline jelly) superiorly then posteriorly and inferiorly with the help of nasal packing forceps.

- *Anesthesia*: It may be general or local anesthesia (2% Lignocaine with 0.5% Bupivacaine with or without adrenaline) by infiltration. It blocks infratrochlear nerve first which supplies the lacrimal apparatus.
- *Skin incision*: A curved incision along lacrimal crest is made. Angular vessels should be avoided. Orbicularis is split and retracted with skin by a lacrimal retractor (**Fig. 26.9**).
- *Exposure of medial palpebral ligament (MPL) and anterior lacrimal crest*: MPL is exposed and disinserted at the anterior lacrimal crest. It opens up the periosteum which

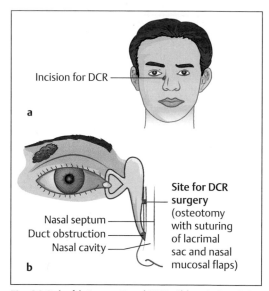

Incision for DCR

a

Nasal septum
Duct obstruction
Nasal cavity

Site for DCR surgery (osteotomy with suturing of lacrimal sac and nasal mucosal flaps)

b

Fig. 26.9 (a, b) Conventional DCR. Abbreviation: DCR, dacryocystorhinostomy.

Table 26.3 Difference between external and endoscopic DCR		
Criteria	**External DCR**	**Endoscopic DCR**
Cutaneous scarring	Yes	No
Bleeding	More	Bloodless surgery
Time consumption	More	Less
Skill requirement	No need for endoscopic skill Easy to perform	Requires skill Better visualization
Success rate	More	Less
Cost factors	Cheap	Expensive
Morbidity	More post-operative morbidity	No post-operative morbidity
Abbreviation: DCR, dacryocystorhinostomy.		

is now separated along the entire length of the incision with periosteum elevator. Periosteum is elevated posteriorly till the lamina papyracea, which is a thin bone.

- *Exposure of nasal mucosa*: Osteotomy (12 × 10 mm) is done with a bone punch, removing the lacrimal crest and lamina papyracea to expose the nasal mucosa.
- *Preparation of flaps of sac*: A probe is introduced into the sac through the lower canaliculus. A vertical incision is made in the medial wall of the lacrimal sac and converted into H-shape to prepare anterior and posterior flaps.
- *Preparation of nasal mucosal flaps*: The two flaps of nasal mucosa are made by an H-shaped incision with the horizontal incision in the middle.
- *Suturing of flaps*: The posterior flaps of the sac and nasal mucosa are sutured. The anterior nasal flap is now sutured to the anterior sac flap with 6–0 vicryl sutures.
- *Closure*: The medial palpebral ligament is reposited and sutured with periosteum. The orbicularis oculi muscle is also sutured with 6–0 vicryl and the skin incision is closed with 6–0 silk suture.
- *Postoperative care*: Complete bed rest for 24 hours:
  ◊ Patients are asked to avoid blowing of nose.
  ◊ Oral antibiotics and nonsteroidal anti-inflammatory drugs (NSAIDs) are given routinely for 5 days.
  ◊ Nasal pack is removed after 24 hours.
  ◊ Local treatment includes otrivin-P nasal drops twice daily, antibiotic ointment on the wound twice daily, and antibiotic with steroid eye drop four times daily.
  ◊ The syringing should be done on third day postoperatively.
  ◊ Sutures are removed after 1 week.

Causes of Failure

- Unrecognized common canalicular obstruction.

- Scarring.
- "Sump syndrome," in which the surgical opening in the lacrimal bone is too small and too high. Thus, there is collection of secretions in lacrimal sac below the level of inferior margin of the ostium, which is unable to gain access to the nasal cavity.

Complications

Bleeding may occur from the vascular nasal mucosa postoperatively. Postoperative infection is rarely seen.

Endoscopic Transnasal DCR

It is indicated in patients of chronic dacryocystitis with associated nasal disorder.

Procedure

A slender light pipe is passed through the lacrimal puncta and canaliculi into the lacrimal sac and viewed from within the nasal cavity with an endoscope. The remainder of the procedure is performed via the nose:

- The mucosa over the frontal process of the maxilla is stripped.
- A part of the nasal process of the maxilla is removed.
- The lacrimal bone is broken off piecemeal.
- The lacrimal sac is opened.
- Silicone tubes are passed through the upper and lower puncta, pulled out through the ostium, and tied within the nose.

Endolaser DCR

It is a relatively rapid procedure and can be performed under local anesthesia. It is therefore particularly suitable for elderly patients. It is performed with a Holmium: YAG laser which is used to ablate the mucosa and thin lacrimal bone. It has a lower success rate (70%) due to smaller bony opening (4–6 mm) in comparison to conventional DCR.

Dacryocystectomy

It is the *removal of lacrimal sac*. Postoperative epiphora is common.

between two hemostats and clamped, after which a section is removed with scissors.

- The wound is now closed.

Disinsertion (or Myectomy)

In disinsertion, a muscle is detached from its insertion but not reattached. Therefore, the technique is identical to recession, except that the muscle is not sutured. It is commonly used to weaken an overacting inferior oblique muscle.

Posterior Fixation Suture (Faden Operation)

The word Faden is German for thread or suture and is derived from the use of sutures to attach the muscle to the sclera. This operation is also designated *posterior fixation suture* or *retropexy* of an extraocular muscle (EOM). In this procedure, the muscle belly is sutured (with a nonabsorbable suture) to the sclera posteriorly, approximately 12 mm behind its insertion. Thus, the pull of the muscle in its field of action is decreased with no effect in the primary position. The Faden procedure may be used:

- On MR in convergence excess esotropia (to reduce convergence).
- On superior rectus in dissociated vertical deviation (DVD).

Strengthening Procedures

These include resection, tucking of a muscle or tendon, and advancement of the muscle.

Resection

It shortens the length of muscle and enhance its effective pull. Excessive resection may mechanically restrict movement of the globe in the opposite direction and, therefore, must be avoided. It is suitable only for a rectus muscle.

The maximum amount of resection for MR is 7 to 8 mm and for LR is 10 mm. When more correction is desired, the muscle is advanced toward the cornea.

Many technical problems occur with the resection of inferior oblique muscle. Therefore, weakening the action of superior rectus muscle in the fellow eye or tenotomy of ipsilateral superior

oblique muscle (in case of inferior oblique paralysis) must be preferred.

Procedure

- A vertical incision in conjunctiva is made in front of the muscle insertion.
- Muscle exposed is covered by Tenon's capsule.
- Slit incisions are made in Tenon's capsule along the upper and lower borders of the muscle. The part of the capsule covering the muscle should be preserved.
- The squint hook is passed under the muscle just behind the insertion.
- The length of muscle and tendon for resection is determined and marked.
- Two absorbable sutures are passed through upper and lower edges of the muscle behind the mark.
- The muscle is held in a muscle clamp and cut at the insertion.
- The needles of suture are passed through the original insertion and the muscle anterior to the suture is excised.
- The muscle is drawn forward, sutures are tied, and conjunctival incision is closed (**Fig. 26.11**).

For resection of vertical recti muscles, the functions of neighboring oblique muscles must be preserved before the procedure is performed and the fascial attachments must be visualized and removed.

> - *Recession of the MR is more effective than recession of the LR.*
> - *Resection of the LR has a relatively greater effect than of the MR.*

Tucking of a Muscle

Tucking (pleating) of the tendon of the superior oblique for its underaction is preferred to resection. Thus, it is usually confined to enhance the action of superior rectus muscle.

Procedure

- An incision is made through the conjunctiva and Tenon's capsule horizontally from the temporal edge of superior rectus.

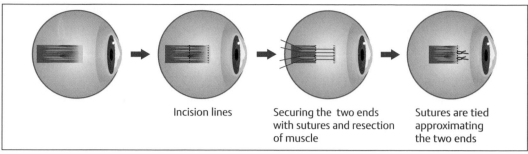

| Incision lines | Securing the two ends with sutures and resection of muscle | Sutures are tied approximating the two ends |

Fig. 26.11 Resection of a muscle.

- A muscle hook is placed under the superior rectus insertion, and the eye is rotated further downward with the hook.
- The temporal border of superior rectus is lifted with the hook, and the superior oblique tendon is exposed with a sweeping motion of a second hook.
- A tendon tucker is introduced beneath the superior oblique tendon. The folded tendon is drawn into the tucker.
- After achieving a desired amount of tucking (usually between 6 and 12 mm), the blades of the instrument are closed.
- Forced ductions are now performed to determine the degree of restriction when elevating the adducted eye. Mild restriction is desirable and should result in a good effect from the operation. Severe restriction necessitates undoing the tuck and tucking a lesser portion of the tendon.
- The wound is then closed with one interrupted stitch of 7–0 vicryl.

Advancement of the Muscle

A previously recessed rectus muscle can be advanced nearer to the limbus to enhance its action.

Transposition/Repositioning Procedures

It is the repositioning of one or more EOMs to substitute the action of a deficient muscle **(Fig. 26.12)**.

Indications

It is indicated in acquired VIth cranial nerve (CN) nerve palsy, resulting in LR weakness, A–V

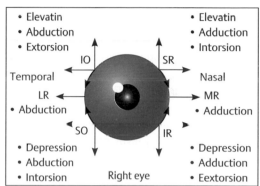

- Elevatin
- Abduction
- Extorsion

- Elevatin
- Adduction
- Intorsion

Temporal

Nasal

- Abduction
- Adduction

- Depression
- Abduction
- Intorsion

- Depression
- Adduction
- Eextorsion

Right eye

Fig. 26.12 Actions of EOMs. Abbreviation: EOM, extraocular muscle; IO, inferior oblique; IR, inferior rectus; LR, lateral rectus; SO, superior oblique; SR, superior rectus.

patterns, Duane syndrome, and monocular elevation deficit.

Procedures

- Vertical rectus muscles in the treatment of horizontal strabismus: Transposition of strips of the superior rectus and inferior rectus muscles are used in the correction of total LR and MR paralyses. It is also necessary to recess the ipsilateral opponent of the paralyzed muscle. For esotropia (total LR palsy), temporal transposition of vertical rectus muscles is recommended. The superior rectus and inferior rectus are split along their length and join to the adjacent halves of the similarly split LR. A suture ties the half muscles together at the level of equator. Similarly, the vertical muscles are transposed nasally for exotropia (total MR palsy).

For Paralytic Strabismus

In long-standing paralysis, the following changes takes place:

- The contracture of ipsilateral antagonist muscle.
- Overaction of contralateral synergist.
- Inhibitional palsy of contralateral antagonists.

For example, in case of left LR palsy: Contracture of left MR, overaction of right MR muscle, and inhibitional palsy of right LR muscle are encountered.

In paralytic strabismus, the treatment with prisms is rarely of much use due to variation in the amount of deviation in the different positions of eyes. Therefore, surgery is done when the deviation has become stabilized.

A unilateral EOM palsy may be treated by one or several of the operations listed in **Table 26.6**.

Often, it seems necessary to plan the surgical treatment in more than one stage to assess the effects of each.

■ Complications of Squint Surgery

Complications following strabismus surgery include:

- Anterior segment ischemia.
- Undercorrection or overcorrection.
- Postoperative diplopia.
- Scleral perforation.
- Postoperative infections.
- Foreign body granuloma.
- Conjunctival inclusion cysts.
- Slipped or lost muscle.

- Suture reactions.
- Corneal dellen.

> Particular caution is required in patients with thin sclera (such as in myopes or having a history of scleritis). The surgeon must be aware of the location of vortex vein, especially during oblique muscle surgery.

■ Corneal and Refractive Surgery

Corneal and refractive surgery include keratoplasty, keratoprostheses and refractive surgery.

■ Keratoplasty (OP4.6)

Synonyms: corneal grafting or corneal transplantation.

It refers to the replacement of patient's diseased cornea by healthy and clear donor cornea.

Donor Tissue

The **donor eye** should be removed within 6 hours of death.

Preservation (Eye banking) (OP4.9)

The donor corneas are stored in *eye bank* prior to transplantation. Corneas are preserved by various methods as follows:

- *Short-term storage*: Globe can be preserved up to 48 hours by the moist chamber technique at 4°.
- *Intermediate term storage*: The cornea can be preserved up to a period of 2 weeks, employing tissue culture technique. McCarey–Kaufman medium (MK medium) could store cornea at 4° for 4 days. Later, a new media was introduced which had chondroitin sulfate added to the tissue

Table 26.6 Operations on Extraocular muscles for long standing paralysis	
Changes in long standing paralysis	**Operations on extraocular muscle**
• The contracture of ipsilateral antagonist muscle. • Over action of contralateral synergist. • Inhibitional palsy of contralateral antagonists.	• Recession of the overacting and subsequently contracted direct (ipsilateral) antagonist. • Recession of the overacting contralateral synergist. • Resection of the contralateral antagonist, particularly if it is affected by disuse palsy. • Resection of the weak and stretched palsied muscle.

culture medium. These can store cornea for up to 2 weeks. These media are K-SOL, CSM, DEXSOL and OPTISOL.

- *Long term storage*: This includes organ culture media and cryopreservation. Organ culture media can preserve the cornea at 34° for 35 days, while cryopreservation can preserve the cornea for an indefinite time at−160 but it can produce endothelial damage.

Contraindications

If any of the following conditions are known to be present in the donor, these eyes are not offered for surgery, either because it could transmit a health threatening condition to the recipient or because the corneal quality is not good. These are as follows:

- Death from unknown cause.
- AIDS.
- Viral hepatitis.
- Syphilis.
- Congenital rubella.
- Rabies.
- Septicemia.
- Ocular diseases (such as retinoblastoma and corneal refractive surgery).
- Leukemia (blast form) and other hematological malignancy.

Evaluation of Donor Cornea

The donor eye requires a careful slit lamp examination. A specular microscopic examination, if possible, has an added advantage. Specular microscopy helps to screen out poor quality donor tissues. It is employed to examine the endothelial cells in terms of their shape, size, uniformity, pleomorphism, polymegathism, cell density, presence of cornea guttata, and keratic precipitates. *Any cornea which shows an endothelial cell count of less than 1500 cells/mm², extreme polymegathism and pleomorphism, significant corneal guttata, or inflammatory cells on the endothelium is considered unsatisfactory.*

Indications

The following indications suffice the purpose of keratoplasty:

- Optical: To improve vision as in keratoconus, corneal opacity, corneal degenerations, corneal dystrophies, or bullous keratopathy.
- Therapeutic: To remove infected corneal tissue unresponsive to antimicrobial therapy.
- Tectonic graft: To restore integrity of eyeball as in thinned cornea with descemetocele or after corneal perforation.
- Cosmetic: To improve the appearance of the eye.

Types

Keratoplasty may be:

- Partial thickness keratoplasty (lamellar keratoplasty): It may be anterior or posterior lamellar keratoplasty.
- Full-thickness keratoplasty (penetrating keratoplasty).
- Endothelial keratoplasty (**Fig. 26.13**).

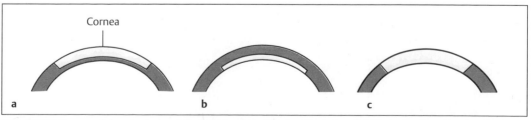

Fig. 26.13 Types of keratoplasty. **(a)** Anterior lamellar keratoplasty. **(b)** Posterior lamellar keratoplasty. **(c)** Penetrating keratoplasty.

- No gross posterior segment disorders on ultrasonography.
- Normal electrophysiological test.

Basic Design of Keratoprostheses

Keratoprostheses basically consists of a central optical cylinder made of polymethylmethacrylate (PMMA) with a surrounding fixation device. The materials used for fixation device include:

- Patients' own tooth root and alveolar bone (*osteo-odonto-keratoprosthesis*).
- Cartilage (*chondro-keratoprothesis*).
- Patient's nail (*onycho-keratoprothesis*).
- Teflon.
- Dacron mesh.
- Polycarbon.

Complications

These include glaucoma, tilting or extrusion, retroprosthetic membrane formation, retinal detachment (RD), uveitis, and endophthalmitis.

■ Refractive Surgery (OP1.4)

The refractive power of the eye can be modified by:

- Modifying the curvature of cornea (keratorefractive procedures).
- Changing the refractive status of eye by implanting an implantable contact lens (ICL).

- Removing the natural crystalline lens with or without implanting an intraocular lens (IOL).

Modification of Corneal Curvature (Keratorefractive Procedures)

Approximately ⅔rd of refraction occurs at the anterior surface of cornea whose curvature can be modified by:

- Procedures over **central cornea** (optical zone).
- Procedures over **peripheral cornea.**

The **central cornea** may be modified either on surface or intrastromally. The procedures over central cornea modify its thickness.

The procedures over **peripheral cornea** change the shape of central cornea through their action on the former. This is achieved without changing the thickness over central cornea (**Flowchart 26.1**).

Keratomileusis refers to carving the cornea. It may be classical keratomileusis or laser keratomileusis. Classic keratomileusis involves *excision of lamellar button* from cornea with microkeratome, followed by its *freezing*. Lamellar button is *reshaped* (a lenticule of predetermined power is removed *from the stromal side* with a lathe) and *sutured back* in place.

Freezing corneal tissue results in severe damage to keratocytes and the lamellar

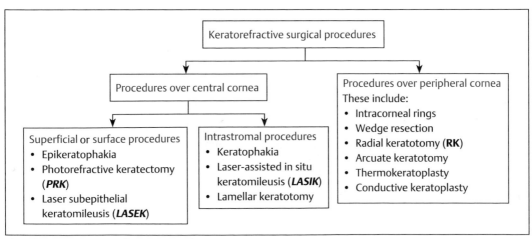

Flowchart 26.1 Keratorefractive procedures.

architecture of cornea. The fact that corneal cap (lamellar button) does not have to be modified led to the use of hinged flap instead of a free cap. This, in turn, led to the sutureless repositioning of flap which simplified the procedure further and came to be known as laser keratomileusis.

Laser keratomileusis involves ablation and resculpting of cornea with excimer laser to correct refractive error. It

- May be: *Laser subepithelial keratomileusis* (**LASEK**)–a surface procedure.
- *Laser-assisted in situ keratomileusis* (**LASIK**)–an intrastromal procedure.

Corneal Surface Procedures

Epikeratophakia

It involves removal of epithelium from central cornea, whereby donor corneal tissue is attached to the host cornea. This procedure has been abandoned largely due to the potential loss of best-corrected visual acuity.

Photorefractive Keratectomy (PRK)

PRK was the first type of laser eye surgery for vision correction and is the predecessor to the LASIK procedure. PRK corrects high degree of myopia (– 1.5 to – 8.0D), low to moderate hypermetropia and astigmatism. Pain is the most compelling drawback of PRK. PRK is done with an excimer laser to reshape the cornea without creating a flap in the cornea.

Steps

- Removal of corneal epithelium with excimer laser or alcohol (18% ethanol).
- Excimer laser (193 nm ultraviolet laser) ablation of superficial layer of cornea. (*Myopia* is treated by ablating the central cornea, so that it becomes flatter. *Hypermetropia* is treated by ablation of the midperiphery of cornea and the center of cornea is left untreated. Therefore, the center becomes steeper. For *astigmatism*, the excimer laser can be used to flatten or differentially steepen the corneal meridians and hence treat the astigmatism).

PRK corrects high degree of myopia (– 1.5 to – 8.0D), low to moderate hypermetropia and astigmatism.

> **Excimer laser:** LASER stands for light amplification by stimulated emission of radiations. Excimer laser is an ultraviolet laser which uses 193 nm wavelength. The 193 nm wavelength is totally absorbed by the cornea, causing the breakage of molecular bonds and making it uniquely applicable for corneal treatment. Hence, an excimer laser can be used to ablate the corneal tissue. **Gas media used in excimer laser is ArF.**

Complications

Delayed visual recovery, faint corneal haze, glare, infectious keratitis, and corneal scar formation are some of the complications seen after PRK.

Laser Subepithelial Keratomileusis (LASEK)

LASEK is indicated in patients having thin cornea and low myopia.

Steps

- *Creation of epithelial flap with 18% ethanol or a microkeratome*: In LASEK, dilute alcohol (18% ethanol) is applied, loosened epithelium is peeled as a single sheet and a hinged epithelial flap is created, while in LASIK, a 120 to 150 μm flap of cornea (epithelium and stroma), leaving an attachment on one side, is cut with a microkeratome (an automated sharp blade), that is, *lamellar dissection of cornea* is done.
- *Laser ablation*: The hinged flap (attached on one side) is lifted up and the *stromal bed is ablated with an* excimer laser.
- *Repositioning of epithelium: Flap* with its intact epithelium *is reposited* onto the stromal bed without sutures. As the flap drapes over the modified stromal surface, the refractive power of anterior corneal surface is modified.

Advantages

- LASEK offers the advantage of avoiding flap complications of LASIK.

clarithromycin, oral clarithromycin and topical amikacin, while the fungal keratitis is treated with natamycin and amphotericin B.

Keratophakia (Kerato = Corneal; Phakia = Lens)

It is a technique by which a corneal lens is inserted to change the shape of cornea and modify its refractive power. Lamellar keratectomy of donor cornea is done and stromal lens is created. The lamellar dissection (lamellar keratectomy) of recipient's cornea is performed with microkeratome and stromal lens from donor cornea is placed intrastromally in the recipient.

Lamellar Keratotomy

Deep keratectomy is performed with microkeratome to elevate a corneal flap and replaced without additional surgery. Stromal bed subsequently develops ectasia under flap. It works for low hyperopia.

Peripheral Corneal Procedures

Intracorneal Rings (ICR)

Intracorneal rings are placed in peripheral cornea (**Fig. 26.16**). The main advantage of ICR is that it is a reversible process. Its main drawback is limited range of correction. Myopia is corrected up to –3D and hyperopia is corrected up to + 2D.

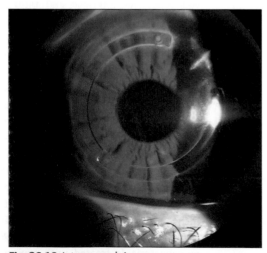

Fig. 26.16 Intracorneal rings.

Steps

Peripheral circular lamellar dissection is done. Two PMMA rings segments of predetermined diameter and thickness are inserted. The midperipheral anterior lamellae are lifted focally by ring segments with compensatory flattening of central cornea. It results in the decrease in refractive power of cornea (**Fig. 26.17**).

Complications

Complications are rare as ICR implantation is a reversible procedure, no corneal tissue is removed, and the central optical zone is not invaded.

Radial Keratotomy (RK)

In radial keratotomy (RK), deep and radial incisions (80% depth) are made with a diamond knife in peripheral cornea, sparing the central optical zone (3–4 mm), and incisions are allowed to heal spontaneously. It weakens paracentral and peripheral cornea, resulting in ectasia with compensatory flattening of central cornea. Thus, refractive power is reduced. Range of myopia corrected is 1 to 6D (**Fig. 26.18**).

Complications

Common complications include perforation, infection, glare, irregular astigmatism and chances of globe rupture following trauma. Stability of refraction after RK is lower than with many other refractive surgical procedures. RK has been largely replaced by excimer laser procedures.

Astigmatism Keratotomy

It is performed to correct astigmatism. The transverse midperipheral incisions (*transverse keratotomy*) or arcuate midperipheral incisions (*arcuate keratotomy*) are made perpendicular to the steep meridian of astigmatism. It results in localized ectasia of peripheral cornea and central flattening of incised meridian. Thus, astigmatism is reduced. It can be performed for astigmatism only or along with RK for associated myopia.

Closer the incision to the center of cornea, the greater is the correction of astigmatism.

Astigmatism keratotomy does not, as a general rule, benefit patients who have hyperopic

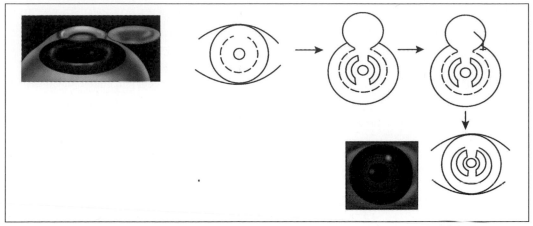

Fig. 26.17 Steps of intra corneal ring (ICR) procedure.

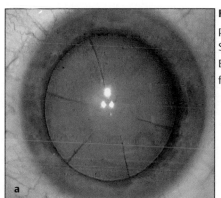

Fig. 26.18 (a) Partial thickness incisions result in ectasia of paracentral cornea. Source: Background. In: Dick B, Gerste R, Schultz T, ed. Femtosecond Laser Surgery in Ophthalmology. 1st Edition. Thieme; 2008. **(b)** Radial keratotomy. **(c)** Compensatory flattening of central cornea.

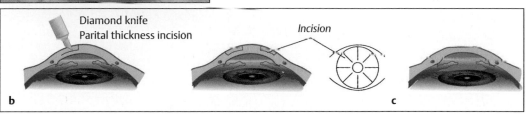

Diamond knife
Parital thickness incision

Incision

b

c

astigmatism in which it is associated with a further hyperopic shift. Therefore, this technique has been replaced by LASIK.

Laser Thermal Keratoplasty (LTK)

LTK is a procedure which involves using laser energy to heat the cornea and altering its curvature. It involves the use of **Holmium: YAG Laser–an infrared laser.** Elevation of the temperature of corneal collagen fibers results in the contraction and subsequent flattening of the area of heating (**Flowchart 26.2**).

For astigmatic corrections, peripheral heating is done along a flatter meridian, resulting in central steepening along the meridian of treatment.

Regression of refractive effects is the main problem. Corneal penetration depth of this laser

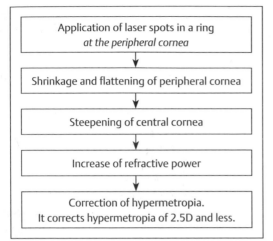

Flowchart 26.2 Mechanism of correction of hypermetropia through LTK. Abbreviation: LTK, laser thermal keratoplasty.

light is 480 to 530 μm. It is ideal for stromal heating with minimum damage to the adjacent tissue.

Conductive Keratoplasty (CK)

It is a **nonlaser procedure** (i.e., nonablative and nonincisional procedure). CK steepens the cornea using high-radio frequency currents.

In CK, the low-energy, high-frequency current is applied through a keratoplasty tip inserted into the peripheral corneal stroma in a circular fashion. It results in shrinkage of peripheral collagen fibers and flattening of peripheral cornea. The steepening of central cornea corrects hypermetropia up to + 3D. To correct astigmatism, extra spots are added to the flat meridian. Its major advantage is greater stability of refractive effect.

Phakic Implantable Contact Lenses (Phakic ICLs)

In this technique, a lens is inserted in the anterior or posterior chamber, anterior to the natural crystalline lens, which is called **phakic ICL.**

Mild-to-moderate refractive errors are treated surgically by PRK and LASIK, but for high-refractive errors, these options are limited, and phakic ICLs are used to correct refractive error. The lens is composed of collagen copolymer. Its refractive index is 1.45 at 35°C.

Criteria for phakic ICL implantation
- Endothelial cell count should be normal (at least 2500 cells/mm²).
- Anterior chamber depth must be adequate (≥3 mm).

Contraindications
- Inflammation of anterior or posterior segment.
- Iris atrophy.
- Aniridia.
- Cataract.
- Glaucoma.

Posterior surface of phakic ICL for posterior chamber is concave to vault over the anterior capsule.

With posterior chamber phakic ICL, laser iridotomies are performed before surgery to reduce the incidence of postoperative pupillary block.

Complications of phakic ICLs
- Elevated IOP.
- Uveitis.
- Cataract.
- Endothelial cell damage.
- Corneal edema.
- Endophthalmitis.

Extraction of Clear Lens

It corrects myopia of about −21D but carries a small risk of RD.

■ Cataract Surgery (OP7.4)

Cataract extraction may be intracapsular or extracapsular (**Table 26.7**). Intracapsular cataract extraction (**ICCE**) is now becoming obsolete. Different methods of extracapsular cataract extraction (**ECCE**) are as follows:
- Conventional ECCE.
- Small incision cataract surgery (SICS).
- Phacoemulsification.

Table 26.7 Differentiating features of ECCE and ICCE

	ECCE	ICCE
Advantages of ECCE over ICCE		
1. Age	Can be performed at all ages	Cannot be performed below 40 years of age
2. Incision	Medium 7-8 mm	Large 10-12 mm
3. Posterior chamber IOL implantation	Can be done	Can't be done
4. Post-operative astigmatism	Relatively low	High
5. Complication rate	Low	High
Disadvantages of ECCE over ICCE		
6. Posterior capsular opacification (PCO)	PCO is main drawback of ECCE as posterior capsule is left behind	No post operative PCO as intact lens is removed
7. Need of operating microscope	Needs operating microscope	Not required
8. Learning curve	Relatively longer	Small
9. Time consumption during surgery	Relatively more time consuming	Quick and less time consuming

Nowadays, phacoemulsification is the most popular and preferred method.

■ Intracapsular Cataract Extraction (ICCE)

ICCE involves removal of entire lens with intact capsule by rupturing the zonules. It is now becoming obsolete because of the high-rate of complications. ICCE is indicated only in:

- Lens dislocation.
- Zonular dialysis affecting >180 degree.

In young patients, zonules are strong, so ICCE cannot be employed.

Extraction of Lens

Lens delivery can be done by:

Forceps delivery: It is done with special lens forceps (Arruga's capsule holding forceps).

Cryoextraction: In this method, a cryoprobe is applied to freeze and hold the lens at −35° C.

Indian Smith method: In this method, the lens is tumbled out by applying pressure at 6 o'clock and counter pressure at 12 o'clock positions. With this method, the lower pole is delivered first. In patients between 40 to 45 years of age, zonules are relatively strong, so zonules are dissolved by the use of chymotrypsin (*a proteolytic enzyme*) to extract the lens by one of the above methods.

Advantages of ICCE

- No posterior opacification as capsule is removed.
- Learning curve is small.
- Simple and quick.
- Does not need operating microscope.

Disadvantages of ICCE

- Large incision is needed.
- Cannot be performed before 40 years of age.
- Postoperative astigmatism is high because of large incision.
- Wound healing is delayed.
- High-rate of complications, particularly vitreous loss, RD and cystoid macular edema (CME).
- Posterior chamber IOL cannot be implanted.

■ Extracapsular Cataract Extraction (ECCE)

It has replaced ICCE and involves removal of a major portion of anterior capsule, nucleus and cortical substance.

In ECCE, the *capsular bag (peripheral part of anterior capsule and entire posterior capsule)* is left in the eye and held in position by zonules. Surgical removal of crystalline lens results in loss of refracting power (*approx. 20D*) and aphakic eye becomes grossly hypermetropic. Modern cataract surgery, therefore, involves implantation of an IOL. Currently, ECCE with IOL implantation is the most preferred surgery.

Techniques of ECCE

There are three techniques of ECCE, namely, conventional ECCE, SICS and phacoemulsification.

Conventional ECCE

The pupils must be dilated preoperatively. Surgical steps include:

1. *Anesthesia* by a mixture used for infiltration anesthesia.
2. *Lid retraction* by speculum or sutures.
3. *Superior rectus suture* is passed to fix the eye in downward gaze.
4. *Fornix-based conjunctival flap* is prepared.
5. *Wet field cautery* for hemostasis, as fashioning of conjunctival flap causes bleeding.
6. *Limbal incision:* 7 to 8 mm partial thickness incision is made, and 2 to 3 sutures are placed at the limbus after making the groove. Now, the anterior chamber with 3.2 mm keratome is opened. These steps are similar to that of ICCE.
7. Viscoelastic substance is injected into the anterior chamber to reform it and protect the endothelium. If the pupil is small during surgery, use high-molecular weight *cohesive viscoelastics.* It pushes the iris away from the lens and *induces mydriasis.* If small posterior capsular tear occurs during surgery, use dispersive viscoelastics. It will push the vitreous back into the posterior chamber and *plug the capsular defect.*
8. *Anterior capsulotomy* is performed with a bent 26 gauge disposable needle. *Trypan blue dye* can be used to stain the lens capsule for better visibility.
9. *Removal of anterior capsule* with McPherson forceps.
10. *Completion of limbal incision* from 10 to 2 o'clock position.

> **Techniques of anterior capsulotomy**
> - **"Can opener" capsulotomy:** In it multiple, close, pinpoint perforations are made in a circular tract in the anterior capsule, and centripetal traction on the central piece of capsule creates a tear along perforations.
> - **Linear capsulotomy (envelope technique):** A linear or curvilinear incision is made in ⅓rd of the anterior capsule, followed by removal of nucleus with cortical matter, and IOL is inserted into the capsular bag. Now, the rest of capsulotomy is performed by a continuous curvilinear capsulorrhexis to make the central circular opening. Thus, in this technique anterior capsule protects the corneal endothelium during the removal of cortical matter.
> - **Continuous curvilinear capsulotomy (capsulorrhexis):** It is the most commonly performed technique for anterior capsule removal. Initial capsulotomy is done by making a nick with a bent 26 gauge needle in the center, and the flap is torn off in a continuous curvilinear fashion by needle or capsulorrhexis forceps. Thus, a round opening is achieved in the anterior capsule (**Fig. 26.19**).

11. *Hydrodissection* with BSS, which is injected in difficult quadrants under the edge of the anterior capsule to separate the cortex from capsule.
12. *Removal of nucleus:* Scleral lip of incision is depressed (posterior Lip) and counter pressure is exerted at the 6 o'clock position with lens expressor.
13. *Cortical aspiration* is done by two-way irrigation aspiration cannula.
14. *IOL implantation*: Capsular bag is inflated with viscoelastic substance and IOL is inserted into the capsular bag (posterior chamber IOL).
15. *Incision is sutured* with 10–0 monofilament nylon suture.
16. *Aspiration of residual viscoelastic substance.*
17. *Anterior chamber is filled with BSS.*
18. *Reposition of conjunctival flap.*
19. *Subconjunctival injection (1 mL)* of *dexamethasone 0.5 mg in 0.5 mL + gentamicin 10 mg in 0.5 mL.*
20. *Patching of eye.*

Small Incision Cataract Surgery (SICS)

It is a *sutureless* ECCE. The steps of SICS are similar to conventional ECCE with some modifications in incision and nucleus delivery (**Table 26.8**).

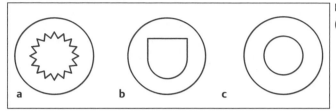

Fig. 26.19 (a) Can opener capsulotomy. **(b)** Linear capsulotomy. **(c)** Capsulorrhexis.

Table 26.8 Advantages of SICS over conventional ECCE		
	SICS	**Conventional ECCE**
1. **Incision**	Small	Medium
2. **Suture**	Sutureless	Sutures required
3. **Post-operative astigmatism**	Low	Relatively high
4. **Wound problems** such as • Wound leak • Iris prolapse • Shallowing of anterior chamber	Generally not encountered	May be present

1. *Incision*: A self-sealing sclerocorneal tunnel is dissected with (**Fig. 26.20**):
   - An external scleral incision (5.5–6.5 mm in length and 2 mm behind limbus). It may be *straight, frown-shaped* or *chevron in configuration* (**Fig. 26.21**).
   - A partial thickness scleral tunnel is made with a crescent knife. It extends 1 to 1.5 mm into the clear cornea.
   - An internal corneal incision made with sharp 3.2 mm-angled keratome. It is larger than the external scleral incision.
2. A *side port entry* is made to inject viscoelastics in the anterior chamber to aspirate cortex at 12 o'clock position (i.e., subincisional cortex) and deepen the anterior chamber at the end of surgery.
3. *Anterior capsulotomy*: Capsulorrhexis is preferred.
4. *Hydrodissection*: BSS is injected under the lens capsule to separate the cortex from the lens capsule. BSS is also injected at the junction of the central dense core of nucleus to separate the hard nucleus from

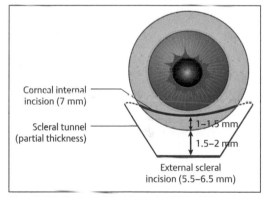

Corneal internal incision (7 mm)

Scleral tunnel (partial thickness)

1–1.5 mm

1.5–2 mm

External scleral incision (5.5–6.5 mm)

Fig. 26.20 Types of incisions in SICS. Abbreviation: SICS, small incision cataract surgery.

the relatively softer epinucleus. This is termed hydrodelineation.
5. *Nucleus* is prolapsed in the anterior chamber and delivered through the corneoscleral tunnel with an irrigating vectis or a small hook inserted between the postcapsule and nucleus (**Blumenthal technique**).
6. *Aspiration of epinucleus and residual cortex* with irrigation aspiration cannula (simcoe cannula) is done.

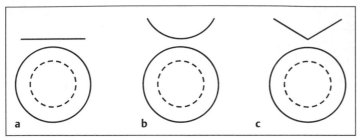

Fig. 26.21 External scleral incision type in SICS. **(a)** Straight. **(b)** Frown shaped. **(c)** Chevron in configuration. Abbreviation: SICS, small incision cataract surgery.

7. *IOL* is implanted.
8. *Viscoelastic is removed* and the *anterior chamber is formed* with BSS (**Fig. 26.22**).

Phacoemulsification (Phaco)

It is the most preferred method and has now replaced all other techniques. It is an *ECCE performed with* a machine, the phacoemulsifier. A phacoemulsifier breaks the nucleus into small pieces and even into fine emulsion of material (*i.e., emulsifies the nucleus*), which is removed by suction as the machine generates a vacuum for aspiration.

Steps

1. A *side port entry* is made for bimanual control and filling of anterior chamber with viscoelastic substance.
2. *Corneal incision* is made by using a keratome. It may be a clear corneal or limbal incision. Incision of 3 to 3.5 mm size is made superotemporally. *Temporal* incision is preferred *for topical* anesthesia.
3. *Viscoelastic* is injected into the anterior chamber.
4. *Capsulorrhexis* or continuous curvilinear capsulotomy (CCC) of 5 to 6 mm is performed with a bent needle.
5. *Hydrodissection* is performed to separate the nucleus and cortex from the capsule. BSS is injected beneath the edge of capsulorrhexis at three to four places. BSS is also injected into the substance of the nucleus to separate the hard nucleus from the relatively softer epinucleus,

which is termed **hydrodelineation**. Thus, the nucleus can be more easily and safely rotated (**Fig. 26.23**).

6. *Nucleus removal*: Phaco probe is inserted to aspirate the superficial cortex and epinucleus. To remove the nucleus through a small circular capsulorrhexis, it is necessary to crack the nucleus within the capsule bag. The nucleus is removed by emulsifying with the phaco machine (*nuclear emulsification*). Common techniques used for nuclear emulsification are as follows:

- Divide and conquer technique (4-quadrant technique): It utilizes sculpting and grooving with ultrasound energy *prior to cracking* the nucleus. It is well-suited for trainee surgeons. A linear groove is sculpted in the nucleus and rotated to. The second groove is made at a right angle to the first. The nucleus is divided into four quadrants by engaging the probe and secondary instrument (chopper) in opposite walls of the groove. Each of the four quadrants is emulsified and aspirated in turn (**Fig. 26.24**).
- Nuclear chop technique: This technique relies instead on high-vacuum and mechanical force for disassembly. It takes greater experience but has an advantage of requiring much less expenditure of energy. A chopper is placed beneath the capsulorrhexis and used to stabilize the nucleus by

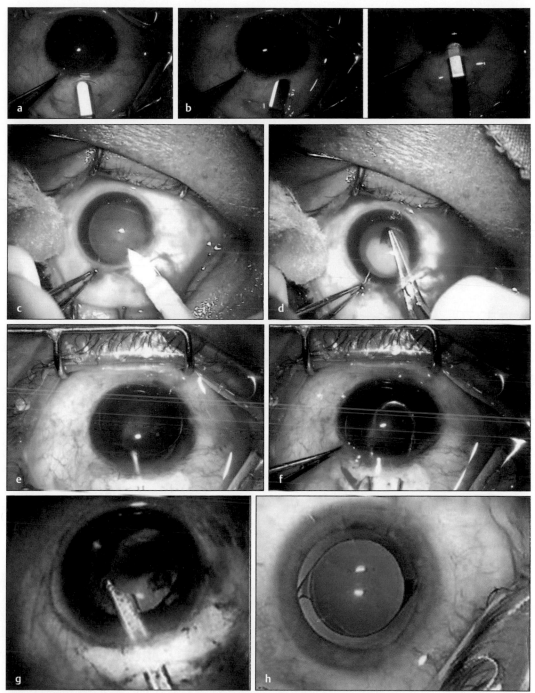

Fig. 26.22 Steps of SICS. **(a)** Scleral incision. **(b)** Formation of tunnel. **(c)** Entry into anterior chamber. **(d)** Capsulorrhexis. **(e)** Prolapse of nucleus into AC. **(f)** Extraction of nucleus. **(g)** Cortical irrigation and aspiration. **(h)** IOL in the bag. Abbreviation: AC, anterior chamber; IOL, intraocular lens; SICS, small incision cataract surgery.

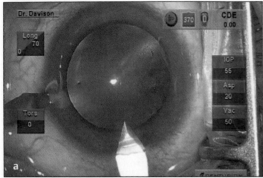

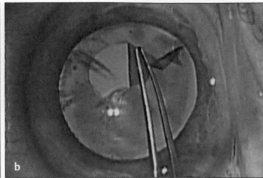

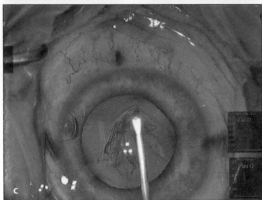

Fig. 26.23 Steps of phacoemulsification. **(a)** Corneal incision. Source: Divide-and-Conquer Technique. In: Fishkind W, ed. Phacoemulsification and Intraocular Lens Implantation: Matering Techniques and Complications in Cataract Surgery. 2nd Edition. Thieme; 2017. **(b)** Capsulorrhexis. Source: Phacoemulsification Cataract Extraction. In: Francis B, Sarkisian, Jr. S, Tan J, ed. Minimally Invasive Glaucoma Surgery: A Practical Guide. 1st Edition. Thieme; 2016. **(c)** Hydrodissection. Source: Fishkind W, ed. Phacoemulsification and Intraocular Lens Implantation: Matering Techniques and Complications in Cataract Surgery. 2nd Edition. Thieme; 2017.

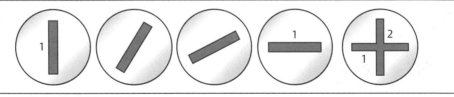

Fig. 26.24 Divide and conquer technique.

lifting and slightly pulling toward the incision. The nucleus is grooved with a phaco probe and the chop instrument is brought to the side of probe to crack the nucleus by pulling them apart. The nucleus is divided into two heminuclei and is rotated. The nucleus is again stabilized with chop instrument and the heminuclei is subdivided into small pieces (pie-shaped segment). The pie-shaped segment is emulsified and aspirated. The nucleus is continually rotated, so that pie-shaped segments can be scored, chopped and removed.

After evacuation of first heminucleus, second heminucleus is chopped, emulsified and aspirated in the same manner (**Fig. 26.25**).

Other techniques described are chip and flip technique and chop and flip technique.

Initial chop nucleus is cracked. Commencing of completion of pie-shaped segment into two heminuclei. Second chop is adherent to phaco and pulling them apart at the tip for mobilization.

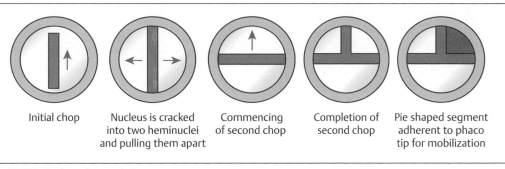

| Initial chop | Nucleus is cracked into two heminuclei and pulling them apart | Commencing of second chop | Completion of second chop | Pie shaped segment adherent to phaco tip for mobilization |

Fig. 26.25 Nuclear chop technique.

Table 26.9 Advantages of SICS over Phaco

		SICS	Phacoemulsification
1.	Surgery on dense cataract	Can be performed on grade V	Difficult to perform on hard cataracts because of the risk of corneal complications.
2.	Instrumentation	Inexpensive	Requires phacoemulsifier. So expensive.
3.	Learning curve	Small	Considerable training is required.
4.	Complications	Low rate of complications	Complication like nucleus drop (into vitreous) during surgery is potentially serious.

Table 26.10 Advantages of phaco over SICS

		SICS	Phacoemulsification
1.	Anesthesia	Required	Can be done under surface (Topical) anaesthesia
2.	Incision	6-7 mm	Small (3.2 mm)
3.	Postoperative congestion	Persists for few days at the site of incision	Minimal
4.	Postoperative astigmatism	More because of larger incision	Minimal because of small incision
5.	Postcapsular opacification (PCO)	High incidence because round edge PMMA IOLs are used in SICS and is a major disadvantage	Relativity low incidence
6.	Visual rehabilitation	Takes more time than phaco	Quicker

7. *Cortical cleaning* is done with irrigation aspiration cannula.

8. *IOL implantation*: The capsular bag is filled with viscoelastic, and posterior chamber IOL (PC IOL) is implanted into the capsular bag.

9. Viscoelastic is aspirated and the side port incision is sealed with saline. It is a sutureless surgery.

Tables 26.9 and 26.10 highlight the advantages of SICS over phacoemulsification and vice versa.

■ Postoperative Management in Cataract Surgery

Following surgery, the patient is *reviewed* the next day and then subsequently after 1 week, depending on surgeon's assessment of his or her progress.

Postoperative Medication

Steroid antibiotic eye drops are instilled (one drop four times daily) for 6 to 8 weeks in ECCE or SICS and for 3–4 weeks in phacoemulsification.

Mydriatic cycloplegic eye drops for 1 to 2 weeks.

Eye drops to reduce IOP for 1 to 2 weeks.

Refraction and prescription of glasses with ECCE after 6 to 8 weeks and with phaco after 3 to 4 weeks.

Instructions

Give general instructions to the patient about restriction of physical activity.

■ Complications of Cataract Surgery (OP7.4)

- Complications may be: Due to local anesthesia.
- Intraoperative (during surgery).
- Postoperative (**Fig. 26.26**).

Complications due to Local Anesthesia (LA)

- Retrobulbar hemorrhage (RBH) follows retrobulbar block. Eye becomes proptosed. It takes approximately 2 weeks to resolve. Postponement of operation is advised.
- Ocular cardiac reflex manifests as bradycardia. I.V. atropine is helpful.
- Perforation of globe.

Intraoperative Complications

- *Detachment of Descemet's membrane* results in persistent corneal edema and decreased visual acuity. To reattach Descemet's membrane postoperatively, an incision is made and air or an expansive gas (e.g. HF_6) is injected into the anterior chamber after drainage of 50% aqueous.
- *Damage to corneal endothelium: To protect corneal endothelium* during surgery, use viscoelastics.
- *Posterior capsular rupture (PCR)* may result in vitreous loss and nucleus drop in vitreous. PCR may occur before nucleus removal during irrigation–aspiration of cortical matter, or during IOL insertion. Vitreous loss almost always accompanies PCR which occurs before nucleus removal. *Early signs of PCR* are:
  - ◊ Sudden deepening of anterior chamber.
  - ◊ Decentration of nucleus.
  - ◊ Loss of efficiency of aspiration which suggests occlusion of tip with vitreous.

Management of PCR depends on the magnitude of tear and the presence or absence of vitreous prolapse.

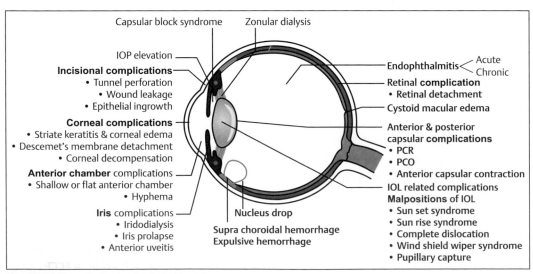

Fig. 26.26 Complications of cataract surgery.

- *Nucleus drop into vitreous* can be avoided by recognizing early signs of PCR. *It is the most potential sight-threatening complication of cataract surgery.* Once nucleus has dropped into vitreous, refer to a vitreoretinal surgeon.
- *Suprachoroidal hemorrhage:* It is the bleeding into the suprachoroidal space from a ruptured long or short postciliary artery. *Risk factors for suprachoroidal hemorrhage* are:
  ◊ Glaucoma.
  ◊ Hypertension.
  ◊ Vitreous loss, resulting in sudden hypotony.

It may result in the expulsion of intraocular contents through a wound (**expulsive hemorrhage**).

Self-sealing incisions resist expulsion of intraocular contents. So, expulsive hemorrhage is much less likely with phacoemulsification. Clinical signs for this are shallowing of anterior chamber, increased IOP resulting in iris prolapse or vitreous prolapse, and loss of red reflex.

- Trauma to iris: Tear of iris from root leads to iridodialysis.
- Zonular dialysis due to undue pressure on zonules (tearing of zonules), resulting in *subluxation of lens.*

Postoperative Complications

Early postoperative complications:
- Striate keratitis and corneal edema.
- Iris prolapse.
- Flat or shallow anterior chamber.
- Hyphema.
- Secondary glaucoma.
- Acute endophthalmitis (**early onset**).
- Anterior uveitis.

Late postoperative complications:
- **CME.**
- Posterior capsule opacification (**PCO**).
- Anterior capsule contraction (**phimosis**).
- Corneal endothelial decompensation.
- RD.

- Delayed onset endophthalmitis.
- Pupillary capture.
- Epithelial ingrowth.
- Malpositions of IOL:
  ◊ Sun set syndrome.
  ◊ Sun rise syndrome.
  ◊ Complete dislocation of IOL.
  ◊ Windshield wiper syndrome.

Early Postoperative Complications

Striate keratitis and corneal edema: It is characterized by Descemet's membrane folds with corneal edema and caused by Intraoperative trauma to corneal endothelium.
- Preexisting endothelial disease (e.g., Fuchs endothelial dystrophy) or cell loss.
- Raised IOP.
- Prolonged surgery.

To minimize the risk of corneal injury, the use of appropriate viscoelastic is advised.

During sleep, in patients with marginal corneal endothelial function, overnight hypoxia results in corneal edema, and the patient may complain of poorer vision in the morning.

Management: IOP should be controlled below 20 mm Hg. For symptomatic relief, Hypertonic saline drops (**5%**) and ointment may be used along with topical steroids.

Iris prolapse: It may be caused by inadequate suturing after ICCE and conventional ECCE. The incidence of iris prolapse is grossly reduced in SICS and phacoemulsification due to self-sealing incisions.

Management: If prolapse occurs within 24 hours, iris is reposited back and wound sutured. Prolapse of long duration needs excision of iris and wound suturing.

Flat or shallow anterior chamber: It is caused by wound leak, ciliochoroidal detachment due to choroidal effusion or suprachoroidal hemorrhage, and pupil block due to vitreous in ICCE.

If it is due to wound leak, and it is managed by pressure patching of eye and suturing of wound if leak persists after 5 to 7 days.

If it is due to ciliochoroidal detachment, management includes the following:

- Topical and systemic steroids are given to reduce intraocular inflammation.
- Ultrasonography is done to assess the severity.
- If condition persists, posterior sclerotomy is done for suprachoroidal drainage with injection of air in the anterior chamber.

If it is due to pupillary block, lower the IOP with hyperosmotic agents. If not relieved, peripheral iridectomy is done to bypass the pupillary block.

Hyphema (collection of blood in anterior chamber): It occurs due to leakage from vessels in the wound or the iris. To minimize the risk of bleeding, discontinue anticoagulant therapy before surgery if it does not pose a significant medical risk to patient.

If hyphema is large and associated with raised IOP, it must be lowered by oral acetazolamide, otherwise blood staining of cornea may develop.

If blood does not get absorbed, paracentesis should be done to drain the blood.

Topical steroids, oral serratio peptidase, and mydriatic eye drops help in absorption of blood.

Secondary glaucoma: Acute IOP elevation postoperatively may be due to retention of viscoelastic substances, obstruction of trabecular meshwork with inflammatory debris, pupillary block, or preexisting glaucoma.

Chronic IOP elevation can be caused by corticosteroid use, chronic inflammation and peripheral anterior synechiae (PAS) formation.

Management: For appropriate therapy, correct diagnosis of underlying cause is required.

Early onset postoperative endophthalmitis (acute form): It develops generally within 2 to 5 days of surgery. A major percentage (90%) of the infection is due to Gram +ve and in 10% of cases due to Gram −ve pathogens.

Common gram + ve causative organisms (in order of frequency) are Coagulase −ve staphylococci (S epidermidis), Staphylococcus aureus and Streptococcus species.

Gram −ve organisms are pseudomonas and proteus.

Source of infection: Flora of eyelids and conjunctiva, contaminated solutions and instruments, and air in operation theatre.

Clinical features:
- Ciliary congestion.
- Decreased visual acuity.
- Conjunctival chemosis.
- Ocular pain.
- Hypopyon.

Management includes the following:
- Culture of aqueous and vitreous aspirates.
- Antibiotics are given which may be intravitreal, subconjunctival, topical, or systemic.
- Steroids: To limit the destructive complications of inflammatory process, steroids are administered through systemic route and subconjunctival injections.
- Pars plana vitrectomy (PPV).

Postoperative anterior uveitis: It is caused by:
- Undue mechanical trauma to uveal tissue during surgery.
- Residual cortical lens matter.
- Viscoelastics etc.

It is managed by topical mydriatic and steroids. If fibrinous reaction occurs, systemic steroids may be required.

Late Postoperative Complications

CME: It is the accumulation of fluid in the outer plexiform layer (Henle's layer) of macula. CME after cataract surgery (**Irvin–Gass syndrome**) is the most common complication. *On ophthalmoscopy,* multiple cystoid spaces are seen in the macular area (honeycomb appearance). *Fluorescein angiography* shows typical "flower petal" pattern due to leakage of dye from perifoveal capillaries.

Predisposing factors: Incidence of CME is highest with ICCE and lowest with ECCE and intact posterior capsule. It occurs more often after–

- Neodymium: Yttrium–aluminium–garnet laser (Nd: YAG laser capsulotomy).
- Intraoperative vitreous loss following PCR.
- Vitreous traction due to incarceration in the incision.
- Diabetic retinopathy.
- History of CME in fellow eye.
- Pre-existing epiretinal membrane (ERM).

Treatment involves the correction of underlying causes. Most cases resolve spontaneously over the course of several weeks.

- In persistent cases, topical steroid drops and nonsteroidal (antiprostaglandin) drops are given.

If there is no improvement, posterior subtenon injection of a long-acting steroids such as *triamcinolone* can be given.

- If vitreous incarceration in incision occurs, disrupt the adhesions with Nd: YAG laser. Anterior vitrectomy may be useful.
- If CME is due to macular ERM–surgical excision of membrane may be beneficial.

PCO: It is also known as "after cataract" or **secondary cataract.** It is the most common late complication of ECCE.

After ECCE, the lens is composed of the peripheral part of anterior capsule, residual epithelial cells, and posterior capsule.

Residual lens epithelial cells still possess the capacity to proliferate, differentiate, and undergo fibrous metaplasia.

PCO *results from* the proliferation and migration of these cells toward the center of the previously acellular posterior capsule together with the synthesis of matrix.

Proliferative capacity of lens: Epithelial cells in children are more than in adults, so PCO after ECCE is extremely common in children than in adults.

Incidence of PCO:

- With PMMA and silicone lenses, incidence is more with acrylic IOLs.
- With round-edged IOLs, incidence is more with square-edged to optic of IOLs.

Morphological forms of PCO: PCO can occur as fibrosis, pearl type (**Elschnig's pearls**) or Soemmerring's ring.

Fibrosis type PCO is due to the fibrous metaplasia of epithelial cells (**Fig. 26.27a**).

Pearl type PCO: Pearls were observed by Elschnig and referred to as Elschnig's pearls.

Elschnig's pearls represent aberrant attempt of residual epithelial cells to form the lens fibers. The cells proliferate and instead of forming lens fibers, form mass of large and globular cells, giving the vacuolated appearance of posterior capsule. It is best visualized on retroillumination (**Fig. 26.27b**).

Soemmerring's ring is the proliferation of cells and synthesis of matrix within the space between the anterior and posterior capsule. It normally *does not encroach on the visual axis* and needs no treatment.

Treatment of PCO: Posterior capsulotomy–It is the creation of an opening in the posterior capsule with Nd: YAG laser.

Indications for capsulotomy:

- Diminished visual acuity.
- Impaired visualization of fundus for diagnostic or therapeutic purposes.

Complications of capsulotomy:

- IOP elevation.
- CME.
- Uveitis.
- RD (rare).

Anterior capsular contraction (**capsulophimosis**): Contraction of anterior capsular opening can occur after surgery and is accompanied by subcapsular fibrosis. Fibrous metaplasia of residual epithelial cells can cause opacification of anterior capsule and fibrosis. Anterior capsular

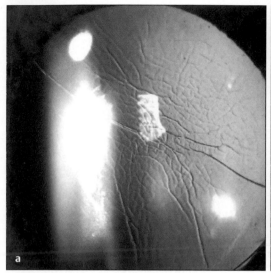 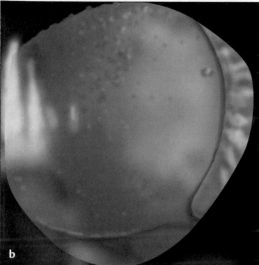

Fig. 26.27 (a) Fibrosis type PCO. Source: Introduction. In: Dick B, Gerste R, Schultz T, ed. Femtosecond Laser Surgery in Ophthalmology. 1st Edition. Thieme; 2018. **(b)** Elschnig's pearls. Abbreviation: PCO, posterior capsule opacification.

contraction is normally centripetal and causes capsulophimosis. It is more with capsulorrhexis than with "can opener" capsulotomy.

If severe, it may require Nd: YAG laser capsulotomy. It is a late complication of cataract surgery.

Corneal endothelial decompensation: It is a rare and late complication of cataract surgery.

Predisposing factors:
- Preexisting endothelial disease.
- Mechanical endothelial injury during surgery.
- Vitreous touch syndrome (contact of formed vitreous with endothelial cells following ICCE).

Endothelial cells decompensate by prolonged contact of vitreous, resulting in corneal edema and bullous keratopathy. If corneal edema is progressive, excision of vitreous in anterior chamber is done.

RD is uncommon following uneventful ECCE or phacoemulsification. It may be associated with the following risk factors:

Preoperative:
- Lattice degeneration.
- High myopia.
- History of RD in fellow eye.

Operative:
- Disruption of posterior capsule.
- Vitreous loss.
- *Postoperative*: If laser capsulotomy is performed within first year following cataract surgery it may predispose to RD.

Delayed onset endophthalmitis: A chronic form of endophthalmitis is diagnosed several weeks or longer after surgery and caused by organisms of low virulence such as Propionibacterium acnes and Staphylococcus epidermidis. The offending **microorganisms** become trapped in residual lenticular tissue in the capsular bag. It presents with decreased visual acuity and chronic uveitis with or without hypopyon.

Malposition in IOL: *Common causes* of malposition of IOL include zonulodialysis, posterior capsular rupture (PCR) and asymmetric loop placement (one haptic of IOL is inserted into the capsular bag and the other into the ciliary sulcus).

The different malpositions of IOL are as follows (**Fig. 26.28**):

- **Inferior subluxation of IOL** (sunset syndrome): It occurs when a sulcus fixated PC IOL decenters through a peripheral break in zonules.
- **Superior subluxation of IOL** (sunrise syndrome).
- **Complete dislocation of IOL:** It may be into pupil/anterior camber (anterior dislocation) or into vitreous (posterior dislocation).
- **Wind shield wiper syndrome:** When small IOL is placed in the sulcus, the upper haptic (loop) of IOL moves to the left and right, with movements of the eye like a wiper on wind shield, that is, pseudophacodonesis (pseudo =false; phaco = lens; donesis = tremulousness).
- **Pupillary capture:** In pupillary capture, some portion of the iris lies posterior to the IOL optic. It can produce acute and chronic iritis and posterior synechiae formation.

Capsular block syndrome: If viscoelastic substance is not removed from the bag at the end of surgery, viscoelastic is entrapped in the capsular bag because of the apposition of the anterior rim of capsulorrhexis with the anterior face of IOL. It is called *capsular block syndrome* and more common with acrylic IOLs because of their slightly "stickier" surface (**Flowchart 26.3**).

Prevention: It is prevented by the meticulous removal of viscoelastics from the bag at the end of surgery.

Treatment: Nd: YAG laser puncture of anterior capsule, peripheral to the edge of capsulorrhexis, results in escape of viscoelastics into the anterior chamber.

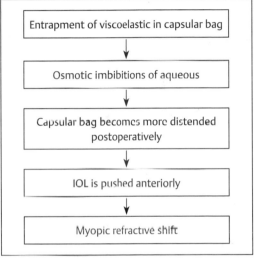

Entrapment of viscoelastic in capsular bag

↓

Osmotic imbibitions of aqueous

↓

Capsular bag becomes more distended postoperatively

↓

IOL is pushed anteriorly

↓

Myopic refractive shift

Flowchart 26.3 Mechanism of development of capsular block syndrome

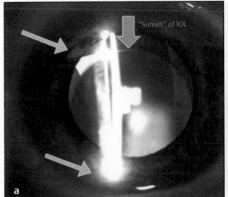

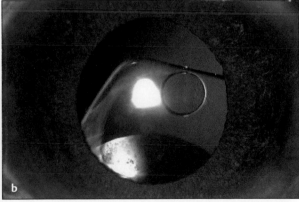

Fig. 26.28 (a) Sun set syndrome. Source: Introduction. In: Randleman J, Ahmed I, ed. Intraocular lens surgery: selection, complications, and complex cases. 1st edition. Thieme; 2016. **(b)** Decentration of PC IOL. Source: Malpositioned intraocular lens. In: Narang P, Trattler W, ed. Optimizing suboptimal results following cataract surgery. 1st edition. Thieme; 2018. Abbreviations: IOL, intraocular lens; PC, posterior chamber.

Epithelial ingrowth: It is common after ICCE and extremely rare after phacoemulsification. The surface epithelium invades intraocular structures such as cornea, anterior chamber angle, iris, ciliary body. It can cause corneal decompensation, chronic anterior uveitis or secondary angle closure glaucoma.

> **"UGH" syndrome** (**U**veitis **G**laucoma **H**yphema): So, UGH syndrome refers to the concurrent occurrence of uveitis, glaucoma and hyphema. It is more common with anterior chamber IOLs. Now, it is relatively rare as anterior chamber IOLs are not used now.

■ Aphakia

Refer to chapter 10 for details on "aphakia."

■ Surgical Treatment of Glaucoma (OP 6.7)

The aim of glaucoma therapy is to preserve visual function and includes:

- Medical treatment (Refer to Chapter 11 on glaucoma).
- Laser treatment.
- Filtering surgery.

■ Laser Treatment

Laser treatment in glaucoma includes:

- Laser trabeculoplasty, which includes the following:
  ◊ Selective laser trabeculoplasty (SLT): The laser energy is applied to the drainage tissue in the eye which starts a chemical and biological change in the tissue which results in better drainage of fluid through the drainage system. It is called selective because the laser used has minimal heat energy absorption, which is only taken up by selective pigmented tissue in the eye. Because of this, the procedure produces less scar tissue and has minimal pain. It is used for the treatment of primary open angle glaucoma (POAG).
  ◊ Argon laser trabeculoplasty (ALT): Another similar procedure is ALT. It uses a thermal laser and may cause more scarring in the drainage angle than SLT which may also limit its ability to be repeated. It is used for the treatment of POAG. The laser opens the fluid channels of the eye and the drainage system works better.

- Laser iridotomy: It is done for the treatment of narrow angle glaucoma. Narrow angle causes the iris to block fluid drainage, precipitating the narrow angle glaucoma. The laser iridotomy makes a small hole in the iris and allow the iris to fall back from the fluid channel. Thus, it helps the fluid drainage in narrow angle glaucoma.

- Laser iridoplasty: It uses the low-energy laser burns to the peripheral iris in order to widen the anterior chamber angle and/or break PAS.

- Cyclophotocoagulation: It is the most common procedure to perform cyclodestruction. The laser can be used to hamper the ciliary body's ability to make fluid, thus lowering IOP. This surgery is done for people who already have eye damage caused by glaucoma and help control glaucoma.

- Laser goniopunctures: Laser goniopuncture is an efficient IOP-lowering procedure after nonpenetrating deep sclerotomy (NPDS), when it is indicated. NPDS avoids full-thickness penetration into anterior chamber and minimizes the risk of complications commonly encountered with the standard trabeculectomy. In NPDS, removal of deep scleral flap leads to the formation of an empty scleral space where the aqueous humor gets collected before its drainage. Laser goniopuncture converts deep sclerotomy from being a nonpenetrating procedure to a penetrating one with fewer complications.

■ Trabeculectomy (Filtering Surgery)

Aim of Glaucoma Surgery

In some patients, despite the normalization of IOP, vision continues to decrease and visual field shows progressive loss. Therefore, glaucoma surgery is undertaken to reduce IOP to a level to halt the progression of the disease.

Procedures

Trabeculectomy is the surgical procedure most commonly performed for POAG. It is a glaucoma filtration surgery that establishes communication between the anterior chamber and subtenon space (by creating a fistula protected by a superficial scleral flap) and passing the obstructed trabecular meshwork. Thus, the aqueous is drained underneath the superficial scleral flap in subtenon space. It gives a well-protected bleb.

Indications

The indications for trabeculectomy are as follows:
- Failure of conservative therapy to reduce IOP to a target level.
- Progression of visual field defects and optic neuropathy despite adequate IOP control.
- Increased IOP which is unlikely to be controlled by medical therapy alone.
- Noncompliant patients.
- Poor follow-up of patient.

Surgical Steps of Procedure

- Topical and infiltration *anesthesia* is given.
- A *bridle suture* is inserted in the superior rectus muscle to expose superior limbus.
- A limbal or fornix-based *flap of conjunctiva and Tenon capsule* is fashioned, and the underlying sclera is exposed.
- The major vessels are cauterized.
- A rectangular (3 mm) or triangular *lamellar scleral flap* is created by making incision in approximately 50% of scleral thickness.
- The superficial *flap is dissected anteriorly* until the clear cornea is reached.
- *Paracentesis* is done for gradual lowering of pressure.
- Anterior chamber is entered and a *block of deep sclera containing the trabecular meshwork is excised* with Kelly's punch.
- *Peripheral iridectomy* is performed to prevent blockage of sclerotomy by iris.

- The superficial *scleral flap is reposited and sutured* at its posterior corners.
- Anterior chamber is deepened by injecting BSS, and patency of the fistula is tested.
- Conjunctival flap is sutured (two interrupted sutures at the limbus in a fornix-based flap or continuous sutures in a limbus-based flap).
- A subconjunctival injection of steroid and antibiotic is given under inferior conjunctiva and the eye is patched (**Fig. 26.29**).

Use of Antimetabolites

Antimetabolites inhibit the natural healing response but because of potential complications they are advocated for high risk patients with surgical failure. The anti-metabolite agents are 5-fluorouracil (5-FU) and Mitomycin C (MMC). Both agents inhibit fibroblast proliferation but 5-FU is less aggressive antimetabolite than MMC.

Complications

Complications of filtering surgery may be early or late. Early complications (Within 3 months of surgery) include shallow anterior chamber, hyphemia and uveitis. Late complications include bleb leakage, bleb failure, blebitis, cataract and bleb related endophthalmitis.

■ Vitreoretinal Surgery

■ Pars Plana Vitrectomy (PPV) (OP8.4)

It is the removal of vitreous through a small incision in the region of pars plana. It may be:
- **Anterior vitrectomy** (removal of anterior part of vitreous).
- **Core vitrectomy** (removal of central bulk of vitreous).
- **Total vitrectomy** (removal of whole vitreous).

PPV could be therapeutic or diagnostic. Therapeutic is done for the removal of pus, blood and pathogenic microorganisms, while diagnostic is done for obtaining samples for culture and sensitivity in endophthalmitis.

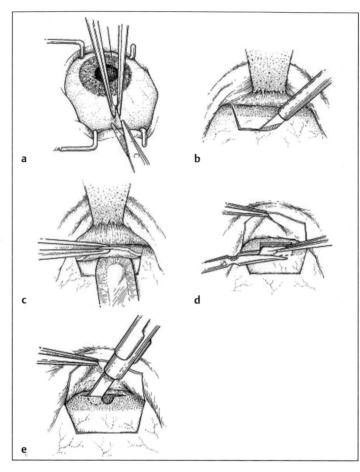

Fig. 26.29 Steps of trabeculectomy. **(a)** Fornix-based conjunctival flap. Source: Angle-Closure Glaucoma. In: Agarwal A, Jacob S, ed. Color Atlas of Ophthalmology. The Quick-Reference Manual for Diagnosis and Treatment. 2nd Edition. Thieme; 2009; **(b)** Dissection of scleral flap. **(c)** Trabeculectomy and peripheral iridectomy. **(d)** Reposition of scleral flap. **(e)** Suturing of scleral flap. Source: Filtration Surgery. In: Morrison J, Pollack I, ed. Glaucoma: Science and Practice. 1st Edition. Thieme; 2002.

Indications

It is commonly indicated for:
- Vitreous hemorrhage.
- Vitreoretinal traction.
- Tractional RD (a complication of diabetic retinopathy).
- Rhegmatogenous RD.
- Intraocular foreign bodies.
- ERM.
- Macular hole.
- Endophthalmitis.

■ Retinal Detachment (RD) Surgery

An acute symptomatic RD should be surgically repaired urgently. Presence of superior or large break, advanced syneresis as in myopia or fresh vitreous hemorrhage with an underlying RD is demonstrated by B-scan ultrasonography which requires urgent surgical intervention.

RD may be rhegmatogenous, tractional or exudative.

Preoperative Evaluation

Operations for RD can be performed only after accurate localization of retinal breaks. It can be performed by:
- Binocular indirect ophthalmoscopy with scleral indentation.
- Goldmann 3-mirror examination
- Ultrasonography (B-scan) is a two-dimensional imaging system which utilizes high-frequency sound waves ranging from 8 to 10 MHz. "**B**" stands for **bright** echoes.

These high frequencies produce shorter wavelengths which allow good resolution of minute ocular and orbital structures.

- Optical coherence tomography (OCT) to detect subretinal fluid (SRF).

> Ultrasound: Low frequency for orbital tissues; medium frequency (7–10 MHz) for retina, vitreous and optic nerve; and high frequency (30–50 MHz) for anterior chamber structures up to 5 mm.

Localization of Primary Retinal Break

The superotemporal (ST) quadrant is by far the most common site (60%) for retinal break followed by inferotemporal (IT, 15%), superonasal (SN, 15%) and inferonasal (IN, 10%) quadrants, that is,

$$ST > IT > SN > IN \text{ quadrants}$$

The location of primary retinal break can be predicted by the configuration of SRF and the shape of RD. SRF usually spreads in a gravitation fashion. If retinal break is located superiorly, SRF first spread inferiorly on the same side as the break and then spreads superiorly on the opposite side of the fundus. The anatomical barriers to the spread of SRF are optic disc and ora serrata.

- If the RD is bullous and inferior, the primary break usually lies above the horizontal meridian.
- When SRF crosses the vertical midline above, the primary break is near 12 o'clock.
- A primary break at 6 o'clock will cause an inferior RD with equal fluid levels.

Surgical Principles

The following principles need to be considered while performing surgery for RD:

- Scleral buckling with or without drainage.
- Sealing of all retinal breaks.
- Drainage of SRF.
- Intravitreal injection (air/BSS/ silicone oil).
- PPV (**Table 26.11**).

Scleral Buckling

It is a surgical procedure to create an inward indentation of the sclera ("buckle"). The material is sutured directly onto the sclera to create a buckle. This is done to close retinal breaks by apposing retinal pigment epithelium (RPE) to the sensory retina and release vitreoretinal traction. Its configuration may be radial (placed at right angle to the limbus) or circumferential placed circumferentially segmentally [segmental circumferential] or around the entire circumference of the globe to create a 360° buckle [encircling circumferential]). It is made of soft or hard silicone. The soft silicone sponge can be used for both radial and circumferential buckling, while the hard silicone straps are used only for 360° buckling (**Fig. 26.30**). The entire break should ideally be surrounded by approximately 2 mm of buckle. It is indicated in the following conditions:

- Large U-shaped tears particularly when "fish mouthing" is anticipated.
- Multiple breaks located in one or two quadrants.
- Anterior breaks.
- It is done when the breaks involve three or more quadrants.
- Extensive RD without detectable breaks.

Sealing of all Retinal Breaks

The break can be sealed by cryotherapy or laser photocoagulation. **Cryotherapy** induces chorioretinal inflammation around the edges of retinal break, and chorioretinal adhesions are formed in 2 to 6 weeks.

Laser photocoagulation requires close chorioretinal apposition and cannot be used in very peripheral retinal breaks.

Pneumatic retinopexy can be used in RD having a single retinal break. In this procedure, an intravitreal gas bubble is injected together with cryotherapy or laser to seal the retinal break and reattach the retina without scleral buckling. The patient is positioned so that the bubble tamponades the retinal break against the pigment epithelium.

Drainage of SRF

It is indicated in the following conditions:

- Difficulty in localization in retinal breaks.
- Immobile retina: If the detached retina is rendered relatively immobile by proliferative vitreoretinopathy (**PVR**), a

Table 26.11 Surgical steps for detachment surgery

Surgical step	Technique
Peritomy (incision of conjunctiva and Tenon's capsule)	• Conjunctiva and Tenon's capsule are picked up near the limbus (as both are fused at the limbus so both will be incised together); cut down to the sclera and undermine. Now these two layers are cut circumferentially with the limbus. The least extent of peritomy is about i.e. one quadrant and two rectus muscles must be included. Now relaxing incisions (6 mm) are made at right angle with the limbus.
Bridle sutures **Purpose** The purpose of bridle sutures is to stabilize the globe and to manipulate it during surgery.	• A squint hook is inserted under a rectus muscle and a silk suture is passed under (not through) the muscle tendon and the suture is secured. These steps are repeated for other tendons as required.
Localization of break **Purpose** The purpose of localization of break is to place the buckle in the correct position. Most breaks are located near the equator (13 mm behind the limbus).	• Sclera is inspected and vortex veins are detected to prevent damage during cryotherapy, scleral buckling or drainage of SRF. While viewing with the indirect ophthalmoscope, scleral indentation is done to achieve accurate localization of the break.
Cryotherapy **Purpose** It creates an inflammatory chorioretinal lesion around the edges of retinal break and chorioretinal adhesions are formed in 2-6 weeks.	• Sclera is indented with the tip of cryoprobe to bring the RPE as close as possible to the break and freezing is commenced until the sensory retina has just turned white. Cryotherapy is repeated until the entire break has been surrounded by a 2 mm margin. *The retinal break will appear dark due to the increased contrast between the frozen retina and underlying choroid.* The assistant should not irrigate the cornea during activation of the cryoprobe. Two heavy freezing is undesirable as it predisposes to post operative vitritis and exudative RD.
Scleral buckling **Purpose** It will close retinal breaks by apposing the RPE to the sensory retina and also will release vitreoretinal traction. **Complications** • Diplopia (due to mechanical effect of the buckle) • Cystoid macular oedema • Anterior segment ischaemia • Infection of buckle (Dip the sponge into antibiotic, gentamicin, to prevent post operative sponge infection). • Elevated IOP – Angle closure can occur. • 'Fish-mouthing' of a retinal tear- it refers to the tendency of a tear (typically large superior equatorial U-shaped tear in a bullous RD) to open widely following scleral buckling.	• Select the appropriate- sized sponge. • Dip the sponge into antibiotic (gentamicin) to prevent post operative sponge infection. • The material is sutured directly onto the sclera to create a buckle. • Check the position of the buckle in relation to the retinal break with the indirect ophthalmoscope. • Trim the edges of sponge so that they will not erode through the conjunctiva postoperatively. • The technique is essentially similar for both a strap (used for buckling) and a sponge. The one end of strap is grasped with curved forceps to feed it under the four recti and the two ends of strap are tightened.
Drainage of SRF Intraocular pressure must be not elevated as drainage of SRF when IOP is high may cause retinal incarceration. Do not drain immediately under the horizontal recti to avoid damage to long posterior ciliary arteries and nerves. **Complications** • Choroidal hamorrhage (due to damage to a large choroidal vessel). • Ocular hypotony. • Iatrogenic break. • Retinal incarceration into the sclerotomy. • Vitreous prolapse.	• Chose the sclerotomy site. • A 3 mm sclerotomy (radial incision) is performed down to the choroid and a mattress suture is passed across the lips of the sclerotomy. • Apply low intensity diathermy to the choroidal knuckle and perforate it with a 25- gauge needle. • Gradually tighten the sutures while the SRF is draining to prevent hypotony. • Knot the sclerotomy suture.

(Continued)

Table 26.11 *(Continued)* Surgical steps for detachment surgery

Surgical step	Technique
Intravitreal injection **Purpose** • To counter act ocular hypotony after SRF drainage. • To prevent 'fish-mouthing' of a U-shaped tear. *BSS must not be used to temponade a retinal tear because it will pass through the tear into the sub-retinal space.*	• Insert the needle 4mm behind the limbus to avoid the vitreous base. Inject the air / BSS. • Check the IOP by depressing the cornea with the squint hook. Excessive elevation of IOP may result in corneal oedema, loss of buckle height and anterior displacement of iris-lens diaphragm.

high buckle is required to seal the break which can be achieved only if the eye is first softened by draining the SRF.

- Long standing RD: Eyes with long-standing RD tend to have viscous SRF which takes a long time to absorb. Therefore, drainage is essential.
- Inferior tears: RD associated with inferior tears are better drained because any residual SRF gravitates inferiorly on assuming upright position postoperatively. It may reopen the tear.

Advantage of drainage is that it provides immediate contact between RPE and sensory retina with flattening of the fovea. If this contact is delayed for more than 5 days, a satisfactory adhesion will not develop around the retinal break because the "stickiness" of the RPE will have worn off.

Intravitreal Injection (Air/BSS/ Silicone Oil)

Intravitreal air injection: indications for intra-vitreal air injection are as follows:

- To prevent excessive hypotony following SRF drainage.
- "Fish mouthing" of a large retinal tear.
- Giant retinal tears.
- Posterior breaks.

Usually by the fifth postoperative day, the air will have completely absorbed. A mixture of 60% of air and 40% sulphurhexafluoride (SF_6) is used because the SF_6 component of the bubble takes up the nitrogen of the air and actually expands as the air is absorbed.

Intravitreal BSS injection: It does not impair the visualization of fundus as may occur with air bubbles. It must not be used in eyes with "fish mouthing" tears because it will pass through the tear into the subretinal space and increase the RD.

Intravitreal silicone oil injection: It is used only in eyes with very complicated RDs. It is a highly viscous substance which will push an immobile retina against the RPE. Unless removed, silicone oil remains permanent in the eye.

Pars Plana Vitrectomy (PPV)

Indication

It is indicated in tractional RD and giant tears to mobilize the detached retina by segmenting ERMs and transvitreal bands.

Surgical Techniques

Before making the incision, the careful examina-tion of fundus using scleral indentation is performed.

- The retinal mobility is assessed by moving the eye with a squint hook; the good retinal mobility (free and undulating movement of detached retina) signifies the absence of significant PVR.
- If retinal break is apposed to the RPE with ease on indenting the sclera, drainage of SRF may not be necessary.
- The retinal breaks must be identified before surgery. Patient is advised bed rest with head turned, so that the retinal break is in the most dependent position. It lessens the amount of SRF and facilitates the surgery. SRF will spread more quickly due to the influence of gravity, if the break is located superiorly. If the vitreous gel is healthy and solid, even giant retinal tears may not lead to RD. If, however, synchysis is advanced (as in myopia and aphakia), progression is usually rapid.

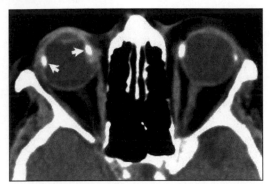

Fig. 26.30 Scleral buckling. Source: Globe. In: Runge V, Smoker W, Valavanis A, ed. Neuroradiology. The essentials with MR and CT. 1st edition. Thieme; 2014.

■ Surgery on the Eyeball

■ Evisceration

It is the removal of the intraocular contents retaining the sclera and optic nerve.

Indications
- Panophthalmitis.
- Very rarely expulsive hemorrhage.

Anesthesia
- General anesthesia (GA) is preferable and local anesthesia is given when GA is contraindicated.

Steps of Operation

- An informed written consent has to be taken prior to surgery.
- An eye speculum is applied.
- The eye is fixed and conjunctival dissection around the limbus is done.
- Cornea is excised with knife and scissors.
- Intraocular contents are removed with an evisceration scoop. The scoop is inserted between the sclera and the uveal tract and swept circumferentially. Thus, uveal tissue is separated from sclera and optic nerve. The intraocular contents are scooped out. All uveal tract must be thoroughly removed, especially around the vortex veins and optic nerve. Retained fragments are a potential danger for sympathetic ophthalmitis.

- Appropriate antibiotics are applied and a pressure bandage with pad is applied for 48 hours.

Variations of Evisceration
- *Frill excision:* When a frill of scleral tissue is left behind around the optic nerve to ensure that the nerve sheath is not opened, it is called a frill excision. If the greater part of sclera is left behind, there is considerable reaction and delayed wound healing. These disadvantages may be avoided by frill excision.
- *Insertion of an Acrylic Ball Implant:* If there is no active inflammation in the eye for evisceration for the year or more, a small acrylic or silicone ball (~14–16mm in diameter) is placed within the scleral cup to achieve the satisfactory cosmetic result. The sclera is sutured over the implant.

■ Enucleation (OP4.9)

Enucleation is the surgical removal of the eyeball with preservation of all other periorbital and orbital structures.

Indications
- Intraocular malignancy (most commonly uveal melanoma and retinoblastoma).
- Trauma: Severely traumatized eye with no perception of light (PL) to prevent sympathetic ophthalmitis of contra lateral eye.
- Painful, blind eye.

Anesthesia
- GA is preferable. A retrobulbar block of local anesthetic with epinephrine is given to aid in hemostasis and postoperative pain management.

Steps of Operation

- An informed written consent has to be taken prior to surgery.
- Universal eye speculum is applied.
- Conjunctiva is dissected all around the limbus. Blunt dissection in the subtenon's plane is then performed, and each rectus

muscle is identified and hooked with a squint hook, secured with suture and cut at the insertion to the globe.

- Once the globe is determined to rotate freely, the optic nerve is identified and cut with enucleation scissors. An attempt should be made to cut a long segment of the optic nerve (at least 10 mm behind the globe), particularly in situations of intraocular malignancy where histologic examination of the optic nerve is crucial.
- Tenon's capsule and conjunctiva are sutured separately, and pressure bandage is applied for 48 hours.

Enucleation with Implants

The aims are:
- To provide a mobile base for the prosthesis to pivot upon.
- To prevent bony deformity of the orbital wall (i.e., contracted socket) in children.

Types of Implants

A **prosthesis** (or an artificial eye) may be fitted in the third or fourth week after the operation. The prosthetic eye is generally made of hard, plastic acrylic, and shaped like a shell. The prosthetic eye fits over an ocular implant. The ocular implant is a separate hard, rounded device that is a surgically and permanently embedded dipper in the eye socket to fill the space previously occupied by an eye. The implant of appropriate size is selected to achieve symmetry with the fellow eye. The orbital implant can be divided into two main groups:
- Nonintegrated (nonporous).
- Integrated (porous).

Nonintegrated implants: It is an acrylic sphere. Nonintegrated implants contain no unique apparatus for attachments to the extraocular muscles and do not allow ingrowth of organic tissue into their inorganic substance. These are inexpensive with very low risk of exposure but have less movement. Usually, these implants are covered with a material that permits fixation of the extraocular recti muscles, such as donor sclera or polyester gauze which improve implant motility. These include acrylic (PMMA) and silicone spheres.

Integrated (porous) implants: The porous nature of integrated implants allows anchoring of the extraocular muscles with proliferation of fibrovascular tissues into the implant itself. These include hydroxyapatite (choral like), porous polyethylene. These afford the excellent mobility. In majority of cases, there is more risk of infection and the extrusion of implant than nonintegrated.

Hydroxyapatite implants: Because of their rough surface, they are typically wrapped with material such as donor sclera, acellular dermis, or pericardium. The extraocular muscles may be then sutured to the wrapping material for enhanced motility of the implant.

Porous polyethylene implants: They have a smoother surface and do not require wrapping. Other advantages of porous polyethylene over hydroxyapatite implants include cheaper cost and ability to suture the extraocular muscles directly to the implant.

Dermis fat graft implants: Fat from buttock is used to fill space formerly occupied by the eye. Muscle cannot be attached to a fat graft. There is no risk of rejection, as this graft uses the patient's own tissue. These provide less movement. When done in adulthood, they often atrophy with time, with a less satisfactory cosmetic result.

Ocular Symptoms and Examination

Ocular Symptoms...708
Ocular Examination..714

■ Ocular Symptoms

Ocular symptoms can be categorized as follows:
- Symptoms due to ocular surface anomalies.
- Visual symptoms.
- Symptoms caused by anomalies of ocular motility.

■ Symptoms due to Ocular Surface Anomalies

Diseases affecting ocular surface (i.e., conjunctiva and cornea) present with symptoms like red eye, foreign body sensation, ocular irritation or burning, photophobia (light sensitivity), discharge, and itching (itchy eyes).

Red Eye

It is a symptom of anterior segment diseases. It has multiple causes as mentioned below:

Conjunctival causes:
- Conjunctivitis (due to any cause).
- Subconjunctival hemorrhage.
- Conjunctival foreign body.
- Toxic or chemical reaction.
- Conjunctival neoplasia.

Corneal causes:
- Corneal foreign body.
- Corneal abrasion.
- Recurrent corneal erosions.
- Infectious keratitis (due to any cause).

Uveal causes:
- Anterior uveitis.

Adnexal causes:
- Trichiasis.

- Distichiasis.
- Blepharitis.
- Dacryocystitis.
- Canaliculitis.

Other causes:
- Chemical or UV burn.
- Angle-closure glaucoma.
- Carotid-cavernous fistula.
- Dry eye syndrome.
- Scleritis.
- Episcleritis.
- Pharmacologic (prostaglandin analogues, miotics and other vasodilatory medication, and brimonidine).
- Trauma.

Foreign Body Sensation

It may be due to:
- Dry eye syndrome.
- Conjunctivitis.
- Corneal abrasion.
- Foreign body (conjunctival or corneal).
- Recurrent corneal erosions.
- Trichiasis.
- Superficial punctate keratopathy (SPK).
- Blepharitis.
- Pterygium.
- Contact lens-related problems.

Ocular Irritation or Burning

Patient may complain of burning or gritty sensations in the eyes which may be caused by:
- Dry eye syndrome.
- Blepharitis.
- Meibominitis.

- Conjunctivitis.
- Medication.
- Contact lens.
- Episcleritis.

Photophobia (Light Sensitivity)

It is the inability to tolerate light and causes discomfort or pain to the eyes due to light exposure. It may be found without visible ocular diseases or may be associated with ocular diseases.

In ocular diseases: Nearly all inflammatory diseases of eye have an associated photophobia, for example:

- Conjunctiva: Conjunctivitis.
- Cornea: Abrasion, edema, foreign body, and ulcer.
- Uvea: Anterior uveitis.
- Sclera: Acleritis.
- Mydriasis due to drugs or trauma.
- Acute angle-closure glaucoma.
- Total color blindness (achromatopsia).

Without visible ocular disease: If photophobia is present with normal eye examination, patient should be investigated for the following:

- Migraine.
- Retrobulbar neuritis (RBN).
- Subarachnoid hemorrhage.
- Trigeminal neuralgia.
- Meningitis.

Discharge

It may be:

- Mucoid.
- Mucopurulent.
- Purulent.
- Ropy.
- Serosanguinous.

It is seen in different types of inflammations, for example, conjunctivitis, keratitis (corneal ulcers), stye, blepharitis, meibominitis, dacryocystitis, etc.

Itching (Itchy Eyes)

Itching may be due to:

- Allergic conjunctivitis.
- Vernal conjunctivitis.

- Blepharitis.
- Topical drug allergy or contact dermatitis.
- Giant papillary conjunctivitis.

■ Visual Symptoms

Common visual symptoms include diminution of vision, distortion of vision (metamorphopsia), micropsia, colored halos, floaters (spots in front of the eyes) and photopsia (flashes of light), glare (excessive awareness of light), diplopia (Double vision), night blindness (nyctalopia), day blindness (hemeralopia), and color blindness.

Diminution of Vision

It is one of the commonest complaints of an ophthalmic patient. It may be:

- Sudden or gradual.
- Transient or permanent.
- Painless or painful.
- Unilateral or bilateral.
- Progressive or stationary.

So, patient is always asked the following questions related to decreased vision (**Flowchart 27.1**):

- Onset: Whether it is sudden or gradual?
- Duration: If the diminution of vision is transient and returns to normal within 24 hours, usually within 1 hour or it lasts longer than 24 hours?
- Progression: Ask the patient whether the diminution of vision is static, steadily worsening, or improving?
- Pattern: Whether it is constant or intermittent?
- Frequency of occurrence: Whether it is episodic or periodic?
- Unilateral (U/L) or Bilateral (B/L): If bilateral, were both the eyes affected simultaneously or sequentially?
- Whether it is more for distance or nearness?
- If the diminution of vision is associated with pain or it is painless?
- Ask about the associated symptoms such as redness, watering, photophobia, floaters, and diplopia.

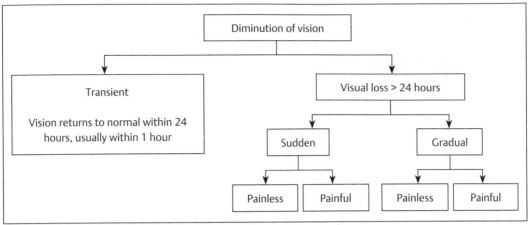

Flowchart 27.1 Algorithm for assessment of decreased vision.

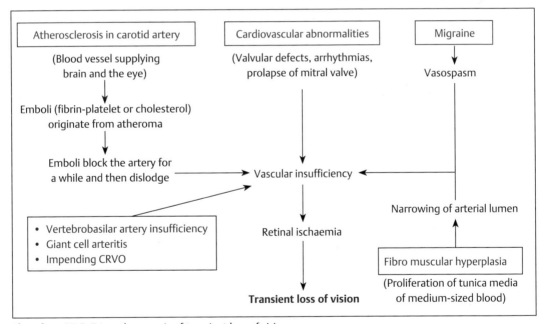

Flowchart 27.2 Etiopathogenesis of transient loss of vision.

Generally, the posterior segment conditions are associated with painless diminution of vision.

Causes of **sudden and painless** diminution of vision are:

- **Unilateral:** It is seen in:
  ◇ Retinal vein occlusion.
  ◇ Retinal artery occlusion.
  ◇ Retinal detachment.
  ◇ Vitreous hemorrhage.
  ◇ Central serous retinopathy (CSR).
  ◇ Central choroiditis.
  ◇ Papillitis.
- **Bilateral:** It is due to:
  ◇ Bilateral occipital infarction.

◊ Toxic optic neuropathy.
  – Ethambutol toxicity.
  – Methanol poisoning.
◊ Diabetic retinopathy.

Causes of **sudden painful** diminution of vision are:

- Acute anterior uveitis.
- Acute angle-closure glaucoma.
- Corneal ulcer.
- RBN: Diminution of vision is associated with pain on eye movements.
- Endophthalmitis.
- Ocular injury (mechanical, chemical, or thermal).

Causes of **gradual, painless and progressive** diminution of vision are:

- Cataract.
- Refractive error.
- Open-angle glaucoma.
- Corneal dystrophy.
- Keratoconus.
- Diabetic retinopathy.
- Retinitis pigmentosa.
- Optic neuropathy.
- Age-related macular degeneration (ARMD)–dry type
- Inferior retinal detachment: Subretinal fluid detaches the retina against gravity. So, detachment occurs gradually causing marked diminution of vision.
- Hereditary macular degeneration.

Causes of **gradual painful** diminution of vision are:

- Chronic anterior uveitis.
- Corneal dystrophy causing corneal edema.
- Aphakic/pseudophakic bullous keratopathy.

Cause of **transient diminution of vision** is amaurosis.

Amaurosis

It is the vision loss or weakness that occurs without an apparent lesion affecting the eye. It may affect one or both the eyes. It is due to temporary lack of blood flow either to retina or the brain. Its causes are as follows:

- Amaurosis fugax: It is unilateral loss of vision due to transient ischemic attack lasting few minutes to 1–2 hours.
- Vertebrobasilar artery insufficiency–bilateral.
- Migraine: With or without a subsequent headache.
- Giant cell arteritis.
- Impending central retinal vein occlusion (CRVO).
- Carotid occlusive disease (atherosclerosis of carotid artery).
- Functional (hysteria and malingering).

Gaze-evoked Amaurosis

It is the transient unilateral loss of vision in a particular direction of the eccentric gaze. It is *pathognomonic of* orbital disease, for example, optic nerve sheath meningioma. Orbital disease causes compression of optic nerve leading to transient optic nerve ischemia which, in turn, causes transient blurring of vision.

Defective vision for distance is seen in myopia and nuclear sclerosis, while defective vision for near is seen in presbyopia, hypermetropia, and cycloplegia.

Distortion of Vision (Metamorphopsia)

In metamorphopsia, patient perceives irregular and distorted shape of objects. It can be reviewed with the Amsler grid. It is associated with diseases affecting macula, for example:

- CSR.
- ARMD.
- Diabetic macular edema.
- Macular hole.

Micropsia

When the retinal elements (cones) at fovea get separated due to collection of subretinal fluid, the objects look smaller than normal. This is termed **micropsia** and it is seen in CSR.

Colored Halos

These are the rings of rainbow color around lights at night. It is associated with angle-closure glaucoma, corneal edema, and incipient or early cataract. Due to accumulation of fluid in all these conditions, refractive condition of the eye alters, causing prismatic dispersion of light. This leads to formation of colored halos with red outside and blue innermost.

Halos due to incipient cataract and corneal diseases may be differentiated by the *Fincham test*. During this test, a stenopeic slit is passed before the eye across the line of vision. Glaucomatous halo (due to corneal edema) remains intact but lenticular halo is broken up into segments. These segments revolve with the movement of the slit.

Floaters (Spots in Front of the Eyes) and Photopsia (Flashes of Light)

Normal vitreous is a transparent gel attached to the retina at places. Two changes, liquefaction and shrinkage, occur (due to age or any other cause) in vitreous (**Flowchart 27.3**).

> If photopsia is accompanied by floaters, look for peripheral retinal degeneration by indirect ophthalmoscope, which may be prone to retinal tear after retinal traction.

Glare (Excessive Awareness of Light)

It is excessive awareness to the light within the field of vision which is brighter than the brightness to which the eyes are adapted.

Causes

- Conditions which allow excess light to enter the eye:
  ◇ Aniridia.
  ◇ Ocular albinism.
- Conditions which produce excessive scattering of light in the eye:
  ◇ Posterior subcapsular cataract.
  ◇ Corneal edema.
  ◇ Corneal opacity.

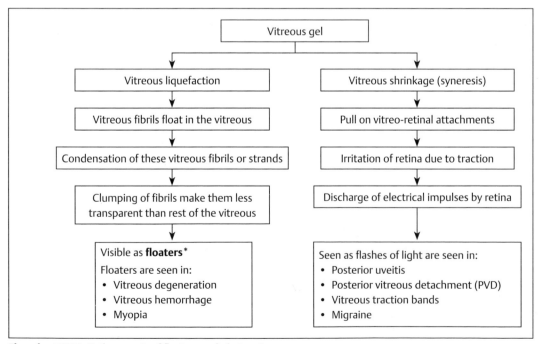

Flowchart 27.3 Pathogenesis of floaters and photopsia.
*Note: In floaters, patient complains of seeing black dots, black rings, strands and spider-like shapes. These move with the eye and are more noticeable against a bright background.

◊ Postrefractive surgery.

◊ Posterior vitreous detachment.

Diplopia (Double Vision)

It may be monocular or binocular.

Monocular diplopia: It is the subjective perception of two images of an object with one eye (either eye). It remains when the uninvolved eye is occluded. It is found in:

- Cataract.
- Dislocation of lens (two images are perceived; one through the aphakic zone and other through the phakic zone).
- Large iridotomies/iridectomy.

Binocular diplopia: It is the perception of two images of an object with both eyes open. It is eliminated when either eye is occluded. It is due to the loss of synchronous movement of both eyes and may be intermittent or constant.

Polyopia means multiple images are seen and it may happen due to cataract.

Night Blindness (Nyctalopia)

It is due to the interference with the functions of retinal rods. It is seen in:

- Vitamin A deficiency in children.
- Pigmentary retinal dystrophy (retinitis pigmentosa).
- Gyrate atrophy.
- Choroideremia.

Day Blindness (Hemeralopia)

It is due to:

- Congenital cone deficiency.
- Central cataract (posterior subcapsular cataract).

Color Blindness

Color blindness is either congenital or acquired; both the types could be partial or complete.

Complete Congenital Color Blindness

It is rare and generally caused by a central defect. All colors appear gray but with differing brightness.

Partial Congenital Color Blindness

It is inherited as X-linked recessive trait, so it is more common in males than females. Three types of photopigments (sensitive for red, green, and blue colors) are found in foveal cones and the absence of one of the photo pigments results in partial congenital color blindness. The red and green defect is more common, while the absence of blue sensation is very rare.

In **protanopes** the *red sensation* is defective; in **deuteranopes,** the *green sensation* is defective, while in **tritanopes**, the *blue sensation* is absent. If the defect is not complete, then these are called **protanomalous, deuteranomalous,** and **tritanomalous** respectively.

■ Symptoms due to Anomalies of Ocular Motility

These include eyestrain or asthenopia, binocular diplopia, "jumping" eyes, and deviation of eyes.

Asthenopia

It is defined as fatigue of the eyes commonly following prolonged close work and watching TV or film. It increases toward the evening. Symptoms of eyestrain may be absent if near work is avoided. *Asthenopic symptoms* (eyestrain) include eye ache, burning, watering, frontal headache, and eye fatigue.

Asthenopia is generally due to the following causes:

- Extraocular (EOM) muscle imbalance.
- Uncorrected refractive error.
- Incorrect refractive correction.
- Convergence insufficiency.

Inadvertent rubbing of eyes (due to eye strain) with dirty fingers may result in recurrent stye, chalazia, or blepharitis.

Binocular Diplopia

It is the perception of two images of an object with both eyes open. It is eliminated when either eye is occluded. It is due to the loss of synchronous movement of both eyes and may be intermittent or constant.

Intermittent binocular diplopia is seen in myasthenia gravis and intermittent decompensation of existing phoria.

Constant binocular diplopia is seen in:
- EOM paresis (isolated 6th, 3rd, or 4th nerve palsy).
- Thyroid eye disease (due to restrictive movements).
- Orbital pseudotumor.
- Orbital wall fracture with EOM entrapment.
- Postsquint surgery.

■ Ocular Examination

■ History Taking

It includes presenting complaints, history of illness, occupation and past and family history.

Chief Presenting Complaints

All the complaints of the patients must be recorded before starting the ocular examination. The common complaints of the patient are:
- Defective vision (for distance, near or both).
- Discharge from the eyes.
- Watering.
- Redness.
- Photophobia.
- Itching.
- Burning.
- Foreign body sensation.
- Headache.
- Asthenopic symptoms.

- Ocular pain.
- Deviation of eye.
- Black spots in front of eyes.
- Colored halos.
- Distorted vision.
- Diplopia.
- Flashes.

History of Present Illness

- Enquire about the mode of onset (acute or insidious) and duration of the ailment.
- Progression of the complaint (whether it is stationary/improving/worsening).
- Nature of discharge (watery/mucopurulent/purulent/ropy/sanguinous).
- Ask about the association of itching and climate/season.

Occupation

Information about the patient's occupation is helpful because of occupational hazards (**Table 27.1**).

Past History

Patient must be asked about:
- Trauma in the past (for posterior subcapsular cataract and retinal detachment).
- Past medical and surgical history.
- History of similar ocular complaints in the past (for recurrent diseases such as uveitis, herpes simplex keratitis, and recurrent corneal erosions).
- History of systemic illness, for example, diabetes, hypertension, thyroid dysfunction, and joint pains.
- Drug allergies.

Table 27.1 Important occupational hazards

Occupation	Occupational hazards
• Computer professionals • Glass blowers • Welders • Agricultural workers • Factory workers • Sport persons	• Computer vision syndrome • Cataract • Photophthalmitis • Microbial keratitis • Foreign body • Ocular injuries and trauma

Family History

Family history is important as certain ocular diseases are genetically transmitted such as:

- Ptosis.
- Strabismus.
- Glaucoma.
- Retinitis pigmentosa.
- Retinoblastoma.
- Refractive error.
- Cataract.

Maternal history regarding any infection (toxoplasmosis, rubella, venereal disease, herpes infection, and HIV infection), drug abuse, smoking, tobacco chewing, alcohol, and sexual history must be taken during the first trimester of pregnancy.

■ Examination of the Eye (Outline)

It is examined by the slit-lamp biomicroscope (with or without +90D), direct ophthalmoscope, retinoscope, indirect ophthalmoscope, and Goldmann 3-mirror contact lens. The examination of the eye requires:

- Testing of **visual acuity** (both for distance and near).
- Examination of **head posture** (in patients afflicted with strabismus, particularly vertical muscles palsies to avoid diplopia).
- Examination of **forehead for wrinkling:**
  ◊ Present due to over action of frontalis muscle as in ptosis.
  ◊ Absent on one side in lower motor neuron facial palsy.
- Examination of **eyelids** for their position, movement, lid crease, lid margins (entropion/ectropion), and direction of eye lashes.
- Examination of **palpebral aperture**: It measures 28 to 30 mm horizontally and approximately 10 mm vertically in the center. *Narrow* palpebral aperture is seen in blepharospasm or inflammatory conditions of conjunctiva/cornea. *Wide* palpebral aperture is seen in retraction of upper lid (upper limbus is visible), proptosis (lower limbus is exposed), facial nerve palsy, and buphthalmos.
- Examination of **eye balls** for:
  ◊ Their position (proptosis or enophthalmos).
  ◊ Their movements (restricted in paralytic strabismus or fibrosis).
  ◊ Position of eye balls (for strabismus).
  ◊ Rhythmic oscillations (nystagmus), indicating that fixation reflex is not well-developed.
- Examination of **lacrimal apparatus:**
  ◊ *Lacrimal sac* is inspected for swelling (dacryocystitis) or any fistula.
  ◊ Inspection of *lacrimal gland* for its size (enlarged in inflammatory and neoplastic conditions).
  ◊ Look for *lower puncta* for its patency/obstruction/narrowing/eversion/any foreign body such as eyelash obstructing it.
  ◊ Look for *regurgitation* on pressing over the lacrimal sac area.
  ◊ Lacrimal *syringing* is done (to locate the site of obstruction).
  ◊ *Dacryocystography* (which is radiological visualization of lacrimal passage after injecting radio-opaque dye).
- Examination of **conjunctiva** (bulbar, palpebral, and forniceal conjunctiva) for:
  ◊ Congestion of vessels (conjunctiva or ciliary congestion).
  ◊ Edema (chemosis).
  ◊ Presence of follicles.
  ◊ Papillary hypertrophy.
  ◊ Any membrane.
  ◊ Concretions.
  ◊ For its luster (it is lusterless in vitamin A deficiency).
  ◊ Foreign body.
  ◊ Degenerative conditions (pinguecula and pterygium).
  ◊ Any conjunctival tumor.

- Examination of **cornea**– Cornea is examined for:
  ◊ Corneal size (microcornea or megalocornea)
  ◊ Corneal curvature (normal/ keratoglobus/keratoconus) by Placido's keratoscopic disc, corneal topography, or keratometery.
  ◊ Corneal abrasions/ulcers by staining with fluorescein (2%) or rose Bengal dye (1%).
  ◊ Corneal transparency (look for corneal edema and corneal opacity).
  ◊ Corneal vascularization (superficial or deep).
  ◊ Corneal sensations (diminished in herpes, leprosy, neuroparalytic keratitis, and absolute glaucoma).
  ◊ Corneal endothelium for keratic precipitates (KPs), and size and shape of endothelial cells by specular biomicroscope.
  ◊ Corneal thickness by pachymeter (for accurate intraocular pressure [IOP] measurement and preoperative evaluation of refractive surgery).
- Examination of **sclera**: Sclera is examined for:
  ◊ Pigmentation (in naevus of ota, which is also known as melanosis bulbi).
  ◊ Blue discoloration (which may be associated with osteitis deformans).
  ◊ Localized ectasia (intercalary, ciliary, equatorial or posterior).
  ◊ Ciliary congestion (suggestive of scleritis).
  ◊ Localized, congested nodule (suggests episcleritis).
- Examination of **anterior chamber** (OP6.6 for:
  ◊ Depth of anterior chamber:
    i. *Deep* anterior chamber is seen in aphakia, myopia, buphthalmos, keratoglobus, and posterior dislocation of lens.

    ii. *Shallow* anterior chamber is seen in primary narrow angle glaucoma, hypermetropia, malignant glaucoma, intumescent (swollen) lens, and anterior subluxation of lens.
    iii. *Unequal depth* (or irregular) anterior chamber is seen in adherent leucoma, tilting of lens in subluxation, and iris bombe formation due to annular synechiae in iridocyclitis.
  ◊ Aqueous flare.
  ◊ Aqueous cells.
  ◊ Hypopyon.
  ◊ Foreign body.
  ◊ Blood in anterior chambers/hyphema– seen after ocular trauma, surgery, gonococcal iridocyclitis, intraocular tumors, and blood dyscrasias.
  ◊ Angle of anterior chamber (examined with gonioscope and slit lamp).
- Examination of the **iris**: Iris is examined for:
  ◊ Color of iris (lighter/darker).
  ◊ Pattern of iris (e.g., muddy iris in iridocyclitis).
  ◊ Adhesions of iris (anterior or posterior synechiae).
  ◊ Tremulousness of iris (iridodonesis): It is seen when the posterior support of iris is lost, as in aphakia or subluxation of lens.
  ◊ Nodules on iris (Koeppe's and Busacca nodules in granulomatous iridocyclitis/ gumma of iris/tuberculoma).
  ◊ Neovascularization of iris (rubeosis iridis): It is seen in:
    – Diabetic retinopathy
    – CRVO.
    – Branch retinal vein occlusion (BRVO).
    – Retinoblastoma.
    – Ocular ischemic syndrome.
    – Coloboma/iridectomy/iridodialysis.
- Examination of **pupil**: Pupil is examined with reference to:
  ◊ Number of pupil (1 or more).
  ◊ Location of pupil (central or eccentric).
  ◊ Size of pupil (miotic or mydriatic).

◇ Shape of pupil (**Table 27.2**).
◇ Color of pupil (**Table 27.3**).

The term **leukocoria** means whitish pupil. Its causes are classified into:

- Retinoblastoma.
- Congenital cataract.
- Cyclitic membrane.
- Retinopathy of prematurity.
- Retinal detachment.
- Endophthalmitis and panophthalmitis.
- Toxocariasis.
- Coat's disease.
- Persistent hyperplastic primary vitreous (PHPV).
- Coloboma.
- Retinal dysplasia.
- Norrie's disease.

◇ Pupillary reaction: this includes.
- Direct light reaction.
- Consensual light reaction.
- Swinging-flash light test.
- Near reflex.

- Any abnormal pupillary reactions (Argyll Robertson pupil, Marcus Gunn pupil, Wernicke's hemianopic pupil, and tonic pupil).

• Examination of the **lens**: Note the following points regarding lens:
◇ Position of lens: Normal
◇ Dislocation (anterior or posterior).
◇ Subluxation.
◇ Aphakia/pseudophakia
◇ Shape of lens
  - Spherophakia
  - Lenticonus anterior.
  - Lenticonus posterior.
  - Coloboma of lens.
◇ Any abnormality in transparency (cataract).
◇ Deposits on the anterior surface of lens:
  - Iris pigments in iridocyclitis.
  - Vossius ring after blunt trauma.
  - Rusty deposits in siderosis bulbi.
  - Green deposits of copper in chalcosis.

• Measurement of **IOP** by tonometer.

Table 27.2 Conditions associated with pupillary shape

Shape	Condition
Circular shape	Normal pupil
D-shape (**Fig. 27.1a**)	Found in iridodialysis
Pear shaped	Found in cases of leucoma adherent
Oval shaped	Found in acute congestive glaucoma and severe brain diseases.
Festooned pupil (on dilatation, **Fig. 27.1b**)	When posterior synechiae are present.

Table 27.3 Pupillary color imparted by different conditions

Color	Condition
Grayish black	Normal
Jet black	Aphakia
Grayish white	Cataract
Whitish	Retinoblastoma and pseudogliomas
Brown	Nuclear cataract
Yellowish	Vitreous abscess (endophthalmitis and panophthalmitis)
Reddish	Albinism

- **Fundus** examination: The details of fundus are recorded in a systematic way as follows:
  ◇ Observe media (opacities in media look black against the red glow on distant direct ophthalmoscopy).
  ◇ Optic disc: Look for its:
    – Size (normal/smaller/larger).
    – Shape (circular or oval): In high-astigmatism, optic disc looks oval in shape.
    – Margins: Well-defined or blurred.
    – Color: Normal pink color/hyperemia/pallor/chalky white/waxy pale.
    – Optic cup: Normal or large/shallow or deep/obliterated.
    – Cup-disc ratio (CDR): Normal or large.
    – Venous pulsations.
    – Splinter hemorrhages.
    – Neovascularization of disc (NVD).
  ◇ Macula: Look for foveal reflex, macular hole, macular hemorrhage, macular edema, cherry-red spot, scar, and dystrophy or degeneration.
  ◇ Retinal blood vessels: Look for narrowing of arterioles, tortuosity of veins, and sheathing of vessels.
  ◇ Look for:
    – Microaneurysms.
    – Retinal hemorrhages (superficial and deep).
    – Cotton wool spots.
    – Hard exudates.
    – Drusen at posterior pole.
    – Neovascularization (NVE).
    – Peripheral retinal degeneration.
    – Retinal holes/retinal tears.
    – Retinal detachment.
    – Myelinated nerve fibers.
    – Tumors.
    – Color of background which may be normally pinkish red in color or tessellated or tigroid fundus due to excessive pigment in the choroid.
- Estimation of **refractive error** by retinoscope or autorefractometer.
- Estimation of **color vision.**
- **Macular function tests (refer to Chapter 10 "The Lens" for details).**
- **Diagnostic tests–**
  ◇ Visual field examination by perimeter (refer to chapter 2).
  ◇ Fluorescein angiography (FA) (refer to chapter 13).
  ◇ Indocyanine green angiography (ICGA) (refer to chapter 13).
  ◇ Electrophysiological tests (electroretinography [ERG], electrooculogram [EOG], visual evoke potential [VEP]) (refer to chapter 2).
  ◇ Optical coherence tomography (OCT) (refer to chapter 13).
  ◇ Ultrasonography (A-scan and B-scan).
  ◇ Exophthalmometry by Hertel's exophthalmometer (refer to chapter 22).
  ◇ Radiography:
    – Noninvasive (plain X-ray, CT scan, MRI, and carotid Doppler).
    – Invasive (arteriography and venography).

■ Determination of the Refraction (OP1.2)

The refractive errors are determined by two examinations: objective and subjective. Objective examination can be done by retinoscopy and refractometry. Corneal astigmatism is objectively measured by a keratometer. After the refraction has been estimated objectively, the values are verified subjectively by testing the patient's visual acuity with suitable lenses to be prescribed.

Objective Verification of Refraction

Retinoscopy (Skiascopy or Shadow Test)

Principle of Retinoscopy

When the light is directed into the patient's eye, the rays of light from the patient's retina travel across the pupil, forming an image at the far point of the patient's eye which varies with the refractive status of the eye.

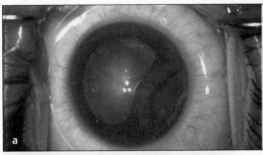

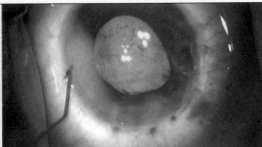

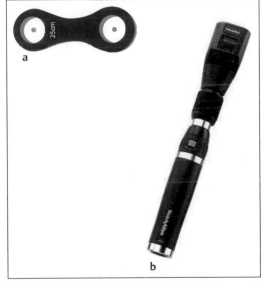

Fig. 27.1 (a) D-shaped pupil. Source: Goniosynechialysis and iris reconstruction. In: Agarwal A, Narang P, ed. Video atlas of anterior segment repair and reconstruction: managing challenges in cornea, glaucoma, and lens surgery. 1st edition. Thieme; 2019. **(b)** Festooned pupil. Source: Antiinflammatories. In: Agarwal A, Jacob S, ed. Color atlas of ophthalmology. The quick-reference manual for diagnosis and treatment. 2nd edition. Thieme; 2019.

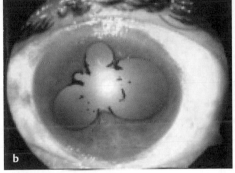

Fig. 27.2 (a) Mirror retinoscope. **(b)** Streak retinoscope.

Methods of Retinoscopy

It can be performed by retinoscope which is of two types: mirror retinoscope (**Fig. 27.2a**) and streak retinoscope (**Fig. 27.2b** and **Table 27.4**).

In practice, plane mirror is used for retinoscopy.

Procedure of Retinoscopy

- The examiner sits at a distance of 1 m from the patient in a dark room.
- The patient is asked to look at a far point to relax the accommodation.
- Light is reflected into the patient's eye with the help of a retinoscope (mirror/streak).
- Now, the retinoscope is moved horizontally and vertically.
- The red reflex also moves when the retinoscope is moved, and the direction of movement of red reflex is noted.

The red reflex is dull and moves slowly in high-refractive errors, while it is bright and moves rapidly in low-refractive errors.

- The movement of red reflex is neutralized by the lenses from the trial set. At the point of reversal or neutral point of retinoscopy, the examiner sees a diffuse bright red reflex in the patient's pupil.
- Each principal meridian should be neutralized separately. In regular astigmatism, the reflex movements vary in different meridians. In astigmatism, one meridian is neutralized and the mirror is then moved

Table 27.4 Difference between mirror and streak retinoscopes

Mirror retinoscope	Spot /Streak retinoscope
• It needs an external source of light which is kept above and behind the head of the patient. It contains plane mirror at one end and concave mirror at the other with a central hole (Priestley–Smith retinoscope). • It projects a circle of light into the patients eye through the pupil.	• It is self-illuminated retinoscope as it contains the bulb inside it. • It projects a spot/streak rather than a circle of light. In streak retinoscope, a circular beam of light is converted into a linear streak of light by a planocylindrical mirror in the retinoscope.

Table 27.5 Interpretation of retinoscopy

Retinoscopic mirror used	In case of with movement	In case of against movement
If a **plane mirror** is used for retinoscopy	The conditions may be: • Emmetropia • Hypermetropia • Myopia of less than 1D	The refractive error is myopia of more than 1D
If a **concave mirror** is used *instead of a plane mirror*	The refractive error is myopia of more than 1D	The conditions may be: • Emmetropia • Hypermetropia • Myopia of less than 1D

at right angle to the neutralized meridian. The point of reversal is obtained by adding the lenses in the trial frame. When a simple spherical refractive error alone is present, the movements of red reflex will be neutralized in both meridia with the same lens in the trial set.

Interpretation

The movement of the reflex with the movement of mirror depends upon the nature of refractive status of the eye. If a plane/concave mirror is used for retinoscopy at a working distance of 1 m, the movement of the red reflex may be in the same direction (**with movement**) or in the opposite direction (**against movement**) to the movement of the mirror. The aim of retinoscopy is to neutralize "with" or "against" movement of red reflex by adding a lens of the required power from the trial set (**Table 27.5**).

If an eye has myopia of 1D, there is no movement of retinoscopic reflex at a distance of 1 m with a plane mirror. The pupil will be either completely illuminated or completely dark. The method, therefore, consists of placing the lenses in front of the eye until no shadow is seen. This is called neutral point.

Generally, −1D is added to the power of trial lenses to calculate the actual refractive error (**reason**: at a distance of 1 m from the patient, the patient has myopia of 1D and there is no movement of reflex. Hence, the patient's refractive state will be 1D less than the lenses used to neutralize the movement). For example, in a hypermetropic individual, if the neutral point is achieved with +3D sphere, the actual error is +2 D sphere (+3 + [−1] = +2). Similarly, in a myopic individual, if the neutral point is achieved with a −3D sphere. The actual error is −4D (−3 + [−1] = −4).

- Equal retinoscopic values along horizontal and vertical meridia means that there is no astigmatism, and a spherical lens is required to correct the refractive error.
- Unequal retinoscopic values along horizontal and vertical meridia means the presence of astigmatism, which is corrected by the cylindrical lens alone or in combination with spherical lens.

Cycloplegic Retinoscopy

In young children and hypermetropes, when accommodation is abnormally exerted, retinoscopy is performed under cycloplegic drugs (**wet retinoscopy**), which cause paralysis of accommodation with mydriasis. In elderly patients, retinoscopy is generally done without the use of any cycloplegic drug (**dry retinoscopy**). The commonly used cycloplegic drugs are:

- Atropine (1% ointment).
- Homatropine (2% drops).
- Cyclopentolate (1% drops).

Atropine is not used as drops, as systemic toxicity occurs due to its absorption from conjunctival and nasal mucosae. Tropicamide (1%) and phenylephrine (5%, 10%) are used as mydriatics.

When refraction is performed under cycloplegia, a correction must be made to compensate for the normal physiological tone of ciliary muscle (deduct 1D for atropine and 0.5D for other cycloplegics).

The cycloplegic/mydriatic drug must be used with caution in patients with shallow anterior chamber, owing to the risk of acute angle-closure glaucoma. In such cases, gonioscopy and prophylactic laser iridotomy must be performed prior to dilatation, if pupillary dilatation is necessary.

Difficulties in Retinoscopy

- "Scissors" shadows (two shadows appear to meet each other and cross as the light is moved in a given direction) may be seen in regular astigmatism, owing chiefly to differences in curvature of the different parts of cornea. These difficulties are diminished with the undilated pupil.
- Shadows move in various directions in different parts of pupillary area in irregular astigmatism and create a problem in accurate correction.
- A triangular shadow with its apex at the apex of the cone may be seen in keratoconus (conical cornea), which swirl around its apex on moving the retinoscopic mirror.

Refractometry

It is the objective estimation of refractive error with an equipment called the refractometer. The autorefractometers are automated computerized instruments which determine the refractive error objectively using infrared light. Autorefractometers measure quickly the far point of the eye and give information about the refractive error of patient in terms of sphere, cylinder, axis, and interpupillary distance. It is advantageous for mass screening (**Fig. 27.3**).

Keratometry (Ophthalmometry)

Keratometry is an objective method of estimating the curvature of the cornea with the help of a keratometer (ophthalmometer). *It assesses the corneal astigmatism.* Since astigmatism may occur due to lenticular factors, so the technique is not reliable in estimating the full astigmatism except in aphakia.

Principle

It is based on the fact that the cornea acts as a convex mirror and the size of image reflected by it varies inversely with its curvature, that is, greater the curvature of the mirror, the smaller is the image.

Instruments

The two types of keratometers used are Javal–Schiotz keratometer and Bausch and Lomb keratometer.

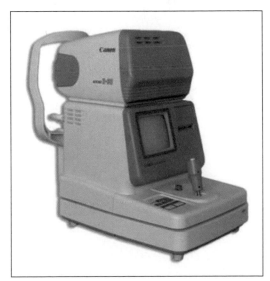

Fig. 27.3 Autorefractometer.

Javal-Schiotz Keratometer

The instrument consists of two illuminated mires disposed on a rotatable circular arc and an attached viewing telescope. The double images (ab and a'b') of the mires (A and B) are formed on the cornea. A and B are adjusted on the arc, so that the two images a' and b just touch each other. The readings are noted from a graduated scale attached to the arc. The arc is now rotated through 90° and a similar reading is made. If the image of the mires remains unchanged (i.e., if a' and b still touch), there is no astigmatism. If mires overlap or separate, there is presence of astigmatism and readjustment is required (**Fig. 27.4a**).

Bausch and Lomb Keratometer

This instrument has two maneuverable prisms aligned vertically and horizontally. In it, the mires are in the form of circles, one of a fixed original size and two adjustable images (one above and one to the left of the original). The adjustable images are moved toward/away from the original. It measures the corneal curvature in horizontal and vertical meridian simultaneously without rotating the mires (**Fig. 27.4b**).

Subjective Verification of Refraction

The refraction is always verified subjectively after the objective estimation. It is carried out by testing the visual acuity of a patient by the most suitable lenses in the trial frame. Each eye is tested separately and then the two eyes are tested together. If cycloplegic has been used, a postmydriatic test is performed after 2 weeks (if atropine is used) or 72 hours (in case of homatropine/cyclopentolate).

Procedure

- Put the trial frame on the face of the patient.
- Put the occluder in the trial frame in front of one eye.
- Put the appropriate lenses in the trial frame (measured by objective test) in front of the other eye.
- The patient is asked to read the test-types by using Snellen's chart, and the power of lenses is gradually increased or decreased to obtain the best visual acuity.
- The same procedure is repeated for the occluded eye. Now, the acceptance is verified binocularly.

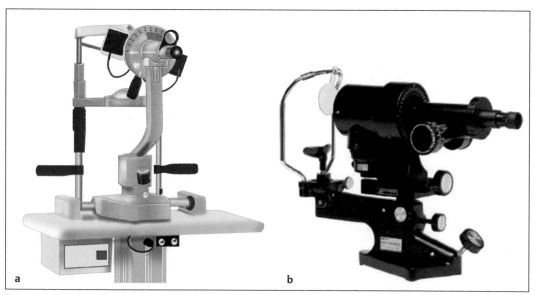

Fig. 27.4 (a) Javal-Schiotz keratometer. **(b)** Bausch and Lomb keratometer.

The over or undercorrection of refractive error can be verified by the **duochrome test** (**Fig. 27.5a**) which is based on the principle of chromatic aberration. In this test, the patient is asked to read red and green letters on the vision drum. The green rays have short wavelength and are focused earlier than the red rays having longer wavelength.

- In *emmetropia*, letters of both colors look equally sharp, as green rays are focused slightly anterior and red rays are focused slightly posterior to the retina.
- In *myopia*, red letters are more clear than green.
- In *hypermetropia*, green letters are sharper than red.

Therefore, if a myopic patient tells that the red colors are clearer than the green, it means that overcorrection has not been done, but if the green letters are more distinct than the red to a myopic patient, he is overcorrected and his/her spherical lenses should be adjusted, so that he/she sees letters of both colors equally sharp.

If the visual acuity does not improve with the optical correction, a **pinhole test** (**Fig. 27.5b**) must be performed. A pinhole (occluder with a small, central hole) is placed in the trial frame. An improvement in visual acuity with pinhole indicates that optical correction is incorrect and the refraction should be rechecked. No improvement in visual acuity even with pinhole, indicates an organic lesion.

Some ophthalmologists use the **fogging method** to relax the ciliary muscle. This method is more useful in hypermetropia. In this method, the patient is made myopic by inserting + 3 or + 4D spherical lens over the previously verified spherical correction, and the patient is asked to see the distant test types. Then, gradually the convex lens is reduced until the maximum visual acuity is obtained.

The modifications in the power and axis of cylindrical lenses can be made by use of cross cylinder (**Fig. 27.6a**) and astigmatic fan (**Fig. 27.6b**).

Use of Cross Cylinder

A Jackson's cross cylinder is a combination of two equal cylinders of opposite signs, with their axis at right angles to each other. The handle of cross cylinder is at angle to both axes. The most common combinations are ± 0.25D and ± 0.5D. It is used to verify the strength and axis of the prescribed cylinder.

To Check the Strength of the Cylindrical Correction

First, hold the cross cylinder of same sign with its axis in the same direction as to the axis of the

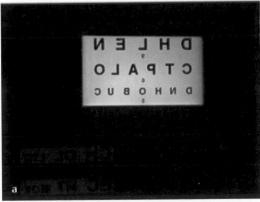
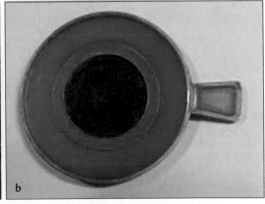

Fig. 27.5 (a) Duochrome test. **(b)** Pinhole.

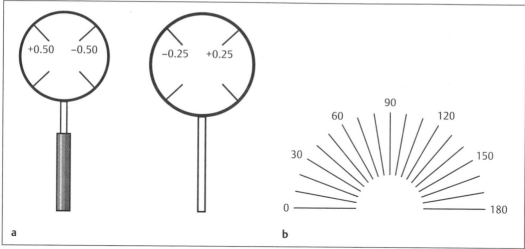

Fig. 27.6 (a) Cross-cylinders. **(b)** Astigmatic fan.

cylinder in the trial frame and ask the patient about the visual acuity. In this position, the cylindrical correction is increased by the 0.25D.

Now, the cross cylinder with opposite sign is held with its axis parallel to the axis in the cylinder in the trial frame. In this position, the cylindrical correction is decreased by the 0.25D or 0.5D.

If the visual acuity remains unchanged, the cylinder in the trial frame is correct.

To Check the Axis of the Cylindrical Correction

Place the cross cylinder with its axis at 45° to the axis of correcting cylinder in the trial frame.

Cross cylinder (± 0.5D) is placed before the eye with its axis at 45° to the axis of cylinder in the trial frame. Now, the cross cylinder is flipped over, so that each side of the cross cylinder lies alternately 45° to either side of the axis of the cylinder in the trial frame. If the patient notices no difference between the two positions, the axis of the correcting cylinder in the trial frame is correct. If visual improvement is attained in one of the positions, the correcting cylinder is rotated in the direction of the cylindrical component of same sign in the cross cylinder. The test is then repeated several times until the letters appear equally clear and rotation of the cross cylinder gives no alteration in clarity.

By Astigmatic Fan

The degree and axis of astigmatism can also be determined by an astigmatic fan. The astigmatic fan consists of radiating black lines in different meridians separated by 10° interval to one another. The test is performed after fogging by + 0.5D is added over the trial lens. The patient is asked to look at the fan.

- If all the lines appear equally clear to the patient, there is no astigmatism.
- If some of the lines are seen more clearly than the others, astigmatism must be present.

Now, add concave cylinder with its axis at right angles to the clearest line until all the lines appear equally sharp. The cylinder which thus renders the outline of the whole fan equally sharp is a measure of the amount of astigmatism. The axis of the cylinder is at right angles to the line which was initially the most clearly defined.

Correction for Near Vision

Correction for near vision is usually needed after the age of 40 years. With the distant correction in place, the correction for near is done. Near vision can be estimated by using Jaeger's chart, Snellen's reading test-types, number point types standardized by the faculty of ophthalmologist

(N5 to N48), or broken C. The patient is asked to hold the reading test types at a distance at which he or she is accustomed to work or read. If the letters are not distinctly seen, appropriate convex lens are added to the distant correction, so that the near point is brought within the working distance. Now, the near point should be determined, which is measured by using the smallest test-types and moving it toward the ear until they can no longer be easily read. The last position at which it can be read gives the near point, which can be measured from the eye in millimeter. The correction given should be such that approximately 1/3rd of the amplitude of accommodation is kept in reserve. In general, it is better to undercorrect than to overcorrect the near correction because difficulties will be experienced with convergence and the range of near vision will be limited. In any case, lenses (power of 3.5D) bringing the near point closer than 28 cm are rarely well-tolerated. If the higher correction is required on occupational ground, prisms are incorporated to facilitate the convergence.

Near correction is required in:
- Both eyes (as in presbyopia).
- One eye (as in unilateral aphakia, unilateral pseudophakia, and unilateral paralysis of accommodation).

■ Fundus Examination (Ophthalmoscopy) (OP8.3)

It is performed in a dark room and the routine of ophthalmoscopic examination should be as follows:
- Preliminary examination with a mirror at a distance of approximately 22 cm from the patient (distant direct ophthalmoscopy).
- Ophthalmoscopic examination by direct method (direct ophthalmoscopy).
- Ophthalmoscopic examination by indirect method (indirect ophthalmoscopy).
- Slit-lamp biomicroscopy with a + 90D lens.

Distant Direct Ophthalmoscopy

It is performed by a plane mirror or an ophthalmoscope at 22 cm distance in a dark room.

When the light is thrown with a plane mirror, a red fundus reflex is seen normally. When there is blood in the vitreous, the fundus reflex may be black. It gives the information about:
- Opacities in refractive media.
- Status of retina (whether it is detached or not).
- Conformation of findings found by external examinations.

Opacities in Refractive Media

If there are opacities in the media, they appear as black against red background. The exact position of the opacity may be determined by observing its *parallactic displacement*. The opacity may be stationary or floating. When the eyes are moved in different directions, a floating opacity will continue to move after the eye is brought to rest.

The eye is moved slightly in a given direction and the position of the opacity is determined as follows:
- If the opacity is in the pupillary plane, it will appear stationary.
- If the opacities move in the same direction, it is in front of pupillary plane, that is, cornea and anterior chamber.
- If the opacities move in the opposite direction, it is behind the pupillary plane, that is, posterior surface of lens and vitreous.

Status of Retina

When light is thrown by the mirror/with self-illuminated ophthalmoscope, the reflex from different directions show difference of colors. The presence of whitish or grayish uneven surface with retinal vessels, seen as black wavy lines, suggests a detached retina or a tumor arising from the retina.

Conformation of Findings found by External Examinations

Distant direct ophthalmoscopy may clearly distinguish between an iris hole and a mole. This black spot in the iris may allow a red reflex through it and thus appear as a hole. Similarly, a black patch at the ciliary margin of the iris may be a melanotic tumor of a ciliary body or it may be a separation of the iris from its ciliary attachment (iridodialysis). If a reflex is obtained through it by the mirror, it is iridodialysis, whereas in melanotic tumor of ciliary body, it will be opaque.

Direct Ophthalmoscopy

The direct ophthalmoscopy allows visualization of posterior pole of the retina up to the equator. An erect, virtual, and magnified image of the fundus is obtained. Direct ophthalmoscopy in emmetropic eye gives about a **15 times** magnified image of the fundus; the magnification is more in myopia and less in hypermetropia. In astigmatism, the magnification is greatest in more myopic meridian and least in more hypermetropic meridian, so the image is not clear in astigmatism.

To examine the fundus, dilate the pupil with a mydriatic-like phenylephrine-tropicamide combination. The right eye of the patient is examined by the right eye of the examiner. In direct ophthalmoscopy, the patient's eye is examined as closely as possible by the examiner. If ametropia is present, the refractive error is corrected with the help of lenses incorporated in the ophthalmoscope to get a clear image.

To examine the optic disc, ask the patient to look straight ahead.

To examine the macula, ask the patient to look at the light of the ophthalmoscope (**Fig. 27.7**).

To examine retinal blood vessels, examine the fundus from the disc toward the periphery in all the sectors.

To examine the peripheral parts of the fundus, ask the patient to look in different directions of gaze.

If there is a difference in level between the two points on the fundus, it can be accurately measured. **1 mm difference of level ≡ difference of 3D**.

Indirect Ophthalmoscopy

It is an important procedure, particularly to examine the periphery of the fundus. In indirect

ophthalmoscopy, a strong convex lens (+20D spherical) is held approximately 10 cm in front of the eyes and a real and inverted image of the fundus is obtained. The lens is held between the thumb and fore finger of the left hand, with the curved surface to the examiner and parallel to the plane of the iris. It gives about a **three times** magnified image of the fundus. The amount of magnification depends upon the refraction of the eye, strength of the lens, and its distance from the eye. With a lens of + 14D, the fundus of an emmetropic eye is magnified about five times (**Fig. 27.8**).

The examination requires practice; the optic disc of right eye can easily be focused by asking the patient to look toward right, and for the left optic disc, he or she should fix the gaze on his or her left side. The macula is examined by asking the patient to look into the light of ophthalmoscope, and the periphery of the fundus can be examined by asking the patient to look in different directions of gaze. Ora serrata can be

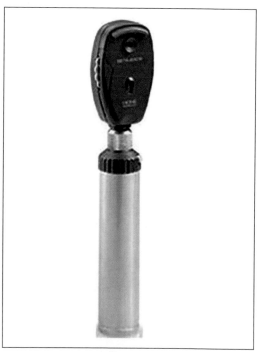

Fig. 27.7 Ophthalmoscope.

visualized by scleral indentation. The advantages of indirect ophthalmoscopy are large field of view and brighter illumination. The disadvantage of indirect ophthalmology is that image is inverted both vertically and laterally and requires orientation during surgery.

Slit-lamp Biomicroscopy

The slit-lamp explores the eye up to the anterior parts of the vitreous because of the convergence of the cornea. However, if the beam is made more divergent by using a contact lens (Goldmann contact lens, Hruby lens, and high-aspherical lenses) in front of the cornea, the posterior part of the vitreous and the central area of the fundus can be examined with the help of slit-lamp. The lenses are of two types, contact and noncontact.

Double aspheric lens (+60D, +78D, and +90D) and highly concave **Hruby lens** (–55D) are noncontact lenses. These lenses form the real and inverted (laterally as well as vertically) image which is useful in the diagnosis of optic nerve lesions and macular lesions such as edema, hole and cyst.

The Goldmann 3-mirror is a contact lens that has three mirrors placed in the cone, each with a different angle of inclination (73°, 67° and 59°). The central part of the contact lens allows a direct view of the posterior fundus. Other mirrors bring into focus the different parts of the peripheral fundus (**Fig. 27.9**).

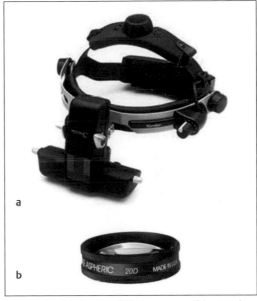

a

b

Fig. 27.8 (a) Indirect ophthalmoscope. **(b)** +20D lens used in indirect ophthalmoscopy.

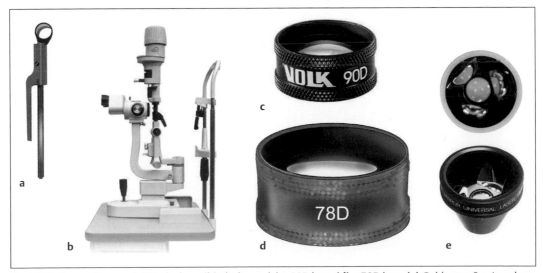

a

b

c

d

e

Fig. 27.9 Types of lenses. **(a)** Hruby lens. **(b)** Slit-lamp. **(c)** + 90D lens. **(d)** + 78D lens. **(e)** Goldmann 3-mirror lens.

Community Ophthalmology

Importance of Community Ophthalmology 728

Definition of Blindness 728

Magnitude of Blindness 728

Causes of Blindness 729

Prevention and Control of Blindness 730

National Program for Control of Blindness in India 734

Proposed NPCBVI Plan for Next 5 Years 737

Community ophthalmology is described as a new discipline in medicine, promoting eye health and blindness prevention through programs utilizing methodologies of public health, community medicine and ophthalmology.

It is the application of the knowledge of ophthalmology for the benefit of the community and the study of how ophthalmic speciality care can reach the last person in the community.

■ Importance of Community Ophthalmology

Community ophthalmology is beneficial for the community due to:

- Out reach at mass level.
- Treatment in remote areas.
- Screening of patients who are other wise missed and at times may land up into blindness.
- Health education and health system strengthening
- Early diagnosis and treatment of eye ailments e.g. school eye camps for refractive error, squint.

Blindness from birth or early childhood has unique problems. The branch of community ophthalmology deals with combating the blindness. It utilizes the ophthalmic knowledge to protect/promote ocular health, methodologies of public health, and community medicine to prevent blindness at the community level.

Prevention of blindness needs ample knowing and understanding of various aspects like:

- Definition of blindness.
- Magnitude of blindness.
- Causes of blindness.
- Control of blindness.

■ Definition of Blindness (OP9.4)

According to WHO, a person having visual acuity of less than 3/60 with correcting glasses in the better eye in day light is defined as blind. A concentric contraction of visual field to an average radius of 10 degree is considered equally disabling. Patients with visual field less than 10° are also considered blind.

■ Categories of Visual Impairment (OP9.4)

The visual impairment varies and may range from mild to severe. According to WHO, visual impairment can be classified as given in **Table 28.1**.

Table 28.1 Visual impairment as per WHO

Category of visual impairment	Best corrected visual acuity in the better eye
Normal vision	6/6 to 6/18
Moderate visual impairment (low vision)	Less than 6/18 to 6/60 (i.e., cannot see 6/18)
Severe visual impairment (low vision)	Less than 6/60 to 3/60 (i.e., cannot see 6/60)
Blindness	• Less than 3/60 to 1/60 (i.e., cannot see 3/60) or • Visual field <10° but >5° (i.e., between 5°–10°) • <1/60 to only light perception (i.e., cannot see 3/60) or visual field <5°. • No light perception

Abbreviation: WHO, World Health Organisation.

Table 28.2 Statistics of blindness

Cause of blindness	Number of people (in millions)
Blindness due to eye disease	37
Blindness due to refractive errors	08
(A) Total blindness due to all causes	45
Low vision due to eye diseases	124
Low vision due to refractive errors	145
(B) Total visual impairment due to all causes	269
Total visual impairment **(A + B)**	**314** (45 + 269)

Table 28.3 Global data on etiology of blindness

Cause of blindness	Percentage of blinds
Cataract	43%
Glaucoma	15%
Diabetic retinopathy	8%
Trachoma	11%
Vitamin A deficiency	6%
Onchocerciasis	1%

Magnitude of Blindness (OP9.4)

Geographic Distribution of Blindness

The problem of blindness is a worldwide phenomenon. Developing countries have more than 90% of all the blind and visually disabled people in the world because people in developing countries are deprived of adequate healthcare to prevent blindness (**Table 28.2**). On the other hand, in developed countries (Europe and North America), effective measures are taken to prevent blindness and eliminate the "avoidable" blindness ("preventable" and "curable" blindness).

Causes of Blindness

According to WHO, the six major causes of blindness are:
• Cataract.
• Glaucoma.
• Diabetic retinopathy.
• Trachoma.
• Vitamin A deficiency.
• Onchocerciasis.

The estimated number of blinds (%) due to the above causes are as given in **Table 28.3**.

Cataract, glaucoma, and diabetic retinopathy occur globally and require surgery or laser treatment. These also need an ophthalmologist for treatment. Trachoma, vitamin A deficiency, and onchocerciasis are focal diseases and occur regionally. These can be controlled with the medicine and do not necessarily require an ophthalmologist for treatment.

The causes of blindness in childhood and adults are given below.

Childhood Blindness

Causes of blindness during childhood vary according to the age group, as listed below.

In newborns:

- Congenital cataract.
- Congenital rubella (intrauterine).
- Nystagmus.
- Ophthalmia neonatorum.
- Retinopathy of prematurity.

In preschool and school-going children:

- Vitamin A deficiency.
- Measles.
- Trauma.
- Amblyopia.
- Strabismus.
- Refractive errors.

The causes of childhood blindness are different in the developed and developing countries too.

In developed countries:

- Retinopathy of prematurity.
- Congenital cataract.
- Congenital malformations.
- Nystagmus.

In developing countries:

- Corneal scarring.
- Vitamin A deficiency.
- Congenital cataract.
- Ophthalmia neonatorum.
- Congenital anomalies.

■ Adulthood Blindness

The common **causes** of visual impairments in adults are:

- Cataract.
- Glaucoma.
- High myopia.
- Trauma.
- Diabetic retinopathy.
- Retinal vascular disorders.
- Microbial keratitis.
- Age related macular degeneration.
- Neurological disorders (multiple sclerosis and brain tumors).
- AIDS (due to opportunist infections such as cytomegalovirus, herpetic, mycobacterial, fungal, syphilitic, or protozoal retinitis).

■ Prevention and Control of Blindness (OP9.4)

Measures to control blindness can be planned at various levels and should be based on:

- **Strategies to control the blindness:** It includes the following:
  ◇ Prevention of the disease before it occurs (primary prevention).
  ◇ Prevention of visual loss if the disease has occurred (secondary prevention).
  ◇ Restoration of sight of a blind person (tertiary prevention).
- **Approach to diseases causing blindness:** To restore and maintain good health in the community, the healthcare must include education, control of endemic diseases, good quality of food, water, and clean environment. There must be provision of services for cataract surgery, vitamin A supplementation, control of trachoma, and distribution of ivermectin for onchocerciasis.
- **Approach to provide services:** The services must be organized at the community level (primary eye care services) to promote, prevent, and treat the eye diseases. To make the services effective, education at various levels, adequate referral system and regular refresher training courses for primary care workers must be included. A willing person is selected and trained as a primary care worker. Education is aimed at making the people aware and general information (both environmental and personal) and measure of eye protection at work must be made known to the community.

The primary healthcare worker must be trained regarding the diseases such as ophthalmia neonatorum, trachoma, vitamin A deficiency, etc., who must recognize and treat the diseases. He must recognize and refer immediately for treatment in relation to conditions such as painful red eye with visual loss, cataract, entropion and trichiasis, corneal ulcers, penetrating injuries, vision-affecting pterygium, etc. The activities related to primary healthcare workers in the community must be supervised for a better healthcare delivery.

The secondary eye care services are provided by the general medical practitioners, ophthalmic assistants, or general medical officers trained in eye care. It comprises an adequate infrastructure (instruments and equipment) to handle common blinding conditions and also includes screening for open-angle glaucoma and diabetic retinopathy.

For diseases that need specialized treatment such as corneal grafting, retinal detachment surgery, etc., the patients are referred to large institutes in urban centers which have all the state-of-the-art diagnostic and therapeutic facilities (tertiary eye care services) as well as eye specialists.

In certain countries, a mobile ophthalmic unit (mobile eye services) is formed which conducts eye camps in the periphery and remote rural areas. These mobile ophthalmic units are supported by the government to provide the comprehensive eye care facilities and health education.

- **A community approach for blindness control:** It is directed at the target population at risk and concentrates on increasing awareness, assessment, and management of the disease to prevent the blindness.

■ Vision 2020: Right to Sight (OP9.4)

It is a global initiative of WHO and IAPB (International Agency for Prevention of Blindness) launched in the year 1999. It is a project to combat the problem of blindness in the world and eliminate the avoidable blindness by the year 2020. It is based on the concept that every living person has a right to sight. It is estimated that one person goes blind every 5 seconds and one child goes blind every minute. Approximately, 80% of global blindness is treatable and/or preventable; to eliminate this unnecessary blindness from the

world, WHO and IAPB are working in collaboration with various international nongovernmental organizations (NGOs).

Objectives of Vision 2020

The objective of this global initiative is to eradicate the avoidable blindness by the year 2020 which can be achieved by:

- Implementing specific programs to control the major causes of blindness.
- Creating adequate eye care facilities in under privileged areas.
- Creating well-trained eye care workers.

To implement Right to Sight (Vision 2020), WHO has focused on five main priorities:

- Cataract.
- Trachoma.
- Onchocerciasis.
- Childhood blindness.
- Refractive errors and low vision.

However, priorities are decided by a country, depending on the specific blinding conditions in that country. The Vision 2020 program was adopted by the government of India, and other diseases of national importance such as glaucoma, diabetic retinopathy, and corneal blindness are also to be tackled as priority.

■ Prevention and Control of the Causes of Blindness

Cataract

It is the main cause of blindness. The high-prevalence of blindness from cataract in developing countries is due to absence of effective high eye healthcare system and poor surgical care for cataract. Cataract may develop at an earlier age due to exposure to UV rays, X-rays, corticosteroids (oral and topical), malnutrition, and dehydration.

Prevention and Treatment

It includes:

- Screening for cataract by health worker and motivation of the affected people to undergo surgery at the primary level.

- Cataract surgery must be performed with intraocular lens implantation. There must be provision of facilities for cataract surgery of complicated cases and provision of trained staff at centers.

Trachoma

According to WHO, approximately 150 million people are affected by trachoma worldwide and nearly 6 million people are believed to be blind due to trachoma. Trachoma is potentially a blinding disease seen worldwide but mostly in developing countries. The disease results in more scarring and consequent blinding complications such as entropion and trichiasis with corneal opacity. To prevent visual loss and blindness from the disease, trachoma must be controlled.

The trachoma is associated with poverty, overcrowding, inadequate face-washing, improper sanitation, and nonavailability of clean water. The active trachoma decreases in severity/prevalence in developed countries. In India, blindness due to trachoma is on the decline.

Prevention and Treatment

In developing communities, the **SAFE** strategy is employed for control of trachoma.

S–**S**urgery (to correct entropion and trichiasis in order to prevent blindness)

A–**A**ntibiotic treatment (to reduce the severity of active trachoma, scarring and blinding complications). The effective antibiotics are topical and oral tetracycline, oral erythromycin, and sulphonamides. Oral sulphonamides have too many side effects but oral azithromycin is now recommended as single dose therapy due to its prolonged effect. Tetracycline eye ointment is applied twice daily for 6 weeks in active trachoma.

F–**F**acial cleanliness.

E–**E**nvironmental improvement (access to clean water and sanitation).

WHO established an alliance for the **G**lobal **E**limination of **T**rachoma by the end of year 2020 (**GET 2020**).

Onchocerciasis (River Blindness)

The disease is endemic in Africa, South and Central America, and Yemen. In Africa, the disease is more severe in countries along the major rivers which lie between 12° north and 15° south of the equator. The black fly (Simulium) is the intermediate host which lays its egg in fast-running water and lives near rivers. About 20 million people are affected with onchocerciasis and 25,000 are blind.

Prevention and Treatment

The goal of the treatment is to eliminate both the adult form and microfilariae from the body. Ivermectin is distributed to the affected population in endemic areas. The community-directed treatment with annual doses of ivermectin (150 µg /kg) is given as a single dose. The target is to develop "National Onchocerciasis Control Program" in endemic areas with the aim to eliminate the blindness due to onchocerciasis by the year 2020. WHO has sponsored a program to control the fly population and has been successful.

Childhood Blindness

Regional Distribution of Childhood Blindness

Approximately, 1.5 million children suffer from visual impairment and blindness in the world. Out of these, 1 million blind children live in Asia. **Table 28.4** shows the global prevalence of childhood blindness.

Table 28.4 Global prevalence of childhood blindness		
Region	**Prevalence per 1000 children**	**Estimated no. of blind children**
Africa	1.1	2,64,000
Asia	0.9	1,080,000
South and Central America	0.6	78,000
Europe, Japan and USA	0.3	72,000
Total		1,494,000

It is estimated that approximately 500,000 children in the world become blind each year; 50% of the childhood blindness is preventable. The aim of the project is to eliminate avoidable causes of childhood blindness by the year 2020.

Prevention and Treatment

To reduce the childhood blindness population at risk, which vary from place to place, causes of childhood blindness are identified. The eye disorders in children must first be identified by screening programs and then timely intervention must be conducted.

The main causes include Vitamin A deficiency, measles, ophthalmia neonatorum, congenital cataract, and retinopathy of prematurity.

Under the global initiative, Vision 2020 includes:

- Vitamin A supplementation.
- Immunization against measles and vaccination against rubella in all children at one year of age and in prepubertal girls.
- Cleansing the eyes of newborn babies after birth to prevent ophthalmia neonatorum, followed by application of 1% tetracycline eye ointment.
- Surgically avoidable causes of childhood blindness such as congenital cataract, glaucoma, and complicated cases of eye trauma are managed.
- Screening and treatment of retinopathy of prematurity is performed.
- School screening programs for diagnosis and management of common conditions like refractive errors, trachoma in endemic area, and health education in school must be promoted.

Prophylactic vitamin A administration in areas with endemic vitamin A deficiency is as given in **Table 28.5**.

Refractive Errors and Low Vision (IM24.15)

Refractive errors cause worldwide visual disability. A global initiative to combat refractive errors and low vision is required. Refractive errors are corrected by spectacles to prevent amblyopia, while the patient with low vision needs low-vision devices. The aim is to eliminate visual impairment (visual acuity less than 6/18) and blindness due to refractive errors or other causes of low vision. Refractive errors are on the priority of the Vision 2020 project. Strategies recommended under "Vision 2020" initiative include:

- Refractive services and dispensing of glasses.
- School eye health programs.
- Low vision service centers to be established at 150 tertiary level eye care institutions.

Glaucoma

Approximately, 15% of all blindness is due to glaucoma, whether it is congenital, primary open-angle, primary angle-closure, or secondary glaucoma. Primary open-angle is more common. Glaucoma is an important cause of blindness in developed and developing countries. It is estimated that nearly 600,000 people per year go blind from glaucoma globally. Vision loss due to glaucoma cannot be recovered, so to prevent blindness from this disease, early detection and proper treatment is important. The risk factors determined by epidemiological studies include age, intraocular pressure (IOP), positive family history, diabetes, hypertension, myopia, smoking, and alcohol intake.

Table 28.5 Prophylactic vitamin A administration	
In infants 6–12 months	100,000 IU of vitamin A orally every 3–6 months.
In children 1–6 years	200,000 IU of vitamin A orally every 3–6 months.
Lactating mothers	200,000 IU of vitamin A orally once a delivery or during the first 8 weeks after delivery if breast feeding.
Infants <6 months not on breast feeding	50,000 IU of vitamin A orally as a single dose.

Prevention and Treatment

A glaucoma scanning program is recommended for early detection and treatment of glaucoma which include tonometry and fundus examination. Visual field examination is conducted in persons with elevated IOP or fundus changes. Compared with open-angle glaucoma, acute angle-closure glaucoma is easier to diagnose. The primary healthcare workers must be trained to recognize acute red eye with pain, decreased vision, and dilated pupil, so that they immediately refer to a higher center. The patients at risk should be tested periodically by a qualified ophthalmologist.

Diabetic Retinopathy

It is a leading cause of blindness in adults both in developed and developing countries. To prevent visual loss from diabetic retinopathy, a periodic follow-up is very important because lost vision due to diabetic retinopathy cannot be recovered. It is uncommon in patients with duration of less than 10 years of diabetes but common after 20 years of diabetes.

Prevention and Treatment

It includes:
- Regular screening.
- Awareness by health workers.
- Referral to eye surgeon.
- Fundus fluorescein angiography and laser photocoagulation.
- Changes in lifestyle of individuals at risk.

Corneal Blindness

Corneal diseases are the leading cause of visual impairment. The major causes of corneal blindness are corneal ulcers which may be secondary to infections, injuries, and nutritional deficiencies. Microbial keratitis mostly affects agriculture workers in developing countries.

Prevention and Treatment

To reduce the prevalence of corneal blindness, the strategies include:
- Protective measures include use of goggles.

- Prevention and control of vitamin A deficiency to prevent xerophthalmia.
- Education of people regarding avoidance of ocular trauma.
- Health education and improvement in personal hygiene to reduce eye infections.
- Promotion of eye donation and establishment of eye banks.
- Keratoplasty to restore vision in cases of corneal blindness.

■ National Program for Control of Blindness in India (OP9.4)

The national program for control of blindness (NPCB) was launched by the government of India in the year 1976 as a 100% centrally sponsored program with the goal of reducing the prevalence of blindness from 1.4 to 0.3% by the year 2000. However, due to constraints at various levels, the target could not be achieved. As per a survey in 2001–02, prevalence of blindness was estimated to be 1.1%, which reduced to 1% in 2006–07, as per another survey on avoidable blindness conducted under NPCB. Therefore, NPCB set the objective to reduce the prevalence of blindness by the year 2020.

Later this was merged with vision 2020 program with a target to achieve blindness prevalence 0.3% by 2020. Currently 13th plan (2017–2020) is going on which has been renamed as "National program for control of blindness and visual impairment (NPCBVI)". Now part of funding is shared by states as well.

■ Objectives of NPCBVI

- To reduce the backlog of blindness through identification and treatment of the blind.
- To provide comprehensive eye care services.
- To improve quality service delivery to the affected population.
- To develop human resources for eye care.
- To enhance community awareness on eye care.

- To secure participation of voluntary organizations and private practitioners in eye care.
- To provide best possible treatment for curable blindness available in the district/region.
- To set up the mechanism for referral coordination and feedback between organizations dedicated to prevention, treatment and rehabilitation.

■ Strategies to Achieve the Objectives

The implementation of the program was decentralized with the formation of the State Health Society (blindness division) and District Health Society (**DHS**) in each district of the country.

State Health Society

Purpose

The purpose of state health society is to plan, implement, and monitor blindness control activities in all the districts of the state.

Functions

- To coordinate and monitor with all the district health societies.
- To receive and monitor the use of funds for equipment and material from the government.
- Repair and renovation of existing equipment.
- To secure participation of voluntary organizations and private practitioners in eye care.
- To promote eye donation through various media and monitor the districts for collection and utilization of eyes collected by eye banks.

DHS

Composition

It has a maximum of 15 members, consisting of not more than 8 ex-officio and seven other members as follows:
- Chairman: District magistrate

- Vice chairman: Chief medical officer/district health officer.
- Member secretary: Officer of the level of deputy CMO (preferably an ophthalmologist), may be designated as District Program Manager (DPM), who would also be the member secretary of the society.
- Technical advisor: Chief ophthalmic surgeon of district hospital. If medical college is located in the district, then Head of Department (HOD) of ophthalmology may be designated as technical advisor to the society.
- Members: Medical superintendent/civil surgeon of district hospital
  ◇ District education officer
  ◇ President local IMA branch
  ◇ Representatives from NGOs engaged in eye care services.
  ◇ Prominent practicing eye surgeons.

The membership of nonofficials should be for one year only and renewable as per the general body decisions for a further period. The ex-officio members shall be members as long as they hold the office.

Functions

The primary purpose of DHS is to plan, implement, and monitor blindness control activities in the district. The important functions of the DHS are:
- To assess the magnitude and spread of blindness village-wise in the district.
- Reduction in the backlog of blind persons– It is achieved by screening of population above 50 years, organizing screening eye camps, and transporting the operable cases.
- To train community level workers and ophthalmic assistants/nurses involved in eye care services.
- To receive and monitor use of funds, equipment, and materials.
- Screening of school age group children to identify and treat the refractive errors especially in underserved areas.
- To promote eye donation through various media, and monitor the districts for

collection and utilization of eyes collected by eye banks.

- Public awareness to prevent and treat the eye diseases.
- To involve voluntary and private hospitals.
- Development of mobile ophthalmic units in the district level for screening and transportation of patients.
- Establishment of vision centers in all PHCs.

The NPCB funds are released by the government of India to the state blindness control society, or state health and family welfare society, based on the annual action plan submitted. India has received technical and financial assistance from World Bank, WHO, DANIDA (Danish International Development Agency), and other international NGOs to control blindness in the country, but currently the program is not dependent on any external funding.

■ Achievements of NPCB

- Higher success rates following cataract surgery with intraocular lens (IOL) implantation as compared with conventional surgery. There has been a significant increase in cataract surgery with IOL implantation from <9% in 1994 to 93% in 2006–07.
- 307 dedicated eye operation theaters and eye wards built in district level hospitals.
- More than 2000 eye surgeons trained in eye surgery and other super specialties.
- Supply of ophthalmic equipment for diagnosis and treatment of common eye disorders.
- Training of teachers, screening of school children, and distribution of free glass in children with refractive errors under school eye screening programs during the year 2009–2010.

■ New Initiatives (Proposed) during 11th Five Year Plan (2007–2012)

Under the program, the following new initiatives are proposed:

- Construction of dedicated eye wards and eye operation theaters in district and subdistrict hospitals.
- Appointment of ophthalmic surgeons and ophthalmic assistant in new district and subdistrict hospitals.
- Appointment of ophthalmic assistants in PHCs/vision centers.
- Appointment of eye donation counsellors.
- Development of mobile ophthalmic units.
- Special attention to clear cataract backlog.
- Telemedicine in ophthalmology (eye care management information and communication network).
- Involvement of private practitioners in subdistrict, blocks, and village level.

A provision of Rs 1550 crore has been proposed for implementation of NPCB during the 11th five-year plan.

■ Initiative during 12th Five Year Plan (NPCB) (2013–2018)

Goals

- To reduce the prevalence of blindness to less than 0.3%.
- To establish infrastructure and efficiency levels in the program to be able to cater to new cases of blindness each year in order to prevent future backlog.

Objectives

- To reduce the backlog of blindness through identification and treatment of blind at primary, secondary, and tertiary levels, based on assessment of the overall burden of visual impairment in the country.
- Develop and strengthen the strategy of NPCB for "eye health" and prevention of visual impairment through provision of comprehensive eye care services and quality service delivery.
- Strengthening and upgradation of RIOs to become centers of excellence in various subspecialities of ophthalmology.

- Strengthening the existing and developing additional human resources and infrastructure facilities for providing high-quality comprehensive eye care in all districts of the country.
- To enhance community awareness on eye care and lay stress on preventive measures.
- Increase and expand research for prevention of blindness and visual impairment.
- To secure participation of voluntary organizations/private practitioners in eye care.

■ Proposed NPCBVI Plan for Next 5 Years

- To clear backlog of cataract blindness.
- Emphasis on quality of surgery.
- Main focus is upon- free cataract surgery, school eye screening, keratoplasties.

In an endeavor to enhance its action plan to hit the blindness, government of India encourages participation by non-government organizations (NGOs) by offering financial support (Grant-in-aid) to meet out expenses incurred. Grant-in-aid is given in **Table 28.6**.

Categorization of visual disability: The persons with visual disability get some government privileges. A categorization of visual disability for that purpose is required which is done by a board with specialists at district hospitals. **Fig. 28.1** is used to know the percentage of visual disability.

Table 28.6 NPCVI grants-in-aid: recurring

	Recurring grant per unit
Cataract surgery	• NGO: Rs 2000
	• NGO/Pvt using govt.
	• OT: Rs 1200
	• Govt.: Rs 1000
Diabetic retinopathy	• Rs 2000
Childhood blindness	• Rs 2000
Glaucoma	• Rs 2000
Keratoplasty	• Rs 7500
Vitreoretinal surgery	• Rs 10000
Spectacles	• Rs 350/pair of spectacles
Cornea collection	• Eye bank: Rs 2000
	• Collection centre: Rs 1000
Information	• Large states: Rs 20 lakh
Education	• Small states: Rs 10 lakh
Communication	

NPCBVI grants-in-aid: Non-recurring	
	Non-ecurring grant/unit
District hospital	Rs 40 lakh
Sub-district hospital	Rs 20 lakh
Vision centre/PHC for govt./NGO	Rs 01 lakh
Eye bank	Rs 40 lakh
Eye donation centres	Rs 01 lakh
Multipurpose district mobile ophthalmic units	Rs 30 lakh
Fixed Tele-ophthalmology network	Rs 25 lakh

Abbreviations: PHC, primary health care; NGO, non-government organization.

	6/6 to 6/18	6/24	6/36	6/60	3/60	2/60	1/60	HMCF to PL
Left eye vision (Best corrected visual acuity (BCVA))								
6/6 to 6/18	0%	10%	10%	10%	20%	30%	30%	30%
6/24	10%	40%	40%	40%	50%	60%	60%	60%
6/36	10%	40%	40%	40%	50%	60%	60%	60%
6/60	20%	40%	40%	40%	50%	60%	60%	60%
3/60	20%	50%	50%	50%	70%	80%	80%	80%
2/60	30%	60%	60%	60%	80%	90%	90%	90%
1/60	30%	60%	60%	60%	80%	90%	90%	90%
HMCF to PL	30%	60%	60%	60%	80%	90%	90%	100%

Row labels are Right eye vision (Best corrected visual acuity (BCVA)); column header above table is Left eye vision (Best corrected visual acuity (BCVA))

Yellow- Right eye is better eye   Brown- Left eye is better eye
Percentage disability is marked inside the box corresponding to the visual acuity for both eyes

Under Rights of persons with Disabilities Act, 2016 (RPWD Act, also known as Divyangjan Adhikaar Kanoon 2016). Low vision is considered to be one of 21 disabilities. A person having benchmark disability (40%), can avail disability benefits from the government.

Fig. 28.1 Categorization of visual disability.

Index

A

Abducens nerve and its lesions, 598–601
Acanthamoeba keratitis, 143–144
Accessory lacrimal glands, 84, 545–546
Accommodation
  amplitude of, 43
  anomalies of, 43
  insufficiency of, 43–45
  mechanism of, 41–43
  physiology of, 41
  spasm of, 45
Accommodative esotropia, 453–454
Acid burns, 497–498
Acne rosacea, 153–154
Acquired cataract, 235–244
Acquired immune deficiency syndrome (AIDS), 643, 646
Acquired non-accommodative esotropia, 455
Acquired nystagmus, 610
Acquired retinoschisis See Senile retinoschisis
Acquired toxoplasmosis, 200
Active secretion, 260
Acute corneal edema, 505
Acute disseminated encephalomyelitis, 621
Acute hemorrhagic conjunctivitis, 96
Acute mucopurulent and purulent conjunctivitis, 90
Acute posterior multifocal placoid pigment epitheliopathy (APMPPE), 363
Acute pseudomembranous and membranous conjunctivitis, 90–91
Acute purulent retinitis, 359
Acute retinal necrosis (ARN), 196
Acute systemic herpes zoster treatment, 143
Acyclovir, 141, 143
Adaptations in strabismus, 465
  head posture, 469
  motor, 468–469
  sensory, 466–468
Adenoviral infections, 94–95
Adie's tonic pupil, 595
Adrenaline, 75
Adrenergic agonists, 283–284
Adulthood blindness, 730
Adult inclusion conjunctivitis, 97–98
Advanced diabetic eye disease, 349
Advanced glaucomatous field defects, 278

Afferent pathway of pupil, 213–214
Afferent pupillary defect, 591–592
Age-related macular degeneration (ARMD), 372–375
Albinism, 649
Alcian blue dye, 126
Alkali burns, 496–497
Alkylating agents, 77
Allergic conjunctivitis, 104
  atopic keratoconjunctivitis (AKC), 109–110
  clinical features and symptoms of, 105
  contact allergic (toxic) conjunctivitis, 111
  giant papillary conjunctivitis (GPC), 110–111
  phlyctenular conjunctivitis, 111–112
  seasonal and perennial, 107–108
  treatment of, 105–106
  vernal keratoconjunctivitis (VKC), 108–109
Allergic edema, 518
Alzheimer disease, 628
Amaurosis fugax, 615–616
Amaurotic pupil, 591
Amblyopia, 449–450
Ameobicides, 144
Ametropia, 45–46
Aminoglycosides, 144
Amiodarone induced optic neuropathy, 415
Amyloid degeneration, 319
Anatomical (pupillary) axis, 449
Anemia, retinopathy in, 358
Anesthesia, for cataract surgery, 246–248
Aneurysm of ICA, 429
Angioid streaks, 375–376
Angiomatosis retinae, 384
Angle closure
  mechanism, 294–295
  types, 295–298
Angle kappa, 449
Angle of deviation, 471–473
Angular conjunctivitis, 93–94
Aniridia, 212
Anisometropia, 56–57, 449
Ankyloblepharon, 537
Ankylosing spondylitis, 202, 639
Anomaloscope, 30
Anopia, 424–425
Anterior capsular cataract, 135
Anterior chamber
  examination, 716
  lenses, 252

Anterior ischemic optic neuropathy (AION), 407–409
Anterior necrotizing scleritis, 168–169
Anterior non-necrotizing scleritis, 168
Anterior polar cataract, 233
Anterior scleritis, 168–169
Anterior segment, 2–3
Anterior staphyloma, 170
Anterior subcapsular lens opacities, 507
Anterior synechiae, 135
Anterior uveitis, 180, 182–190
  anterior chamber signs, 183–185
  anterior vitreous sign, 185
  circum corneal (ciliary) congestion, 182
  complications, 190
  corneal signs, 182, 184
  differential diagnosis, 187
  investigations, 187
  lenticular signs, 185
  pupillary signs, 185
  symptoms, 180, 182
  treatment
    corticosteroids, 188–189
    cycloplegics and mydriatics, 187–188
    cytotoxic agents, 189–190
Antiallergic drugs
  antihistamines, 74
  dual action agents, 74
  mast cell stabilizers, 73–74
Antifungal agents, 69
  azoles, 70–71
  classification, 70
  flucytosine (5-FC), 71
  polyene antibiotics, 70
Antiglaucoma drugs, 280–288
Antiherpes agents, 67
  acyclovir, 67–68
  famciclovir, 69
  ganciclovir, 68–69
  idoxuridine (IDU), 67
  trifluorothymidine (TFT/F3T), 67
  valacyclovir, 69
  vidarabine, 69
Antihistamines, 106
Anti-inflammatory drugs
  corticosteroids, 72–73
  NSAIDs, 73
Antimetabolites, 76–77
Antimicrobial drugs
  aminoglycosides, 64–65
  cephalosporins, 64
  chloramphenicol, 65
  classification, 62–63
  fluoroquinolones, 66
  macrolides, 65–66

penicillins, 63–64
polypeptides, 65
sulphonamides, 67
tetracyclines, 66
vancomycin (glycopeptide), 64
Antiretroviral agents, 69
Anti-vascular endothelial growth factor, 75
Anti-vascular endothelial growth factor (Anti-VEGF) agents, 75
Antiviral agents, 67
"A" patterns, 457–459
Aphakia, 249–252, 309
Aphakic correction choice, in children, 255
Apparent squint See Pseudostrabismus
Applanation tonometry, 267–269
Aqueous formation, 259–260
Aqueous humor, 257–261, 261–262
Aqueous misdirection syndrome See Malignant glaucoma
Aqueous outflow, 260–261
Arcuate NFB defects, 277
Arcus senilis (gerontoxon), 154
Argon laser trabeculoplasty (ALT), 291
Argyll Robertson (AR) pupil, 594
Argyrosis, 124
Aromatic diamidines, 144
Arterial supply of eyeball, 3, 4
Arteriolar–venular shunts, 330
Ascending optic atrophy, 416
Asteroid hyalosis, 319
Asthenopia, 713
Astigmatic power and axis, 54
Astigmatism, 52–56
  etiology, 52
  keratotomy, 684–685
  optics in, 53
  symptoms, 53–54
  treatment, 56
  types, 53, 55
Atheroma of carotids, 429–430
Atheromatous corneal ulcer, 153
Atopic keratoconjunctivitis (AKC), 109–110
Atrophic papilloedema, 401
Atropine, 74
Axial hypermetropia, 50
Azathioprine, 76–77
Azithromycin, 66
Azoles, 70–71, 144

B

Bacterial cell wall, 62

Bacterial conjunctivitis, 89–94
  acute mucopurulent and
    purulent conjunctivitis, 90
  acute pseudomembranous
    and membranous
    conjunctivitis, 90–91
  angular conjunctivitis, 93–94
  chronic, 92–93
  gonorrhoeal (hyperacute)
    conjunctivitis, 91–93
  pathophysiology of, 89
  types of, 89
Bacterial endophthalmitis,
  205–206
Bacterial keratitis, 128–135
  causative organisms, 129
  clinical features, 130
  corneal ulcer
    complications, 134–135
    management, 132
  pathogenesis of, 129–130
    treatment, 132–134
  defence mechanisms, 128
  hypopyon corneal ulcer, 131
  predisposing factors, 128–129
Bacterial uveitis, 193–194
Bagolini striated glasses test,
  473–474
Band keratopathy, 190
Band shaped keratopathy, 155
Baring of blind spot, 278
Basal cell carcinoma (BCC),
  541–542
β-blockers, 281–283
Behçet syndrome, 203
Bergmeister papilla, 420
Best's disease See Best's
  vitelliform macular dystrophy
Best's vitelliform macular
  dystrophy, 382, 383
Bilateral cataracts, 235
Binasal hemianopia, 428
Binocular diplopia, 713–714
Binocular vision, 32, 421, 475
  advantages of, 34
  conditions necessary for, 33
  development of, 33
  disorders of, 34
  grades, 33–34
Bipolar cells, 14–15
Bird shot retinochoroidopathy,
  363–364
Bitemporal hemianopia, 428
Blepharitis, 519–522
Blepharochalasis, 538
Blepharophimosis, 537–538
Blepharospasm, 538–539
Blindness
  adulthood, 730
  causes of, 729–730
  childhood, 729–730, 732–733
  definition of, 728–729
  magnitude of, 729
  prevention and control, 730
    cataract, 731–732
    corneal blindness, 734
    diabetic retinopathy, 734
    glaucoma, 733–734
    onchocerciasis, 732

  refractive errors and low
    vision, 733
  trachoma, 732
  Vision 2020, 731
Blinking act, 550
Blood disorders, vascular
  retinopathies in, 358–359
Blow-out fracture of medial
  wall, 590
Blow-out fracture of orbital
  floor, 589
Blue-dot cataract, 232–233
Blue sclera, 172
Blunt trauma, 503–508, 506
Bourneville disease See
  Tuberous sclerosis
Bowen intra epithelial
  epithelioma, 483
Bowman layer dystrophies, 157
Brain abscess, 622
Branch retinal artery occlusion
  (BRAO), 341
Branch retinal vein occlusion
  (BRVO), 343–344
Brown's syndrome, 465
Brun's nystagmus, 611
Bull's eye maculopathy, 371
Butterfly-shaped macular
  dystrophy, 382

C
Calcific degeneration See Band
  shaped keratopathy
Campimetry, 26
Canaliculi, 547
Canaliculitis, 552
Candidiasis, 199
Capillaropathy, 346
Carbonic anhydrase inhibitors
  (CAIs), 284–285
Carotid artery occlusive disease,
  616
Cataract, 228–230, 238
  acquired, 235–244
  developmental, 230–235
  management, 244–249
  prevention and control,
    731–732
Cataract surgery, 686
  anesthesia for, 246–248
  cataract extraction, 248–249
  complications
    due to local anesthesia, 694
    intraoperative, 694–695
    postoperative, 695–700
  extracapsular cataract
    extraction, 687–688
  intracapsular cataract
    extraction, 687
  nuclear chop technique, 693
  phacoemulsification, 690, 692
  postoperative management
    in, 693–694
  small incision cataract
    surgery, 688–690, 691, 693
Catarrhal ulcer See Marginal
  ulcer
Caterpillar hair conjunctivitis
  See Ophthalmia nodosa

Cationic antiseptics, 144
Cavernous sinus thrombosis
  (CST), 578
Central areolar choroidal
  atrophy, 209
Central chorioretinitis, 361
Central corneal thickness (CCT),
  126, 269
Central guttate choroidal
  atrophy, 209
Central retinal artery occlusion
  (CRAO), 340–341
Central retinal vein occlusion
  (CRVO), 342–343
Central serous
  chorioretinopathy (CSR),
  365–366
Cerebellopontine angle, tumors
  of, 626
Cerebellum, tumors of, 626
Cerebral areas, 443
Cerebral contusion, 627
Chalazion, 523
Chalcosis, 124
Chemical injuries, 496–499
Chemosis, 86–87
Chiasma
  nerve fiber arrangement
    within, 422
  and pituitary gland, tumors
    of, 626
Childhood blindness, 729–730,
  732–733
Childhood glaucoma, 311–315
Childhood metastatic tumors,
  587
Chin elevation, 469
Chlamydial conjunctivitis,
  97–101
  adult inclusion conjunctivitis,
    97–98
  neonatal chlamydial
    conjunctivitis, 98
  trachoma, 98–101
  transmission of, 97
Chlamydia species, 97
Chlamydia trachomatis, 97
Chlorambucil, 77
Chloroquine toxicity, 371
Choroid
  degenerative changes in,
    209–211
  detachment of, 211–212
Choroidal lesions following
  blunt trauma, 507
Choroideremia, 210–211
Chromatic aberration, 38
Chronic chiasmal arachnoiditis,
  429
Chronic conjunctivitis, 92–93
Chronic papilloedema, 401
Chronic posterior cyclitis See
  Intermediate uveitis
Chronic progressive external
  ophthalmoplegia (CPEO), 629
Chronic serpiginous ulcer See
  Mooren's ulcer
Chrysiasis, 124

Ciliary block glaucoma See
  Malignant glaucoma
Ciliary body, 257
Ciliary ganglion, 6
Ciliary muscle, 74
Ciliary staphyloma, 171
City university test, 30
Climatic droplet keratopathy
  See Spheroidal degeneration
Clotrimazole, 71
Cluster headache, 631
Cockayne's syndrome, 380
Coloboma
  of lens, 225
  of lids, 544
  of optic disc, 418–419
  of retina, 338
  of uveal tract, 212
Color blindness, 713
Colored halos, 712
Color sense, 19–20
Color vision, theories of, 21
Comitant convergent squint,
  453–455
Comitant divergent squint,
  455–457
Comitant strabismus, 452–459
Community ophthalmology,
  728
Concave lenses, 37–38
Concretions, 114
Concussion, 626–627
Concussion/contusion injury,
  503–504
Conductive keratoplasty (CK),
  686
Confocal microscope, 127
Confrontation test, 25–26
Congenital glaucoma, 312–315
Congenital myopia, 47
Congenital toxoplasmosis,
  199–200
Conjunctiva
  anatomy of, 83, 84
  blood supply, 85
  bulbar, 83
  degenerative changes in
    concretions, 114
    pinguecula, 114
    pterygium, 115, 116
  examination, 715
  forniceal, 83
  glands, 84
  histology, 83–84
  inflammation of See
    Conjunctivitis
  lymphatic drainage, 85
  nerve supply, 84–85
  palpebral, 83
Conjunctival disorders
  clinical features of, 85–86
  conjunctival inflammatory
    reactions, 86–89
  eye discharge, 86
  lymphadenopathy, 89
Conjunctival epithelial
  melanosis, 483
Conjunctival flora of eye, 85

Conjunctival inflammatory
reactions, 86–89
Conjunctival injection *See*
Hyperemia of conjunctiva
Conjunctival naevus
(conjunctival mole), 482
Conjunctival papilloma, 483
Conjunctivitis
in blistering mucocutaneous
diseases
ocular cicatricial
pemphigoid, 112–113
Stevens–Johnson
syndrome, 113–114
definition, 89
infective, 89–104
bacterial conjunctivitis,
89–94
chlamydial conjunctivitis,
97–101
granulomatous
conjunctivitis, 103–104
neonatal conjunctivitis,
101–103
viral conjunctivitis, 94–97
noninfective, 104–114
Conjunctivodacryocysto-
rhinostomy, 670
Connective tissue disorders
Ehlers–Danlos syndrome, 638
giant cell arteritis, 637
Marfan syndrome, 638
pseudoxanthoma elasticum,
638
rheumatoid arthritis, 636
sarcoidosis, 637–638
systemic lupus
erythematosus, 636–637
Vogt–Koyanagi–Harada
syndrome, 638
Wegener's granulomatosis,
638
Connective tissue system of
orbit, 567–568
Contact allergic (toxic)
conjunctivitis, 111
Contact lenses, 50, 52, 56,
57–59, 58
aphakic correction with,
251–252
side effects, 59
types, 58–59
Contrast sensitivity *See* Sense
of contrast
Convergence-retraction
nystagmus, 611
Convex lens, 37, 38
Copper deposition, 124
Coralliform cataract, 232
Cornea, 117
anatomy of, 117, 118
blood supply of, 119
Bowman's membrane, 118
Descemet's membrane, 119
endothelium, 119
epithelium, 117–118
examination, 716
metabolism of, 119–120
nerve supply of, 119, 120

pathological changes in,
120, 121
corneal edema, 121–122
corneal filaments, 124
corneal opacity, 122–123
deep vascularization, 123
infiltrates, 124
pigmentation of cornea,
123–124
prominent corneal nerves,
124
superficial vascularization,
123
and sclera, development
of, 11
stroma, 118–119
Corneal abrasion, 504
Corneal aesthesiometer, 126
Corneal blindness prevention
and control, 734
Corneal curvature modification,
680–681
Corneal degenerations
arcus senilis (gerontoxon),
154
band shaped keratopathy, 155
classification, 154
etiology, 154
hassell–henle bodies, 154
Salzmann nodular
degeneration, 156
spheroidal degeneration,
155–156
Terrien's marginal
degeneration, 154–155
Vogt limbal girdle, 154
Corneal diseases
evaluation of, 124–127
symptoms of, 124
Corneal dystrophies, 156–161
Corneal edema, 121–122
Corneal filaments, 124
Corneal opacity, 122–123
Corneal sensations, 126
Corneal sensitivity, 126
Corneal staining, 126
Corneal stromal procedures,
682–684
Corneal surface procedures,
681–682
Corneal surgery, 50
keratoplasty, 676–679
keratoprostheses, 679–680
Corneal topography, 125
Corneal ulcer, topical
corticosteroids in, 133–134
Coronary cataract, 232
Cortical blindness, 618
Cortical senile cataract,
235–237
Corticosteroids, 72–73
for allergic conjunctivitis,
106, 107
for anterior uveitis, 188–189
for bacterial endophthalmitis,
206
Cotton-wool spots, 330
Cover tests, 470–471

Cranial nerve nuclei and
respective nerves, lesions
of, 448
Cranial nerves, disorders of
abducens nerve and its
lesions, 598–601
facial nerve and its lesions,
603–607
neuroophthalmological
significance, 595
oculomotor nerve and its
lesions, 596–597
trigeminal nerve and its
lesions, 601–603
trochlear nerve and its
lesions, 597–598
Craniopharyngioma, 428–429
Cryotherapy, 654–655
Cryptophthalmos, 544
Crypts of Henle, 84
Curvature hypermetropia, 50
Cushing's syndrome, 641
Cyclitic membrane, 190
Cyclopentolate, 75
Cyclophoria, 451
Cyclophosphamide, 77
Cycloplegia *See* Paralysis of
accommodation
Cycloplegics, 133, 187–188
Cyclosporine, 77
Cylindrical lenses, 38
Cysticercosis, 201–202, 577, 647
Cystoid macular edema (CME),
190, 366–368
Cysts of iris, 212
Cytomegalovirus (CMV)
retinitis, 197
Cytotoxic agents, anterior
uveitis, 189–190

D

Dacryoadenitis, 564
Dacryocystectomy, 669–670
Dacryocystitis
acquired, 558–559
congenital, 558
Dacryocystorhinostomy (DCR),
667–670
Dacryops, 564
Dark adaptation, 19, 29
Day blindness, 713
Deep vascularization, 123
Deformities of eye lashes,
524–525
Degenerative changes in uveal
tract, 208
degenerative changes in
choroid, 209–211
detachment of choroid,
211–212
essential atrophy of iris,
208–209
Demyelinating disease, 618
acute disseminated
encephalomyelitis, 621
diffuse sclerosis, 621
multiple sclerosis, 619–620
neuromyelitis optica,
620–621

Dendritic ulcer, 138
Dermatochalasis, 538
Dermatogenic cataract, 242
Dermoid, 481–482, 582
Dermolipoma, 482, 582
Descemetocele, 134
Descemet's membrane, 134
Descending (retrograde) optic
atrophy, 416
Deutranopia, 20
Developmental cataract,
230–235
Devic's disease *See*
Neuromyelitis optica
Diabetes mellitus (DM), 238,
346, 640
Diabetic maculopathy, 349–351
Diabetic papillopathy, 409–411
Diabetic retinopathy (DR),
346–351, 734
Diffuse chorioretinal atrophy,
378
Diffuse scleritis, 168
Diffuse sclerosis, 621
Diminution of vision, 709–711
Diplopia, 461–462, 477–480,
713
Direct ophthalmoscopy, 726
Disc edema, 396–397
Disciform keratitis, 139
Disinfection of tonometers, 270
Disseminated or diffuse
choroiditis, 191–192
Distant direct ophthalmoscopy,
725–726
Distortion of vision, 711
Districhiasis, 525
Double elevator palsy, 461
Down beat nystagmus, 610
Down syndrome, 241–242, 649
Drug-induced maculopathy, 371
Drusen of optic disc, 401
Dry eye, 559–562
Dual action drugs, for allergic
conjunctivitis, 106
Duane's retraction syndrome
(DRS), 465
Duochrome test, 723
Dyes, in ophthalmology, 79–82
Dynamic contour tonometer
(DCT), 270
Dystrophia myotonica, 241
Dystrophies of retina
macular dystrophies
Best's vitelliform macular
dystrophy, 382, 383
butterfly-shaped macular
dystrophy, 382
familial dominant drusen,
381–382
juvenile retinoschisis, 380
Leber congenital amaurosis,
382
progressive cone dystrophy,
382
sphingolipidoses, 382–383
stargardt disease and
fundus flavimaculatus,
381

Tay–Sachs disease, 383
retinitis pigmentosa, 378–380

E
Eales' disease, 360–361
Early onset nystagmus, 609
Early papilloedema, 401
Eccentric fixation, 450
Econazole, 71
Ectatic cicatrix, 134
Ectatic conditions of cornea,
161–163
Ectopia lentis, 225–228
Ectropion, 535–536, 662–663
Edema of lids, 518–519
Efferent ocular motor pathway,
434
Efferent pathway of pupil,
214–215
Efferent pupillary defect, 592
Ehlers–Danlos syndrome, 638
Electrical injuries, 511–512
Electromagnetic spectrum, 35
Electro-oculography (EOG),
31, 332
Electrophysiological tests, 332
Electroretinography (ERG),
30–31, 332
Emmetropia, 45, 46
Emmetropic eye, refraction
in, 46
Encephalitis, 622
Encephalofacial angiomatosis,
385
End-gaze nystagmus, 608
Endocrine disorders
Cushing's syndrome, 641
diabetes mellitus, 640
homocystinuria, 641
hyperthyroidism, 640
hypoparathyroidism,
640–641
Endolaser DCR, 669
Endophthalmitis, 135, 205–207,
207–208
Endoscopic transnasal DCR, 669
endothelial cell count, 126–127
Endothelial corneal dystrophies,
158–161
Enlargement of blind spot, 278
Entropion, 532–535
lid surgery for, 660–662
Enucleation, 706–707
Epibulbar tumors, 481–483
Epicanthus, 543–544
Epidemic keratoconjunctivitis
(EKC), 94–95
Epikeratophakia, 681
Epiphora, 551–553
Epiretinal membrane (ERM),
370
Episcleral tissue, 164
Episcleritis, 165–167, 166
Epithelial basement membrane
dystrophy, 156–157
Epithelial dystrophies, 156–157
Epithelial keratitis treatment,
140
Equatorial staphyloma, 171–172

Erythromycin, 65–66
Esophoria, 450
Esotropia See Comitant
convergent squint
Essential atrophy of iris,
208–209
Essential infantile esotropia,
454–455
Ethambutol optic neuropathy,
415
Evisceration, 706
Exophoria, 450
Exophthalmos, 581
Exotropia See Comitant
divergent squint
Exposure keratitis, 151–153
External ophthalmoplegia, 460
Extracapsular cataract
extraction (ECCE), 687–688
Extraocular (superficial) foreign
bodies, 499–500
Extraocular muscles (EOMs)
actions of, 437–438
blood supply, 438–439
central nervous control, 434
course of, 436–437
insertion, 435
nerve supply, 435
origin, 434–435
Eye
and fundus examination, 470
light damage to, 495–496
optical system of, 39
reduced, 39–41, 40
Eyeballs
accessory structures of, 12–13
anatomy, 1
arterial supply, 3
blood supply of, 3–5, 4
embryology of, 6–13
differentiation, 7–8
embryogenesis, 7
important events in, 13
ocular structures, 9–13
organogenesis, 7
examination, 715
injuries to, 503
innervation of, 5–6
segments, 2–3
structure, 1–2
surgery on
enucleation, 706–707
evisceration, 706
Eye discharge, 86
Eye drops, systemic reactions
to, 79, 80
Eyelids
benign tumors of, 539–541
blood supply, 516–517
congenital anomalies of,
543–544
disorders of
ankyloblepharon, 537
blepharochalasis, 538
blepharophimosis, 537–538
blepharospasm, 538–539
deformities of eye lashes,
524–525
dermatochalasis, 538

disorders of lid margins
and palpebral aperture,
526–532
ectropion, 535–536
edema of lids, 518–519
entropion, 532–535
eyelid retraction, 532
inflammation of lid glands,
522–524
inflammation of lids,
519–522
lagophthalmos, 539
symblepharon, 536–537
glands, 517
injuries, 543
lymphatic drainage, 516
malignant tumors of,
541–543
margin, 513
nerve supply, 516
retraction, 532
structure, 513–515

F
Face turn, 468
Facial angioma, 386
Facial nerve and its lesions,
603–607
Facultative hypermetropia, 51
Familial dominant drusen,
381–382
Farnsworth-Munsell 100-Hue
test, 30
Favre–Goldmann syndrome,
322
Ferry's line, 123
Field defects
in lesions of optic radiations,
431
in LGB, 431
in optic chiasma lesions, 428
in optic nerve lesions,
427–428
in optic tract lesions, 430–431
in visual cortex lesions,
431–433
Filamentary keratitis, 149–150
Filtering bleb, 123
Filtering surgery See
Trabeculectomy
Fixation types, 473
Floaters, 712
Floriform cataract, 232
Flucytosine (5-FC), 71
Fluorescein and Rose Bengal
dyes, 126
Fluorescein sodium, 81
5-Fluorouracil (5-FU), 78
Focal choroiditis, 191
Focal pigment clumps, 378
Follicular reaction, 87, 88
Foreign body sensation, 708
Form sense, 19
Foscarnet, 69
Foster–Kennedy syndrome,
397, 398
Fracture of base of skull, 429
Frontal lobe, tumors of, 624

Fuchs' endothelial dystrophy,
158–160
Fuchs heterochromic
iridocyclitis, 204
Fundus angiography, 332–335
Fundus examination, 718,
725–727
Fungal endophthalmitis,
206–207
Fungal keratitis, 135–137
clinical features, 136
diagnosis, 136
etiology, 136
risk factors for, 135–136
treatment, 136–137
Fungal orbital cellulitis, 577
Fungal uveitis, 198–199
Fungi, 69
Fusional reserve, 450

G
Galactosemia and cataract,
238–239
Ganglion cells, 15
Gaze centers, 443–444,
446–448
Gaze-paretic nystagmus,
610–611
Generalized constriction of
visual field, 278
Geographical choroidopathy See
Serpiginous choroidopathy
Ghost cell glaucoma, 308
Giant cell arteritis, 637
Giant papillary conjunctivitis
(GPC), 110–111
Glare, 712–713
Glaucoma, 189
childhood, 311–315
classification, 265
clinical examination
gonioscopy, 270–273
optic nerve head analysis,
273–275
RNFL analysis, 279–280
tonography, 270
tonometry, 265–270
visual field analysis,
275–279
laser treatment, 700
normal-tension, 265, 292
optic nerve damage in,
289–290
prevention and control,
733–734
primary angle-closure,
293–298
primary open-angle, 288–292
secondary, 134, 298–311
trabeculectomy, 700–701
"Glaucoma suspect," 292
Glaucomatocyclitic crisis, 204,
304
Glaucomatous field defect,
278–279
Glaucomatous optic atrophy,
417
Goblet cells, 84
Gold deposition, 124

Goniolenses, 272
Gonioscopic identification of angle structures, 272
Gonioscopy, 270–273
Goniotomy, 314–315
Gonorrhoeal (hyperacute) conjunctivitis, 91–92, 93
Granular dystrophy, 157–158
Granuloma, 483
Granulomatous chronic anterior uveitis, 196
Granulomatous conjunctivitis, 103–104
Graves' ophthalmopathy, 578–582
Gullstrand See Schematic eye
Gyrate atrophy of choroid, 209–210

H
Hansen disease See Leprosy
Hard exudates, 329–330
Hassell–Henle bodies, 154
Headache, 623, 630–635
Head injury
  cerebral contusion, 627
  concussion, 626–627
  skull base fractures, 627–628
Head posture
  abnormal, 462, 477
  in ocular paralysis, 469
Head tilt, 468–469
Hemangioma, 540
Hematological diseases, 647–648
Hemeralopia See Day blindness
Hemianopia, 425–426
Hemolytic glaucoma, 308
Hemosiderotic glaucoma, 308
Hepatolenticular degeneration See Wilson disease
Hereditary optic neuropathy, 412–413
Hering theory, 21
Herpes simplex, 643
Herpes simplex conjunctivitis, 96
Herpes simplex keratitis
  complications, 139
  diagnosis, 140
  disciform keratitis, 139
  neonatal infection, 137
  primary infection, 137–138
  recurrent infection, 138–139
  stromal necrotizing keratitis, 139
  treatment, 140–141
Herpes zoster, 643
Herpes zoster ophthalmicus (HZO), 141–143
Herpetic eye disease, 139
Herpetic uveitis, 196–197
Heterochromia of iris, 212
Heteronymous hemianopia, 426
Heterophoria, 450–451
Heterotropia, 450–452
High myopia, 47, 48
Hirschberg test, 471
Holmgren wool's test, 30

Homatropine, 75
Homocystinuria, 641
Homonymous hemianopia, 425–426
Hordeolum internum, 522–523
Horner's syndrome, 593
HSV iridocyclitis treatment, 141
Hudson–Stahli line, 123
Hyperemia of conjunctiva, 86
Hypermetropia, 50–52
Hyperosmotic agents, 287–288
Hyperphoria, 450
Hypersecretion of tears, 550
Hypertensive iridocyclitis, 189
Hypertensive retinopathy, 351–353
Hyperthyroidism, 640
Hypertropia, 457
Hyphema, 123, 505–506
Hypoparathyroidism, 238, 640–641

I
Idiopathic orbital inflammation, 575–576
Imidazoles, 71
Immune modulators, for allergic conjunctivitis, 106
Immunologically mediated keratitis, 146–148
Immunological uveitis, 202–204
Immunomodulators, 77–78
Immunosuppressant drugs, 76–78
Implants, 707
Incomitant strabismus, 459–465
Indentation gonioscopy (pressure gonioscopy), 271
Indentation tonometry, 265–267
Index hypermetropia, 50
Indirect ophthalmoscopy, 726–727
Indocyanine green (ICG), 81
Indocyanine green angiography, 335–336
Infections, 509–510
Infectious keratitis, 127
  bacterial keratitis, 128–135
  fungal keratitis, 135–137
  parasitic keratitis, 143–144
  viral keratitis, 137–143
Infective conjunctivitis, 89–104
  bacterial conjunctivitis, 89–94
  chlamydial conjunctivitis, 97–101
  granulomatous conjunctivitis, 103–104
  neonatal conjunctivitis, 101–103
  viral conjunctivitis, 94–97
Infective diseases, eye in, 641
  AIDS, 643, 646
  cytomegalovirus, 643
  herpes simplex, 643
  herpes zoster, 643
  leprosy, 642
  measles, 643
  mumps, 643

rubella, 643
syphilis, 643
tuberculosis (TB), 642
Inferior orbital fissure, 567
Infiltrates, 124
Inflammation of cornea see Keratitis
Inflammation of lid glands, 522–524
Inflammation of lids, 519–522
Inflammation of optic nerve, 403–407
Inflammation of sclera
  episcleritis, 165–167, 166
  scleritis, 167–170
Inflammatory edema, 518
Inherited disorders, in eyes, 649–650
Installation, 60–61
Intercalary staphyloma, 170–171
Intermediate uveitis, 190–191
Internal ophthalmoplegia, 461
Internuclear pathways, lesions of, 444, 446–448
Interstitial keratitis (IK), 144–146
Intracapsular cataract extraction (ICCE), 687
Intracorneal rings (ICR), 684
Intracranial aneurysms, 613–614
Intracranial infections
  brain abscess, 622
  encephalitis, 622
  meningitis, 621–622
Intracranial space occupying lesions (ICSOLs), 397
  categorization of, 623
  cerebellopontine angle, tumors of, 626
  cerebellum, tumors of, 626
  chiasma and pituitary gland, tumors of, 626
  frontal lobe, tumors of, 624
  headache, 623
  midbrain, tumors of, 625–626
  occipital lobe, tumors of, 624
  papilloedema, 623
  parietal lobe, tumors of, 624
  pons, tumors of, 626
  posterior fossa, tumors of, 624–625
  temporal lobe, tumors of, 624
Intraocular/expulsive hemorrhage, 135
Intraocular foreign body (IOFB), 500–503
Intraocular injections, 61
Intraocular lenses (IOLs), 35
  anterior chamber, 252
  aphakic correction with, 252
  haptics, 254
  iris-supported, 252
  magnification by, 253
  optical transmission, 254–255
  optics, 253–254
  parts, 253
  posterior chamber, 252–253

power, 255
selection, 255–256
Intraocular muscles, drugs acting on
  parasympatholytic drugs, 74–75
  sympathomimetic drugs, 75
Intraocular pressure
  diurnal variation of, 264
  factors affecting, 262–263
  postural variation of, 264
Intraocular tumors, 483–495
Intraretinal microvascular abnormalities (IRMA), 330
Intravitreal antibiotics, 206
Intravitreal anti-VEGF agents, 351
Intravitreal steroids, 351
Irideremia See Aniridia
Iridocorneal endothelial (ICE) syndrome, 209
Iridocyclitis See Anterior uveitis
Iridoschisis, 209
Iris
  anatomy, 187
  examination, 716
  heterochromia of, 212
  pathological changes in, 186
  prolapse, 135
Iris supported IOLs, 252
Iron deposition, 123
Irrigating solutions, 78
Ischemic optic neuropathy, 407–409
Ishihara's charts, 29, 30
Isolated muscle palsy, 461
Itching (itchy eyes), 709

J
Junctional scotoma, 426
Juvenile chronic arthritis (JCA), 202
Juvenile epithelial dystrophy See Meesmann's dystrophy
Juvenile glaucoma, 315
Juvenile retinoschisis, 380

K
Kaposi's sarcoma, 543
Kayser–Fleischer ring, 124
Kearns–Sayre syndrome, 380, 649
Keratitis
  associated with skin diseases, 153–154
  classification of, 127
  infectious, 127
    bacterial keratitis, 128–135
    fungal keratitis, 135–137
    parasitic keratitis, 143–144
    viral keratitis, 137–143
  noninfectious, 128
    immunologically mediated keratitis, 146–148
    interstitial keratitis (IK), 144–146
  source of, 127
  superficial, 148–151
  trophic, 151–153

Keratoconus, 123
Keratoconus (conical cornea), 161–163, 162
Keratoglobus, 163
Keratometry, 721–722
Keratophakia, 684
Keratoplasty, 676–679
Keratoprostheses, 679–680
Keratorefractive procedures, 680–681
Kinetic perimetry, 26

L

Lacrimal apparatus
  anatomy of, 545–547
  examination, 715
  physiology, 547–550
Lacrimal drainage system, 546–547
Lacrimal gland
  carcinoma, 564
Lacrimal glands, 545
  diseases of, 564
Lacrimal sac, 547
Lacrimal sac surgery, 667
Lagophthalmos, 539
Lamellar (zonular) cataract, 231
Lamellar keratotomy, 684
Lamina fusca, 165
Lantern test, 30
Laser-assisted in situ keratomileusis (LASIK), 682–684
Laser beam production, 655
Laser interferometer, 24
Laser light
  delivery system, 655–656
  properties of, 655
Lasers
  classification of, 656
  laser-assisted in situ keratomileusis, 659
  mode of operation, 657
  photocoagulation, 351
  uses, 657–658
  wavelength and tissue interactions, 656
Laser subepithelial keratomileusis (LASEK), 681–682
Laser thermal keratoplasty (LTK), 685–686
Laser trabeculoplasty, 291
Laser treatment of glaucoma, 700
Latent strabismus See Heterophoria
Lateral orbital wall, 565
Lattice degeneration, 377
Lattice dystrophy, 158
Laurence–Moon–Bardet–Biedl syndrome, 380
Leber congenital amaurosis, 382
Lens
  abnormalities
    abnormal position, 225–226
    abnormal shape/size, 225

abnormal transparency, 228–230
  anatomy, 219–222
  changes with age, 225
  composition, 222
  cylindrical, 38
  development of, 11, 12
  examination, 717
  fitting of, 57
  material of, 57
  metabolism, 223–225
  placode, 9
  spherical, 37–38
  surgery, 50
  transport of amino acids, 223
  transport of ions, 223
  types of, 57
Lens-induced uveitis, 204
Lenticonus and lentiglobus, 225
Leprosy, 642
Leprotic uveitis, 194
Leukemia, retinopathy in, 358–359
Leukocoria, 717
LGB process, 21, 431
Lid margins and palpebral aperture, disorders of, 526–532
Lid surgery
  for ectropion, 662–663
  for entropion, 660–662
  for ptosis, 663–667
  See also Eyelids
Light
  adaptation, 19
  properties of, 36
Light reflex, 215
Light sense, 19
Light sensitivity See Photophobia
Limbal region, 257–258
Long sightedness See Hypermetropia
Long standing paralysis, changes in, 463
Lowe's syndrome, 240
Lymphadenopathy, 89
Lymphocytic leukemia, 647
Lymphoid tumors, 586
Lymphosarcoma See Malignant orbital lymphoma

M

Macula lutea, 325–326
Macular disorders
  central serous chorioretinopathy, 365–366
  cystoid macular edema, 366–368
  drug-induced maculopathy, 371
  epiretinal membrane, 370
  macular hole, 368–369
Macular dystrophies, 158
  Best's vitelliform macular dystrophy, 382, 383
  butterfly-shaped macular dystrophy, 382

familial dominant drusen, 381–382
  juvenile retinoschisis, 380
  Leber congenital amaurosis, 382
  progressive cone dystrophy, 382
  sphingolipidoses, 382–383
  stargardt disease and fundus flavimaculatus, 381
  Tay–Sachs disease, 383
Macular hole, 368–369
Macular inflammations, 361–362
Madarosis, 525
Maddox rod test, 472–473
Maddox wing, 472
Malignant glaucoma, 310–311
Malignant melanoma, 483, 543
Malignant orbital lymphoma, 586
Manifest hypermetropia, 51
Manifest strabismus See Heterotropia
Marcus Gunn pupil, 218
Marfan syndrome, 638
Marginal keratitis, 127
Marginal ulcer, 147
Mast cell stabilizers, for allergic conjunctivitis, 106
Maxillary carcinoma, 586
Measles, 643
Medial orbital wall, 566
Meesmann's dystrophy, 157
Meibomian cyst See Chalazion
Melanin deposition, 124
Membranes, 87–88
Membranous cataract, 233
Meningeal angioma, 386
Meningitis, 621–622
Mesenchymal tumors, 586
Mesoderm, 9
Metabolic cataract, 238–240
Metaherpetic ulcers, 140
Metamorphopsia See Distortion of vision
Metastatic orbital tumors, 587
Methotrexate, 77
Methyl alcohol optic neuropathy, 414–415
Microaneurysms, 328
Microblepharon, 544
Micropsia, 711
Microspherophakia, 225
Midbrain, tumors of, 625–626
Migraine, 631–632
Mitomycin C (MMC), 78
Molluscum contagiosum, 524
Molluscum contagiosum conjunctivitis, 96–97
Mooren's ulcer, 147
Morning glory disc anomaly, 419
Motility tests, 476–477
Motor adaptations to strabismus, 468–469
Motor defect nystagmus, 609
Motor nerve supply of eyeball, 5–6

Mucin secretors, 84
Multifocal choroiditis, 191
Multiple myeloma, 648
Multiple sclerosis (MS), 619–620
Mumps, 643
Muscular disorders, 648–649
Myasthenia gravis, 648
Mycotic keratitis See Fungal keratitis
Mydriatics, 187–188
Myelinated nerve fibers, 338–339
Myeloid leukemia, 647
Myeloid sarcoma, 587
Myopia, 46–50
  clinical types, 47
  complications of, 50
  etiological types, 46–47
  grades, 47
  signs and symptoms, 47–48
  treatment, 48–50
Myopic chorioretinal degeneration, 209, 375
Myotonic dystrophy, 649

N

Naevi, 541
Nasal NFB defects, 278
Nasolacrimal duct (NLD), 547
Nasopharyngeal carcinoma, 586
National Program for Control of Blindness (NPCB)
  achievements, 736
  implementation strategies, 735–736
  initiatives during 11th Five Year Plan, 736
  initiatives during 12th Five Year Plan, 736–737
  launch of, 734
  merger with Vision 2020, 734
  NPCBVI objectives, 734–735
"National Program for Control of Blindness and Visual Impairment (NPCBVI)", 734–735, 737
Near reflex, 215–217
Near reflex test, 218
Near response, pathway of, 42–43
Near vision, correction for, 724–725
Necrotizing scleritis, 170
Neomycin and miconazole, 144
Neonatal chlamydial conjunctivitis, 98
Neonatal conjunctivitis, 101–103
Neovascularization, 330
Nerve fiber bundle (NFB) field defects, 276–278, 426–427
Nerve fibers, arrangement of, 421–424
Nerve supply
  of extrinsic muscles, 5–6
  of intrinsic muscles, 6
Neural tumors, 583–585
Neuroblastoma, 587

Neurofibroma, 540
Neurofibromatosis, 385, 649
Neuromyelitis optica, 620–621
Neuroretinal rim (NRR), 274
Neurosyphilis, 622
Neurotrophic keratitis, 151
Night blindness, 713
Nodular scleritis, 168
Non-accommodative esotropia, 454–455
Noncontact tonometer (NCT), 269
Nongranulomatous uveitis and granulomatous uveitis, 180
Nonhealing corneal ulcer
local causes of, 134
treatment of, 134
Noninfectious keratitis, 128
immunologically mediated keratitis, 146–148
interstitial keratitis (IK), 144–146
Non-necrotizing scleritis, 170
Nonproliferative diabetic retinopathy (NPDR), 347–348
Nonrefractive accommodative esotropia, 453–454
Nonsteroidal anti-inflammatory drugs (NSAIDS), 73, 106, 107, 143
Nonsuppurative keratitis, 144
Normal retinal correspondence, 33
Normal-tension glaucoma (NTG), 265, 292
Nuclear cataract, 231
Nuclear chop technique, 693
Nuclear senile cataract, 237
Nutritional deficiencies, 650–653
Nutritional optic neuropathy
See Toxic or nutritional optic neuropathy
Nyctalopia See Night blindness
Nystagmus
description, 607
management, 612
pathological, 609–612
physiological, 608–609

O
Occipital cortex, nerve fiber arrangement within, 424, 425
Occipital lobe, tumors of, 624
Occlusive vasculopathies, 614–615
Ocular cicatricial pemphigoid, 112–113
Ocular damage, 497
Ocular diseases
cataract associated with, 241
drugs for treatment of, 60
Ocular examination
eye examination, 715–718
fundus examination, 725–727
history taking, 714–715
refraction determination
objective verification, 718–722

subjective verification, 722–725
Ocular foreign bodies, 499–503
Ocular hypertension, 292–293
Ocular irritation, 708–709
Ocular light damage, 496
Ocular manifestations in HZO, 142
Ocular motility, disorders of, 446–448
Ocular movements, 462, 581
ductions, 440
examination of, 475–476
laws of ocular motility, 442
monocular or binocular, 439
nervous control, 442–444
positions of gaze, 440–441
vergences, 440
versions, 440
Ocular paralysis, 460–461, 469
Ocular preservatives, 78–79
Ocular symptoms
due to anomalies of ocular motility, 713–714
due to ocular surface anomalies, 708–709
visual, 709–713
Ocular tumors, 481
astrocytoma, 491
Bowen intra epithelial epithelioma, 483
choroidal hemangioma, 485–486
choroidal melanoma, 488–490
choroidal naevus, 485
choroidal osteoma, 486
ciliary body melanoma, 487
conjunctival epithelial melanosis, 483
conjunctival naevus, 482–483
conjunctival papilloma, 483
dermoid, 481
dermolipoma, 482
granuloma, 483
iris melanoma, 486–487
malignant melanoma, 483
medulloepithelioma, 485
metastatic tumors, 490
naevus of iris, 484–485
retinoblastoma, 491–495
squamous cell carcinoma, 483
uveal naevus, 483–484
Oculo cerebrorenal syndrome
See Lowe's syndrome
Oculomotor nerve and its lesions, 596–597
Oculosympathetic paresis See Horner's syndrome
Onchocerciasis, 201, 647
Onchocerciasis prevention and control, 732
Ophthalmia neonatorum, 101–103, 102
Ophthalmia nodosa, 104
Ophthalmic artery, 4
Ophthalmoscopy See Fundus examination
Optical aberrations, 38–39

Optical coherence tomography (OCT), 336
Optic atrophy, 415–418
Optic chiasma lesions, field defects in, 428
Optic cup
changes in, 274–275
with choroidal fissure, 8
derivatives of, 9
layers of, 9, 10
Optic disc, 325
Optic disc pit, 419–420
Optic foramen, 567
Optic nerve
blood supply, 394
congenital anomalies of, 418–420
damage in glaucoma, 289–290
damage to, 508
development of, 10, 11
nerve fiber arrangement within, 422
parts, 393–394
physiology, 394
sheaths, 394
venous drainage, 394
Optic nerve dysfunction, 394
clinical features of, 394–395
inflammation of optic nerve, 403–407
ischemic optic neuropathy, 407–409
pseudotumor cerebri, 403
swollen optic disc or disc edema, 395–403
Optic nerve glioma, 583, 585
Optic nerve head (ONH)
analysis, 273–275
nerve fiber arrangement within, 422
Optic nerve hypoplasia, 418–420
Optic nerve lesions
field defects in, 427–428
Optic nerve sheath meningioma, 585
Optic neuritis See Inflammation of optic nerve
Optic neuropathies, 581
ocular manifestations, 411–412
pathogenesis, 411–412
types, 411
Optic radiations
field defects in lesions of, 431
nerve fiber arrangement within, 423–424
Optic tract and LGB, nerve fiber arrangement within, 423
Optic tract lesions, field defects in, 430–431
Optokinetic nystagmus (OKN), 24, 608
Ora serrata, 386
Orbit
apertures, 567
blood supply of, 568

connective tissue system of, 567–568
surgical spaces of, 568–569
walls and relations of, 564–566
Orbital cellulitis, 574–575
Orbital diseases
cavernous sinus thrombosis (CST), 578
clinical features and investigations in, 569–570
Graves' ophthalmopathy, 578–582
orbital inflammation, 573–577
orbital injuries
orbital fractures, 588–590
orbital hemorrhage, 587–588
orbital tumors
metastatic, 587
primary, 582–586
secondary, 586
proptosis, 570–573
Orbital floor, 565–566
Orbital roof, 565
Orbscan, 125
Orneal aesthesiometer, 126
Orthophoria, 450
Outer fibrous coat, 1

P
Panophthalmitis, 207–208
Panuveitis and retinal complications, 190
Papillary reaction, 87, 88
Papillitis, 401–402, 405, 406
Papilloedema, 395, 397–403, 623
Papillomacular bundle defects, 276–277, 427
Paralysis of accommodation, 44–45
Paralysis of IIIrd nerve, 460
Paralytic strabismus, 459–460
Parasitic diseases, in eye, 646–647
Parasitic keratitis, 143–144
Parasitic uveitis, 199–202
Parasympathetic pathway, 214
Parasympatholytic drugs, 74–75
Parasympathomimetic drugs, 285–286
Paretic muscle, diagnosis of, 463–464
Paretic squint, 461
Parietal lobe, tumors of, 624
Parinaud's oculoglandular syndrome (POS), 104
Parkinson disease, 629
Pars plana vitrectomy (PPV), 206, 701–702
Pars planitis See Intermediate uveitis
Partially accommodative esotropia, 454
Passive edema, 518
Pathological insufficiency of accommodation, 44

Index

Pathological myopia, 47, 48
Pathological vestibular nystagmus, 610
Pelli–Robson chart, 29
Pellucid marginal degeneration, 163
Penetrating injury, 508–509
Penetrating keratoplasty (PKP), 137, 141
Perennial allergic conjunctivitis (PAC), 107–108
Perforated corneal ulcer treatment, 133
Perforating injury, 508–509
Peri bulbar injections, 61
Perimeter, 26
Perimetry, 25–26
Periocular injections, 61
Periodic alternating nystagmus, 610
Periostitis, 576–577
Peripheral anterior chamber depth, 293–294
Peripheral corneal procedures, 684–686
Peripheral cortical vitreous, 316–317
Peripheral retinal degenerations, 376–378
Periphlebitis retinae See Eales' disease
Perkin's tonometer, 269
Persistent hyper plastic primary vitreous (PHPV), 320
Persistent pupillary membrane, 212
Phacoemulsification, 690, 692
Phakic implantable contact lenses (Phakic ICLs), 686
Phakomatoses, 384–386
Pharyngoconjunctival fever (PCF), 95
Phenylephrine, 75
Phlyctenular conjunctivitis, 111–112
Phlyctenular keratitis, 146
Photochemical changes, 15–16
Photocoagulation burns, 351
Photodynamic therapy (PDT), 659
Photophobia, 709
Photophthalmia, 150–151
Photoreceptors, 15
Photorefractive keratectomy (PRK), 681
Photoretinitis, 362
Phototransduction, 16
Physical agents, injuries due to, 511–512
Physiological diplopia, 33
Physiological insufficiency of accommodation See Presbyopia
Pigmentation of cornea, 123–124
Pigment dispersion syndrome, 208
Pinguecula, 114
Pinhole test, 23–24

Pituitary adenoma, 428
Pituitary gland, 428
Placido keratoscope, 125
Pleomorphic adenoma, 564
Plexiform neurofibroma, 585–586
Pneumotonometer, 269
Poliosis, 525
Polycythemia, 647–648
Polyene antibiotics, 70
Polymegathism, 127
Pons, tumors of, 626
Positional hypermetropia, 50
Posner–Schlossman syndrome See Glaucomatocyclitic crisis
Posterior chamber lenses, 252–253
Posterior fossa, tumors of, 624–625
Posterior ischemic optic neuropathy (PION), 409
Posterior polar cataract, 233, 234
Posterior polymorphous dystrophy, 160–161
Posterior scleritis, 169–170
Posterior segment, 3
Posterior staphyloma, 172
Posterior uveitis, 191–193
Posterior vitreous detachment (PVD), 317–318
Postherpetic neuralgia, 142, 143
Postinfectious ulcer See Metaherpetic ulcers
Postoperative management, 693–694
Potential acuity meter (PAM), 24
Presbyopia, 43–44
Preseptal cellulitis, 574
Presumed ocular histoplasmosis syndrome (POHS), 198–199
Primary angle-closure glaucoma (PACG), 293–298
Primary choroidal degenerations, 209
Primary colors, 20
Primary congenital glaucoma (PCG), 312–315
Primary deviation, 449
Primary exotropia, 455–456
Primary open-angle glaucoma (POAG), 288–292
Primary optic atrophy, 416
Primary retinal telangiectasia, 344–345
Prism bar test, 472
Prisms, 36–37
Progressive cone dystrophy, 382
Progressive outer retinal necrosis (PORN), 196–197
Proliferative DR (PDR), 348–349
Prominent corneal nerves, 124
Prophylaxis
  for allergic conjunctivitis, 106
  for neonatal conjunctivitis, 103
Proptosis, 570–573

Prostaglandin and prostamide analogues, 286–287
Protanopia, 20
Pseudoesotropia, 452
Pseudoexfoliation glaucoma, 311
Pseudomyopia, 45
Pseudopapillitis, 52
Pseudopapilloedema, 401
Pseudophakia, glaucoma in, 309
Pseudopolycoria, 208
Pseudoptosis, 529
Pseudostrabismus, 452
Pseudotumor See Idiopathic orbital inflammation
Pseudotumor cerebri, 403
Pseudoxanthoma elasticum, 638
Psycho sensory reflex, 217
Pterygium, 115, 116, 123
Ptosis, 525–532
  lid surgery for, 663–667
Puncta, 546–547
Pupil
  afferent pathway of, 213–214
  anomalies of, 212
  and anterior uveal injury, 506
  characteristic features, 213
  efferent pathway of, 214–215
  examination, 218, 716–717
Pupil anomalies
  afferent pupillary defect, 591–592
  efferent pupillary defect, 592
  Horner's syndrome, 593
  pupillary light-near dissociation, 594–595
Pupillary light-near dissociation, 594–595
Pupillary muscle, 74
Pupillary reflexes, 215–217
Purine derivatives, 67
Pyrimethamine, 201
Pyrimidine derivatives, 67

Q

Quadrantanopia, 426
Quinine neuropathy, 415

R

Radial keratotomy (RK), 684
Radiation cataract, 243
Radiation injuries, 512
Reactions to medicines, 79
Reactive arthritis See Reiter's syndrome
Recurrent corneal erosion, 504
Recurrent corneal erosions, 150
Recurrent herpetic eye disease, 141
Red cell glaucoma, 308
Red eye, 708
Reduced eye, 39–41, 40
Reflection, 36
Refraction, 36
  objective verification, 718–722
  subjective verification, 722–725

Refractive accommodative esotropia, 453
Refractive errors, 470
  ametropia, 45–46
  anisometropia, 56–57
  astigmatism, 52–56
  correction of
    contact lenses, 57–59
    refractive surgeries, 59
    spectacles, 57
  emmetropia, 45, 46
  hypermetropia, 50–52
  and low vision, 733
  myopia, 46–50
Refractive index of media, 36
Refractive surgeries, 59
  corneal curvature modification, 680–681
  corneal stromal procedures, 682–684
  corneal surface procedures, 681–682
  peripheral corneal procedures, 684–686
  phakic implantable contact lenses, 686
Refsum's syndrome, 380
Reiter's syndrome, 202–203, 639–640
Relative afferent pupillary defect (RAPD), 218, 404, 591–592
Restrictive strabismus, 464–465
Retina, 2
  blood supply of, 326–327
  degenerations of, 371
    age-related macular degeneration (ARMD), 372–375
    angioid streaks, 375–376
    myopic chorioretinal degeneration, 375
    peripheral retinal degenerations, 376–378
  development of, 9, 10
  division of, 325–326
  dystrophies of See Dystrophies of retina
  inflammation of, 359
  layers of, 14
  light focused in front of, 46
  microscopic structure, 323, 325
  nerve fiber arrangement within, 422
Retinal artery occlusion, 339–341
Retinal breaks, 386–387
Retinal detachment (RD), 386–392, 702–705
Retinal diseases
  coloboma of retina, 338
  evaluation, 331–337
  myelinated nerve fibers, 338–339
  symptoms and signs in, 327–331
Retinal edema, 328–329
Retinal hemorrhages, 328

Retinal lesions following blunt trauma, 507
Retinal nerve fiber layer (RNFL) analysis, 279–280
Retinal photocoagulation, 337–338
Retinal surgery, glaucoma associated with, 309
Retinal vasculitis, 360
Retinal vein occlusion, 341–344
Retinal vessels, changes in, 331
Retinitis, 359–360
Retinochoroidopathies, 362–363
Retinopathy of prematurity (ROP), 354–357
Retinoscopy, 718–721
Retrobulbar neuritis, 405
Rhabdomyosarcoma, 586
Rhegmatogenous RD, 387
Rheumatoid arthritis, 636
Rhodopsin, photochemical changes in, 16
Riddoch phenomenon, 433
River blindness See Onchocerciasis
Rodent ulcer See Mooren's ulcer
Rods and cones, 14, 15
Rosacea keratitis, 153–154
Rose Bengal, 81–82
Rubella, 643
Rubeola See Measles

S
"SAFE" strategy for trachoma control, 101
Salzmann nodular degeneration, 156
Sarcoidosis, 637–638
Schematic eye, 39
Schilder's disease See Diffuse sclerosis
Schiotz tonometer, 266–267
Schnyder crystalline dystrophy, 158
Sclera
    anatomy, 164–165
    examination, 716
    inflammation of See Inflammation of sclera
    rupture of, 508
Scleral stroma (sclera proper), 164–165
Scleritis, 167–170
Seasonal allergic conjunctivitis (SAC), 107–108
Sebaceous gland carcinoma (SGC), 542
Secondary cataract, 241–244
Secondary choroidal degenerations, 211
Secondary deviation, 449
Secondary esotropia, 455
Secondary exotropia, 456–457
Secondary glaucoma, 134, 189, 298–311
    EVP elevation, 306–307
    inflammatory glaucoma, 304

intraocular hemorrhage, 307–308
IOP elevation, 304–305
iridocorneal endothelial (ICE) syndrome, 299
neovascular glaucoma, 301–304
ocular trauma, 307
phacoanaphylactic glaucoma, 301
phacolytic glaucoma, 300–301
phacomorphic glaucoma, 301
phacotopic glaucoma, 300
pigmentary glaucoma, 299–300
steroid administration and, 305–306
Secondary keratectasia See Ectatic cicatrix
Secondary optic atrophy, 416–417
See-saw nystagmus, 610
Selective laser trabeculoplasty (SLT), 291
Senile (age-related) cataract, 235–238
Senile retinoschisis, 378
Sense of contrast, 19, 20, 29
Sensory anomalies, tests for, 473–475
Sensory deficit nystagmus, 609
Sensory nerve endings, regional variations of, 15
Sensory nerve supply of eyeball, 5
Serpiginous choroidopathy, 364
Shaffer grading system, 273
Short sightedness See Myopia
Sickle-cell disease, 648
Sickle-cell retinopathy, 357–358
Silver deposition, 124
Sinus headache, 631
Skin disease, cataract associated with, 242
Slit-lamp biomicroscopy, 727
Small incision cataract surgery (SICS), 688–690, 691, 693
Snail track degeneration, 377
Snellen's test types, 22–23
Spasmus nutans, 609–610
Spectacles, 49, 52, 56, 57, 250–251
Specular microscope, 126
Speed of light, 36
Spherical aberration, 38
Spherical lenses, 37–38
Spheroidal degeneration, 155–156
Sphingolipidoses, 382–383
Spirochaetal uveitis, 197–198
Spondyloarthropathies
    ankylosing spondylitis, 639
    reactive arthritis, 639–640
Squamous cell carcinoma (SCC), 483, 542
Staphyloma, 170–172
Stargardt disease and fundus flavimaculatus, 381

Static perimetry, 27–28
Stevens–Johnson syndrome, 113–114
Stickler syndrome, 322
Strabismus, clinical evaluation of case of, 469
    abnormal head posture, 477
    angle of deviation, 471–473
    cover tests, 470–471
    diplopia, 477–480
    eyes and fundus, 470
    history, 470
    motility tests, 476–477
    refractive error, 470
    sensory anomalies, tests for, 473–475
    type of fixation, 473
    visual acuity, 470
Strabismus fixus, 465
Strabismus (squint) surgery, 670–676
Stromal corneal dystrophies, 157–158
Stromal keratitis treatment, 140–141
Stromal necrotizing keratitis, 139
Stromal scarring and opacity treatment, 141
Sturge–Weber syndrome, 385–386, 649
Subacute infective retinitis, 359–360
Subcapsular senile cataract, 237–238
Subconjunctival hemorrhage, 87
Subconjunctival injections, 61
Subconjunctival scarring, 88–89
Subtenon injections, 61
Superficial keratitis, 148–151
Superficial punctate keratitis (SPK), 148–149
Superficial vascularization, 123
Superior limbic keratoconjunctivitis (SLK), 149
Superior orbital fissure, 567
Supranuclear disorders, 446
Supranuclear pathways, 443–444
Sutural (stellate) cataract, 231–232
Swinging flashlight test, 218, 592
Swollen optic disc or disc edema, 395–403
Sylvian aqueduct syndrome, 611–612
Symblepharon, 536–537
Sympathetic ophthalmitis, 510
Sympathetic pathway, 214
Sympathomimetic drugs, 75
Synchysis scintillans, 319
Synoptophore examination, 474–475
Syphilis, 197–198, 643
Syphilitic and tubercular IK, 145
Systemic administration, 61

Systemic disorders, cataract associated with, 241–242
Systemic lupus erythematosus, 636–637
Systemic reactions to eye drops, 79, 80
Systemic steroids, 143
Systemic therapy, neonatal conjunctivitis, 103

T
Tacrolimus, 77–78
Tay choroiditis See Central guttate choroidal atrophy
Tay–Sachs disease, 383
Tear film, spread of, 549–550
Tears
    elimination of, 550
    hypersecretion of, 550
    secretion of, 547–549
Tear-secreting glands, 545–546
Telecanthus, 544
Temporal lobe, tumors of, 624
Tension headache, 631
Teratoma, 583
Terrien's marginal degeneration, 154–155
Thyrotoxicosis See Hyperthyroidism
Tobacco–alcohol amblyopia, 413–414
Tolosa–Hunt syndrome, 576
Tonography, 270
Tonometry, 265–270
Total ophthalmoplegia, 460
Toxemia of pregnancy (TOP), 353–354
Toxic cataract, 243–244
Toxic maculopathy See Drug-induced maculopathy
Toxic or nutritional optic neuropathy
    amiodarone induced optic neuropathy, 415
    causes of, 412–413
    ethambutol optic neuropathy, 415
    methyl alcohol optic neuropathy, 414–415
    ocular manifestations, 411–412
    quinine neuropathy, 415
    tobacco–alcohol amblyopia, 413–414
Toxocariasis, 201, 647
Toxoplasmosis, 199–201, 646–647
Trabecular outflow, 260–261
Trabeculectomy, 291–292, 700–701
Trachoma, 98–101, 100, 732
Transparency of cornea, 121–123
Trauma and brain See Head injury
Traumatic cataract, 242–243
Traumatic edema, 519
Traumatic optic neuropathy, 508

Triazoles, 71
Trichiasis, 524–525
Trichromats, 20
Trigeminal nerve and its lesions, 601–603
Trisomy 21 See Down syndrome
Tritanopia, 20
Trochlear nerve and its lesions, 597–598
Trophic keratitis, 151–153
Tropicamide, 75
Trypan blue, 82
Tubercular uveitis, 193–194
Tuberculosis (TB), 642
Tuberous sclerosis, 384–385
Tunics (coats) of eyeball, 1

U
Uhthoff's phenomenon, 404
Ultrasonography, 336–337
Unilateral cataracts, 235
Usher syndrome, 380
Uveal effusion syndrome, 392
Uveal tissue, 2, 11, 12
Uveal tract
    blood supply of, 177
    choroid, 176
    ciliary body, 174–176, 175, 176
    coloboma of, 212
    congenital anomalies of, 212
    degenerative changes in See Degenerative changes in uveal tract
    inflammation See Uveitis
    iris, 173–174
Uveitis, 177
    anatomical classification, 177–178
    anterior uveitis (iridocyclitis), 180, 182–190
    bacterial, 193–194
    clinical classification, 178
    etiological classification, 178–179
    fungal, 198–199
    immunological, 202–204
    intermediate uveitis, 190–191
    investigations, 179–180, 181
    parasitic, 199–202
    pathological classification, 179
    posterior uveitis, 191–193
    in sarcoidosis, 194–196, 195
    spirochaetal, 197–198
    viral, 196–197
Uveoscleral outflow, 261
UV radiation damage, biochemical mechanism of, 495–496
UV spectrum, 495

V
Vascular changes, 275
Vascular disorders, 612–618
    amaurosis fugax, 615–616

carotid artery occlusive disease, 616
cortical blindness, 618
intracranial aneurysms, 613–614
mechanism of vascular lesion, 612–613
occlusive vasculopathies, 614–615
vertebro-basilar insufficiency (VBI), 616–618
Vascular disorders of retina
    primary retinal telangiectasia, 344–345
    retinal artery occlusion, 339–341
    retinal vein occlusion, 341–344
Vascularization of cornea, 123, 126
Vascular retinopathies, 345
    in blood disorders, 358–359
    diabetic retinopathy (DR), 346–351
    hypertensive retinopathy, 351–353
    retinopathy of prematurity (ROP), 354–357
    sickle-cell retinopathy, 357–358
    toxemia of pregnancy (TOP), 353–354
Vascular tumors, 583
Vasoconstrictors, for allergic conjunctivitis, 106
Venous drainage, 3–5
VER (visually evoked response), 32
Vernal keratitis, 146
Vernal keratoconjunctivitis (VKC), 108–109
Vertebro-basilar insufficiency (VBI), 616–618
Verteporfin, 82
Vertical deviation See Hypertropia
Vertigo, 462–463
Vestibular nystagmus, 608–609
Vestibular pathway, 444–446
Vestibuloocular reflexes (VORs), 444
Viral conjunctivitis, 94–97
    acute hemorrhagic conjunctivitis, 96
    adenoviral infections, 94–95
    clinical presentation of, 94
    herpes simplex conjunctivitis, 96
    molluscum contagiosum conjunctivitis, 96–97
    transmission of, 94
Viral keratitis, 137–143
    herpes simplex keratitis
        complications, 139
        diagnosis, 140
        disciform keratitis, 139

neonatal infection, 137
    primary infection, 137–138
    recurrent infection, 138–139
    stromal necrotizing keratitis, 139
    treatment, 140–141
    varicella-zoster virus keratitis (VZV keratitis), 141–143
Viral uveitis, 196–197
Viscoelastic substances, 75–76
Vision 2020, 731
Visual acuity assessment, 418, 470
    in hard/dense cataract, 24
    in infants and young children, 24
    pinhole test, 23–24
    Snellen's test types, 22–23
Visual axis, 449
Visual cortex lesions, field defects in, 431–433
Visual disability, 738
Visual field, 24–28
    analysis, 275–279
    defects, 405
    divisions of, 24–25, 26
    measurement, 25–28
    monocular, 24
    physiologic influences on, 28
Visual function assessment, 21
    contrast sensitivity assessment, 29
    dark adaptation assessment, 29
    electrooculography (EOG), 31
    electro retinography (ERG), 30–31
    field of vision, assessment of, 24–28
        monocular visual field, 24, 25
        visual fields, 24–28
    VER (visually evoked response), 32
    visual acuity assessment See Visual acuity assessment
Visual impairment, 728–729
Visually evoked potential (VEP), 332
Visual pathway
    anatomy of, 421–424
    blood supply of, 424
    lesions of, 424–433
Visual process
    definition, 15
    visual cortex, 18
    visual impulse transmission, 16
        at lateral geniculate body, 17–18
        at retina, 17
    visual sensation initiation, 15–16
    visual sensations, 19–21
Visudyne See Verteporfin

Vitamin A
    absorption, 650
    daily requirements, 650
    deficiency, 651–653
    functions, 650–651
    sources, 650
Vitamin A deficiency, 153
Vitamin B deficiency, 653
Vitamin C deficiency, 653
Vitamin D deficiency, 653
Vitiliginous retinochoroiditis See Bird shot retinochoroidopathy
Vitreoretinal degenerations, 321–322
Vitreoretinal surgery
    pars plana vitrectomy (PPV), 701–702
    retinal detachment (RD) surgery, 702–705
Vitreo retinal traction, 386
Vitreous
    anatomy of, 316–317
    bands and membranes, 319–320
    detachment, 317–318
    development of, 12
    hemorrhage, 320–321
    humor, 3
    injuries on, 507
    opacities, 318–319
    persistent hyper plastic primary, 320
Vogt–Koyanagi–Harada (VKH) syndrome, 203–204, 638
Vogt limbal girdle, 154
Von Hippel-Lindau disease (VHL), 384, 650
von Recklinghausen's disease See Neurofibromatosis
"V" patterns, 457–459

W
Wagner disease, 321–322
Watering eye
    epiphora, 551–553
    evaluation of case with, 553–558
    hypersecretion of tears, 550
Wegener's granulomatosis, 638
Wernicke's hemianopic pupil, 595
White without pressure, 377
Wilson disease, 240, 629–630
Worth's 4-dot test, 474

X
Xanthelasma, 540
Xerosis, 88

Y
Young-Helmholtz theory, 21

Z
Zidovudine, 69